Nursing Research

METHODS, CRITICAL APPRAISAL AND UTILISATION

2nd edition

Nursing Research

METHODS, CRITICAL APPRAISAL AND UTILISATION

2nd edition

Zevia Schneider
Doug Elliott

Christine Beanland

Geri LoBiondo-Wood

Judith Haber

Mosby

Sydney Edinburgh London New York Philadelphia St Louis Toronto

Mosby
is an imprint of Elsevier Science

Elsevier (Australia) Pty Limited
30–52 Smidmore Street, Marrickville, NSW 2204

Published by Elsevier (Australia) Pty Limited
ACN 000 910 583

National Library of Australia Cataloguing-in-Publication Data

Nursing research: methods, critical appraisal and utilisation.

2nd ed.
Includes index.
ISBN 0 7295 3665 3.

1. Nursing—Research. I. Schneider, Zevia.

610.73072

Publishing Editor: Meg O'Hanlon
Publishing Services Manager: Helena Klijn
Edited by Rebecca Henson
Cover and internal design by Darben Design
Index by Max McMaster
Typeset by Sun Photoset Pty Ltd, Brisbane
Printed in Australia by Southwood Press

Foreword

This second edition of *Nursing Research: Methods, Critical Appraisal and Utilisation* embodies the art and the science of contemporary nursing research in this region. Where the first edition focused on portraying a broadly based introduction to nursing research, its foundations and strategies, this volume advances our thinking towards critical appraisal in all nursing actions, and the many ways this is linked to wider bodies of knowledge. It is a pleasure to find that the structural elements that made the first edition so reader-friendly are retained. Each chapter sets out the advance organisers, the key terms and learning outcomes, which are then examined in depth. These are articulated in a scholarly yet creative manner and culminate in a set of critical thinking challenges.

A number of features illustrate the book's usefulness to all researchers interested in healthcare. It encompasses the many ways nursing research contributes to health, firmly grounding us in a wide range of strategies for generating evidence and providing the linkages between this body of evidence and the personal and social contexts of people's lives. From the fundamental argument for scholarly work in nursing, to the various methodological approaches, the authors go beyond a mere collection of studies to blend their knowledge into a coherent pattern. The first chapter provides an overview of the rationale and progress in the field, whetting the appetite for web-based resources for future studies. Subsequent chapters in the first section take the reader through the initial stages of research, constructing pathways for analysing existing knowledge and articulating the series of steps that can be used to accomplish both personal learning and the advancement of clinical practice. Web-based resources for further reading are presented throughout. The second and third sections provide specific guidelines for conducting research, presenting first qualitative, then quantitative approaches. Methodological information is demarcated in a way that allows the reader to better understand the nexus between the study itself and its conceptual foundations. Each chapter guides the researcher from rationale to findings, then connects the body of work to a larger agenda in disseminating this information to the professional community and beyond.

The major element that makes this book invaluable to all scholars is the presentation of exemplary studies, each as a separate appendix, as was done in the first edition. These works illustrate conventions of method and distinctive ways of representing the findings. The studies highlight the synergies achieved between learning to research, situating the research in a body of knowledge, and providing inspiration for others to undertake the next increments. This text is a pleasure to read, a source of pride for the nursing research community and an invitation to the future.

Anne McMurray
August, 2002

Preface

In the three years since the first edition of this book appeared, nurses, midwives and other health professionals have continued to embrace the need for research utilisation and primary research activities as a basis for enhancing clinical practice and quality patient care. Despite the challenges of continuing staffing and budget crises, and yet more government reviews into nursing, nursing education and tertiary education in general, nurses and midwives continue to recognise the need to question traditional practices and processes by developing skills in critical appraisal of the research literature.

We gratefully acknowledge comments and suggestions from our colleagues and nursing students and have accordingly modified and revised this edition to better support the contemporary process of enquiry. This 2nd edition has a completely revised structure of 23 chapters divided into three sections: Research and practice; Qualitative research methods; and Quantitative research methods. All chapters have been either re-structured or newly written by experts in the field, to better reflect the current knowledge base and application of clinical nursing and midwifery research. We hope that these inclusions and modifications will have relevance for undergraduate, beginning graduate students, and nurses in a variety of clinical settings.

As well as the factors listed above, there are other major initiatives influencing education and research. Preparation for midwifery practice in particular is undergoing fundamental change, and is reclaiming its separateness as a profession from nursing. Midwives and students of midwifery should find this text a useful resource for their learning and practice.

Professional nurses and midwives believe that evidence-informed practice will achieve best practice. In recent years, there has been an increasing contribution to the international nursing research literature and knowledge base of the discipline by Australian and New Zealand nurses and midwives. We have therefore presented the major research methodologies used by Australasian nurses and midwives. With an emphasis on qualitative approaches to understanding human experience in Australasian research, we have made the qualitative content in the text more explicit. The text also uses many examples of clinical research that can influence and inform practice. The appendices include papers published by local authors in journals based in Australia, Britain and the United States.

The explosion of internet-based sources for accessing research and other information is reflected in the text, with the inclusion of a variety of websites. However, a limitation of citing online resources in a text is that web addresses are constantly evolving and changing. At the time of writing, all cited addresses were correct, but these may change over the life of the text. Our suggestion is to use a search engine if the link listed in the text is not functional.

We hope that you enjoy using this text and that it stimulates and encourages you to read and think about research and its place in your professional practice. We also hope it assists in the development of your skills and confidence in critically appraising the research literature. Most importantly, we hope that you will share your information about research with your colleagues and use research findings to inform the care that you deliver to your patients.

The delivery of quality nursing and midwifery care is a challenge in our dynamic healthcare environment. We hope that this text will be a valuable tool to assist you in that process.

Zevia Schneider and Doug Elliott
August, 2002

Contents

Contributors

Merilyn Annells, RN, DipAppSc, BN (Ed), MNS, PhD, Chair in Community Nursing, La Trobe University, Melbourne, Vic

Sanchia Aranda, RN, PhD, MN, BAppSci (Adv Nurs), Oncology Cert, Professor/Director of Cancer Nursing Research, Peter MacCallum Cancer Institute, Melbourne, Vic

Esther Chang, RN, PhD, Professor of Nursing, School of Nursing, Family and Community Health, College of Social and Health Sciences, University of Western Sydney, Sydney, NSW

Judith Clare, RN, MA (Hons), PhD, FCNA, Foundation Professor of Nursing in the School of Nursing and Midwifery at Flinders University, Adelaide, SA

John Daly, RN, PhD, FRCNA, FINE, FCN (NSW), Professor of Nursing and Head, School of Nursing, Family and Community Health, College of Social and Health Sciences, University of Western Sydney, Sydney, NSW

Doug Elliott, RN, PhD, ICCert, BAppSc (Nurs), MAppSc (Nurs), MCN (NSW), Professor of Nursing (Critical Care), Prince of Wales Hospital and the Department of Clinical Nursing, University of Sydney, Sydney, NSW

Judith Finn, RN, RM, PhD, ICCert, DipAppSc (Nurs), BSc, GradDipPubHlth, MEdStud, Senior Lecturer in Clinical Epidemiology within the Department of Public Health at the University of Western Australia and Adjunct Senior Research Fellow in Nursing at Royal Perth Hospital, Perth, WA

Sue Forsyth, RN, PhD, MA (with merit), BA, Lecturer, Department of Family and Community Nursing, Faculty of Nursing, University of Sydney, Sydney, NSW

Judith Godden, BA (Hons), PhD, DipEd, Senior Lecturer, Department of Clinical Nursing, Faculty of Nursing, University of Sydney, Sydney, NSW

Lillian Hayes, RN, PhD, MPH, DipEd, BA, Lecturer, Faculty of Nursing, Department of Family and Community Nursing, University of Sydney, Sydney, NSW

Debra Jackson, RN, PhD, Associate Professor of Nursing, School of Nursing, Family and Community Health, College of Social and Health Sciences, University of Western Sydney, Sydney, NSW

Tina Koch, RN, BA, PhD, Professor and Director, RDNS Research Unit, Royal District Nursing Service, SA

Gavin Leslie, RN, PhD, ICCert, BAppSc, GradDip (ClinNurs), FRCNA, Associate Professor, Critical Care Nursing, Edith Cowan University, Director, Nursing Professional Development Unit, Royal Perth Hospital, Perth, WA

Judy Mannix, RN, MN (Hons), MCNA, Lecturer, School of Nursing, Family and Community Health, College of Social Health Sciences, University of Western Sydney, Sydney, NSW

Louise O'Brien, RN, PhD, FRCMHN, MRCNA, Senior Lecturer, University of Western Sydney, Sydney, NSW

Annabel Pollard, RN, BA, GradDip (AppPsych), CritCCert, Coordinator—Patient Support, Peter MacCallum Cancer Institute, Melbourne, Vic

Zevia Schneider, RN, RM, PhD, MEd, MAppSc, FRCNA, Consultant, formerly Associate Professor, Research, Faculty of Nursing, RMIT University, Melbourne, Vic

Annette F. Street, TPTC, TTCTD, BEd (Hons), PhD, Professor of Cancer and Palliative Care Studies, La Trobe University, Melbourne, Vic

Grace Tham, BAppSc (ChinMed), Master AppSc (Acup), RN, BAppSc (NsgEd), MEdStud, formerly Senior Lecturer, Faculty of Nursing, RMIT, Melbourne, Vic., Practitioner of Chinese Medicine and Acupuncture

Reviewers

Jackie Crisp, Professor of Child and Adolescent Nursing, Sydney Children's Hospital, South East Health; and Faculty of Nursing, Midwifery and Health, University of Technology, Sydney; Conjoint Professor, University of New South Wales, Sydney, NSW.

Christina Bobrowski, School of Nursing, University of Tasmania, Hobart, Tas.

Carol Windsor, School of Nursing, Queensland University of Technology, Brisbane, Qld.

Judy Wollin, School of Nursing, Queensland University of Technology, Brisbane, Qld.

Note from the publisher

We at Elsevier Science hope you will find this text challenging and rewarding. A number of ancillaries are available at **www.elsevier.com.au** and we trust they will make this book more useful to you whether you are a student or a lecturer.

All students purchasing this book will have access to the following online ancillaries, compiled by the authors and contributors:

- student activities and answers for all chapters
- selected additional research papers for further reading.

Lecturers adopting this book will receive free access to the above, plus, to assist with teaching:

- a testbank
- PowerPoint slides.

The lecturer materials have been written by Dr Lynne Barnes and Ms Marie Heartfield, both from the School of Nursing and Midwifery, University of South Australia.

There is a separate passcode for each of the student and lecturer sections of the website—lecturers should contact their Elsevier Science representative for both of these passcodes, and students should be advised of their passcodes by their lecturers.

We wish you success in your studying and teaching.

Acknowledgments

This second edition has moved substantially from the content and structure of the first Australasian edition, itself an adaptation of the fourth edition of the United States text. Despite this evolution, we gratefully acknowledge the contributors of those editions for a strong base from which to work. Our sincere appreciation goes to the chapter contributors for this edition—19 in all—for their collegial and scholarly work within a challenging time frame.

Thanks also to the publishing team from Elsevier (Australia) Pty Limited: Vaughn Curtis for his vision and ongoing support; Meg O'Hanlon for her project management, contributor liaison and editorial support activities; Helena Klijn for managing the manuscript-to-publication process; and Rhiain Hull for managing the copyright and figure typesetting issues. A special thanks to Rebecca Henson for her copy editing skills, attention to detail, and supportive approach at the end of a long writing and editing process.

We also wish to thank the manuscript reviewers, as well as our colleagues and students, for providing feedback and constructive criticism in preparing this edition. We gratefully acknowledge the various copyright holders for their generosity in allowing us to use their works in the text.

Most importantly, thank you to our families for their love and support as we worked on this project.

Zevia Schneider and Doug Elliott

SECTION ONE

Research and practice

1
CHAPTER

Research and professional practice

Doug Elliott

LEARNING OUTCOMES

After reading this chapter the student should be able to:

- State the significance of research to the practice of nursing.
- Discuss the development of nursing research internationally over the last 100 years.
- Describe Australasian perspectives of the relationships between research, education and practice.
- Identify the role of the consumer of nursing research.
- Evaluate the nurse's role in the research process as it relates to their level of educational preparation.
- Recognise the value of evidence-based practice (EBP).
- Identify the future trends in nursing research.

Key terms

clinical governance

consumer

critical review

research utilisation

systematic review

theory

INTRODUCTION

Students of nursing may initially wonder why a research course is part of their nursing curriculum. What has research to do with the practice of nursing? How will research help nurses practise in a better way, or how will it help patients or clients? In answer to these questions, the research course you are taking has *everything* to do with the practice of professional nursing. As the ability to appraise research studies develops, the complexity of nursing and the associated critical thinking skills will become more appreciated. This, in turn, will help to refine clinical judgment and decision-making skills; the ultimate beneficiaries will be the recipients of nursing care and nursing practice. Many nurses share the belief that a knowledge of and involvement in nursing research can have a significant effect on the depth and breadth of the professional practice of every nurse. The purpose of this chapter is to help to develop an appreciation of the significance of research in nursing and the research roles of nurses through historical and futuristic views.

Nursing research encompasses the full range of philosophical and methodological pursuits—from studying an 'n of one' (an in-depth study of one participant) through to large epidemiological studies; from in-depth understanding of unique personal experiences through to survey findings. Nursing is a diverse discipline in an epistemological sense—that is, the philosophical examination of human knowledge in terms of its origins, nature, methods and limits. The important consideration is to match the research question being asked to an appropriate method. For example, a question about identifying the most effective clinical intervention needs to be answered using a design and method that allow comparison of the different interventions or treatments available. Similarly, if the research aim is to gain better understanding of the health problems for a particular population, then a design and method that facilitates exploration of the experiences of individuals with a specific condition are warranted.

The aim of this book is to assist nurses, midwives and other health professionals in developing critical appraisal skills and research consumer expertise, as well as to provide some beginning skills in conducting research. There are of course many resources for this learning available in a variety of settings: journals, websites, reports and texts. This book acts as an organiser of this learning in conjunction with formal research courses undertaken primarily at the undergraduate level. This edition has three sections—Section 1 primarily examines the key aspects of critical appraisal skills and their links to practice and professional development; and Sections 2 and 3 discuss specific aspects of qualitative and quantitative research approaches respectively.

This chapter explores the relationships between research, practice and professional development, including a brief examination of developments in nursing and midwifery, particularly in terms of professional organisations and journals. Chapter 2 introduces the concepts of qualitative and quantitative research approaches as a prelude to more in-depth discussion in Sections 2 and 3. Triangulation of methods is also examined in Chapter 2. Chapter 3 discusses literature search skills, and Chapter 4 provides some beginning generic critical appraisal skills as preparation for further examination of specific research methods in Sections 2 and 3. Chapter 5 examines review (secondary research) papers, while evidence-based practice (EBP) is discussed in Chapter 6, and an example of implementing research into practice is presented in Chapter 7. Chapter 8 moves away from the research consumer theme to discuss the issues in preparing a proposal for conducting primary research.

SIGNIFICANCE OF RESEARCH IN NURSING

As the healthcare environment evolves at an unprecedented pace, nurses are continuously challenged to expand their 'comfort zone' by considering creative approaches to old and new health problems (Davidson & Elliott, 2001), and designing new and innovative programs that make a difference to the health status of our patients and community (e.g. Stewart, Vendenbroek, Pearson & Horowitz, 1999). This challenge can best be met by integrating the rapidly expanding knowledge bases of environmental, behavioural and biological influences on health and nursing practice. In addition, nursing research provides a specialised scientific knowledge base that empowers the nursing profession to participate actively in these constantly shifting challenges and maintain our societal relevance. Nursing is practised in a highly complex and structured environment with many competing influences, and hence nurses must continue to lead in communication, cooperation, collaboration and coordination within the clinical environment, despite the political and power structures inherent in such complex healthcare and education organisations.

A number of professional organisations have identified the importance of nursing research within the Australasian region. The Australian Nursing Council (ANC), in developing a set of national competencies for registered nurses, identified research as a core competency of a professional nurse. The elements relating to this core competency state that an RN acknowledges the importance of research in improving nursing outcomes; incorporates research findings into nursing practice; and contributes to the process of nursing research. The Royal College of Nursing Australia (RCNA, 1998) statement on nursing research proposed that all nurses should be committed to advancing nursing science through the conduct of research and utilisation of research findings in practice. The statement noted that scientific investigation promotes accountability, which is one of the hallmarks of a profession. The RCNA also has a research network to support members interested in research.

Speciality nursing groups also highlight the importance of research in their practice settings. For example, the Australian College of Critical Care Nurses (ACCCN) developed a set of competencies for specialist critical care nurses, which included promoting research designed to improve practice, participating in collaborative research within the multidisciplinary team, and incorporating research findings into nursing practice (ACCCN, 2002). The College also has a research advisory panel to support members and advise the National Executive. Other professional colleges have similar statements relating to the importance of research in their practice. The Australian and New Zealand College of Mental Health Nurses Incorporated also has a research board to support professional practice development. The Australian College of Midwives, Incorporated (ACMI) recognises that midwifery practice, as an independent discipline, requires demonstration of evidence-based knowledge (ACMI, 1998). The New Zealand Nurses Organisation (NZNO) recognises research as an integral component of nursing practice, and fosters research through their nursing research section. Similarly, the East Asian Forum of Nurse Scholars (EAFONS) convened in 1997 to promote research and scholarship among its university members from Hong Kong, South Korea, Taiwan, Thailand and the Philippines, particularly in terms of doctoral education and support.

Table 1.1 lists examples of professional nursing organisations and journals that have formed to advance the nursing discipline through various activities, including research and publishing. The listing is for illustrative purposes only, and does not encompass all organisations or journals associated with nursing or midwifery. For example, journals with a predominantly industrial focus are not included (such as *Australian Nursing Journal* and *The Lamp*).

TABLE 1.1 Sample of professional nursing organisations and journals in Australasia

NURSING ORGANISATION	AFFILIATED JOURNAL	FURTHER DETAILS—WEBSITE
Association for Australian Rural Nurses	newsletter	http://www.aarn.asn.au
Australasian Neuroscience Nurses' Association	*Australian Journal of Neuroscience*	http://www.users.bigpond.com/annaexecutive
Australian and New Zealand College of Mental Health Nurses	*Australian and New Zealand Journal of Mental Health Nursing*	http://healthsci.utas.edu.au/nursing/college/index
Australian College of Critical Care Nurses	*Australian Critical Care*	http://www.acccn.com.au
Australian Confederation of Operating Room Nurses	*ACORN: the Journal of Perioperative Nursing in Australia*	http://www.acornjournalcjb.net.au
Australian College of Midwives, Incorporated	*Australian Journal of Midwifery*	http://acmi.org.au
Australian Nursing Federation	*Australian Journal of Advanced Nursing*	http://www.anf.org.au
Congress of Aboriginal and Torres Strait Islander Nurses	newsletter	http://www.indiginet.com.au/catsin
Joanna Briggs Institute for Evidence Based Nursing and Midwifery	*Changing Practice information sheets*	http://www.joannabriggs.edu.au
Royal College of Nursing, Australia	*Collegian*	http://www.rcna.org.au
New Zealand Nursing Organisation	*Kaitiaki: the New Zealand Nursing Journal*	http://www.nzno.org.nz
New South Wales College of Nursing	*Nursing.Aust*	http://www.nursing.aust.edu.au
South East Asian Forum of Nursing Scholars	*Asian Journal of Nursing Studies*	http://nhs.polyu.edu.hk/nhs/scacht/schact-asian
Transplant Nurses Association	*Transplant Nurses Journal*	http://www.tna.asn.au
INDEPENDENT AND OTHER PROFESSIONAL PUBLICATIONS		
Australian Journal of Rural Health		
Contemporary Nurse		

Hong Kong Nursing Journal

International Journal of Nursing Practice

Journal of Korean Academy of Nursing

Nursing Inquiry

Singapore Nursing Journal

There are also many other intra-disciplinary and inter-disciplinary professional groups promoting education, research and practice development throughout the Asia Pacific region and elsewhere, e.g. Australian Cardiac Rehabilitation Association (http://www.acra.net.au); Renal Society of Australasia (http://www.renalsociety.org).

There is general consensus that the research role for nursing graduates (from a Bachelor of Nursing) calls for the skills of critical appraisal. That is, the nurse must be a knowledgeable research consumer, one who can critique research and use existing standards to determine the merit and readiness of research for utilisation in clinical practice. This reflects the '4 As of research' (Crookes & Davies, 1998, p. xi; Daly, Elliott & Chang, 1999):

- awareness
- appreciation
- application
- ability.

All nurses, (whether formal students or not) need to be aware of the available evidence which impacts on their nursing practice (awareness), have the necessary skills and experiences to critically review the methods and findings (appreciation), and decide whether the findings should be applied to their own clinical setting (application). These first three categories (awareness, appreciation and application) require broad knowledge and skills to critique nursing research, regardless of the philosophy and methods of the primary researcher. In contrast, the fourth 'A' is the ability to undertake independent primary research. These skills are usually refined within an honours or higher research degree, or as a member of a clinical research team. The focus here is on an in-depth study using a defined and specific method.

Therefore, not all nurses need to conduct research, but all nurses need to be able to critically appraise research in order to use the findings appropriately in their clinical practice. Think of research utilisation as the actual systematic implementation of a scientifically sound, research-based innovation in a healthcare setting with an accompanying process to assess the outcome(s) of change (see Chapter 7 as an example of using research findings and knowledge to improve nursing practice). Through research utilisation efforts, knowledge obtained from primary research is translated into improving clinical practice. This relates to the goal of evidence-based nursing (EBN): 'The process by which nurses make clinical decisions using the best available research evidence, their clinical expertise and patient preferences, in the context of available resources' (DiCenso, Cullum & Ciliska, 1998, p. 38; see Chapter 6).

As we progress through this new century, nurses will continue to be accountable for the quality of the care they deliver. Adding to the complexity of maintaining and improving the quality of nursing care are issues such as managing the nursing workforce and ongoing recruitment and retention staffing crises. In addition, increasing government and consumer questioning of the quality and increasing costs of healthcare has resulted in health professionals being continually asked to demonstrate the effectiveness of their care. Essentially we are asked, 'How do nurses make a difference?'. The way that society, consumers and employers, in both the public and private healthcare sectors, perceive the value of nurses' contributions will ultimately determine the profession's role in any future healthcare delivery system across the globe (Buerhaus, 1996; Buerhaus, Staiger & Auerbach, 2000a; Buerhaus, Staiger & Auerbach, 2000b). This is indeed a challenge for nursing, but as with any challenge, there are also great opportunities for practice and professional development. The use of research findings from rigorous, high quality studies to justify nursing practice and knowledge is one way of meeting these challenges.

RESEARCH: LINKING THEORY, EDUCATION AND PRACTICE

Research links theory, education and practice. Theory supported by research findings becomes the foundation of theory-based practice in nursing. The educational setting provides an environment in which students can learn about the research process. In this setting, they can also explore different theories and begin to evaluate them in light of research findings. All primary research adheres to a set of principles and guidelines regarding the ethical conduct of research—see, for example, the Australian Vice-Chancellors Committee and National Health and Medical Research Council guidelines (http://www.avcc.edu.au/news/publications). These issues are also discussed in more detail in Chapter 8.

Examples of linking research to practice are outlined below, and discussed further throughout the book. A study by Barclay, Everitt, Rogan, Schmied and Wyllie (1997), which explored men's experiences during their partners' first pregnancy, illustrates a theory-developing investigation that has societal relevance and is clinically oriented. It appears from the study that men often experienced confusion, ambivalence, anxiety and adjustment as their partner carried their first child. The findings of the study confirm the work of other researchers and raise issues regarding the planning of antenatal care and education for couples during their first pregnancy. In an intervention study, Small and colleagues (2000) examined the prevalence of depression in postnatal women who had an operative birth (see Appendix D), and found that one session of midwife-led debriefing was ineffective in reducing maternal depression at six months postpartum. The findings of this study supported an earlier systematic review that there is no evidence to support the view that debriefing has any benefits on psychological morbidity (Kenardy, 2000). The theory generated by this study supported the increasing body of knowledge regarding the minimal or possibly deleterious effects of debriefing in certain clinical settings. Conversely, another intervention study demonstrated reduced re-admissions and out-of-hospital deaths for patients with congestive heart failure who received an outreach home visit by a nurse and pharmacist (Stewart et al., 1999; Stewart, Pearson & Horowitz, 1998). This study continues to generate interest in the cardiac rehabilitation field, including the need for an economic analysis (Farmer, 1999), and for comparison of specialist outreach or generalist community delivery approaches.

At this point it could be asked how education in nursing research links theory and practice. The answer is twofold. First, knowledge about research methods provides an appreciation and an understanding of the research process to encourage participation in research activities. Second, it should enable students to become intelligent research consumers. A research consumer uses and applies research to practice in an active and systematic manner. To be a knowledgeable consumer, a nurse must have knowledge about the relevant research process, the ability to evaluate information logically and the skills to apply the knowledge gained. It is not necessary to undertake research studies to be able to appreciate and use research findings in practice.

ROLES IN THE RESEARCH PROCESS

There are many roles for nurses, midwives and other health professionals in clinical research (e.g. Dunn & Yates, 2000; Ocker & Pawlick Plank, 2000). Academic nurses and senior clinical nurses are commonly involved as both primary researchers and in the utilisation of research into clinical practice (research consumers). As noted earlier, all registered nurses are expected to be proactive consumers of research within the domain of their clinical practice. Thus, the role of the Bachelor of Nursing graduate in the research process is primarily that of a knowledgeable consumer, a role that promotes the integration of research and clinical practice. Both registered nurses with direct patient care responsibilities and more senior positions within the healthcare and tertiary sector need skills and experience in critical reading.

Through critical appraisal skills that use specific criteria to judge all aspects of the research, a professional nurse interprets, evaluates and determines the credibility of research findings. The nurse must be able to discriminate between research that is interesting but requires further investigation before implementation in practice, and findings that have sufficient support to be considered for utilisation and application (Beyea, Farley & Williams-Burgess, 1996).

In this context, understanding the research process and acquiring critical appraisal skills opens a broad realm of information that can contribute to the professional nurse's body of knowledge, and in a number of ways can improve patient care (Shorten, Wallace & Crookes, 2001; Thede, 2001). In particular, clinical nurses are involved in the development or revision of clinical guidelines to reflect the current evidence base. Specific activities may include joining the healthcare agency's quality improvement (QI) program, where research findings are evaluated for evidence-based clinical decision-making and dissemination of clinical guidelines (Cook et al., 1997). It may also involve sharing with colleagues the findings of a research report that has been reviewed and has merit and potential applicability to local practice. As members of a profession, it is also incumbent on nurses to share research findings with colleagues, through local education sessions, conference presentations and publications.

Generating clinical research questions

Questions about clinical practice form the basis for examining the literature, and there are many resources now available for finding answers through previous reviews of published findings or as a prelude to conducting a new review of the literature. The evolution of the EBN movement continues to influence how nurses think about and use research in their daily practice. Evidence-based practice (EBP) is a clinical activity with the premise that decisions about patient care should be informed by the best available current scientific evidence (Sackett et al., 1996; Shorten & Wallace, 1997; Droogan & Cullum, 1998). The multidisciplinary process is also now labelled evidence-based clinical decision-making, or as single disciplines (e.g. nursing, medicine, physiotherapy). Evidence-based nurses ask whether there is a scientific basis for the care that they deliver, in order to provide the best quality, effective care for their clients and their families.

The concept of 'clinical governance' is integral to nurses' goal to provide the most effective and best quality care for their clients. Clinical governance was first described in the United Kingdom as a system designed to ensure that clinical standards are met and that strategies are present to ensure continuous improvement of clinical practice. The major elements of clinical governance are: 'education, clinical audit, clinical effectiveness, risk management, research and development, and openness' (Starey, 2001, p. 2). Nursing and other professional primary healthcare agencies champion the need for continuing education and recognise it as necessary if their goal of providing best quality care to their clients is to be achieved.

'Clinical audit' or measuring clinical performance against a profession's performance indicators has long been a feature of nurse education. While necessary, clinical experience and expertise are no longer sufficient for ensuring the best care; clinical expertise must be informed by evidence from quality research studies. Ultimately, evidence from research studies should determine clinical practice. Chapter 7 provides an example of some difficulties encountered when nurses tried to introduce a different treatment of oral care for clients with mucositis-based on research findings. The nurses persevered and were successful in changing the regime for oral care.

The Joanna Briggs Institute for Evidence Based Nursing and Midwifery (see Table 1.1 on pages 6–7) is one centre established to support EBN practice in the Australasian region by producing and disseminating evidence-based guidelines for clinical practice. There are also numerous other entities promoting EBP through their activities which impact on nursing, e.g. Cochrane Collaboration, York Centre for Evidence-Based Nursing, and other UK National Health Service centres. However, there are issues to be considered regarding the relationships between nursing, evidence and EBP (e.g. Carnwell, 2000; Closs & Cheater, 1999; Smith & Sutton, 1999). See Chapter 6 for additional resources and further discussion and critique of EBN.

In addition to research utilisation, it is often nurse clinicians or midwives who generate research ideas or questions, based on hunches, gut feelings, intuition, observations of patients, or nursing care or quality assurance programs in their healthcare environment. These ideas are often the seeds of further research investigations or quality improvement projects. For example, a nurse working in a cardiac catheterisation laboratory questioned whether the practice of applying pressure bandages to patients' puncture sites following coronary angiography was an effective practice in reducing complications such as bleeding and haematoma formation. Through a well designed clinical trial, the nurses were able to demonstrate the effects of bandaging compared to no bandaging on patient comfort and the incidence of post-angiography complications. These findings have influenced nursing practice in this clinical area (Botti et al., 1998). Other examples of 'bottom-up' projects resulting from clinical questions are detailed in a paper from Hong Kong (French, 1999). Three vignettes are discussed—time interval for urethral catheter replacement in long-term patients; effectiveness of nurses in delivering a secondary prevention cardiac rehabilitation program; and the lived experience of the therapeutic relationship of nurses and doctors with female clients experiencing perinatal loss.

Collaborative research teams

Nurses and midwives also participate in primary or secondary research projects as members of an inter-disciplinary or intra-disciplinary research team in one or more phases of such a project. Primary research is where original data are being collected as part of a defined research project. For example, a nurse may work on a clinical research unit where a particular type of nursing care is part of an established research protocol, such as for nurse-initiated analgesia in the emergency department, management of decubitus ulcers (pressure sores), or urinary incontinence. In such a situation, the nurse manages the care according to the format described in the protocol. The protocol may be substantiated by a systematic review developed by the unit staff, or available from a data repository (Cook et al., 1997) (e.g. http://cochrane.hcn.net.au/clib). The nurse may also be involved in the design of the study, collection and recording of data relevant to nursing care delivery, and evaluation of that care, including clients' responses. Secondary research refers to the collection and new synthesis and analysis of findings, as in a review of previous studies. In this case, a collaborative team of multidisciplinary stakeholders may form to establish the best available evidence for a specific clinical practice (e.g. the management of mucositis for individuals with cancer). These activities inform the development of clinical guidelines and other documents to guide clinical practice.

Educational preparation for conducting research

As noted earlier, a Bachelor of Nursing (or equivalent) qualification prepares the graduate for using research findings (awareness, appreciation, application) to inform their clinical practice. The *ability* to conduct research is learned at a bachelor honours or graduate research level. In particular, nurses and midwives are educationally prepared at the research master's and doctoral levels to conduct independent primary research. At the master's level, nurses and midwives are prepared to be active members of research teams. They are able to assume the role of clinical expert, collaborating with an experienced researcher in proposal development, data collection, data analysis and interpretation. Master's prepared nurses enhance the quality and relevance of nursing research by providing clinical expertise about problems and by providing knowledge about the way the clinical services are delivered. They facilitate the investigation of clinical problems by providing a climate favourable to conducting research and provide leadership by assisting colleagues in applying research-based knowledge to nursing practice.

Nurses or midwives who have a PhD (Doctor of Philosophy, an advanced higher research degree) have the greatest amount of expertise in appraising, designing and conducting research. They develop theoretical explanations of phenomena relevant to nursing, methods of scientific enquiry and use analytical and empirical methods to discover ways to extend the knowledge base of the discipline. In addition to their role as producers of research, doctoral-prepared nurses act as role models and mentors who guide, stimulate and encourage other nurses who are developing their research skills. They also collaborate with and serve as consultants to social, educational or healthcare institutions or governmental agencies in their research endeavours. Doctoral-prepared nurses are expected to disseminate their research findings to the scientific community, to clinicians and, as appropriate, to the lay public. Scientific journals, professional conferences and the news media are among the avenues for dissemination (Dunn & Yates, 2000). The most important implication of the delineation of research activities according to educational preparation is the necessity of having a collaborative research relationship within the nursing profession. Nursing education programs affiliated with universities enable the study of research through to the doctoral level. Nurses at all educational levels, whether they are consumers or producers of research or both, need to view the research process as something of integral value to the growing professionalism in nursing.

HISTORY OF NURSING RESEARCH

The development of nursing, and therefore nursing research, has a long and interesting history which has included many theories, models and innovations. The groundwork for what has blossomed into an international research-based discipline was laid in the late nineteenth century and the first half of the twentieth century, and is intimately related to the development of clinical practice, education and disciplinary knowledge.

Post-1850

In the mid-nineteenth century, nursing as a formal discipline began evolving with the ideas and practices of Florence Nightingale. Her concepts have contributed to and are congruent with the present priorities of nursing research, particularly epidemiological methods. The promotion of health, prevention of disease and care of the sick were central ideas of her system. Nightingale believed that the systematic collection and exploration of data were necessary for nursing. Her collection and analysis of data on the health status of British soldiers during the Crimean War led to a variety of reforms in healthcare (Palmer, 1977). Nightingale also noted the need for measuring outcomes of nursing and medical care (Nightingale, 1863) and she had an expertise in statistics and epidemiology. Nightingale stated, 'Statistics are history in repose, history is statistics in motion' (Keith, 1988, p. 147).

Other than Nightingale's work, there appears to have been little documented research during the early years of the development of nursing, perhaps in part because schools of nursing had just begun to be established internationally and nursing leadership was beginning to develop independently of medicine. Osborn introduced the Nightingale model of nurse training to Australia in 1868 (Godden & Forsyth, 2000)—this was a formalised apprenticeship where student nurses provided the majority of direct nursing care in hospitals while undertaking the course (Russell, 2000). The Japanese Red Cross established a similar model in 1890 (Hisama, 2001), as did other countries in the Western Pacific region.

1900–1950

The Australasian Trained Nurses Association was formed at the turn of the century, with the *Australian Nurses Journal* (ANJ) first published in 1903. But it was not until the 1920s that nursing training and practice began to be regulated and standardised within the States of Australia (Russell, 2000).

In the United States, development and documentation of nursing research focused mainly on nursing education, but some patient- and technique-oriented research was evident. That is, nurses were predominantly the subjects of study, not patients. This was later reflected in initial nursing research in Australia. The early efforts in nursing education research in the US were made by such leaders as Dock (1900), Goodrich (1932), Nutting (1912; 1926), Robb (1906) and Wald (1915). These pioneering works were for the purpose of reforming education in nursing and establishing it as a viable profession in the US. Some clinical research emerged in the US in the early half of the twentieth century and mainly centred on the morbidity and mortality rates associated with such problems as pneumonia and contaminated milk (Carnegie, 1976). A few of these projects were instrumental in the development of patient care protocols and the employment of nurses in community settings.

Social change and World War II affected all aspects of nursing, including research. There was an urgent need for more nurses; increased hospital admissions and military needs created a shortage of personnel. After the war, nursing, like the rest of the world, began to reassess itself and its goals. A number of reports from the US continued to highlight the inconsistencies in educational preparation in the US, and demonstrated the need for nursing to enter the university setting and to update the description of nursing practices. A number of studies on nursing roles and needs followed, including exploration of nursing needs and resources (Simmons & Henderson, 1964).

1950–2000

In Australia, by the 1960s there were six separate areas of nursing: general, psychiatric, geriatric, mental retardation, midwifery and mothercraft (Russell, 2000). The 1970s saw the enrolled nurse (EN) role introduced to improve the supply of nursing-related personnel (services). While not the cause of introducing ENs, poor wages for registered nurses (RNs) and the requirement for trainees to live-in under strict regulations were issues that impacted on the supply of student nurses and registered nurses. A period of industrial and professional changes coincided with changes in societal factors (including the role of women and increased general education). This ultimately resulted in undergraduate nursing education transferring from hospital-based certificate programs into higher education diploma programs (1985–1993). The *Australian Journal of Advanced Nursing* commenced publication in 1983, and postgraduate programs in research and speciality coursework developed from the late 1980s. Doctoral studies in nursing were possible following implementation of the unified national tertiary education system in 1993. Prior to this time, nurse academics had qualifications predominantly from education, arts and social sciences.

A full examination of the development of nursing research globally and the works of so many excellent researchers, especially in the 1980s and 1990s, is beyond the scope of this chapter, but is discussed elsewhere from Australian (Russell, 2000; Wiles & Daffurn, 2002), New Zealand (NRSNZNO, 2001),

British (Crookes & Davies, 1998) and United States perspectives (NINR, 2001).

A review of the many active professional nursing organisations provides further support for the efforts of nurses throughout Australasia and globally. As the profession developed during the 1990s, a number of peer-reviewed Australian nursing research journals commenced publication (see Table 1.1). Both the RCNA and NSW College of Nursing were producing professional journals, and the development of clinical chairs in nursing became a relatively Australian approach to creating effective links between the healthcare sector and tertiary education sectors. A study of a number of clinical professors found that their role involved research, education and politics. A number of research centres also developed to support the professors, included programs which joined education and practice, and provided support and guidance for research efforts in the clinical environment (Dunn & Yates, 2000). In New Zealand the NZ Nurses Organisation was developing along a similar path, and the East Asian Forum of Nursing Scholars formed for cross-national support of academic nursing. Currently both national-based and State-based nursing professional groups and organisations are developing priorities for nursing research and strategies for promoting EBN practice in Australasia (see Chapter 6).

Nursing in the US continued to develop earlier than in Australasia. In the 1950s, nursing schools at the undergraduate and graduate levels were growing in number and graduate programs were including courses related to research. The worth and benefit of research were acknowledged by nursing leadership and were beginning to filter to the various levels of nursing. This period saw the inception of the *Journal of Nursing Research*, which was dedicated to the promotion of research in nursing. In the late 1950s nursing studies began to focus on patient or clinical problems. In a guest editorial featured in *Nursing Research* (1956), Henderson commented that studies about nurses outnumbered clinical studies ten to one, and reiterated that an essential characteristic of a profession was its ability to design its own methods for research and development of the discipline.

A reordering of research priorities and a targeting of practice-oriented research occurred in the 1960s in the US. However, even with support from major nursing organisations, research did not flourish. This may be partly attributed to the continued lack of educational preparation in research activities for the majority of nurses. Where research education did exist, nurses had not yet developed sufficient expertise in research design and methodology to teach their own research courses. Therefore nurses were, until recently, dependent on others from related disciplines such as psychology, education and sociology, who had the expertise to teach these courses. Today this is not usually the case. During the 1960s, studies on nurses and nursing continued, but at the same time the pioneers in the development of nursing theories and models, such as Orlando (1961), Peplau (1952) and Wiedenbach (1964), called for the development of nursing practice based on theory. Although their theories and those of others have only begun to be tested, the early development of those theories has spurred nurses on to a more critical level of thinking regarding nursing practice. Consistent with the increased numbers of nurses with advanced training, Federal funding and support for research increased not only in universities but also in practice settings. Many centres for nursing research grew in educational settings and in hospitals.

The 1970s also saw extended growth among US graduate programs in nursing, especially at the doctoral level. Many nurses from Australia went to the United States to complete higher degree programs as none were available locally at the time. These programs, along with the American Nurses Association (ANA) and Sigma Theta Tau (the international honour society for nurses—see (http://www.nursingsociety.org), clearly supported nurses learning the research process as well as producing research that could be used to enhance care quality. Sigma Theta Tau has over 400 chapters throughout the world, including Australia, Hong Kong, Korea, Taiwan and Pakistan. Alliances with this and other international organisations committed to the goal of health for all will create natural research partnerships. The International Council of Nurses (ICN), to which the RCNA is affiliated, and groups such as the American Academy of Nursing (http://www.nursingworld.org/aan), and other organisations and associated conferences are examples of international nursing research forums designed to inform nurses of the global breadth of health issues. Additional journals such as *Advances in Nursing Sciences*, *Nurse Researcher*, *Journal of Advanced Nursing*, *Research in Nursing and Health*, *Western Journal of Nursing Research*, and *Journal of Nursing Scholarship*, were established and promoted the generation of nursing theory and research.

The efforts in the last 20 years have been aimed at the refinement and development of research and the utilisation of research findings in clinical practice in Western healthcare delivery. Adoption of research findings to practice should be based on findings from a systematic review (SR) of a series of related studies. There are now many resources available to assist clinical nurses to provide best practice. The Joanna Briggs Institute for Evidence Based Nursing and Midwifery (http://www.joannabriggs.edu.au) was formed to examine the literature in relation to practice. Elsewhere, the EBP movement was to the fore (e.g. Cochrane Collaboration; York Centre for Evidence-Based Nursing; see Chapter 6).

Such forums for dissemination of research and clinical practice development will continue to increase, challenging nurse researchers in all regions of the world to form collaborative research relationships in which they share research expertise, educational opportunities and the ability to conduct research projects of mutual interest and, perhaps, ultimately create an international research agenda.

FUTURE DIRECTIONS: 2001–

The future of nursing research in the Australasian region looks to be an exciting one in which all nurses will have the opportunity to participate. Research continues to grow and flourish despite the difficulties being experienced by the profession within the evolving healthcare environment. In Australia, New Zealand and the Western Pacific region there are increasing numbers of doctoral-prepared nurses and higher degree programs are available within most universities. All new nurses graduate with a Bachelor of Nursing degree in Australia, and previously registered nurses are upgrading their qualifications to degree level and above in other countries. Development in midwifery as a separate and unique health discipline continues, with direct-entry programs being implemented.

As more nurses graduate from university programs, the growth in research conduct and utilisation will continue in the clinical setting at both the undergraduate and postgraduate level. In complex, health-oriented societies such as Australia (http://www.aihw.gov.au), New Zealand (http://www.health.gov.nz), Singapore (http://www.moh.gov.sg) and other Asian Pacific countries, there are increasing responses to the public's concerns related to the cost, quality, availability and accessibility of healthcare. It is of paramount importance to define the future direction of nursing research and establish research priorities (Hinshaw, 1988; 1990). Equity of access to appropriate healthcare services for all members of society will continue to challenge the collective consciousness of nurses and other stakeholders at the practice and policy-making levels, as well as providing opportunities for research. With the discipline's emphasis on cultural aspects of nursing care and the influence of such factors on practice, increasing international research is a natural futuristic trend. Access to multiple populations as a function of globalisation allows the generation and testing of nursing science from many different perspectives. Interaction with colleagues from other countries provides a rich context for the generation and dissemination of research issues (e.g. McKinley, Moser & Dracup, 2000; Stewart & Jaasma, 2001). Professional speciality organisations will also continue to formalise collaborative networks for mutual benefit, both locally and internationally. For example, in 2001 the World Federation of Critical Care Nurses was formed as an alliance between critical care nursing organisations from Australasia, Europe and North America.

Promoting depth in nursing research

It has been suggested that the nursing profession will be acknowledged as being research-based when every nurse and midwife recognises the need for research and when research becomes incorporated, inherently, into their practice (Cormack, 1996). Programs of research that include a series of studies in a similar area of study, each of which builds on prior investigation, both replicating and adding to the research question being studied, will promote depth in nursing knowledge (Beck, 1994).

Research-based practice reflects the characteristics of the research from which it is derived. The quality of research by which nursing knowledge is generated will be one of the major keys to producing predictable patient outcomes and improving patient care for our own discipline (Bavier, 1995). Essential to the achievement of this goal will be the continuing development of a national and international research environment (Dickenson-Hazard, 1995; Dreher, 1995; Zanotti, 1996). Within this environment an increasing number of nurses who have significant expertise in appraising, designing and conducting research will continue to emerge from within the profession. They will provide a 'critical mass' of investigators who will be at the forefront of the ongoing development and refinement of our scientific knowledge base for nursing practice.

Clinical consortia will help delineate the common and unique aspects of patient care for the various health professions. Cluster studies, multiple site investigations and programs of research will facilitate the accumulation of evidence supporting or refuting an existing theory and thereby contribute to defining the base of nursing practice. Nursing research is increasingly addressing physiological as well as psychological responses to actual and potential health problems (e.g. Boyle et al., 2001; Potger & Elliott, 1994; Sigmon, Amende &

Grady, 1996). Investigations that reflect state-of-the-art science will examine the interface of the biological sciences with the evolving knowledge base of nursing. Nurse researchers will continue to have increased opportunity to participate in clinical trials; this will provide direction to improve aspects of care such as symptom assessment, management and interventions to prevent and reduce physical distress such as pain (Hinshaw, 1991).

Nurse researchers will continue to gain increased methodological expertise across the full range of the paradigm, and are increasingly sophisticated regarding the development and application of computer technology to the research process. A greater emphasis will be placed on measurement issues such as the development of valid tools that accurately measure clinical phenomena. The increasing focus on the need to use multiple measures to assess clinical phenomena accurately is also apparent. Related to the need to measure clinical phenomena accurately will be the development of non-invasive methods to measure physiological parameters of interest in high technology settings (e.g. non-invasive, minimally invasive and invasive haemodynamic measurement). Qualitative research methods will continue to evolve as an increasingly important mode of enquiry, contributing to theory development and providing essential descriptive data that provide direction for clinical practice and future research studies.

The proliferation of outcomes research that is both patient- and delivery system-focused will continue to be stimulated by the need for cost-effective care that makes a difference without compromising quality. Outcome studies will provide an unprecedented opportunity for nurses to pursue research that will contribute to the knowledge base of nursing practice. By verifying the relationship between nursing interventions and patient outcomes, nurse researchers will be adding to the body of nursing interventions that are scientifically sound and document the impact of nursing care. This goal fits with the aims of EBN: to enable nurses to make clinical decisions using the best available research evidence, their clinical expertise and patient preferences, in the context of available resources (DiCenso, Cullum & Ciliska, 1998). Research-based practice guidelines and protocols are becoming benchmarks for cost-effective quality clinical practice. Nurse researchers and nurse leaders are visibly involved at the national level, participating in policy making, representing nursing on expert panels and organisations such as the National Health and Medical Research Council (NHMRC: http://www.nhmrc.gov.au), State health committees, and lobbying for needed funding dollars. Through examination of outcomes related to organisational systems outcomes, the most cost-effective models for the delivery of high quality collaborative care are being identified as health services continue to restructure with a focus towards chronic disease management and seamless care.

Programs of research

Nurses who are prepared to direct the conduct of research will head an expanding number of nursing research departments in clinical settings. Nurse researchers, often clinical professors, who head these centres will increasingly involve clinical nursing staff in generating and conducting research projects, and critically evaluating existing research data to enable improvements in clinical practice. Collaborative centres that link healthcare services and universities in partnership are established focuses for nursing research development in Australasia.

Research training for the scientific role of nurses will increasingly become an essential component of a research career plan. Programs that support a clinician scientist track, such as with the Canadian Institutes of Health Research (http://www.cihr.ca/funding_opportunities/) or the US National Institute of Nursing Research (http://www.nih.gov/ninr/research) will develop more widely. Succession planning for clinical chairs will become more sophisticated, and linked to developing programs of research that are supported by public and private funding sources at national and international levels. They will also subscribe to a lifestyle of periodic education and re-training, supported by awards, grants and fellowships. Research priorities of some groups of clinical nurses have been examined (e.g. Bell, Daly & Chang, 1997; Daly & Chang, 1996; Daly, Chang & Bell, 1996), and will continue with support from the various professional organisations. However, there is currently minimal documentation or systematic examination of specific priority areas for nursing research within Australasia. Some organisations (e.g. Joanna Briggs Institute for Evidence Based Nursing and Midwifery; NZNO) maintain registers of projects submitted by individual researchers, but in the case of the RCNA, a directory of research ceased publication in 1994. Readers are therefore directed to publications from Australasian professional nursing organisations (listed in Table 1.1) and the NHMRC for current or future opportunities for primary research in priority areas.

In the US, research priorities are much more established as a result of the National Institutes of Health infrastructure and significant funding: the 2002 priority areas include management of chronic pain; cachexia; biobehavioural management and quality of life; informal care giving; infrastructure development in nursing research training and career development; and training opportunities in clinical genetics research (http://www.nih.gov/ninr/research/dea).

KEY POINTS

- Nursing research provides the basis for expanding the body of scientific knowledge that forms the foundation of nursing practice. Research links education, theory and practice.
- Nurses become knowledgeable consumers of research through continuing education and practical experiences. As consumers of research, nurses must have a basic understanding of the research process and critical appraisal skills that provide a standard for evaluating the strengths and weaknesses of research studies before applying them in clinical practice.
- As the discipline developed through the twentieth century, research focused mainly on studies related to nursing education, although some clinical studies related to nursing care were evident. Nursing research has now an increasing emphasis on research related to patient outcomes and improving nursing practice, and understanding the nature of nursing.
- Nurses at all levels of educational preparation have a responsibility to participate in the research process. A role of the Bachelor of Nursing graduate is to be a research consumer.
- A collaborative research relationship within the nursing profession will extend and refine the scientific body of knowledge that provides the grounding for theory and evidence-based practice (EBP).

- The future of nursing research will continue to be the extension of the scientific knowledge base for nursing expertise in appraising, designing and conducting research and will provide leadership in both academic and clinical settings. Collaborative research relationships between education and industry will increase. Replication of studies will be encouraged.
- Multi-site multidisciplinary research studies will emphasise clinical issues, problems and outcomes. Priority will be given to research studies that focus on promoting health, diminishing the negative impact of health problems, ensuring care for the health needs of vulnerable groups and developing cost-effective healthcare systems.
- Both consumers and producers of research will engage in a collaborative effort to further the growth of nursing research and accomplish the research objectives of the profession.

CRITICAL THINKING CHALLENGES

- What is the assumption underlying the recommendation that the role of the degree-prepared nursing graduate in the research process is primarily that of a knowledgeable consumer?
- What effects will patient outcomes studies have on the practice of nursing?
- Is there a difference between research utilisation and evidence-based practice? Discuss.
- Identify some possible areas for nursing research that arise from your clinical practice. How might nursing research improve your practice in these areas?

Additional resources

Abdellah, F.G. (1970a). Overview of nursing research 1955–1968, part I. *Nurse Researcher*, 19(6), 17.

Abdellah, F.G. (1970b). Overview of nursing research 1955–1968, part II. *Nurse Researcher*, 19, 151–62.

Abdellah, F.G. (1970c). Overview of nursing research 1955–1968, part III. *Nurse Researcher*, 19, 239–52.

Australian and New Zealand College of Mental Health Nurses (ANZCMHN). http://www.healthsci.utas.edu.au/nursing/college/

Australian College of Critical Care Nurses (ACCCN). http://www.acccn.com.au/

Australian College of Midwives, Incorporated (ACMI). http://www.acmi.org.au/

Australian Nursing Council (ANC). http://anc.org.au/

Cochrane Collaboration. http://www.cochrane.edu.au

Dickoff, J. & James, P. (1968). A theory of theories: a position paper. *Nurse Researcher*, 17, 197–203.

East Asian Forum of Nurse Scholars (EAFONS). http://nhs.polu.edu.hk/nhs/schact/schact_eafons.html

Fawcett, J. et al. (2001). On nursing theories and evidence. *Journal of Nursing Scholarship*, 22, 115–19.

Gray, G. & Pratt, R. (1995). *Issues in Australian nursing* (4th ed.). Melbourne, Churchill Livingstone.

Gray, G. & Pratt, R. (1992). *Issues in Australian nursing* (3rd ed.). Melbourne, Churchill Livingstone.

Haber, J. et al. (1994). Shaping nursing practice through research-based protocols. *JNY State Nursing Association*, 25(3), 4–12.

Haller, K., Reynolds, M. & Horsley, J. (1979). Developing research-based innovative protocols: process, criteria and issues. *Research in Nursing & Health*, 2, 45.

Joanna Briggs Institute for Evidence Based Nursing and Midwifery. http://www.joannabriggs.edu.au/

McCormick, K. (1992). Areas of outcome research for nursing. *Journal of Professional Nursing*, 8, 71.

Middleton, S. & Lumby, J. (1999). Comparing professional and patient outcomes for the same period of care. *Australian Journal of Advanced Nursing*, 17, 22–27.

National Health Service (NHS) Centre for Reviews and Dissemination. http://www.york.ac.uk/inst/crd

New Zealand Nurses Organisation (NZNO). http://www.nzno.org.nz/

Riegal, B. et al. (1992). Moving beyond: a generative philosophy of science. *Image: The Journal of Nursing Scholarship*, 24(2), 115–20.

Royal College of Nursing, Australia. (1996). *Directory of higher education nursing courses.* RCNA, Melbourne.

Russell, R.L. (1990). From Nightingale to now: nurse education in Australia. Sydney, Saunders.

Silva, M.C. (1986). Research testing nursing theory: state of the art. *Advances in Nursing Science*, 9, 1–11.

Stetler, C.B. & Marram, G. (1976). Evaluating research findings for applicability in practice. *Nursing Outlook*, 24, 559–63.

Taylor, N. et al. (1989). Comparison of normal versus heparinized saline for flushing infusion devices. *Journal of Nursing Quality Assurance*, 3(4), 49–55.

Thompson, C. et al. (2001). Research information in nurses' clinical decision-making: what is useful? *Journal of Advanced Nursing*, 36, 376–88.

Tracy, S., Barclay, L. & Brodie, P. (2000). Contemporary issues in the workforce and education of Australian midwives. *Australian Health Review*, 23, 78–88.

2
CHAPTER

Approaches to research

Doug Elliott

LEARNING OUTCOMES

After reading this chapter the student should be able to:

- Discuss briefly the various approaches to the research process.
- Describe the process of identifying and refining a research problem, question or hypothesis.
- Identify the issues in matching a research question to an appropriate method.
- Identify the criteria for determining the significance of a research problem.
- Discuss the use of triangulation as a research approach.
- Discuss the case study as a research approach.
- Describe the characteristics and uses of the Delphi technique as a research approach.

Key terms

case study
data
Delphi technique
hypothesis
naturalistic
paradigm
population
problem statement
research problem
testable
theory
triangulation
variable

INTRODUCTION

This chapter introduces the different approaches of quantitative and qualitative research. The basic principles and distinguishing features of quantitative and qualitative designs are explored within the context of differences in philosophical origins, terminology and evaluation criteria. The philosophical basis of a researcher may be from a specific paradigm. A paradigm is a position or view of understanding the world that is shared by a community of scholars or scientists. This world view shapes one's approach to a variety of activities, including research. Whatever method is used, the research process requires the same level of rigour. The use of triangulation of methods, a case study approach and the Delphi technique, are also introduced in this chapter, while more detailed discussion on specific quantitative and qualitative methods appears in Sections 2 and 3.

The formulation of the research problem (research question, problem statement or hypothesis) is the key preliminary step in the research process, regardless of the method used. The reader should examine the consistency between the research problem and the methods used to address that problem. Critical appraisal skills are required to effectively review research studies. Such research studies are often published in academic or professional journal articles. This topic is discussed in Chapter 4.

In generating knowledge, researchers can use methods from fundamentally different paradigms. Selection of the paradigm and the resulting design is dependent upon the following starting points:

- purpose—the questions being asked
- knowledge and experience of the researcher
- need for generalisability—application of findings to larger groups.

The search for knowledge and truth is the study of epistemology, and the related study of existence is termed ontology. These philosophical concepts are discussed further in Chapter 9. From a nursing perspective, the study of individuals' responses to disease, treatment and recovery is paramount. Unique experiences or transferable findings form the basis of the decision-making for a qualitative or quantitative approach. Further delineation is outlined in one classification of paradigms:

- critical—emancipatory
- interpretive—naturalistic
- positivist—reductionist, empirical.

The first two paradigms above use qualitative methods to examine phenomena of interest. Both approaches are viewed as post-positivist in terms of critical research methodologies operating within a social change context, often with a post-modern stance that includes questioning the status quo of social and political institutions. Thus the researcher adopts a position that is free from restraint, especially from the limitations of tradition. Critical approaches seek to enable empowerment, emancipation and equality for research participants, and to challenge and change political and social issues. Interpretive approaches to research aim to describe, explore and generate meaning within a social or practice context. This philosophical position and the related concepts are complex, and may be difficult to comprehend for beginning readers of research. Nevertheless, continuing engagement of the theoretical bases for critical and interpretive approaches is important for understanding research papers that use these processes. Chapters 9 to 16, which deal with historical methods, grounded theory, ethnography, phenomenology, feminist approaches, action research and evaluation, further add to the understanding of qualitative approaches.

The term 'positivism' refers to a philosophical position which reflects the traditional scientific approach of objective observation, and prediction and testing of causal relationships (Maggs-Rapport, 2001). Empirical-analytical or logical positivism are equivalent terms used to describe the origins and belief system of the quantitative research paradigm.

The origins and belief systems for the qualitative and quantitative paradigms are compared in Table 2.1. The decision path for selecting a research approach is outlined in Figure 2.1.

TABLE 2.1 A brief comparison of qualitative and quantitative approaches

CONCEPTS	QUALITATIVE	QUANTITATIVE
Origins	Search for meaning; interactive approach	Search for truth in an objective and controlled manner
Beliefs	Complex beings who attribute unique meanings to situations	Bio-psychosocial beings with measurable components
Truth	Subjective with multiple realities	Objective reality
Basis of knowing	Meaning, discovery	Cause and effect relationships
Focus	Complex and broad	Concise and narrow
Level	Holistic	Reductionist
Reasoning	Dialectic, inductive	Logistic, deductive
Setting	Occurs in uncontrolled naturalistic (social or human) settings	Investigator seeks experiment control of the setting
Purpose	Develops theory by exploring meaning and describing relationships	Tests hypotheses and theories by control and observation
Sample	People in a sample are referred to as participants, or in ethnographic studies, as informants	People in a group are termed the sample, and are referred to as subjects, cases or respondents
Researcher position	An active and interactive participant, immersed in the setting	Uses measuring instruments or tools; e.g. questionnaires
Data elements	Written form (words)	Numerical form (numbers)
Analyses	Interpretive analysis undertaken manually or using software (e.g. NUD*IST, ETHNOGRAPH) that orders and categorises the data	Statistical analysis using software (e.g. SAS, SPSS, Minitab, Statview) to facilitate examination of quantitative data
Outcomes	Are often thematic or conceptual, but not quantifiable	Must be measurable and are reported in numeric terms
Clinical application	Exploration of unique experiences by individuals	Findings are able to be generalised to similar groups

FIGURE 2.1 Decision path for selecting a research process

If your beliefs are:

Researcher beliefs	Humans are biopsychosocial beings, known by their biological, psychological, and social characteristics. Truth is objective reality that can be experienced with the senses and measured by the researcher.	or	Humans are complex beings who attribute unique meaning to their life situations. They are known by their personal expressions. Truth is the subjective expression of reality as perceived by the participant and shared with the researcher. Truth is context laden.

then you'll ask questions, such as:

Example questions	What is the difference in blood pressure and heart rate for adolescents who are angry compared to those who are not angry?	or	What is the structure of the lived experience of anger for adolescents?

and select approaches:

Approaches	**Quantitative/deductive**	or	**Qualitative/inductive**

leading to research activities:

Research activities	Researcher selects a representative (of population) sample and determines size before collecting data. Researcher uses an extensive approach to collect data. Questionnaires and measurement devices are according to a standard protocol administered to control for extraneous variables. Primarily deductive analysis is used, generating a numerical summary that allows the researcher to reject or accept the null hypothesis.	or	Researcher selects participants who are experiencing the phenomenon of interest and collects data until saturation is reached. Researcher uses an intensive approach to collect data. Researcher conducts interviews and participant or nonparticipant observation in environments where participants usually spend their time. Researcher bias is acknowledged and set aside. Primarily inductive analysis is used, leading to a narrative summary which synthesises participant information, creating a description of human experience.

DEVELOPING AND REFINING A RESEARCH PROBLEM

A researcher spends a great deal of time refining a research idea into an examinable research problem. Unfortunately, the reviewer of a research study is not privy to this creative process, because it occurs during the study's conceptualisation. As illustrated in Table 2.2, research problems or topics originate from a variety of sources. Research problems should indicate that practical experience and a critical appraisal of the scientific literature or interest in untested theory have provided the basis for the generation of a research idea. The problem statement should reflect a refinement of the researcher's initial thinking. The reader of a research study should be able to discern that the researcher has:

- defined a specific problem area
- reviewed the relevant literature
- highlighted the potential significance of the problem to nursing or midwifery
- examined the feasibility of studying the research problem.

TABLE 2.2 Factors influencing the development of a research idea

FACTORS	INFLUENCE	EXAMPLE
Practical experience	Clinical practice provides a wealth of experience from which research problems can be derived. The nurse may observe the occurrence of a particular event or pattern and become curious about why it occurs, as well as its relationship to other factors in the patient's environment.	A nurse working with patients who have chronic heart failure observes that patients are often re-admitted because of poor treatment compliance. An outreach service is designed and tested with important results (Stewart, Pearson & Horowitz, 1998; Stewart, Vandenbroek, Pearson & Horowitz, 1999).
Critical appraisal of the scientific literature	A review of studies appearing in journals may indirectly suggest a problem area by stimulating the reader's thinking. A nurse may observe a conflict or inconsistency in the findings of several related research studies and wonder which findings are most valid.	A review of studies which examined the health outcomes of ICU survivors (beyond mortality and morbidity measures) (Elliott, 1999) outlines recommendations for primary research, as well as some methodological concerns.
Gaps in the literature	A review may identify gaps in the literature and suggest areas for future study. Research ideas can also be generated by research reports that suggest the value of replicating a particular study to extend or refine the existing scientific knowledge base.	A nurse who had just begun working on an oncology unit observed that the concerns and well-being of partners of patients with breast cancer were not a focus of attention after diagnosis and during treatment of the patients' breast cancer. He wondered whether the partners' emotional and physical concerns and feelings of well-being as predictors of adjustment had even been examined. A review of the literature identified no studies that provided a scientific basis for determining factors related to adjustment of breast cancer patients and their partners (Hoskins, 1996).

Interest in untested theory	Verification of an untested nursing theory provides a relatively uncharted area from which research problems can be derived. Although theories themselves are not tested, a researcher may investigate a particular concept or concepts related to specific theory. A deductive process would be used to generate the research problem,with questions posed such as, 'If this theory is correct, what kind of behaviour would I expect to observe in particular patients and under which conditions?' or 'If this theory is valid, what kind of supporting evidence would I find?'.	Developments of theoretical models derived from nursing and related literature are conducted to provide empirical support for the accuracy of a specific theoretical model that examines the fit between the hypothesised model and the data. One researcher sought to explain adaptation to the uncertainty of multiple sclerosis (MS) in women. A causal model, developed from the literature and from interviews with four women with MS, was tested. Successful adaptation was measured by self-esteem and mastery. The negative impact of uncertainty was significantly reduced by the women's spiritual and social relationships (Crigger, 1996).

Defining a specific problem area

Researchers generally begin with an interest in some broad topic area, such as pain management, family communication patterns, self-care activities of the aged or management of urinary incontinence. When nurses ask questions such as 'Why are things done this way?', 'I wonder what would happen if…?' or 'What characteristics are associated with…?', they are often well on their way to developing a researchable problem. Using qualitative methods, the research may explore individuals' responses to treatment, or experiences of a clinical condition or health/illness state, and the meanings attached to these experiences. In quantitative designs the research focuses on defined variables of interest and their relationship to each other. Regardless of the approach, the researcher engages in an enquiry process linked to their philosophy of research and experience, as well as the question or topic under consideration. These aspects led to studies which explored, for example, men's experiences during their partner's first pregnancy (Barclay, Donovan & Genovese, 1996), the accuracy of alcohol history-taking by nurses and doctors (Burns & Adams, 1997), women's experiences of breast cancer (Webb & Koch, 1997), or the recovery process for survivors of a myocardial infarction (Daly et al., 2000; Jackson et al., 2000). Figure 2.2 illustrates how the development of a research idea is influenced by practical experience, scientific literature and untested theory.

The research consumer may not see a formal statement of the research problem or hypothesis in a research article because of space constraints or stylistic considerations in particular publications. What does appear more often in published articles is a statement of the aims, purpose or goals of the research study. Nevertheless, it is equally important for both the consumer and producer of research to understand the importance of the problem statement and hypothesis as foundation elements of the study, as they are elements that set the stage for the development of the research study.

FIGURE 2.2 Process of formulating a research problem

Idea emerges

Recovery processes of patients following hospital discharge with a diagnosis of myocardial infarction

↓

Brainstorming

How do survivors from a recent myocardial infarction deal with their illness and recovery?

What factors impact on this recovery process?

How do these factors interrelate?

↓

Review of the literature

The period after discharge following a myocardial infarction is noted as a vulnerable period with psychological morbidity a common phenomenon. The literature suggests that little is known about the process of adjustment for these survivors. Stress and coping are personal experiences, with factors such as age, personality traits and situational factors affecting appraisal and coping. Thus, an examination of issues that influence patients' recovery and compliance with lifestyle changes is necessary in the immediate post-hospitalisation period.

↓

Identify variables

Potential variables:

- age
- disease morbidity
- health status
- health behaviours/risk factors
- coping
- social support
- health support needs

↓

Research problem is formulated

To explore the health status, perceptions of coping and social support among survivors of a recent myocardial infarction in the first three weeks after discharge from hospitals in south-western Sydney (Daly et al., 2000).

Reviewing relevant literature

Consistent with the study design, the review is a systematic and rigorous exploration of the extant (existing) literature related to the concept(s) of interest. An accomplished review provides synthesis of findings from studies and analysis of themes and methods identified from the literature, written in a clear and concise form. There are numerous styles and steps to a literature review, which are discussed more fully in Chapter 5. The literature review should reveal that the literature relevant to the problem area has been critically examined. Often, concluding sections on recommendations and implications for practice in previous articles identify remaining gaps in the literature, the need for replication, or the need for extension of the knowledge base about a particular research focus.

In a previously cited example about women's experience of breast cancer (Webb & Koch, 1997), the researchers would have conducted a preliminary review of papers for theories and research studies on the topic. The psychosocial research examined focused on coping strategies, quality of life and women's participation in the choice of treatment. At this point the researcher could have written the following problem statements:

- How do women experience breast cancer?
- What are the similarities or differences in the way women experience invasive and non-invasive breast cancer?

The reader can identify the interrelatedness of the initial definition of the problem area, the literature review and the refined problem statement. The reader of a research paper examines the end product of this formulation process and should have an appreciation of this time-consuming process. For example, the experience of new motherhood was the research problem for a grounded theory study by Barclay et al. (1997). The data provided a conceptualisation of early motherhood that resulted in the development of strategies for health professionals to assist women at this time in their lives. In a previously cited example about men's experiences during their partner's first pregnancy (Barclay, Donovan & Genovese, 1996), the researchers' purpose was to develop an empirically grounded theory through observations and interviews. Wellard and Palaster (1996) conducted an experiment in the evaluation of two methods of pre-cannulation skin disinfection. The motivation for the study was environmental concern about the disposal of the packs and the benefits of povidone iodine as a skin disinfectant.

Significance to nursing or midwifery

Before proceeding to a final formulation of the problem statement, it is crucial for the researcher to have examined the problem's potential significance to nursing. The research problem should have the potential for contributing to and extending the scientific body of nursing knowledge. The significance should be in relation to:

- potential for patients, nurses, the healthcare community in general and society to benefit from the study
- the results being applicable for extending the knowledge base of nursing practice, education or management
- the results providing theoretical relevance

- the findings supporting previously untested theoretical assumptions, extending or challenging an existing theory or clarifying a conflict in the literature
- the findings informing the formulation or revision of nursing practices or policies.

If the research problem has not met any of these criteria, then the significance is questionable. In a previously cited example (Daly et al., 2000), the problem statement demonstrating the significance of the problem included the following facts:

- admission to hospital for an acute myocardial infarction is a stressful event for individuals and their families
- the impact of decreasing lengths of stay for hospital admissions needs to be examined for specific clinical cohorts (groups), so that adequate support is available to enable optimal post-hospital patient outcomes
- the coping process may be of prime importance as it works to facilitate or impair adaptational outcomes during the immediate post-hospital discharge period.

REFINING THE PROBLEM STATEMENT

The final problem statement may be written in declarative or interrogative forms as illustrated in Table 2.3. The style chosen is largely a function of the researcher's preference, experience and originating paradigm. An effective problem statement exhibits the following three characteristics:

- provides clear identification of the concept of interest (concepts, phenomena or variables under investigation)
- specifies the population being studied
- demonstrates the focus of the study (i.e. examination of experiences, exploration of variables and relationships, or empirical testing).

These components can also be used to develop statements for secondary research approaches such as systematic reviews (SRs) (see Chapter 5).

TABLE 2.3 Problem statements in declarative and interpretive forms

RESEARCH FOCUS	PROBLEM STATEMENT
DECLARATIVE	
Men's experiences during their partner's first pregnancy: a grounded theory analysis.	This study reported interviews with 53 men who were attending antenatal classes with their partners. Experiences were discussed in focus groups run by male midwives who were also fathers (Barclay et al., 1996).
Evaluating two methods of pre-cannulation skin disinfectant.	No previous reports of empirical evaluation of skin disinfection prior to invasive nursing procedures (Wellard & Palaster, 1996).
Investigating the impact of massage therapy on patients' perceptions of post-operative pain.	The study examined the effects of massage on pain. Four of the five basic techniques of Swedish or relaxation massage were used. No studies have previously analysed the relationship between duration of massage and reduction of pain (Nixon et al., 1997).

INTERPRETIVE	
Factors in stress and burnout in paediatric nurses in a general ward.	What is the burnout level of nurses in a multi-specialty paediatric area; what are the causes of stress; and how can stress be prevented on the ward? (Watson & Feld, 1996).
A comparison of the possible similarities or differences in the way women experience invasive and non-invasive breast cancer.	What are women's experiences of invasive and non-invasive breast cancer? (Webb & Koch, 1997).
Factors that contribute to the delay in seeking treatment among patients with an evolving acute myocardial infarction (MI).	What cognitive, emotional, socio-demographic and clinical factors contribute to the delay in seeking treatment among patients with MI? (McKinley, Moser & Dracup, 2000).

Concept of interest

The concepts of major interest in studies are called variables or phenomena, depending on the paradigmatic position of the research. From a quantitative perspective, variables exhibit different values (i.e. the properties of the variable can vary, e.g. pain, anxiety). Properties that differ from each other, such as age, weight, height, religion and ethnicity, are other examples of variables. Quantitative research attempts to understand how and why differences in one variable are related to differences in another variable. In qualitative studies, the phenomenon of interest is explored within a more holistic and humanistic context. Relationships or experiences are explored within the real world setting. The philosophical stance has an interpretive or emancipatory and transformative intent (critical social theory) (see Chapter 14). Interpretive methodologies include ethnography, grounded theory, historical methods and phenomenology. Critical methodologies include action research and feminist research. The experiences of women who survived an acute myocardial infarction (AMI) were examined from a feminist perspective (Jackson et al., 2000), with themes of increasing confidence and optimism highlighted at three weeks post-discharge, after some initial fear and uncertainty. This study focused on providing women's voices to the experiences of an acute health crisis, therefore providing some sense of emancipation, particularly in an area where it was evident from previous research that women were under-represented in studies of AMI.

The concept of interest can also be examined through documentary evidence, as in historical research (see Chapter 10), or other approaches which are discussed in Chapters 11 to 16.

Population of interest

The terms population or sample are commonly used in quantitative studies to identify the societal group of interest. The people being studied need to be specified in the problem statement. If the scope of the problem has been narrowed to a specific focus and the variables have been clearly identified, the nature of the population will be evident to the reader of a research report. For example, Small and colleagues (Small, Lumley, Donohue, Potter & Waldenstrom, 2000) developed a problem statement that evaluated the effect of a midwife-led debriefing session for women undergoing operative birth on postnatal depression and health status. The reader can immediately identify that the population of interest is mothers undergoing operative birth. Similarly, Watson and Feld (1996) aimed to identify factors in stress among paediatric nurses in a general hospital to measure their burnout level and identify new ways of preventing stress on the ward. The sample consisted of 26 nurses working on the ward. The problem statement was 'What are the factors contributing to the high stress and staff turnover on the ward?'.

In qualitative approaches, participants in the study also reflect a particular group of society. For example, in Kermode's (1995) study the research question was 'What are patients' perceptions of nursing interventions that were helpful and unhelpful during their hospitalisation with an AIDS-defining illness?'. The sample was eight male patients hospitalised for an AIDS-defining illness. This phenomenological study sought to examine the participants' experiences of nursing interventions, but not to generalise the findings to a wider population.

Focus of the study

The refined problem statement includes the approaches used to examine the question, aim or hypothesis being posed. The reader should examine the consistency between the aims, methods and results of a study. The specific research methods available to researchers are discussed in more detail in Sections 2 and 3 of the book. Specifically, Chapters 9 and 17 continue on from this chapter in examining the common aspects of qualitative and quantitative approaches, respectively. Each chapter provides further insight into the most common research approaches used in nursing and midwifery research. There is also opportunity for researchers to combine methods of enquiry, and this concept is discussed in the following section.

TRIANGULATION

Triangulation is the expansion of research methods in a single study or multiple studies to enhance diversity, enrich understanding and accomplish specific goals. There are several perspectives about triangulation. Morse (1991) illustrated a combination of methods labelled simultaneous or sequential triangulation. In simultaneous and sequential triangulation each combination is made for distinct reasons (see Table 2.4).

TABLE 2.4 Simultaneous and sequential combinations of quantitative and qualitative research methods

COMBINATION	RATIONALE	EXAMPLE
SIMULTANEOUS		
Qualitative + quantitative	There is a qualitative foundation and quantitative methods are used to provide complementary information.	The research is focused on the experiences of feeling depressed after the loss of a spouse. Phenomenological methods could be used to address the question, and use of a depression scale would provide complementary information.
Quantitative + qualitative	There is a quantitative foundation and qualitative methods are used to provide complementary information.	The research is testing hypotheses about depression after the death of a spouse. The phenomenological method is used to uncover the experience for a select group who acknowledge feelings of depression.

SEQUENTIAL		
Qualitative → quantitative	Findings from qualitative investigation lead to use of the quantitative approach.	The research has described the experience of feeling depressed after the death of a spouse. The themes emerging from the data are then used to create a depression scale, which is tested for reliability and validity.
Quantitative → qualitative	Findings from quantitative investigation lead to use of the qualitative approach.	The research has tested hypotheses linking the death of a spouse with depression and found no significant relationships. A qualitative study is undertaken to uncover the experience of living through the death of one's spouse in an effort to let the data lead to common thoughts and feelings.

Modified from Morse, 1991.

Simultaneous triangulation is the combination of qualitative and quantitative methods in one study at the same time (see Table 2.5). A triangulated methodology was used to explore the experiences, health status and social support of women and men who were recovering from an acute myocardial infarction (Daly et al., 2000; Jackson et al., 2000).

TABLE 2.5 Use of triangulated approach in one study

RESEARCH PROCESS COMPONENTS	QUANTITATIVE APPROACH	QUALITATIVE APPROACH
Design	Descriptive, repeated measures.	Exploratory, informed by feminist principles.
Participants	Thirty-eight survivors of AMI.	Ten women survivors of AMI.
Data collection	Health status, coping, social support during first three weeks post-discharge.	Three semi-structured interviews comprising 10 questions. Each interview was one hour in duration and was audiotaped.
Analysis	*t* test: cardiac recovery, social support (seven and twenty-one days); repeated ANOVA: health status, cardiac symptoms.	Three-step method—moral language, dissonance and logic of narrative/themes.
Findings	Stable health status, attitude, behaviour; optimistic, self-reliant, confrontive coping styles.	Complex response—fear, uncertainty initially; at three weeks more positive, return of energy, increasing confidence.

Modified from Daly et al., 2000; Jackson et al., 2000.

In sequential triangulation, only one approach is used in a study, but the researcher conducts multiple studies using different approaches in each. Beck (1992) used sequential triangulation, beginning with a quantitative approach followed by qualitative work (see Table 2.6). In each of these studies, Beck used a different approach to study the same topic, namely postpartum depression. She was guided by her research questions. In each instance, she embraced a different set of values and activities to add to the body of nursing knowledge of postpartum depression. Although most nurses tend to use one or other research approach repeatedly, their choice of approach is guided by the questions identified. Beck continues to research the field a decade after the cited studies given in the following table (Beck, 1992; Beck & Gable, 2001; Beck, Reynolds & Rutowski, 1992).

TABLE 2.6 Comparison of two linked studies examining postpartum depression: quantitative and qualitative approaches

	MATERNITY BLUES AND POSTPARTUM DEPRESSION (Beck, Reynolds & Rutowski, 1992)	THE LIVED EXPERIENCE OF POSTPARTUM DEPRESSION: A PHENOMENOLOGICAL STUDY (Beck, 1992)
Participants	n = 49 Primiparous American-born women who had uncomplicated pregnancies and vaginal deliveries.	n = 7 Mothers who attended a local postpartum depression support group; 4 were primiparous and and 3 had caesarean deliveries.
Data collectors	Four trained research assistants who had no health-related education to confounding variables.	The researcher was the data collector (see Instruments).
Instruments	Stein's Maternity Blues Scale, a 13-symptom self-rated scale with acceptable reliability and validity; Beck Depression Inventory, measuring 21 categories of symptoms and attitudes and reporting well-established reliability and validity.	Researcher interviewed the subjects and scheduled follow-up interviews to be sure that participants agreed with the researcher's interpretation of their experiences; before each interview the researcher recalled and transcended her biases to capture the participant's reality.
Analysis/summary	Deductive analysis was accomplished through inferential statistics: 'No significant differences were found at 1, 6 and 12 weeks postpartum in the mean depression scores for mothers who were discharged after the customary length of hospital stay.	Inductive analysis was conducted by using the phenomenological approach; the meaning of participants' descriptions was distilled and synthesised into 11 themes, including loneliness, obsessive thoughts of being a bad mother, fear and guilt over pondering harming infant, inability to concentrate and insecurity leading to a need to be mothered herself.

Denzin (1978) provides another perspective, identifying four basic types of triangulation:

- data
- investigator
- theory
- methodological.

Janesick (1994) has expanded Denzin's view to include inter-disciplinary triangulation (see Table 2.7). This perspective is very different from Morse (1991) (see Table 2.4), in proposing other areas of triangulation beyond methodological diversity. These perspectives of triangulation offer frameworks to enrich understanding of human phenomena.

TABLE 2.7 Types of triangulation

TYPE	EXPLANATION
Data triangulation	The use of a variety of data sources in a study.
Investigator triangulation	The use of several different researchers or evaluators.
Theory triangulation	The use of multiple perspectives to interpret a single set of data.
Methodological triangulation	The use of multiple methods to study a single problem.
Multidisciplinary triangulation	The use of multiple disciplines to inform the research process.

Modified from Denzin, 1978; Janesick, 1994.

The Byrne and McMurray study (1997) used triangulation as well as concurrent data collection, analyses and verification of themes (as suggested by Colaizzi, 1978). The interview data were compared with the interviewer's notes of observations and reflections on non-verbal data. This process of data triangulation provided more depth than using a single source of data collection and analysis. Sub-themes were identified and examples of the words of the participants were provided to enable the reader to share in the analyses and discover what caring for the dying meant to the nine nurses. Two examples of comments from the sub-theme 'balancing guilt and compassion' were, 'I felt guilty in the past about making more of an effort, but I now realise it's just different priorities. Guilt means not being committed to what you are doing', and, 'Initially, I used to think, why was I short with that person? I could have done this or that. I could have done more. But not now'. The nurses perceived that they had changed as a result of their palliative care experiences. The researchers concluded from the nurses' comments that care meant 'being receptive and responsive to needs and in knowing the importance of the self in functioning effectively'. This process of data triangulation resulted in more depth and understanding of the issues investigated. The findings also have implications for nursing education programs in this important area of care.

The aim of another triangulated study was to methodologically triangulate the perceptions of family members and intensive care nurses in regard to the needs of families of critically ill patients (Burr, 1998). Both qualitative and quantitative methods were used to collect data from family members of patients admitted to a general intensive care unit and from nurses working on those units. The qualitative component of the study consisted of data obtained through taped interviews. The Critical Care Family Needs Inventory was also used to obtain quantitative data. By converging the data through triangulation, 'a more comprehensive understanding of family needs and experiences was achieved than would have been possible with one method alone' (Burr, 1998).

CASE STUDY APPROACH

Methodological triangulation can also be used in other approaches, such as a case study. The term 'case study' has a variety of meanings within both research and clinical contexts. A case study research approach enables a detailed examination of a single 'case' or 'unit', within a real life and contemporary context using multiple data sources (Bergen & While, 2000; Hewitt-Taylor, 2002). The phenomenon of interest can be an individual, a social group, a community, an organisation or an event. The approach is observational and responsive to the context, and is examined in its own right without regard for generalisation (Keyzer, 2000). Thus, the approach is qualitative in philosophical stance, although the triangulation of methods enables use of the full range of data collection strategies—interviews, field notes, participant observation, and contemporary documents (Bergen & While, 2000). As with other qualitative approaches, the analysis of case study data commonly uses a constant comparative approach (Hewitt-Taylor, 2002; see Chapter 9). This type of research method should not be confused with a 'case presentation' of a particular 'clinical case' (e.g. Dunford, Donoghue & Lazaris, 1999) or a case-control study (an epidemiological design) (see Chapter 19).

DELPHI TECHNIQUE

The Delphi technique is an approach used to gain group consensus on a specific topic. The process involves a group of respondents providing expert opinion on a topic by extracting the viewpoints of all parties, enabling individual responses to the viewpoints, and ultimately achieving consensus (Bowles, 1999; Crisp et al., 1999). The stages of the Delphi process include selection of the expert panel, formulation of the question(s), generation of statements, reduction and categorisation of statements, rating of statements, and analysis and iteration (Mead & Moseley, 2001). The panel size ranges from 10 to 50 (Bowles, 1999).

Content analysis is used to synthesise responses at each survey round and results are reported back to the respondents. Respondents then review all of the responses and submit another response until consensus is reached—usually within two or three rounds. The benefits of the Delphi technique include the ability to harness many opinions across geographical distance, the freedom of individuals to express their opinion without being influenced by other group members, allowing individuals to participate at a convenient time, and with relatively small expense. These benefits overcome the potential limitations of other consensus methods such as focus groups, nominal group technique or consensus conferences (Mead & Moseley, 2001).

The Delphi technique is a useful strategy for examining an area with a scant research base, and has been used in workforce planning, curriculum planning, identifying clinical research priorities, identifying competencies, developing clinical guidelines, and determining best practice standards (Bowles, 1999; Mead & Moseley, 2001). For example, Williams and Clarke (2001) used a consensus method to determine nurse staffing requirements for intensive care units in Australia. Sixteen critical care nurse experts were surveyed on four occasions to develop and refine a number of consensus statements on nursing workforce issues. Another study surveyed 13 experts in three rounds to validate set aims, competencies and objectives for a clinical orientation program (Boyle, Butcher & Kenney, 1998). Other examples are listed in the 'Additional resources' section of this chapter. As noted above, expert opinion on a clinical practice may be the only available evidence when no quality primary research findings are evident (NHMRC, 2000)—see Chapter 6 for further discussion of expert opinion in relation to levels of evidence.

Despite the utility of the Delphi technique for nursing and midwifery research, a recent review highlighted a decreasing trend in publications using this approach (Bowles, 2001). In addition, there are a number of methodological considerations to address, including inadequate descriptions of panellist characteristics, imprecise definitions and measures of consensus, and high wastage of respondents (Bowles, 1999), as well as other fundamental theoretical and methodological concerns, particularly in terms of modifications to the process which may threaten the validity of the study findings (Crisp et al., 1999).

KEY POINTS

- Qualitative and quantitative methods have differing philosophical bases, approaches, terminology and evaluation criteria.
- Formulation of the research problem is an important key preliminary step in the research process; the detail to which the problem is identified is often representative of the overall conceptual development and design of the study.
- Refinement of the research problem includes examination of the previous research literature, and discussion of the potential significance of the problem to nursing or midwifery practice, education or theory.
- Triangulation is a strategy for combining research methods and/or approaches to improve understanding of the research problem.

CRITICAL THINKING CHALLENGES

- If nurses with a Bachelor of Nursing degree are not expected to conduct research, what sense does it make to expect this group of nursing students to be able to critique each step of the research process? Support either a pro or con position.
- What are the advantages of data triangulation over a single method of data collection?

Additional resources

Barrett, S., Kristjanson, L.J., Sinclair, T. & Hyde, S. (2001). Priorities for adult cancer nursing: a West Australian replication. *Cancer Nursing*, 24, 88–98.

Chang, E. & Daly, J. (2000). A Delphi study of clinical research priorities in aged care nursing. *Geriaction*, 18, 7–12.

Crisp, J., Pelletier, D., Duffield, C., Adams, A. & Nagy, S. (1997). The Delphi method? *Nursing Research*, 46, 116–18.

Duffield, C. (1989). The Delphi technique. *Australian Journal of Advanced Nursing*, 6, 41–45.

Duffield, C. (1993). The Delphi technique: a comparison of results obtained using two expert panels. *International Journal of Nursing Studies*, 30, 227–37.
Fry, M. & Burr, G. (2001). Using the Delphi technique to design a self-reporting triage survey tool. *Accident & Emergency Nursing*, 9, 235–41.
Ibrahim, J.E. (2000). Translating quality into research: do we need more research into quality or should quality activities be conducted using the principles and methodological rigour of scientific research? *Journal of Quality in Clinical Practice*, 20, 63–64.
Kenney, S., Hasson, F. & McKenna, H.P. (2001). A critical review of the Delphi technique as a research methodology for nursing. *International Journal of Nursing Studies*, 38, 195–200.
Lincoln, Y.S. (1992). Sympathetic connections between qualitative methods and health research. *Qualitative Health Research*, 2(4), 375–91.
Miller, M.A. & Malcolm, N.S. (1990). Critical thinking in the nursing curriculum, *Nursing & Health Care*, 11(2), 67–73.
Morse, J.M. & Field, P.A. (1995). *Qualitative research methods for health professionals.* (2nd ed.). Thousand Oaks, California, Sage.
Pelletier, D., Duffield, C., Adams, A., Mitten-Lewis, S., Nagy, S. & Crisp, J. (1997). The cardiac nurse's role: an Australian Delphi study perspective. *Clinical Nurse Specialist*, 11, 255–63.
Pelletier, D., Duffield, C., Adams, A., Nagy, S., Crisp, J. & Mitten-Lewis, S. (2000). Australian nurse educators identify gaps in expert practice. *Journal of Continuing Education in Nursing*, 31, 224–31.
Turkel, M.C. & Ray, M.A. (2001). Relational complexity: from grounded theory to instrument development and theoretical testing. *Nursing Science Quarterly*, 14, 281–87.
Williams, P. & Webb, C. (1994). The Delphi technique: a methodological discussion. *Journal of Advanced Nursing*, 19, 180–86.

3

CHAPTER

Searching literature sources

Doug Elliott

LEARNING OUTCOMES

After reading this chapter the student should be able to:

- Differentiate between types of literature.
- Differentiate between primary and secondary sources of professional and scientific information.
- Compare online databases and traditional print database sources for conducting a relevant search of the literature.

Key terms

bibliographic database
Cumulative Index to Nursing and Allied Health Literature (CINAHL)
internet
Medline
online
OVID
primary source
print databases
refereed (peer-reviewed) journals
secondary source
web browser
world wide web (www)

INTRODUCTION

A systematic approach to searching and reviewing the literature enables a review of the state of the science for a particular discipline such as nursing. It is now routine for a researcher to log on to OVID (http://www.ovid.com) through their institutional internet server and examine CINAHL (http://www.cinahl.com), Medline (http://www.medline.com), and other databases using specific key words and a search of publication dates from the last five years (of course, searches are not necessarily restricted to the last five years).

Portals such as OVID or clinician support sites maintained by health departments and other organisations, for example:

- Clinical Information Access Program—CIAP (http://www.clininfo.health.nsw.gov.au)
- Clinicians Health Channel (http://www.clinicians.vic.gov.au)

enable a search across multiple databases rather than users conducting sequential multiple searches. OVID also enables automatic downloading of references to bibliographic databases for reference management and links to word-processing applications. This facility enables the research consumer to undertake a review of the extant (that which exists at the present time) literature on a specific clinical practice question. Readers should examine which portals or other resources are available through their university, health service or other organisations.

A competent research consumer is expected to have information literacy skills, know how to conduct a literature review, critically evaluate it and then write about it in a progressively sophisticated style. This includes the ability to:

- efficiently retrieve an adequate amount of scholarly literature using information technology and CD-ROM or online programs such as OVIDweb, which links to numerous scholarly databases (e.g. Cumulative Index to Nursing and Allied Health Literature—CINAHL), Medline, as well as traditional print resources for material not entered into the common databases
- evaluate material based on accepted criteria for respective literature sources
- synthesise the critically evaluated literature (e.g. the entire compilation of conceptual and data-based literature about patient-controlled analgesia [PCA]).

Table 3.1 presents an overview of the steps for conducting a literature search. In the right-hand column are some useful strategies for successfully and efficiently completing these steps. This process is the same whether the purpose is critiquing or writing a literature review. It reflects the cognitive processes and manual techniques of retrieving and critically reviewing sources from the literature.

This chapter examines sources of academic literature and search strategies (steps 1–3 in Table 3.1) as a prelude to a critical review of the extant literature, primarily from the perspective of the research consumer. Chapters 4 and 5 discuss the critical review of the literature (steps 4–6 in Table 3.1). Chapter 5 specifically examines the literature review as a section of a primary research article, or as the focus in a secondary research paper (literature review; systematic review). Knowledge and skills for both searching the literature and critically reviewing the literature are essential and complementary. In practical terms, searching and reviewing the literature is a continuous and seamless process.

TABLE 3.1 Steps and strategies for searching and reviewing the literature

STEPS OF THE REVIEW PROCESS	STRATEGY
1. Formulation of a review question.	Keep focused on the types of patients/clients you deal with in your work setting. You know what works and doesn't work in the delivery of nursing care.
2. Conducting a comprehensive search of the literature.	Ask your reference librarian for help and read the data-based guide books usually found near the computers used for student searches; include 'research' as one of your variables.
3. Assessing studies for inclusion in the review.	Do it yourself with the help of your librarian; it is important for nurses to use appropriate databases such as those available through the OVID portal.
4. Critically appraising studies.	Scan through your search, read the abstracts provided and highlight or otherwise mark only those that fit your topic; check that 'references' (RF) are included in the print field for your search. Organise by journal type and year and reread abstracts to determine if the articles chosen are relevant. Scan each article to determine if it is worth your time and money to retrieve it.
5. Synthesising the findings from individual studies.	Copy the *entire* article including the references, making sure that you can clearly read the name of the journal, year, volume number and pages; this can save you an immense amount of time when you are word-processing your paper. Review critical reading strategies (see Chapter 4). For example, read the abstract at the beginning of the article (see example in this chapter). Use the critical reading strategies from Chapter 4; take the time to word-process each summary (no more than one page long) include references in APA style at the top or bottom of each summary and staple the copied article to the back of your summary.
6. Reporting results and recommendations.	Decide how you will present your synthesis of the reviewed articles (e.g. chronologically, according to type—conceptual or data-based), and word-process the synthesised material and a reference list.

TYPES OF RESOURCES

Nursing has an ever-growing body of scholarly literature that also focuses on the use of specific nursing theories or models, as well as a range of concepts or variables from other disciplines, which also relate to the nature and practice of nursing. The resources available to assist the conduct of a literature review are practically endless. Common sources of professional nursing literature are journal articles, abstracts, critique reviews, text books, chapters of books, abstracts published in conference proceedings, professional and governmental reports and unpublished doctoral dissertations. Also, there are a growing number of full-text articles or abstracts available through internet sources. Less common and less used sources of scholarly material are audiotapes, videotapes, personal communications (letters or telephone or in-person interviews), unpublished doctoral dissertations and master's theses. Primary and secondary sources, refereed journals, electronic and print databases, and websites are discussed below.

Primary and secondary sources

A credible literature review reflects the use of mainly primary sources. An individual or team who conducted the original research or developed the theory writes a primary source. Most primary sources are found in published literature. (See the section called 'Refereed journals' on pages 42–43 for a discussion and examples of commonly used journals.) A person other than the individual or team who conducted the original research or developed the theory writes a secondary source. Sometimes a secondary source represents a response to or a summary and critique of a theorist's or researcher's work, or an in-depth analysis on an issue, problem or concept (e.g. a review paper).

Journals contain both primary and secondary research articles, and Table 3.2 provides some examples of these print sources. Primary articles are reports on an original piece of research, while secondary research articles are reviews of a series of primary studies on a specific topic (see Chapter 5). Both types of articles are accessible through refereed journals, electronic or print databases, and websites. Experience in working with these knowledge sources is a requirement for nursing graduates in clinical, educational and professional settings.

There are two general reasons for using secondary sources. One reason is that a primary source is literally unavailable. This is rarely the case in this age of computer searches, interlibrary book loans and the ability of libraries to copy an article and send or fax it to the person requesting the information (a charge may occur for this service). Another reason, which is more common, is that a secondary source can provide different ways of looking at an issue or problem. Secondary sources can help students develop the ability to see things from another person's point of view, which is an essential aspect of critical reading (Paul, 1995).

Secondary sources that are published in refereed journals are generally written by experienced nursing scholars. Secondary sources include systematic reviews (SRs) (see Chapters 5 and 6 for further discussion). The advantages of secondary sources are that they are already a review of the state of the science, and form an important component in the application of knowledge to practice. Such articles usually provide a critical evaluation of, or a response to, a theory or research study, and include implications for practice and/or contributions of the work to the development of the science of nursing. Journals such as *Evidence-Based Nursing* (http://www.evidencebasednursing.com) and organisations such as The Joanna Briggs Institute for Evidence Based Nursing and Midwifery (http://www.joannabriggs.edu.au) and The Cochrane Collaboration (http://www.cochrane.org and http://www.cochrane.org.au), are devoted to evidence-based practice (EBP) (see Chapter 6), and generate large volumes of secondary material. Secondary sources should be used in context (e.g. in clinical practice guideline development), and should relate to the purpose of the literature reviews—they can have tremendous value for the beginning research consumer.

TABLE 3.2 Examples of primary and secondary journal articles, books, chapters in books, or documents

PRIMARY	SECONDARY
Journal article Kermode, M. (1995). Patients' experiences of nursing interventions during hospitalisation with an AIDS-defining illness. *Australian Journal of Advanced Nursing* 12(3), 20–30.	Elliott, D. (1999). Measuring the health outcomes of general ICU patients: a systematic review of methods and findings. *Australian Critical Care*, 12,132–40.
Book Lawler, J. (1991). *Behind the screens: nursing, somology and the problem of the body*. Churchill Livingstone, Melbourne.	Johnstone, M. (1999). *Bioethics: a nursing perspective*. (3rd ed.). Sydney, WB Saunders.
Chapter in a book n/a	Russell, R.L. (2000). Milestones in Australian nursing. In Daly, J., Speedy, S. & Jackson, D., eds, *Contexts of nursing: an introduction*. Sydney, MacLennan & Petty.
Doctoral dissertation Bucknall, T.K. (1996). Clinical decision making in critical care nursing practice: decisions, processes and influences. Unpublished doctoral thesis, La Trobe University.	n/a
Document Uyeda, M.L., Farrell, M.J., Schneider, Z. & Millership, R. (1997). *National palliative care education and training needs analysis final report*. Canberra, Commonwealth Department of Health and Family Services.	RCNA. (1998). *Position statement: nursing research*. Canberra, Royal College of Nursing, Australia.

Refereed journals

A major portion of most literature reviews consists of published papers as journal articles. Increasingly, there may be both printed and electronic versions of the journal issues accessible as full-text articles from the publishers. Currently, journals continue to be the preferred mode for communicating the latest theory or results of a study in the written form, but this is being increasingly supported by internet resources with pre-publication articles being released on journal websites (e.g. http://www.bmj.com). Textbooks are now also available on the internet (e.g. http://www.gateway1.ovid.com has *The Lippincott Manual of Nursing Practice* online, as well as other nursing and medical texts). Some of these texts also provide regular web-based updates of their information, rather than waiting for the next edition of the book to be published on a regular three to five year cycle.

As a beginning research consumer, refereed or peer-reviewed journals should be the first source of primary scholarly literature. A refereed journal uses a panel of external and internal reviewers or editors who peer-review submitted manuscripts for possible publication. The external reviewers are drawn from a pool of nurse scholars and practitioners who are experts in various fields. In most cases these reviews are 'blind' to author details, that is, the manuscript to be reviewed does not include the name of the author(s). The review panels use the same set of scholarly criteria to judge whether a manuscript is worthy of publication. The credibility of the reported research is enhanced through this peer review process. Most journals have details of the review process on websites or in certain issues of the journal. For example, the Australian College of Critical Care Nurses has specific information regarding the peer review process at http://www.acccn.com.au

An indicative list of scholarly and professional journals is presented in Table 3.3. This is not an exhaustive list of journals—other disciplinary and professional journals also publish primary research and review papers on the state of current knowledge, as well as articles on practice, theory and education issues.

TABLE 3.3 Examples of nursing journals that publish primary and secondary articles

Australian sourced journals	*Australian Critical Care* *Australian Journal of Advanced Nursing* *Contemporary Nurse* *International Journal of Nursing Practice* *Nursing Inquiry*
North American sourced journals	*Advances in Nursing Science* *American Journal of Critical Care* *AORN (Association of Operating Room Nurses journal)* *Applied Nursing Research* *Archives of Psychiatric Nursing* *Clinical Nursing Research* *Computers in Nursing* *Dimensions of Critical Care Nursing* *Heart & Lung* *Holistic Nursing Practice* *Journal of Nursing Scholarship* *Issues in Mental Health Nursing* *Journal of Neonatal Nursing* *Journal of Nursing Administration* *Journal of Nursing Education* *Journal of Nursing Management* *Journal of Obstetric, Gynecologic and Neonatal Nursing* *Journal of Qualitative Research* *Nurse Educator* *Nursing Clinics of North America* *Nursing & Health Care Research* *Nursing Management* *Nursing Research* *Nursing Science Quarterly* *Research in Nursing Health* *Scholarly Inquiry for Nursing Practice* *Western Journal of Nursing Research*
United Kingdom/European sourced journals	*Intensive and Critical Care Nursing* *International Journal of Nursing Studies* *Journal of Advanced Nursing* *Journal of Clinical Nursing* *Journal of Professional Nursing* *Nursing Outlook* *Nurse Researcher*

Electronic databases

The internet is a global resource, and a rather broad term that describes an international network that links a cadre of participating networks (e.g. commercial, educational and government agencies). These resources share computer power, software and information. The internet's main objective of communication is congruent with the objectives of this chapter. Other internet objectives are to share ideas, provide selected information and to provide entertainment (Hutchinson, 1997; Kaufeld & Kaufeld, 1996; Nicoll & Ouellette, 1997). The research consumer should be aware of the utility of email and the world wide web (www) as resources for conducting a search of the literature. Most internet service providers (ISPs) include a web browser, such as Internet Explorer or Netscape Navigator. Classes are often run in universities and health services, and there are online resources available for the web browsers. In the case of the www, the hypertext interface, in addition to text capabilities, also has video, audio and non-text capabilities.

In the US since the 1980s and now in Australasia almost all libraries of larger universities and healthcare agencies and those near metropolitan areas provide students and healthcare workers with direct access to computer searches. Currently, students are able to access a computer search from their computer centre, library or classroom or remotely via a modem; members of faculties have access from their office; and some healthcare professionals have access from their work stations and offices.

Box 3.1 provides a list of common databases used by nurses, midwives and other health professionals to examine the research literature. The website addresses in Box 3.1 and throughout this book were functional and accurate at the time of publication. However, addresses do change, and if the site address does not work and there is no automatic re-direction, then readers should use a generic search engine, such as <http://www.google.com http://>, <www.askjeeves.com> or <http://www.yahoo.com>. The databases listed below may be best accessed through portals such as OVID via a university or health service server, and may require a password before entry into their search facilities. However, PubMed, at <http://www.ncbi.nlm.nih.gov.au/PubMed/> provides public access to Medline searches.

BOX 3.1 Common databases

Cochrane Collaboration http://www.cochrane.org.au
Prepares, maintains and promotes the accessibility of systematic reviews of the effects of healthcare through a variety of documents and facilities, e.g. systematic reviews, clinical guidelines, databases.

Cumulative Index to Nursing and Allied Health Literature (CINAHL) http://www.cinahl.com
Initially called Cumulative Index to Nursing Literature. Published from 1956, the print version is known as the 'Red Books'. The CD-ROM database became available from 1982. The online service became available from 1995 and includes material published from 1982 onwards. It provides search capabilities in various print, CD-ROM and online services. CINAHLdirect online requires a membership fee. CINAHL has been the best choice for most searches in nursing—at first by using the red print indexes and now by accessing it online. CINAHL's database is excellent for searches by postgraduate nursing students, as well as by practising nurses and members

of faculties. For a review of the literature and research consumer purposes, it contains the most comprehensive nursing information compared to any other databases online.

Index Medicus (IM) http://www.nlm.gov
The oldest health-related index, first published in 1879. It provides information in the fields of medicine, allied health, biophysical sciences, humanities, veterinary medicine and nursing, and is managed by the National Library of Medicine in the US. It is sourced from over 4300 journals, primarily English language or with English translation abstracts. It is produced online or CD-ROM as Medline, and also provides PubMed for public access Medline searches.

International Nursing Index (INI)
A quarterly publication by the American Journal of Nursing Company in cooperation with the National Library of Medicine. It started in 1966, and indexes over 200 journals, in all languages, including nursing publications in non-nursing journals.

Nursing Studies Index
Developed by Virginia Henderson. It includes nursing literature from 1900 to 1959, as well as information from other disciplines (see INI above). Sigma Theta Tau International's (STTI) Registry of Nursing Research and the *Online Journal of Knowledge Synthesis for Nursing* are available online at a cost.

OVID http://gateway1.ovid.com
Provides a portal to scientific literature databases and also provides the dominant portal into a number of important clinical databases. These include the simultaneous searching of multiple databases. journals@ovid abstracts approximately 50 nursing journals, sourced mainly from the US and the UK as full text or abstracts and bibliographic details. The current limitation is a lack of Australasian sourced journals, e.g. *Australian Critical Care and Nursing Inquiry* are not sourced through the nursing collection of OVID.

Psyclit: (online PsycINFO–APA)
This is the psychological database associated with the American Psychological Association (APA). The APA has a widely used reference format which is a variant of the Harvard (author/date) style.

Educational Resources Information Center (ERIC)
First published in 1969 in cooperation with Current Index to Journals in Education (CIJE).

Other databases include AIDSLINE (AIDS literature online); CancerLit (Cancer literature); HealthSTAR (a merger of AHA, Health Planning and Administration [HEALTH] and Health Services/Technology Assessment Research [HSTAR]); EMBASE (international biomedical and drug literature); Australasian Medical Index (indexes over 100 Australasian health and medical journals not abstracted on Medline); and OSH-ROM (occupational health and safety databases).

Abstract reviews
Dissertation Abstracts International, Nursing Abstracts, Psychological Abstracts and Sociological Abstracts all list theses and dissertations from graduate students, primarily from North America.

Print databases

Before the 1980s, a search was usually done by hand using print index databases. This was a tedious and time-consuming process. Print databases consist mainly of indexes, card catalogues and abstract reviews. They are useful for finding sources that have not been entered into electronic databases. Print indexes are used to find journal (periodical) sources of data-based and conceptual articles on a variety of topics, as well as publications of professional organisations and various government agencies. Card catalogues were used to secure books, monographs, conference proceedings, master's theses and doctoral dissertations. Abstract reviews contain summaries of data-based articles and prepared bibliographies. Most CD-ROM and online databases include sources from their particular form's publication date or a few years before that date. For example, CINAHL's computer database sources date from 1982, whereas the print index dates from 1956. The most relevant and frequently used print source for nursing literature remains the CINAHL, also known as the 'Red Books'. CINAHL covers all nursing and related literature from 1956 to the present. Print resources are still relied on if a search requires materials not entered into an electronic database before a certain year (e.g. CINAHL on CD-ROM or online cover literature dated from 1982). Almost all print databases are now available through some type of computer or electronic means.

Websites

Table 3.4 lists selected examples of the hundreds of nursing sites, internet home pages and chat rooms available. Many university schools of nursing, individual nurses and nursing organisations have websites. However, in general these sites do not provide literature search and retrieval capabilities anywhere similar to that of OVID or Cochrane.

TABLE 3.4 Selected examples of Australasian nursing and midwifery websites

Australian College of Critical Care Nurses **http://www.acccn.com.au**
This site provides information on college resources, professional, educational and research activities, members' access to online asynchronous and email communication; and a range of links to related sites. Access this site for information on competency and credentialling, *Australian Critical Care* articles, news from *Critical Times*, or for posing questions to a range of Australian critical care experts.

Australian College of Midwives, Incorporated **http://www.acmi.org.au**
This site provides information on issues such as competency standards, codes of practice, independent practice accreditation, educational preparation, professional development, conferences, and membership.

Australian Nursing Council **http://www.anc.org.au**
This site provides information on professional issues such as codes of conduct and ethics, competency standards, assessment of overseas qualifications, as well as projects, position statements and publications.

Clinical Information Access Program, NSW Health **http://www.clininfo.health.nsw.gov.au**
This site supports practice guideline databases and communication for CNCs, through password access. Individual password access is available through NSW Health. The site is also a portal for access to online literature databases and other resources for clinical nurses.

Joanna Briggs Institute for Evidence Based Nursing and Midwifery **http://www.joannabriggs.edu.au**
This site offers public access to 'Best Practice Information Sheets', executive summaries of systematic reviews, research protocols, a regularly updated noticeboard, a research area to post current research information and a links page to other useful nursing and evidence-based practice websites. Subscription (individual or institutional) provides access to all publications, including full-text systematic reviews.

New South Wales College of Nursing **http://www.nursing.aust.edu.au**
This site provides professional information for members on current news, education, library facilities, research and membership.

New Zealand Nurses Organisation **http://www.nzno.org.nz**
This site provides professional information on the organisation's network of sections and colleges, including the research section with statements on research and ethics, and an index of research. Also included on the site are current issues, services, publications and education pages.

Royal College of Nursing, Australia **http://www.rcna.org.au**
This site provides professional information and access to college resources, including chapters, networks, online forums, publications, policies, scholarships, conferences and membership information.

Other useful websites are listed below in Box 3.2. As noted earlier, these selected examples demonstrate only a fraction of the possible resources available through the internet.

BOX 3.2 Other useful websites

- Australian Vice-Chancellors Committee (AV-CC) http://www.avcc.edu.au
  Includes the joint NHMRC statement and guidelines on research practice, as well as other policies and activities.
- National Institute of Nursing Research (NINR) http://www.nih.gov/ninr/
  This US-based site promotes science for nursing practice, supports inter-disciplinary research, and is linked to a nurse scientist training program.
- Sigma Theta Tau International Nursing Honor Society (STTI)
  http://stti-web.iupui.edu
  Can visit and be updated on the news and activities of the society. A subscription fee is required to access the *Online Journal of Knowledge Synthesis for Nursing* and the *Virginia Henderson International Nursing Library*. Provides links to chapter websites.
- Publisher alerts are available for selected journals after registering free online. The contents of forthcoming issues for nominated journals are then emailed to each registrant. If working through a university or hospital server that subscribes to the journal, it is also possible to gain full-text or abstract downloads. For example, Springer Verlag provides alerts at http://link.springer.de/alert and Elsevier Science has a similar service at http://www.idealibrary.com as well as access to online journals and other materials.
- http://www.nursingcenter.com is a US-based portal by Lippincott publishers, providing a large range of information and online links.

Remember that the quality and accuracy of information available from the internet also needs to be assessed in a systematic manner. Compared to journal articles and textbooks, there may have been no peer review process undertaken prior to the publication of internet material. The reader should therefore consider the source of the website when judging the merits of any information:

- Is it a well known, reputable organisation?
- What is the purpose of the information dissemination?
- Is the information substantiated by references?
- How does this information relate to other published material?
- Is there any inherent bias in the statements?

As with other information sources, the reader should always critically review the material.

SEARCH PROCESSES

In most universities, both students and members of the faculty are able to conduct their own searches, print the results on site, and download or email their results without any charge, using the current information technology. Subject headings are established for many specific types of research variables (e.g. designs, conceptual frameworks, data collection methods and statistical methods of data analysis). In addition, CINAHL provides an instrumentation field that lists all the instruments used in a study (CINAHL, 2002). Designated computers are CD-ROM-ready and have menu driven 'user-friendly' databases. Step-by-step printed guides for the search, as well as search guides for each database, are usually available. These guides provide information about variables/terms, broadening or narrowing a search, marking or eliminating unwanted records and printing the citations (that is, references found at the end of an article).

Prior to the introduction of online or CD-ROM–based indexes, manual searches of printed databases and journals were necessary. However, this was a very time-consuming and costly proposition. It was also conceivable that an important entry was missed during the review of all possible entries of the subject heading. Many libraries conduct sessions on search strategies, and online tutorials are available.

Questions frequently asked by students are 'How many articles do I need?', 'How much is enough?', and 'How far back in the literature do I need to go?'. With the rate of knowledge expansion increasing exponentially, searching beyond five years is probably not required, unless a particular period was known for seminal articles. These would be identified in the reference lists of later papers. If required, CINAHL will recover information dating from 1982, and Medline has earlier data. A general time line for conceptual academic or clinical practice papers/projects is to go back in the literature at least three but preferably five years; a research project may warrant ten years or more. It can be handy if you come across an extensive literature review on a particular topic or a concept clarification methodology study, as this usually means you can begin your search at the date of the last reviewed citation or at least a year or two before that time.

Bibliographic databases are a useful tool in managing the literature search and review processes, as they store bibliographic details of journal articles, reports and other print materials. Bibliographic databases also provide an interaction with word-processors as an integrated package. Examples of these databases include Endnote Plus, Reference Manager, Pro-Cite and Papyrus (Nicoll, Ouellette, Bird, & Harper, 1996).

Keywords

The abstraction process for each computer database has some limitations and the issue of keywords needs to be considered. Each database usually has a specific search guide that provides information on the organisation of the entries and the terminology used. 'Medical Subject Headings' (MeSH) were developed by the US National Library of Medicine (see http://www.nlm.gov/). CINAHL uses nursing specific terms. Finding the right key words (or variables/ concepts/terms) to 'plug in' for a computer search is an important aspect of conducting a search. The current applications have user-friendly interfaces; all have an explode feature for terms, which allows multiple keywords searches with a single command. Another feature is the mapping capability, where the application maps or connects you to a term nearest to your search term.

Box 3.3 provides an example of a search, with a number of helpful hints given through the steps of a search. As indicated, an entry usually consists of the author, title, source (e.g. book or journal) and may include an abstract. The following abbreviations are common across the databases: title (TI), author (AU), source (SO), abstract (AB) if available, document type (DT) and references (RF).

BOX 3.3 Helpful hints for electronic searches

- Highlight your preferred database (e.g. CINAHL) on the computer search menu.
- Type in the search words (e.g. 'nursing research').
- 'nursing research' was mapped as a subject heading. Click 'continue', mark 'include all subheadings' (unless you want to search a specific aspect of the subject) and continue.
- Results were 7781 citations for 'nursing research'.
- Repeat the search strategy for 'mental health nursing'. This maps to the subject heading 'psychiatric nursing'. Include all subheadings and continue.
- Typing '1 and 2' will combine the search to capture all articles with both subject headings as keywords.
- Limit the search to the last five years (e.g. 1996–2001). This will result in an output similar to:

#	Search History	Results
1	Research, Nursing/	7781
2	Psychiatric Nursing/	5432
3	1 and 3	170
4	limit to yr=1996–2001	85

- The search has therefore resulted in 85 articles abstracted to CINAHL with 'nursing research' and mental health ('psychiatric nursing') for the years 1996–2001.
- Examine the 'display' of the results. Read each title and abstract to help you decide whether to keep the article and access a full-text copy for further review.
- To mark the entry or record you want to print at the end, check the box.

- There are numerous facilities available—bibliographic details and abstracts can be emailed, imported into a bibliographic database or printed; full-text articles can be printed in a variety of formats.
- Advantages of downloading include printing as many citations as you wish. You can edit the search document by cutting and pasting each entry and create an instant reference list for your paper. Use a bibliographic database to manage your references and reference format.

Search conducted January 2002 using OVID-based CINAHL, 1982 to December Week 2, 2001.

There are many other aspects related to learning an effective search strategy. The above search was a simple illustration of a complex task that requires good training and experiential learning. The former can be gained from online tutorials and faculty or hospital librarians (Shorten, Wallace & Crookes, 2001), and the latter will occur during academic education courses and clinical practice.

This chapter has discussed the processes involved in conducting a literature search, and should be considered in relation to both the previous chapter and the following chapters: Chapter 4 discusses the critical review process; and Chapter 5 examines review papers. In practice, the search and review processes are seamless and continuous in their execution.

KEY POINTS

- Primary resources are essential for literature reviews.
- Secondary sources, from peer-reviewed journals, are part of a learning strategy for developing critical evaluation skills.
- There are many advantages for using computer databases rather than print databases for retrieving scholarly material.
- Strategies for efficiently retrieving scholarly literature include consulting the reference librarian and using IT OVID databases.

CRITICAL THINKING CHALLENGES

- How does a researcher justify using both conceptual and data-based literature in a literature review; and would you use the same types of literature for research consumer purposes, such as developing an academic scholarly paper?
- The nursing research committee at an acute care institution is developing a research-based practice protocol for inpatient cardiac rehabilitation. One suggestion is to use the National Heart Foundation and another is to conduct a review of the literature from the past six years on rehabilitation programs. How would you settle the question? Which one of these suggestions will contribute most effectively to the goal of a research-based protocol?

Additional resources

Hart, C. (2001). *Doing a literature search: a comprehensive guide for the social sciences.* London, Sage.

Hott, J.R. & Budin, W.C. (1999). *Notter's essentials of nursing research* (6th ed.). New York, Springer.

Larson, E. & Satterthwaite, R. (1989). Searching the literature: a professional imperative. *American Journal of Infection Control*, 17, 359–64.

4

CHAPTER

Strategies for conducting a critical review

Zevia Schneider

LEARNING OUTCOMES

After reading this chapter the student should be able to:

- Identify the reasons why it is necessary to critically review studies.
- List the criteria used to review qualitative studies.
- Recognise the major differences between the various research approaches.
- Discuss the strengths and weaknesses of a research report.
- Discuss the implications of the findings of a research report for nursing practice.
- Construct a critique of a research paper.

Key terms

abstract
criteria
critical reading
critical review
data analysis
data collection
findings
phenomenon
qualitative research approaches
quantitative research approaches
sample
statistical information
structure of a study
synthesis

INTRODUCTION

The critique or critical review is the process of objectively, critically and analytically reading a research report's content for scientific merit and application to practice or theory. It requires some knowledge of the subject matter, knowledge of how to read critically, and how to use appropriate criteria. Never was Sir Arthur Helps' dictum that 'Reading is sometimes an ingenious device for avoiding thought' (*Friends in Council*, Bk II, Ch. I, in Cohen & Cohen, 1980) less fitting for the critique process. It is above all a lucid and stringent cognitive process requiring a basic understanding of the research process and relevant terminology.

Criteria necessary to adequately review an article are any measures, standards, evaluation guides or questions used to judge (critique) a product or behaviour. The reader, in analysing a research report, must evaluate each step of the research process and ask questions about whether the explanation of each step of the process meets or does not meet these criteria. For instance, one of the objectives of a literature review is to determine gaps, consistencies and inconsistencies in the literature about a subject, concept or problem. One question to guide the reviewer is, 'What gaps or conflicts in knowledge about the problem are identified and how does this study intend to fill those gaps?'. Search strategies for accessing the relevant literature are explained in Chapter 3. Once articles have been selected and acquired, the process of review begins.

CRITICAL READING

Critical reading is an active, intellectually engaging process in which the reader participates in an inner dialogue with the writer (Paul, 1995). A critical reader therefore actively looks for assumptions, key concepts and ideas, reasons and justifications, supporting examples, parallel experiences, implications and consequences in the written text. This exercise enables accurate and fair interpretation. Critical reading of research articles is difficult for the beginning research consumer and may be somewhat frustrating at first. To accomplish the purpose of critically reading a research study, the reader must have skilled reading, writing and reasoning abilities. These skills are experiential and cumulative—the more practice and experience, the higher the skill level. It is quite common for a research article to require several readings. A minimum of three or four readings and sometimes as many as six readings, with a research textbook at your side, facilitates an effective review and is necessary to do the following:

- identify concepts
- clarify unfamiliar concepts or terms
- question assumptions and rationale
- determine supporting evidence.

Box 4.1 presents some highlighted strategies for reading and evaluating a research report. No matter how difficult it may seem, read the entire article and reflect on it. Critically read for the levels of understanding described in this chapter. Most importantly, draw on previous knowledge, common sense and the critical thinking skills you already possess.

BOX 4.1 Highlights of critical thinking and reading strategies

1. Read primary research articles from refereed journals.
2. Read secondary research (critique/response/commentary) articles from refereed journals.
3. Obtain primary and secondary articles (photocopy or print copies) and make notations directly on the copy.
4. While reading articles:
   - keep a research text and a dictionary by your side
   - review the chapters in a research text (such as this one) on various steps of the research process, criteria used to critique, unfamiliar terms and so on
   - list key variables at the top of the article
   - highlight or underline new terms, unfamiliar vocabulary and significant sentences
   - look up the definitions of new terms and write them on the article copy
   - review old and new terms before subsequent readings
   - highlight or underline identified steps of the research process
   - identify the main idea or theme of the article—state it in your own words in one or two sentences
   - continue to clarify terms that may be unclear on subsequent readings
   - make sure you understand the main points of each reported step of the research process you identified before you critique the article.
5. Determine how well the study meets the criteria:
   - ask fellow students to analyse the same study using the same criteria and compare results
   - consult faculty members about your evaluation of the study.
6. Type a one-page summary and critical review of each study:
   - cite bibliographical information of the reference at the top of the summary according to relevant reference style (e.g. APA, Harvard, Vancouver)
   - briefly summarise each reported research step in your own words
   - briefly describe strengths and weaknesses in your own words (bibliographical databases allow you to write a narrative for each paper reviewed—see the section called 'Synthesis understanding: putting together' on page 59).

Critical reading can be viewed as a process that involves various levels or stages of understanding, including the following:

- preliminary understanding
- comprehensive understanding
- analysis understanding
- synthesis understanding.

Preliminary understanding: familiarity

Preliminary understanding is gained by quickly or lightly reading an article to familiarise yourself with its content or to get a general sense of the material. During the preliminary reading the title and abstract are read closely, but the content is skimmed. The abstract, a brief overview of a study, keys the reader to the main components of the study while the title keys the reader to the main variables of the study. 'Skimming' includes reading the introduction, major headings, one or two sentences under a heading and the summary or conclusion. The preliminary reading includes use of the following strategies:

- highlighting or underlining the main steps of the research process
- making notes on the copied article
- writing key variables at the top of the copied article
- highlighting or underlining on the photocopy new and unfamiliar terms and significant sentences
- looking up the definitions of new terms and writing them in the margins of the copy
- reviewing old and new terms before the next reading
- writing comments, questions and notes on the copy
- keeping a research text and a dictionary by your side.

Using these strategies enables the reader to identify the main theme or idea of the article and bring this knowledge to the second comprehensive reading. An illustration of how to use a number of these strategies is provided by the example in Box 4.2 (on pages 56–57), which contains an excerpt from the introduction and literature review section of the study by Rudy et al. (1995).

Comprehensive understanding: content in relation to context

Gagne (1985) refers to this level as 'skilled' reading. The purpose of comprehensive understanding is to understand the article—to see the terms in relation to the context or the parts of the study in relation to the whole article. For example, when reading Barclay and colleagues' (1996) study for comprehension, it is essential to understand that the purpose of a grounded theory study is to develop a theory about basic social processes. To simply recall that the major variable in the study was men's experiences during their partner's first pregnancy would be inadequate. At the comprehension level reading, you should be able to discuss the core variables that emerged: 'Confusion in their relationship to their partners, and roles in their relationship to their infant and other people'.

When reading for comprehension, keep your research text and dictionary nearby. Although during the preliminary reading some terms may have seemed clear, on the second reading they may be unclear. Do not hesitate to write cues or key relationship words on the photocopy. If, after this reading, the article still does not make sense, ask for assistance before reading it again. One suggestion is to make another copy and ask your lecturer or supervisor to read it. Indicate on the copy the unclear areas and write out your specific questions. Often what is or is not highlighted or the comments on the copy help your tutor or lecturer to understand your difficulty. The problem may be that further reading on the topic is necessary to comprehend the article. For example, if a student is unfamiliar with Rogers' *Science of Unitary Human Beings* (Rogers, 1990), reading a study testing a proposition of this model may be difficult unless Rogers' model has first been read.

Comprehensive understanding is facilitated by the following strategies:

- reviewing all unfamiliar terms before reading for the second time
- clarifying any additional unclear terms
- reading additional sources as necessary
- writing cues, relationships of concepts and questions on the photocopy
- making another copy of your annotated article and requesting that your lecturer or supervisor read it
- stating the main idea or theme of the article, in your own words, in one or two sentences on an index card or on the photocopy.

BOX 4.2 Example of skimming strategies

Conceptual definition

The original purpose of intensive care units (ICUs) was to locate groups of patients together who had similar needs for specialised monitoring and care so that highly trained health care personnel would be available to meet these specialised needs. As the success of ICUs has grown and expanded, the assumption that a typical ICU patient will require only a short length of stay in the unit during the most acute phase of an illness has given way to the recognition that stays of more than one month are not uncommon (Berenson, 1984; Daly et al., 1991).

Significance of problem

These long-stay ICU patients represent a challenge to the current system, not only because of costs but also because of concern for patient outcomes. These patients are often elderly, have underlying chronic conditions that complicate or exacerbate their acute illness, and often require sustained ventilatory and nutritional support. A prime example of these types of patients are those referred to as 'ventilator dependent', found to varying degrees in nearly every ICU in the country (American Association for Respiratory Care, 1991).

Previous conceptual definition

More significance

Impact on resources

The term 'chronically critically ill' has been previously used (Daly et al., 1991) to describe patients who have extended stays in the ICU. Those patients have become most burdensome to nurses and physicians who see their progress as slow and frustrating, to hospital administrators because of extended bed occupancy in times of high demand, and to hospital financial officers because of costs that usually exceed the diagnosis-related group (DRG) cost allocation. Patients who have ICU stays greater than 21 days account for approximately 3 per cent of the total number of patients admitted to the ICUs, yet they account for approximately 25 per cent to 38 per cent of the patient days (Daly et al., 1991).

While ample evidence confirms that this sub-population of ICU patients represents a drain on hospital resources, few studies have attempted to evaluate the effects of a delivery system outside the ICU setting on patient outcomes, cost and nurse outcomes. The majority of studies that have examined ICU patient outcomes have been limited primarily to mortality and length of stay (Berenson, 1984; Borlase et al., 1991; Madoff et al., 1985). More recently, attention has been given to cost in terms of risk-adjusted ICU lengths of stay, cost, utility of diagnostic and laboratory tests and time on mechanical ventilation (Gundlach & Faulkner, 1991; Kappstein et al., 1992; Roberts et al., 1993; Schapira et al., 1993; Zimmerman et al., 1993).

In studies limited to mechanically ventilated patients, comparisons on length of stay and costs have been examined in 'a before-and-after' design following initiation of a ventilatory management team (Cohen et al., 1991), on overall costs for mechanically ventilated patients cared for in an ICU versus a non-invasive respiratory care unit (Elpern et al., 1991), and on hospital charges and life expectancy for elderly mechanically ventilated ICU patients (Cohen, Lambrinos & Fein, 1993). The lack of randomised trials comparing care delivery systems for these high-cost patients is noteworthy, as are the limitations of outcome measurements to mortality and cost.

The purpose of the current study was to compare the effects of a low-technology environment of care based on a nurse-managed care delivery system (special care unit [SCU] environment) with the traditional high-technology ICU environment based on a primary nursing care delivery system. The two groups were compared on the outcomes of length of stay, mortality, readmission to the hospital, complications, patient and family satisfaction and cost. The complications were defined as number and types of infections, number and types of respiratory complications and number and types of life-threatening complications.

Text from Rudy, E., Daly, B.J., Douglas, S., Montenegro, H.D., Song, R. & Dyer, M.A. (1995). Patient outcomes for the chronically ill: special care unit versus intensive care unit. *Nursing Research*, 44, 324–31.

Comprehensive understanding is necessary to analyse and synthesise the material. Understanding the author's perspective for the study reflects critical thinking (Paul, 1995) and facilitates the analysis of the study according to established criteria. The next reading or two allows for analysis and synthesis of the study.

Analysis understanding: breaking into parts

The purpose of reading for analysis is to break the content into parts to understand each aspect of the study. Some of the questions to ask during analysis of the research article include:

- Can the main idea or theme of this article be captured in one or two sentences?
- How are the major parts of this article organised in relation to the research process?
- What is the purpose of this article?
- How was this study carried out? Can it be explained step by step?
- What are the author's(s') main conclusions?
- Is each section understood and can it be summarised or paraphrased into your own words?

In a sense you are determining how the steps of the research process are presented or organised in the article and what the content related to each step is all about. You are beginning the process of critically analysing the merit of the study. It may require some knowledge of the subject matter, but knowledge of how to critically read is the most important consideration.

The review of the literature section of a study by Burns and Adams (1997) entitled 'Alcohol history taking by nurses and doctors—how accurate are they really?' provides the reader with data on the alcohol consumption habits of Australians from the Commonwealth Department of Health, Housing and Community Services (1993) and the Australian Bureau of Statistics (1989–1990). These data indicate that Australia ranks well above average in alcohol consumption when compared with all English-speaking nations. Two important factors emerge: the paucity of Australian empirical data and the finding in an American study that only 61% of patients were asked about their alcohol consumption and other drugs on admission to hospital. Thus, the need for research into the accuracy of history-taking is made evident. In summary, it appears that little empirical evidence exists as to how nurses and doctors use alcohol withdrawal scales or record alcohol histories, and the findings of two available studies indicate that this is a problematic area.

This statement implies that reading for analysis took place. Understanding gained by reading for analysis is facilitated by the following strategies:

- being familiar with critical review criteria
- reaching the comprehensive reading stage before applying criteria, and re-reading if necessary
- applying the criteria to each step of the research process in the article
- asking whether the content meets the criteria for each step of the research process
- asking fellow students to analyse the same study with the same criteria and comparing results
- writing notes on the copy about how each step of the research process measures up against the established criteria.

Synthesis understanding: putting together

Synthesis is 'the process of combining objects or ideas into a complex whole' (Hanks, 1986, p. 1546). The purpose of reading for synthesis is to pull all the information together to form a new whole (Kerlinger, 1986); to make sense of it; to explain relationships. Although the process of synthesising the material may be taking place as you are analysing the article, another reading is recommended. It is during the synthesis reading that the understanding and critique of the whole study are put together. During this final step you decide how well the study meets the criteria, its contribution to nursing, and how useful it is in practice. It is the point at which the reader decides how well each step of the research process relates to the previous step. Synthesis can be thought of as like looking at a jigsaw puzzle once it is completed. Does it form a comprehensive, cohesive picture, or is there a piece out of place? In the case of reviewing or reading for synthesis of several studies, the interrelationship of the studies is assessed. Reading for high-level synthesis is essential when critically analysing research studies. The previous example of Burns and Adams' (1997) summary statement of their review of the literature also reflects synthesis reading.

Reading for synthesis is facilitated by the following strategies:

- Reviewing your notes on the article on how each step of the research process measured up against the established criteria.
- Briefly summarising the study in your own words, including in your summary:
    - the components of the study
    - the study's overall strengths and weaknesses.
- Following the suggested format of:
    - limiting the summary to one page
    - including the citation at the top of the page in the specified reference style
    - stapling the summary to the top of the photocopied article.

There are also bibliographic databases available which enable categorising and managing of article reviews as well as linking to word-processing programs (e.g. Endnote, Procite) (Nicoll et al., 1996). The type of summary above is viewed as the first draft of a final written critique. It teaches brevity, facilitates easy retrieval of data to support your critical analysis and evaluation, and increases your ability to write a scholarly report. In addition, the ability to synthesise one study prepares you for the task of critically analysing several studies on a similar topic and comparing and contrasting their findings.

AN INTRODUCTION TO READING RESEARCH ARTICLES

When reading, the organisation and format of articles are as important to consider as the content. Many journals publish research, either as the sole type of article in the journal or in addition to clinical or theoretical articles. Although many journals have some common features, they also have unique characteristics. All journals have guidelines for manuscript preparation and submission, which are generally published in each journal or on a related website.

Format and style

All journals contain guidelines for the preparation and submission of manuscripts. An abstract at the beginning of an article is usually required.

Journals may differ with regard to the structure of the abstract and instruct the potential author that manuscripts that fail to conform to their particular specifications will not be reviewed. Examples of different structure requirements for the abstract are evident in a comparison of two journals, for example, the *Australian Journal of Advanced Nursing* (*AJAN*) and *Midwifery*. *AJAN* requires 'a short resume, not exceeding 120 words, of the aims, method, major findings and conclusion' (*AJAN*, Author Guidelines). *Midwifery* specifies that 'an abstract should be in the "Structured Abstract Format" giving objectives, design, setting, participants, interventions (if appropriate), measurements and findings, key conclusion and implications for practice' (*Midwifery*, Instructions to Authors).

A review of these guidelines will provide information on the format and style of articles that appear in specific journals. It is important to remember that even though each step of the research process is discussed at length in this text, only a short paragraph or a sentence in the research article may provide the details of the step in a specific study. Because of the journal's space limitations or other publishing guidelines, the published study that one reads in a journal is a shortened version of the total work done by the researcher(s). Some researchers devote more space in an article to the results, whereas others present a longer discussion of the methods and procedures. In recent years most authors have given more emphasis to the method, results and discussion of implications than to details of assumptions, hypotheses or definitions of terms. Decisions about the amount of information to present on each step of the research process within an article are bound by the following:

- a journal's space limitations
- a journal's author guidelines
- the type or nature of the study
- an individual researcher's evaluation of what is the most important component of the study.

Some suggestions regarding the critique of qualitative and quantitative research approaches follow. It may be useful for you to compare the structure of the critical review process with the structure of a research proposal as explained in Chapter 8.

Critical review of qualitative studies

A careful reading of the qualitative research chapters in Section 2 will identify the factors that distinguish the various approaches; however, the critique of qualitative research studies involves a similar structure, that is:

1. identifying the phenomenon
2. structuring the study
3. gathering the data
4. analysing the data
5. describing the findings.

Notwithstanding the difference in terminology, you will notice that qualitative studies require a different kind of critical analysis. Some suggestions regarding the critique of qualitative research approaches are listed in Box 4.3. In the following text, only three qualitative approaches will be discussed in terms of the research question (or phenomenon) and participants, in order to provide relevant examples that address the critique process. Discussion of the issues, data analysis, interpretation and rigour in qualitative research occurs in Chapter 9. Differences in the purpose of choosing between the qualitative approaches are acknowledged and will be evident in the additional chapters on qualitative research. A review of the qualitative chapters will also add to your understanding of the critical review process. It would be worthwhile to use the above critical review guidelines when analysing the qualitative studies that appear in full in Appendices A and B.

BOX 4.3 Critical review guidelines for qualitative studies

Title and abstract

1. Is the title of the research paper congruent with the text?
2. Were the aims and/or objectives stated? What are they?
3. Did the abstract contain sufficient information about the stages of the research process (e.g. aims, research approach, participants, data collection, data analysis, findings)?

Identifying the phenomenon

1. Is the phenomenon focused on human experience within a natural setting?
2. Is the phenomenon relevant to nursing, midwifery and/or health?

Structuring the study

1. Is it clear that the selected participants are living the phenomenon of interest?
2. How is published literature used in the study?
3. Does the question identify the context (participant/group/place) of the method to be followed?
4. Is the theoretical framework clearly stated?
5. Does the theoretical framework fit the research question?
6. Is the method of data collection and analysis clearly specified?
7. Does the qualitative method of data collection chosen fit the research question (e.g. grounded theory, ethnography)?
8. Are the limitations of the study stated?

Research question and design

1. Was the research question determined by the need for the study? How was this determination made?
2. Are the data collection strategies appropriate for the research question?
3. Do the data collection strategies reflect the purpose and theoretical framework of the study (e.g. in-depth interviewing, focus groups)?
4. Can the data analysis strategy be identified and logically followed?

Participants

1. How were the participants and setting selected (e.g. sampling strategies)?
2. How was confidentiality of the participants assured?
3. How was the anonymity of participants assured?
4. What ethical issues were identified in the study?
5. How were the ethical issues addressed?

Data analyses

1. How were the data analysed?
2. Is the analysis technique congruent with the research question?
3. Is there evidence that the researcher's interpretation captured the participants' meaning?
4. Did the researcher say how the criteria for judging the scientific rigour of the study were maintained in terms of credibility, auditability, fittingness and confirmability?

Describing the findings

1. Does the researcher demonstrate to the reader the method (e.g. audit trial) by which the data were analysed?
2. Does the researcher indicate how the findings are related to theory?
3. Is there a link between the findings to existing theory or literature, or is a new theory generated?

Researcher's perspective

1. Are the biases of the researcher reported (e.g. researcher/participant expectations, researcher bias (objectivity–subjectivity) and power imbalance)?
2. Are the limitations of the study acknowledged?
3. Are recommendations suggested for further research?
4. Are implications for healthcare mentioned?

A number of examples are listed below to elaborate some of the concepts above. Further elaboration is provided in the various qualitative chapters of Section 2. For example, the focus of the phenomenological approach is the lived experience of an individual. This approach is likely to be chosen when studying some dimension of day-to-day existence for a particular group of individuals. An example of a phenomenological approach research question is 'Could you describe in your own words, your experience of caring for the dying?' (Byrne & McMurray, 1997).

A research question appropriate for the grounded theory method is one that addresses basic social processes. They tend to be action-oriented or change-oriented, such as 'How do older women experience "home"?' (Gattuso, 1996) or 'What is the nurse's perspective of the delivery of quality nursing care?' (Williams, 1998). In a grounded theory study, the research question can be a statement or a broad question that permits in-depth explanation of the phenomenon. For instance, Barclay and colleagues' (1996) study aimed 'to identify and explore the social and relationship changes that Australian men experience during their partner's first pregnancy'. The study was designed to address a recognised step in men's psychological development.

When reviewing a report of ethnographic research, note that questions are asked about particular patterns of behaviour within the social context of a culture or sub-culture. Ethnographic nursing studies address questions that concern how cultural knowledge, norms, values and other contextual variables influence one's health experience. Uphall (1992) asked, 'How do nurses from various health care settings (government, private, missions, industrial and non-governmental organisations) perceive collaboration between indigenous and cosmopolitan health care systems?'.

Critical review of quantitative studies

The following review process for quantitative studies (Box 4.4) is not exhaustive. As you read research papers or other chapters in this book, additional pertinent questions may occur to you.

BOX 4.4 Critical review guidelines for quantitative studies

The title and abstract

1. Is the title of the research paper congruent with the text?
2. Were the aims and/or objectives stated? What are they?
3. Did the abstract contain sufficient information about the stages of the research process (e.g. aims, hypothesis, research approach, sample, instruments, findings)?

Structuring the study

1. How was the investigation carried out?
2. Is the hypothesis stated?
3. Which hypothesis is stated: the scientific hypothesis or the null hypothesis?
4. Does the hypothesis indicate that the researcher is interested in testing for differences between groups or in testing for relationships?
5. Is the motivation for the study demonstrated through the literature review?
6. Is the literature review adequate? Are the references recent?
7. Are the stated limitations and gaps in the reviewed literature appropriate and convincing?

The sample

1. Is the sample size large enough to prevent one extreme score (descriptive statistics) from affecting the summary statistics used?
2. How was the sample size determined?
3. Was the sample size appropriate for the analyses used?

Data collection

1. How were the data collected (questionnaires and other data collection tools)?
2. Who collected the data?
3. What is the origin of the measurement instruments?
4. Are the instruments adequately described?
5. How were the data collection instruments validated?
6. How was the reliability of the measurement instruments assessed?

Data analysis

1. Are descriptive or inferential statistics reported?
2. What tests were used to analyse the data: parametric or non-parametric?
3. Were the descriptive statistics/inferential statistics appropriate to the level of measurement for each variable?
4. Were the appropriate tests used to analyse the data?
5. What is the level of measurement chosen for the independent and dependent variables?

6. Were the statistics appropriate for the research question and design?
7. Are there appropriate summary statistics for each major variable?
8. Were the statistics primarily descriptive, correlational or inferential?
9. Identify the outcome of each statistical analysis.
10. Explain the meaning of each outcome.

Findings

1. Were the findings expected? Which findings were not expected?
2. Is there enough information present to judge the results?
3. Are the results clearly and completely stated?
4. Describe the researcher's report of the findings.
5. Identify any limitations or gaps in the study.
6. Were suggestions for further research made?
7. Did the researcher mention the implications of the study for healthcare?
8. Was there sufficient information in the report to permit replication of the study?

As you read the section called 'Methods', consider what level of measurement the author used to measure the important variables. If the level of measurement is interval or ratio, the statistics most likely to be used will be parametric (see Chapter 23). However, if the variables are measured at the nominal or ordinal level, the statistics used should be non-parametric (see Chapter 22). Also consider the size of the sample and remember that samples have to be large enough to permit the assumption of normality. If the sample is quite small, say, five to ten subjects, the assumptions necessary for inferential statistics may have been violated. The important question is whether the researcher has provided enough justification to use the statistics presented.

Finally, consider the results as they are presented. The first place to begin to critique the statistical analysis of a research paper is with the hypothesis. The hypothesis should indicate to you what type of statistics were used. If the hypothesis predicts that a relationship between the variables will be found, you should expect to find indices of correlation. If the study is experimental or quasi-experimental, the hypothesis would indicate that the author is looking for differences between the groups studied and you would expect to find statistical tests of differences between means. There would be serious implications for the study if the stated aims and hypotheses are written in a vague way. There should be enough data presented for each hypothesis studied to determine whether the researcher actually examined each hypothesis. The tables, procedures, analysis and text should be congruent. For example, the text should not indicate that a test reached statistical significance while the tables indicate that the probability value of the test was above 0.05.

There are two other aspects of the data analysis section that the reader should review. The paper should not read as if it were a statistical textbook. The results in the text of the paper should be clear enough to the average reader so that the reader can determine what was done and what the results were. In addition, the author should attempt to make a distinction between practical and statistical significance. Some results may be statistically significant, but their practical importance may be doubtful. If this is so, the author should note it. Alternatively, you may find yourself reading a research report that is elegantly presented, but you come away with a 'so what?' feeling. Such a feeling may indicate that the practical significance of the study and its findings have not been adequately explained.

Note that the critical analysis of a research paper's statistical analysis is not done in a vacuum. The adequacy of the analysis must be judged in relation to the other important aspects of the paper: the problem, the hypothesis, the design, the sample, and data collection methods. For example, a researcher may sometimes use a non-parametric statistic when it appears that a parametric statistic is appropriate. Because parametric statistics are more powerful than non-parametric statistics, the result of the parametric analysis may not have been what the researcher expected. However, the non-parametric result might be in the expected direction, so the researcher reports only that result—this would be misleading.

SAMPLES OF CRITICAL REVIEWS

To assist you further a short critique of two studies follows.

Sample No. 1

The article 'Models of nursing care: a comparative study of patient satisfaction on two orthopaedic wards in Brisbane' by Wu, Courtney and Berger (2000) is critically examined in terms of its quality and the potential usefulness of the findings for application to nursing practice.

Problem and purpose

The authors state that the three purposes of the study were to:

1. conduct a comparative study to determine if levels of patient satisfaction differed when using a patient allocation model or a team approach model
2. investigate the relationship between demographic characteristics and patient satisfaction
3. investigate differences between models and between patients' characteristics.

The purpose specifies a population of orthopaedic patients in a Brisbane hospital, and provides direction for statistical analyses.

The authors identify the significance of the problem as improved patient satisfaction. For this purpose, team nursing (Model 1), was used in one 36-bed orthopaedic ward, and patient allocation (Model 2) was used in another 38-bed orthopaedic ward.

Review of the literature and definitions

This is a comparative study with no obvious conceptual framework. The definition of patient satisfaction with medical care is defined by Pasco (1983, p. 189) as a 'health care recipient's reaction to salient aspects of the context, process and result of their service experience'. In this section, the authors provide an explanation of a comparative approach commonly used by nurses; this involves a subjective process, that is, a matching of the patient's subjective standard to the healthcare received. The justification for the study is the apparent lack of studies focusing on a comparison between team nursing and patient allocation approaches. The majority of studies were based on nurses' professional perceptions. In addition, 'patient satisfaction' instruments developed for Australians do not appear to have been used in recent research studies (Wu, Courtney & Berger, 2000).

Hypotheses and/or research questions

Three hypotheses rather than a research question were used in this study. They are stated as:

1. There will be no significant difference in the level of patient satisfaction between the patient allocation model and the team nursing model.
2. There will be no significant relationship between patients' demographic characteristics and patient satisfaction across the patient allocation model and team nursing model.
3. There will be no difference between Ward 1 (team nursing model) and Ward 2 (patient allocation model) patients' characteristics.

All hypotheses are stated in research form and are testable. The important point in statistical analysis is that we do not actually test the operational/scientific hypothesis but its opposite, the null hypothesis. In other words, we test the hypothesis that there is no statistically significant population correlation or difference between the two models in respect of (a) patient satisfaction, (b) patients' demographic characteristics and patient satisfaction, and (c) patients' characteristics. The independent variables in this study are the two models of care. The dependent variables are patient satisfaction and patient characteristics.

The sample

The sample consisted of 137 patients randomly selected from the hospital computer database of the two orthopaedic wards. These patients were discharged during the previous four weeks.

Research design

The study design was a non-experimental, comparative descriptive design. Since it was not a true experiment the criteria do not apply. The choice of the design is congruent with the stated objectives of the study.

Methods

A self-reported questionnaire or patient satisfaction survey (PSS), a statement requiring informed consent, a letter supporting the study from the director of both wards, and a reply-paid pre-addressed envelope were posted to each patient. Eighty questionnaires were returned and six of them could not be used. A total of 74 (54% response rate) questionnaires was available for analysis: 36 responses from Ward 1, and 38 responses from Ward 2.

Instruments

The patient satisfaction survey (PSS) contained 36 items. The instrument was developed, tested and validated to measure patient satisfaction within an acute hospital setting in a previous study (Greenhill & Henderson, 1997). When discussing the patient satisfaction survey, the report indicates that there were 56 items covering five major areas; the total of items mentioned numbers 38. It is clear that there were more than 36 items, but no mention is made of the 18 items not listed.

Items in the questionnaire were distributed in the following way:

- patients' feelings and perceptions (6 items)
- nurses' skills (9 items)
- nurses' behaviour and attitudes (11 items)
- nurses' communication and education skills (7 items), and
- continuity of care experienced (5 items).

Overall satisfaction levels were also sought. A Likert-type scale required patients to rate the items for patient satisfaction from 1 (best) to 5 (worst) or N/A (not applicable). Demographic data were requested and patients were asked to record any comments they may wish to make at the conclusion of the survey.

Reliability and validity

The authors state that the instrument was tested and validated in a previous study. To establish content validity, volunteer inpatients who were not part of the study participated in focus groups. The groups continued until consensus regarding validity was reached. In addition, a reference group of appropriately informed nurses and clinicians provided ongoing advice on the design and analysis phase of the survey. Reliability of the instrument was tested using Cronbach's Alpha coefficient on each of the five major areas and was found to be high, ranging from 0.82 to 0.93.

Analysis of data

Three statistical tests—Spearman's rho correlation, independent t-tests, and a chi-square test—were used to analyse the data. The authors state the Spearman's rho correlational tests examined the relationship between the demographic data and various aspects of nursing care and overall patient satisfaction on each ward. An independent t-test was used to measure patient satisfaction levels with the particular model on each ward. The chi-square test was used to examine demographic variables and also the significance of different associations in the groups. Alpha was set at 0.05 and using the medium effect, the sample size was found to be sufficiently large (Wu, Courtney & Berger, 2000). However, a question here could be, 'What was the justification for a medium effect size, given the previous comment that minimal research had compared the effects of the different models of nursing care?'.

Demographic information is provided clearly in relation to patient backgrounds, age, female/male distribution, educational level completed and income. Six tables are used to present the information. Means and mean scores (SDs) were calculated from responses on a 5-point Likert-type scale about aspects of nursing care (Table 1). The highest mean is 4.13 (SD 0.71) and the lowest mean is 3.93 (SD 1.07). These results suggest that the patients formerly in Ward 1 and Ward 2 were very satisfied with their nursing care.

Table 2 and Table 3 give the mean and SD for five different responses for each ward. Table 4 calculates differences in patient satisfaction survey scores for Wards 1 and 2 and gives a clear description of the mean, SD, t-value, p-value and df. Table 5 shows the results of patients' overall satisfaction in Ward 1 using Spearman's rho, and Table 6 shows the results of patients' overall satisfaction in Ward 2 using Spearman's rho. All the tables are precisely titled and headed. The non-parametric statistical tests used were appropriate.

Conclusion, implications and recommendations

The null hypothesis was accepted for each hypothesis. The authors state that individual nurse behaviours affect patient satisfaction significantly more than any model of nursing care because there appeared to be no difference in levels of patient satisfaction between the two models tested. It appears that all patients were highly satisfied with the overall quality of nursing care, however, negative written comments were made about lack of information at time of admission and discharge, nurses' lack of availability, level of noise, waiting time and inadequate facilities.

The authors suggest that some negative comments may be related to staff shortages, especially in the patient allocation ward. Patients were especially critical of nurses' skills and continuity of care. The authors argue that patient satisfaction is mainly influenced by what health professionals do together with patients' own characteristics.

The authors suggest two recommendations for further investigation:

1. whether communication problems between team leaders and members exist in the team nursing model, and
2. if the patient allocation model causes a higher workload and greater lack of organisation than the team model.

A suggestion is made that the reliability of the patient satisfaction survey be further established. Seven suggestions for improving practice are made. These include: improvement of nurses' pain management skills; providing more information on discharge; communication; and attention to patient privacy concerns.

Application to nursing practice

The design of the study is appropriate, however, the small sample size appeared to mitigate against more definitive findings, if, in fact, there were differences. Thus, direct application to nursing practice is not supported. This study should be repeated using the authors' suggestions about further establishing the reliability of the instrument, finding a much larger sample, and addressing the question of how patient characteristics relate to patient satisfaction.

Sample No. 2

The article 'A survey of nurses' views on indicators for continuing competence in nursing' by Pearson and FitzGerald (2001) is critically examined in terms of its purpose, quality, and the potential usefulness of the findings for application to the nursing profession.

Study purpose

The study was commissioned by the Australian Nursing Council (ANC). The study aimed to develop an approach to the maintenance of continuing competence in nursing. A number of indicators of continuing competence in nursing were developed. An explanation of the basis for each of the identified indicators, as well as a description of any applications or qualifications in respect of each indicator, was sought. The study design was based on four key stages. The paper reports on Stage 4 of the survey—the development of an options booklet and a national survey of registered nurses (RNs). The options booklet and questionnaire were sent to a sample of RNs in Australia.

Sample and sampling

A stratified random sample of 2% of RNs in each State and Territory (except the Australian Capital Territory [ACT]) was chosen. ACT nurses were not included because the nursing regulatory authority does not release register details. A total of 4133 booklets (containing a questionnaire) were distributed through a random sampling process, and 1005 were returned, representing a 24.35% response rate. This resulted in a final sample size of less than 0.5% of the population. The sampling distribution appears by State in Table 2 of the study.

Method

The research team developed a comprehensive user-friendly Options Booklet. In addition, a structured questionnaire was developed for participants to respond to Optional Instruments described in the booklet. The design of the booklet was reviewed and modified during a one-day expert panel meeting and feedback from the Project Management Committee. The questionnaire was then piloted on six clinical nurses from a variety of backgrounds, with only minor changes resulting. The booklet (including questionnaire) was mailed to a stratified random sample of 2% of the total RN population. Nurses were asked to complete the questionnaire attached to the booklet and to rank the six Optional Instruments according to their ability to:

- provide evidence of continuing competence to regulatory bodies
- provide evidence of professional development.

Optional Instruments were rated from 1 to 6 (with 1 being the most preferred and 6 being the least preferred). Demographic information collected in the questions included State or Territory of residence, age and highest educational qualification.

Data analysis

The mean scores (SD) for each option were calculated (lower scores indicating more preferred) and analysed using one-way analysis of variance with Student-Newman-Keuls post-hoc analysis to determine significant differences between the options (Pagano, 1986).

Results

Responses to Question 1 (58.5%, $n = 538$) indicate that the nurses did not feel that their particular State or Territory addressed the profession's need to guarantee competency. Queensland was the only State to differ: the majority of nurses there felt that the need to guarantee competency was addressed (61%, $n = 98$). Table 3 shows Question 1 by State/Territory.

Question 2 asked participants to rate the Optional Instruments in order of preference. The ranking of options for providing evidence of continuing competence to regulatory authorities appears in the histogram (bar graph) in Figure 1 of the study. Optional Instrument E was the most preferred and Optional Instrument A the least preferred.Question 3 required the ranking of options for providing evidence of professional development (see in Figure 2). Optional Instrument C was the most preferred and Optional Instrument A the least preferred.

Questions 4–6 related to age, State of residence and highest nursing qualification. Table 4 shows preferences to Questions 2 and 3 by qualifications and age. It will be noted that overall Optional Instrument D was the most preferred by qualification, and Optional Instrument A was the least preferred. Answers to Question 3 show that, overall, Optional Instrument C was the most preferred, with Optional Instrument A once again the least preferred.

Discussion

The authors indicate that methods or strategies to assess continuing competence in any of the professions in terms of ease of administration, reliability and acceptability to the profession, have not been articulated. There is intensive interest among the professions (Cady et al., 1998; Borko et al., 1997; Cross, 1997; Chambers et al., 1996; Bradley, 1993) in this area. Nursing has made more progress internationally and nationally in the past decade than many other professions, both in Australia and worldwide, however, much work remains to be done. The main reason for establishing regulatory authorities for the profession is to protect the public through restricting practice to only those individuals considered competent. A summary of Australian States' re-licensing requirements appears in Table 1 of the study.

The present study is important therefore in addressing issues of competency by obtaining nurses' views on the provision of evidence of competence and ongoing professional development Australia-wide.

The sampling strategy was designed to obtain data from nurses in all Australian States (apart from the ACT). The study was limited in its ability to present a comprehensive picture of RNs' views throughout Australia by the poor response rate (24.3%) from the 2% of RNs surveyed, notwithstanding its comparability, according to the researchers, with response rates of most randomised surveys of RNs in Australia. The issue of low response rates should have been considered when calculating the sample size so that the final sample would approximate the 2% of all RNs in Australia. One must wonder just how representative of RNs as a whole are those who did respond. In addition, while it was stipulated that the Options Booklet be sent to RNs, some booklets were sent to Enrolled Nurses (ENs—62 responses). It is unclear, then, why the responses from ENs were included in the analysis. People who respond to surveys are generally different from those who do not and in such cases the sample is likely to be a non-representative group (Hawe, Degeling & Hall, 1990).

Conclusion

The Australian nurses who responded to the questionnaire collectively showed their preference for providing evidence of competence and professional development. When the data were analysed State by State there was no clear consensus regarding preference for providing evidence of competence, however, there is consensus for providing evidence of professional development. The authors recommend a course of action for Australian nurses including:

- a requirement for nurses to submit a signed legal declaration of competence annually when applying for re-licensing
- a random auditing process in which nurses are free to respond to the auditing process
- that auditing is a legitimate role of nursing professional associations, and
- the development of a strategy to assist nurses to find ways to assure regulatory authorities that they can legally sign a declaration of competence.

The authors further suggest that State and Territory regulating bodies introduce a requirement for:

- an annual legal declaration of competence when re-licensing
- a random auditing process as a quality assurance measure, and
- the development of a policy supporting the view that nurses should be free to respond to the auditing process according to the format chosen by the nurse.

Recommendations for further research

The authors recommend that a process of self-declaration of competence be linked with a process of audit by regulatory bodies to monitor the ability of self-declaration to identify those nurses who have not maintained their continuing competence. The policies and processes once developed and implemented should be evaluated. Also suggested is an examination of the support nurses receive with regard to professional development, documentation of such development, and the identification of barriers that prevent nurses from maintaining competence.

KEY POINTS

- The best way to become an intelligent research consumer is to have a good understanding of the research process and the major research approaches.
- The goal of synthesis understanding is to combine the parts of a research study into a whole. During this final stage the reader determines how each step relates to all the steps of the research, how well the study meets the criteria used to critique the study, and the usefulness of the study for practice.
- It is not necessary for every nurse to become a researcher, but it is most important that every nurse becomes an intelligent research consumer.
- Critical and analytical thinking involve active interpretation and objective assessment of an article, looking for key concepts, definitions, objectives, method, and findings.
- Critical reading involves active interpretation and objective assessment of an article, looking for key concepts, ideas and justification.
- The most important point when analysing statistical procedures in a study is the relationship of the statistics used to the research question, design and method.
- Clues to the appropriate statistical test to be used by the researcher should stem from the researcher's hypothesis.
- Data analysis for qualitative methods aims to make meaning from narrative data.
- Ethical issues in qualitative research involve issues related to the naturalistic setting, emergent nature of the design, research–participant interaction and the 'researcher as instrument'.
- Credibility, auditability, fittingness and confirmability are criteria for judging the scientific rigour of a qualitative research study.

CRITICAL THINKING CHALLENGES

- As noted in the key points above, it is important that all nurses are active research consumers. What does this statement mean in terms of having an appropriate knowledge base?
- Discuss the reasons why research is evaluated.
- It is claimed that the critical reading of research articles may require a minimum of three or four readings. Is this always the case? What assumptions underlie this claim?
- Discuss the concepts of applicability, completeness and consistency in terms of a research report.

- What potential problems exist when a nurse decides to replicate a study on the basis of a researcher's report?
- What potential contribution can research make to nursing practice, theory and education?
- Beverley is a part-time final year Bachelor of Nursing conversion student. She works as a full-time theatre nurse. She has decided that she wants to do a research project using a qualitative approach, but has not yet decided on a topic. Discuss her potential options.
- The research question should determine the research approach. Do you agree?

Additional resources

Brown, S.J. (1999). *Knowledge for health care practice: a guide to using research evidence.* Philadelphia, Saunders.

Crabtree, B.F. & Miller, W.L., eds. (1992). *Doing qualitative research.* Newbury Park, California, Sage.

Denzin, N.K. & Lincoln, Y.S. (1994). Introduction: entering the field of qualitative research. In Denzin, N.K. & Lincoln, T.S., eds, *Handbook of qualitative research.* Thousand Oaks, California, Sage.

Glaser, B.G. & Strauss, A.L. (1967). *The discovery of grounded theory: strategies for qualitative research.* Chicago, Aldine.

Guba, E. & Lincoln, Y. (1981). *Effective evaluation.* San Francisco, Jossey-Bass.

Hawe, P., Degeling, D. & Hall, J. (1990). *Evaluating health promotion.* Australia, MacLennan & Petty.

Janesick, V.J. (1994).The dance of qualitative research design: metaphor, methodolatory, and meaning. In Denzin, N.K. & Lincoln, Y.S., eds, *Handbook of qualitative research.* Thousand Oaks, California, Sage.

Johnson, M. (1992). A silent conspiracy: some ethical issues of participant observation in nursing research. *International Journal of Nursing Studies,* 29(2), 213–33.

Kvale, S. (1996). *InterViews: an introduction to qualitative research interviewing.* Thousand Oaks, California, Sage.

Leininger, M.M. (1985). Ethnography and ethnonursing: models and modes of qualitative data analysis. In Leininger, M.M., ed., *Qualitative research methods in nursing.* Orlando, Grune & Stratton.

Lincoln, Y.S. (1992). Sympathetic connections between qualitative methods and health research. *Qualitative Health Research,* 2(4), 375–91.

Lipson, J.G. (1994). Ethical issues in ethnography. In Morse, J.M., ed., *Critical issues in qualitative research methods.* Thousand Oaks, California, Sage.

Morse, J.M. & Field, P.A. (1995). *Qualitative research methods for health professionals.* (2nd ed.). Thousand Oaks, California, Sage.

Sandelowski, M. (1995). Qualitative analysis: what it is and how to begin. *Research in Nursing Health,* 18, 371–75.

Spradley, J.P. (1979). *The ethnographic interview.* New York, Holt, Rinehart & Winston.

Strauss, A. & Corbin, J. (1990). *Basics of qualitative research: grounded theory procedures and techniques.* Newbury Park, California, Sage.

Van Maanen, J. (1988). *Tales of the field: on writing ethnography.* Chicago, University of Chicago Press.

5
CHAPTER

Reading review papers

Doug Elliott

LEARNING OUTCOMES

After reading this chapter the student should be able to:

- Discuss the review of literature in relation to nursing theory, research, education and practice.
- Discuss the use of the literature in relation to specific research designs and methodological approaches.
- Identify the characteristics of a relevant literature review.
- Critically read (summarise and critique) research articles, at a beginning consumer level.
- Apply criteria to the evaluation of selected review papers or the literature review sections of selected research studies.

Key terms

narrative review

research literature

review of the literature

scholarly literature

scientific literature

secondary source

systematic review

theoretical literature

INTRODUCTION

The review of the literature is traditionally considered a systematic and critical review of the most important published scholarly literature on a particular topic (Carroll-Johnson, 1992). The term 'scholarly literature' refers to published and unpublished research literature, as well as conceptual materials found in print and non-print forms.

This chapter introduces the review of literature as a concept essential to the growth of nursing as a discipline, in terms of practice, research, education and theory (see Figure 5.1). In turn, knowledge, generated from theorists, researchers, educators and practitioners, builds the literature through scholarly publications and presentations. In relation to these four concepts, a critical review of the literature presents:

- the extant knowledge in relation to a particular subject, concept, or problem
- new knowledge that can lead to the development, validation or refinement of theories
- appropriate research questions for the discipline to consider
- the latest knowledge for educational activities
- research findings that can lead to changes in clinical practice (e.g. the development of research-based nursing interventions/practice protocols).

FIGURE 5.1 Relationship of the review of literature to theory, research, education and practice

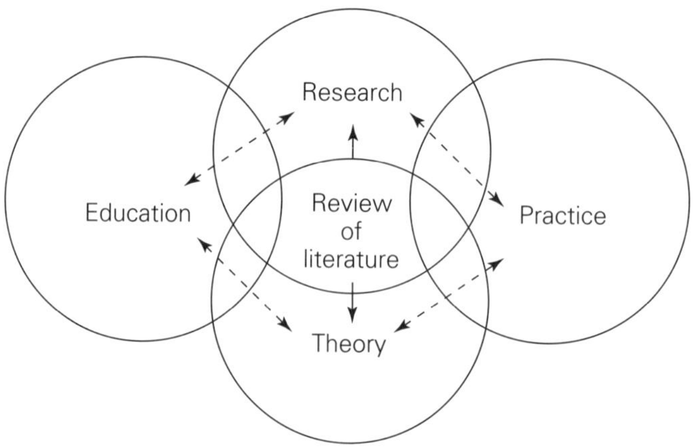

This chapter also introduces the review of the literature in research and scholarly activities, primarily from the perspective of the research consumer rather than the 'conductor of research'. The information provides the essential components for the production of a structured and critical literature review.

PURPOSES OF A LITERATURE REVIEW

The overall purpose of a review of the literature is to develop a strong knowledge base to carry out research and other research consumer scholarly activities in the educational and clinical practice settings (Glass, 1991). The common forms of a review include:

- the background section of an original research paper
- a systematic summary of a series of original research papers (with or without a meta-analysis)
- a literature review which is not systematic (and therefore may be open to bias)
- a supporting literature section of a clinical guideline or evidence-based recommendation.

The objectives listed in Box 5.1 relate to research producer and research consumer purposes. The knowledge uncovered from a critical review of the literature contributes to the development, implementation and results of both quantitative and qualitative studies. Such knowledge enhances the writing of scholarly papers. In the clinical practice arena, the knowledge from a critical literature review contributes to the implementation of research-based practice interventions, protocols and evaluation programs that improve the quality of patient care (see Chapters 6–7).

BOX 5.1 Overall purposes of a review of literature

Major goal—to develop a strong knowledge base to carry out research and other scholarly educational and clinical practice setting activities.

Objectives—a review of the literature does the following:

1. determines what is known and not known about a subject, concept or problem
2. determines gaps, consistencies and inconsistencies in the literature about a subject, concept or problem
3. discovers unanswered questions about a subject, concept or problem
4. discovers conceptual traditions used to examine problems
5. uncovers a new practice intervention(s) or provides evidence for current practice intervention(s)
6. generates useful research questions and hypotheses for the discipline
7. describes the strengths and weaknesses of designs/methods of enquiry and instruments used in earlier works
8. determines an appropriate research design/method (instruments, data collection and analysis methods) for answering the research question(s)
9. determines the need for replication of a well designed study or refinement of a study
10. promotes development of new or revising practice protocols, policies and projects/activities related to nursing practice and the discipline.

The first nine objectives in Box 5.1 represent different ways of thinking about the literature when considering the development of a study. These objectives direct the questions the researcher asks while reading the literature to determine a useful research question(s) and an appropriate design and method and/or the need for replication or refinement of a particular study.

Undertaking a literature review is a common learning and assessment task for undergraduate nursing students. Literature reviews are also undertaken by graduate coursework and research students, and for research proposals submitted to Institutional Ethics Committees (IECs) and funding bodies. The process for completing this challenging task needs to be explicitly modelled and learned within the educational setting. From a clinical perspective, reviews of the literature inform practice guidelines.

The major research consumer focus of the literature review is uncovering knowledge for use in educational and clinical practice settings. Critically reading the literature generates useful projects for these settings. Table 5.1 illustrates a few examples of scholarly activities related to reviews of the literature. Each reviewed source of information reflects critical thinking and scholarly writing, is relevant to the study/topic/project, and the content satisfies the following criteria. The objectives reflect both academic and professional expectations for a beginning research consumer in the nursing profession (see Chapter 1).

TABLE 5.1 Examples of the uses of the literature for research consumer purposes: educational and practice settings

EDUCATIONAL SETTING	CLINICAL/PROFESSIONAL SETTING
Undergraduate students ■ develop academic scholarly papers (on a specific topic, problem or issue) ■ prepare oral presentations or debates of a topic, problem or issue; clinical projects	**Nurses in the clinical setting** ■ implement research-based nursing interventions ■ develop hospital-specific nursing protocols or policies related to patient care ■ develop, implement and evaluate hospital-specific quality improvement (QA*, CQI* or TQM*) projects related to patient outcome data
Graduate students (master's and doctoral): ■ develop research proposals ■ develop research-based practice protocols and other scholarly projects **Faculty:** ■ develop and revise curricula ■ develop theoretical papers for presentations and/or publication ■ develop research proposals	**Professional nursing organisations/government agencies develop documents such as:** ■ position statement on nursing research (RCNA*, 1998) ■ position statement on postgraduate critical care nursing education from ACCCN* (Underwood, Elliott, Aitken et al., 1999) ■ palliative care education and training needs analysis (Uyeda et al., 1997)

*ACCCN Australian College of Critical Care Nurses
CQI continuous quality improvement
QA quality assurance
RCNA Royal College of Nursing, Australia
TQM total quality management

CRITICAL REVIEW

From a student perspective, a critical review of the literature is essential to acquiring knowledge for the development of scholarly papers, presentations and debates. Faculties usually require that students use literature to support their rationale for each nursing intervention. For example, a student assignment might involve retrieving and critically reviewing the primary sources listed for a particular practice protocol to determine the degree of support found for the interventions in the protocol. An effective literature review will have the characteristics listed in Table 5.2 that meet critical review criteria, which are discussed throughout this chapter and the text.

TABLE 5.2 Characteristics of a written review of literature

LEVELS OF REVIEW	CRITERIA
Description	■ purposes of a literature review were met ■ summary is succinct and adequately represents the reviewed source
Analysis	■ critical review (objective critical evaluation) reflects analysis and synthesis of material ■ application of accepted 'criteria' to analyse strengths, weaknesses or limitations and conflicts or gaps in information, as it relates directly and indirectly to the area of interest
Synthesis	■ evidence of synthesis of the critiques of each source of information (may use summary tables*); putting the parts (that is, each critique) together to form a new whole (Kerlinger, 1986) or connecting link for what is to be studied, replicated, developed or implemented
Structure and flow of paper	■ review consists of mainly primary sources ■ sufficient number of sources are used, especially data-based sources ■ summarises/paraphrases material rather than continually quoting content ■ summaries/critiques of studies are presented in a logical flow ending with a conclusion or synthesis of the reviewed material that reflects why the study, project or conceptual stand should be taken

* Summary tables facilitate the critique articles in sections or themes and enable questions and gaps to be identified during the review (see section titled 'Summary tables' on pages 84–85).

Most students preparing an academic paper read the required course materials, as well as additional library materials. Students search the literature to uncover knowledge to prepare an academic paper on a certain topic rather than to uncover knowledge on a specific topic to carry out a research project. From an academic standpoint, the level, type of course and objective of the assignment determines whether a student's literature search needs to be minor, selected, cursory, major, in-depth, extensive or exhaustive. Regardless, discovering knowledge is the goal of any 'search'; therefore a research consumer needs to know how to search the literature. Becoming a competent research consumer requires knowing the way to search the literature quickly and efficiently. Reference librarians are excellent people to ask about various sources of scholarly literature. If you are unfamiliar with the process of conducting a scholarly computer search, your reference librarian can help (Shorten, Wallace & Crookes, 2001).

The review of the literature is usually defined as a step of the research process. When a research study is written as a proposal or is published, the literature review is often written as a separate aspect of the study. However, the actual review of the literature (that is, the results of the review) is used in developing all steps of the process. The review includes a critical evaluation of both primary and secondary literature related to the proposed study, as well as a summary of the overall strengths or weaknesses of the reviewed studies' conflicts and gaps in the literature. It concludes with a statement relating the proposed study to the reviewed research. A critical literature review is central to developing and implementing research consumer activities. A practice protocol or nursing interventions implemented in a healthcare setting should be based on nurses' 'critical' review of research literature. For example, Stetler (1994) incorporates an extensive review of all types of research studies in her nursing model for research utilisation (see Chapter 7).

The literature review is considered essential to all steps of the quantitative research process. From this perspective the review is broad and systematic, as well as in-depth but not usually exhaustive; it is a critical collection and evaluation of the important published scholarly literature in journals, monographs, books and/or book chapters, as well as unpublished scholarly print and computer-accessed materials (e.g. doctoral dissertations and master's theses), information technology materials (e.g. websites, CD-ROMs, doctoral and master's theses), audiovisual materials (audiotapes, videotapes) and personal communications (e.g. conference presentations, one-to-one interviews).

The review in quantitative research

The brief overview in Box 5.2 illustrates the use of the literature review in relation to the steps of the quantitative research process. A critical reading of relevant literature is done in the following steps of the research process.

BOX 5.2 Use of the literature review in relation to the quantitative research process

- Source of knowledge and paradigmatic position
  A review of the position of theoretical or conceptual frameworks within a critical literature review reveals conceptual traditions, concepts and/or theories or conceptual models from nursing and other related fields that can be used to examine problems; it presents the context for studying the problem and can be viewed as a concept map for understanding the relationships between or among the variables in studies. The literature review provides a rationale for the variables and develops propositions about individual variables within the theoretical framework of the study.
- Problem statement and hypothesis
  Determines what is known and not known; to uncover gaps, consistencies or inconsistencies; and/or to reveal unanswered questions in the literature about a subject, concept, theory or problem. The review allows for refinement of research problems and questions and/or hypotheses (see Chapter 2).
- Design and method
  Reveals the strengths and weaknesses of designs and methods of previous research studies. The review is crucial to choosing a feasible and ethical design, data collection method, sample size, valid and reliable instruments and effective data analysis method(s). A critical literature review reveals the appropriateness of a study's design and can help the researcher determine whether a previous study should be replicated and/or refined. It can also identify the need for instrument refinement or development through continued psychometric testing (see Chapter 19).

- Outcome of the analysis (findings, discuss recommendations)
  Interprets and discusses the results/findings related studies. The researcher returns to conceptual and data-based literature to acc instance, findings from a study on the clinical validatio diagnosis of anxiety may indicate that the most common indic to diagnose anxiety is the patient's subjective expression, 'I'm anxiou The research would then indicate in this section of the journal article/report that this particular finding was supported in the literature review. The literature review also helps to develop the implications of the findings for practice, education and further research.

From a quantitative perspective, the review of the literature is used for all designs and levels of observational and interventional approaches. Table 5.3 provides two examples, and illustrates in which sections of the papers specific steps of the research process are located.

TABLE 5.3 Examples of the use of a literature review in quantitative research

STEPS IN THE RESEARCH PROCESS	PRIMARY SOURCE—SECTION HEADINGS IN ARTICLE (Small, Lumley, Donohue et al., 2000)	SECONDARY SOURCE—SECTION HEADINGS IN ARTICLE (Thomas, McColl, Cullum et al., 1999)
Problem, need/significance, question(s)/hypothesi(e)s, theoretical/conceptual framework	Introduction	Introduction
Design/methodology	Participants and methods: aims	Methods of the review: inclusion and exclusion criteria
Measurement issues	Sample size and study power, recruitment, debriefing intervention	Methodological criteria
Data collection method Analytical approach	Data management and analysis	Systematic review
Findings (interpretation)	Results: recruitment and participation, characteristics of study participants, maternal health outcomes, women's view about debriefing and postpartum care, effect of research midwife	Findings: clinical area, nomenclature, sources, evidence base, formats, development, dissemination, implementation of guidelines, consumer involvement, strategies
Implications for practice	Discussion	Discussion
Recommendations for midwife		

eview in qualitative research

A qualitative approach may be used when conceptual knowledge is examined in the review of the literature. The following examples highlight the predominant use of the literature review for the particular qualitative approach:

- Historical (see Chapter 10)—review of literature is a (secondary) source of data (e.g. Godden and Forsyth, 2000; Roberts, 1996)
- Grounded theory (see Chapter 11)—constantly compares literature with data being generated (e.g. Barclay et al., 1996; O'Connell, 2000)
- Ethnographic (see Chapter 12)—more conceptual than data-based, provides framework for study (e.g. Russell, 1996)
- Phenomenological (see Chapter 13)—compare findings with information from the review of the literature (e.g. Kermode, 1995; O'Brien, 2000; Walters, 1995a; Walters, 1995b)
- Feminist (see Chapter 14)—provides a framework for study (e.g. Jackson, Daly, Davidson, et al., 2000)

If, as suggested earlier in steps 3 and 4 of Table 3.1, preliminary reading of available abstracts allowed article entries to be selected or discarded before printing the search, the printed search should then be a list of all articles required for copying. Having a copy of each article allows organisation for priority critical reading, and eventual sorting into themes or categories. Now the truly important aspect of the search begins: the critical reading of the retrieved materials. Critically reading scholarly material, especially research articles, requires several readings and the use of criteria. Do not be discouraged if all the retrieved articles are not as useful as first thought; this happens to the most experienced researcher. If most of the articles are not useful, be prepared to do another search, but discuss the variables to be used next time with an academic and/or a reference librarian. It is also a good idea to review the reference list of articles; if any seem relevant, they can also be retrieved for review.

STYLES FOR LITERATURE REVIEWS

When deciding upon a style for the review, consider the following:

- the purpose of the review
- the research question/topic
- the number of retrieved sources reviewed.

Reviews can be written according to:

- the variables being studied and presented chronologically under each variable
- presentation of material chronologically with sub-categories or variables discussed within each period, and
- the variables and included sub-categories related to the study's types or designs or related sub-variables.

Integrative reviews (Smith & Stullenbarger, 1991), narrative reviews (Cook, Mulrow & Haynes, 1997) and systematic reviews (Droogan & Cullum, 1998), have been discussed in the literature. One comparison noted the following differences between systematic and narrative reviews (see Table 5.4). When

TABLE 5.4 Comparison of narrative and systematic reviews

NARRATIVE REVIEW	COMPONENT	SYSTEMATIC REVIEW
Often broad aim	← Question →	Focused clinical question
Not specified; open to bias	← Strategy →	Explicit process
Not specified; open to bias	← Selection →	Defined criteria; uniform application
Variable quality; open to bias	← Appraisal →	Rigorous and methodical
Subjective; qualitative summary	← Synthesis →	Pooling of quantitative data
Sometimes evidence based	← Inferences →	Usually evidence based

Adapted from Cook, Mulrow & Haynes, 1997; used with permission.

examining a review paper, the reader should consider the components given in the middle column of Table 5.4, and identify whether those issues have been addressed.

Systematic reviews

A systematic review (SR) is a common strategy for examining an explicit issue in clinical practice (Cook, Greenhold, Ellrodt & Weingarten, 1997; Cook, Mulrow & Haynes, 1997; Evans & Chang, 2000). For example, a nurse wanted to know what the health outcomes of survivors of a critical illness were like after ICU discharge. An appropriate SR question has specific components (see also Chapter 6):

- a patient cohort (population) and clinical setting
- exposure to an intervention
- a condition of interest with a measurable outcome (end-point).

A template for a question is: 'What is the effectiveness of ... [a specific intervention] ... for ... [a defined patient type] ..., as measured by ... [a measurable outcome]?'. For example, 'What is the health status of survivors of an emergency admission to a general ICU?' Articles are reviewed according to specified criteria. Additional sources from reference lists are then examined along with a hand or electronic search of journals commonly publishing in the area of interest. The review process then includes sorting of articles for referencing, description, analysis and synthesis. One review paper examined 31 previously published primary studies that measured patient outcomes from adult general ICUs (Elliott, 1999). The search strategy included examination of CINAHL and Medline databases for English language articles. Inclusion criteria for the review process included papers with explicit measurement of patient outcomes beyond mortality rates. Keywords were 'functional status', 'health status', 'health outcomes', 'health-related quality of life' and 'patient outcomes'. The paper included summative descriptions of the reviewed papers, discussion of the various methods, results and limitations, and some synthesis of the pooled findings. Papers were studied using the following assessment process for the literature review (see Table 5.5). The components to be reviewed are identified after a number of readings of the selected papers.

TABLE 5.5 Components of review process: patient outcome studies from general ICU

METHODS	RESULTS
Design ■ prospective ■ retrospective	Sample characteristics ■ respondents/initial sample size ■ losses to follow-up ■ patient type ■ ICU acuity ■ ICU LOS
Instruments ■ unvalidated ■ validated	
Pre-admission status measured ■ self-report/recall ■ proxy ■ proxy—level of agreement measured	**Findings** ■ physiological status ■ mental status ■ social status ■ productivity ■ daily activities/self-care ■ employment status (return to work)
Comparison ■ other clinical sample(s) ■ population norms	
Follow-up period	**Statistical significance measured**

Adapted from Elliott, 1999; used with permission.

Methods and results were examined for comparison across the sample of primary studies, so that pooling or synthesis could be attempted. On average, studies had a 16-month subject recruitment period and a 14-month follow-up data collection period, mostly using a retrospective design (55%). The average subject was 55-years-old with an ICU length of stay of 5.6 days. Sixty-one per cent of studies used unvalidated instruments, and pre-ICU health status measurement was not measured in 52% of studies. Recall by the patient at various follow-up periods was used in 42% of studies, despite the potential for recall bias. All studies were affected by losses to follow-up. Average ICU mortality was 22% and cumulative mortality at follow-up was 24%, although the ranges were extreme. Other non-responses averaged 27%. The average final study sample was 433 subjects (median 159, influenced by the range of 13–3655 patients) (Elliott, 1999).

In this review, a minimum number of studies provided enough data to allow some interpretation of functional status following ICU discharge and convalescence. In general, physiological functioning decreased by 36% in the pooled cohort (range: 5%–70% decrease), while mental health returned to similar pre-ICU states in 65% of subjects. Social functioning and productivity were quite disparate, with some studies reporting a diminished status and others a similar functioning. Daily activities returned to normal in 54% of respondents, and a return to previous work occurred in 45%–70% of subjects. Overall, the findings from the studies reviewed indicated that the majority of survivors who responded to follow-up returned to a somewhat diminished or similar health status and activities as that prior to their critical illness. However, whether these subjects were representative of the general ICU survivors is not conclusive, as lack of control over exclusions and losses to follow-up were evident in a substantial number of studies (Elliott, 1999). Each of these methodological issues will be examined in Chapters 17–19 and 21.

As noted earlier, a variety of databases can be accessed for the conduct of a systematic review, including some online full-text journals and textbooks (see http://www.ovid.com/ovid). For example, in an integrated literature review on the development of inter-disciplinary practice, the databases Medline, Psyclit and Socioabs, and the keywords 'inter-professional practice', 'collaboration', and 'multidisciplinary practice' were used (McCallin, 2001). The review examined the themes of changing interactions, teams and teamwork. One finding was that separate disciplinary education does not foster inter-professional practice. The search strategy could also have examined the Cochrane database (http://www.cochrane.edu.au), and found an SR that assessed the impact of interventions designed to improve nurse–doctor collaboration (Zwarenstein et al., 1998) published in a journal which was not searched using the above databases.

Another SR searched six common electronic databases using the keywords 'falls', 'risk factors', 'systematic review' (Evans, Hodgkinson, Lambert & Wood, 2001). Eighteen papers that satisfied the inclusion criteria of a cohort or case-control design (see Chapter 17) were reviewed. Impaired mental status or mobility, a history of falls or special toileting needs, were the major factors identified. Less evidence was apparent for advanced age and medications.

The SR process is similar to the primary quantitative research process, as indicated in Table 5.6.

TABLE 5.6 Comparison of primary quantitative research and SR processes

PRIMARY RESEARCH	COMPONENT	SYSTEMATIC REVIEW
Rationale Study questions	← Background/objectives →	Rationale Study questions
Population Interventions Outcomes	← Research question →	Population Interventions Outcomes
Methods … Design/sample Study procedure	← Research plan →	Search strategy … Keywords Databases/hand searching
Subject inclusion criteria	← Sampling procedure →	Study inclusion criteria … Participants, designs, interventions, outcomes
IEC submission	← Ethics →	Peer review
Validity Reliability Responsiveness	← Measuring instruments →	Study quality assessment[1]
Data collection/management	← Data collection →	Data abstraction
Analysis Interpretation	← Data analysis →	Data synthesis[2]
Conferences Journal publications	← Reporting →	Professional/public domains Published SR Practice guidelines

1 Assessment of study design in an SR includes allocation to groups, sample size, blinding, adequacy of control, validity of outcome measures, confounders.

2 The data synthesis in an SR attempts to gain standardised scores (e.g. OR, 95% CI), assess heterogeneity (χ^2), with narrative summaries of observational studies.

Summary tables

After an initial review of papers, it may be useful to construct some working summary tables to enable the critique of articles in sections or themes, and to identify questions and gaps in the literature. The summary tables may be used only in the preparation of the literature review, or may evolve into an integral component of the final manuscript. Initially, column headers are selected to allow analysis of the various papers under specific themes (see Table 5.7). The development and sophistication of the table then develops as the review of papers continues.

TABLE 5.7 Example of summary table column headers

AUTHOR	SAMPLE	METHOD	OUTCOME VARIABLES	FINDINGS

Table 5.8 illustrates a simple summary table with four columns, labelled 'Study', 'Sample', 'Method', and 'Major findings'. The summary table allows descriptive information to be noted for each study (description), as well as enabling a reviewer to identify similarities and differences between the studies (synthesis). Limitations can also be identified (analysis). For example, as a collective, the recent studies listed in Table 5.8 examined outcomes from cardiac surgery using validated health-related quality of life (HRQOL) instruments—the most frequently used being the SF-36 Health Survey, Nottingham Health Profile and the Quality of Life Index. Limitations were evident in the studies reviewed, including short follow-up periods (Ross & Ostrow, 2001), small sample sizes (all papers cited in Table 5.8); and no pre-surgery health status measures (Hunt et al., 2000; Skaggs & Yates, 1999).

TABLE 5.8 Example of a summary table: recent outcome studies for cardiac surgery patients

STUDY	SAMPLE	METHOD	MAJOR FINDINGS
Skaggs & Yates, 1999	36 PTCA & 38 CABG patients.	QLI 3 months post-surgery.	No differences between groups.
Edell-Gustafsson et al., 1999	38 CABG patients.	NHP at pre-surgery and 1 month, and at 6 months post-surgery.	Pre-operative scores significantly lower than other scores ($p < 0.01$) for sleep, pain, energy and physical mobility; sleep was significantly worse at 1 month compared to other measures.
Barnason, 2000	47 CABG patients.	SF-36 pre-operatively (by recall) and at 3 months, 6 months and 12 months post-surgery, and modified 7-day activity for post-surgery timepoints.	Pre-operative scores significantly lower than other measures for all subscales ($p < 0.0001$) except role emotional; 3-month scores lower than 6-month and 12-month measures for all subscales except social and general health; no differences between 6-month and 12-month scores. No differences between measures for modified 7-day activity instrument.
Hunt, 2000	108 CABG patients.	SF-36 and pain/sleep ratings at 12 months post-surgery plus separate pre-surgery cohort ($n = 150$).	Significant improvement ($p < 0.05$–0.001) in physical functioning, bodily pain, social functioning and role-emotional at 12 months, compared to equivalent baseline group; 21% severe/very severe pain with significant correlation to poor QOL.
Ross & Ostrow, 2001	30 CABG patients.	SF-36, QLI, POMS pre-operatively and 6 weeks and 12 weeks post-surgery.	Significant improvement in physical functioning, vitality, social functioning, and mood at 12 weeks compared to pre-surgery ($p < 0.05$-0.01); in physical functioning and social functioning at 12 weeks compared to 6 weeks ($p < 0.001$).

CABG coronary artery bypass graft surgery
NHP Nottingham Health Profile
POMS Profile of Mood States
PTCA Percutaneous Transluminal Coronary Angioplasty
QLI Quality of Life Index
SF-36 Short-Form 36 Health Survey

CRITERIA FOR A REVIEW OF THE LITERATURE

The characteristics of a relevant review of the literature (see Table 5.2) and the purposes of the review of the literature (see Box 5.1) provided the framework for the development of literature review evaluation criteria. Difficulties that the research consumer might have regarding this task and related strategies are presented after a discussion of the criteria.

A critical appraisal of the literature review is a challenging task for the research consumer. Criteria have been developed for all aspects of the quantitative research process, for various quantitative designs and qualitative approaches, and for research consumer projects for the educational and clinical settings. Criteria for the review of the literature are usually presented from the quantitative research process perspective. Because the focus of this book is on the nurse in the research consumer role, the criteria incorporate this frame of reference. The important issue is for the reader to determine the overall value of the paper. Does the review of the literature permeate the report? Does the review of the literature contribute to the significance of the report in relation to nursing theory, research, education or practice? The overall question to be answered is, 'Does the review of the literature uncover knowledge?', which is based on the overall purpose of a review (see Box 5.1). The major goal turns into the question, 'Did the review of the literature provide a strong knowledge base to carry out the reported research or scholarly educational or clinical practice setting project?'. Box 5.3 provides questions for the research consumer to ask about a literature review.

BOX 5.3 Important questions to ask about a literature review

1. Does the literature review uncover gaps or inconsistencies in knowledge?
2. How does the review reflect critical thinking?
3. Are all the relevant concepts and variables included in the review?
4. Does the summary of each reviewed study reflect the essential components of the study design, research process and analysis techniques?
5. Does the critique of each reviewed study include strengths, weaknesses or limitations of the design, conflicts, and gaps or inconsistencies in information in relation to the area of interest?
6. Are primary sources mainly used?
7. Is there a synthesis of the reviewed scholarly literature?
8. Does the synthesis summary follow a logical sequence that leads the reader to why there is the need for the particular study?
9. Does the organisation of the reviewed studies (e.g. chronologically, according to concepts/variables or by type/design/level of study) flow logically, enhancing the ability of the reader to evaluate the need for the particular research or project?
10. Does the literature review follow the purpose(s) of the research or project?

Questions related to the logical presentation of the reviewed articles are somewhat more challenging for the beginning research consumer, as the process of learning is based on experiences. The more you read scholarly articles, the easier this question is to answer. At times the type of question being asked in relation to the particular concept lends itself to presenting the reviewed studies chronologically (that is, perhaps beginning with early or landmark data-based or conceptual literature).

Questions must be asked about whether each explanation of a step of the research process met the criteria. For instance, in Box 5.1, the second objective states that the review of the literature is to determine gaps, consistencies and inconsistencies in the literature about a subject, concept or problem. You could ask, 'What gaps or conflicts in knowledge about the problem are identified?' and 'How does this study intend to fill those gaps or resolve those conflicts?'. In this example, the purpose or objective of the literature review became the evaluation question or criterion for critically reviewing of the literature.

Other sets of criteria may phrase these questions differently or more broadly. For instance, the question might be, 'Does the literature search seem adequate?' or 'Does the report demonstrate scholarly writing?'. These questions may seem to be difficult for you to answer, however, one place to begin is by determining whether the source is a refereed journal. It is fairly reasonable to assume that a scholarly refereed journal publishes manuscripts that demonstrate an adequate search of previous literature using mainly primary sources, and are written in a scholarly manner. However, this does not mean that every study reported in a refereed journal will meet all the criteria in an equal manner. Consultation with a colleague may be necessary to develop skills in answering these questions.

Other questions that should be asked are, 'Is there a written summary of each reviewed source?' and 'Does the summary of the study include a critique?'. These questions seem as if they would be easily answered by reading what is reported in the literature review. However, because of style differences and space constraints, each citation is usually briefly summarised and often lacks a critique. In addition to a summary and critique of each source, a literature review requires a complete summary or a synthesis of all reviewed sources. The relationship between and among these studies must be explained.

- The summary should reflect the putting together of the main points or value of all the sources in relation to the research question.
- A synthesis of a written review of the literature usually appears at the end of the review section before the research question or hypothesis-reporting section. If not labelled as such, it is usually evident in the last paragraph.

A relevant literature review demonstrates synthesis of the reviewed sources. Therefore, demonstrating synthesis becomes an essential criterion for the review of the literature.

Articles that are published in a scholarly professional journal usually include an abstract following the title of the article that provides a rationale for the study. Abstracts are concisely written summaries of the main aspects of a research study or conceptual paper. Many published articles have a brief summary or abstract (200–300 words) on the first page, set out at the beginning of the article. Most computer searches have the feature of including the abstract for the reference, as well as all of the references used in the article.

One abstract provided the following rationale: 'Given the continued lack of research and evaluation in relation to antenatal education and the real concern for early parenting influences on childhood development, this research surveyed 705 midwives' (Jackson, Schmierer & Schneider, 1996). Reading the abstract helps to determine whether the paper is relevant to the review question. The complete abstract includes statements on the method, findings, conclusions and clinical implications (see Box 5.4, for example).

BOX 5.4 Example of abstract with headings

Background: The immediate period following discharge from hospital after an acute myocardial infarction (AMI) is noted to be a stressful and vulnerable time. Minimal information is available in this time window.

Objective: To explore the health status, perceptions of coping and social support of survivors of a recent myocardial infarction in the first three weeks following discharge from hospital in south-western Sydney.

Methods: A descriptive, exploratory approach using a triangulated methodology was used to describe the experiences of 38 survivors, reveal patterns in these experiences, explore the health support needs of the participants and document changes in the health status over the initial three-week period post-discharge. Quantitative data were collected using the MOS-SF-36, New York Heart Association Class (NYHA), Canadian Cardiovascular Society Status (CCVS), and the Jalowiec Coping Scale (JCS). A semi-structured interview schedule provided additional qualitative data regarding the experiences of the survivors.

Results: The health status of participants was relatively stable over the three-week period, with the majority having no activity limitation due to dyspnoea or angina. However, the subjects' health status was considerably lower than for their age-matched population. The common and most effective coping strategies adopted during this period were confrontation, optimism and self-reliance. In addition, feelings of anxiety, depression, ambiguity and uncertainty, fear of recurrence of the MI and deterioration in health, and boredom and inertia were elucidated from interviews.

Conclusion: These findings are of use to nurses in hospital and community settings in assisting post-MI patients to prepare for and deal effectively with their experiences during convalescence.

From Daly et al., 2000; used with permission.

The preceding summary synthesis meets the objective of uncovering knowledge, determining what is known and not known and finding gaps and inconsistencies in the literature. This example specifically addresses a number of questions found in the criteria for critical review.

Being able to critique a review of the literature is an acquired skill. Continue reading and re-reading, as well as seeking advice from clinical and academic colleagues. Use the literature review as an essential key in implementing a research-based practice (see Chapter 7).

KEY POINTS

- The review of the literature is defined as a broad, comprehensive, in-depth, systematic and critical review of scholarly publications, unpublished scholarly print materials, internet materials, audiovisual materials and personal communications.
- The review of the literature is for research and research consumer activities. The main objectives for the research consumer in relation to the literature review are to acquire the ability to:
  - conduct a computer data-based search
  - efficiently retrieve a sufficient amount of scholarly materials for a literature review
  - critically evaluate data-based and conceptual material based on accepted reviewing criteria.
- Systematic reviews (SRs) provide an explicit protocol for the search strategy, inclusion criteria for article selection and critical appraisal in the examination of explicit aspects of methodological rigour.
- Criteria for reviewing scholarly literature reflect the purposes and characteristics of a relevant literature review and are presented in the form of questions.
- The ability to critically review data-based literature is necessary for implementing a research-based practice in nursing.

CRITICAL THINKING CHALLENGES

- How is it possible that the review of the literature can be both an individual step of the research process and a research component used in each of the steps of the process? Support your answer with specific examples.
- How does a researcher justify using both conceptual and data-based literature in a literature review; and would you use the same types of literature for research consumer purposes, such as developing an academic scholarly paper?

Additional resources

American Psychological Association. (2001). *Publication manual of the American Psychological Association* (5th ed.). Washington, APA.

JBIEBNM [Joanna Briggs Institute for Evidence Based Nursing and Midwifery]. (2000). Appraising systematic reviews. *Changing Practice*, 1(1), 1–6.

JBIEBNM [Joanna Briggs Institute for Evidence Based Nursing and Midwifery]. (2001). An introduction to systematic reviews. *Changing Practice*, 2(1), 1–6.

Magarey, J. (2001). Elements of a systematic review. *International Journal of Nursing Practice*, 7, 376–82.

McCain, N.L. & Lynn, M.R. (1990). Meta-analysis of a narrative review: studies evaluating patient teaching. *Western Journal of Nursing Research*, 12, 347–58.

NHMRC. (1999). A guide to the development, implementation and evaluation of clinical practice guidelines. Canberra, NHMRC.

NHMRC. (2000). How to use the evidence: assessment and application of scientific evidence. Canberra, NHMRC.
Nicoll, L.H., Ouellette, T.H., Bird, D.C., & Harper, J. (1996). Bibliography database managers. *Computers in Nursing*, 14(1), 45–6.
Strunk, W., & White, E.B. (2000). *The elements of style* (4th ed.). Boston, Allyn & Bacon.
Tornquist, E.M. (1986). *From proposal to publication: an informal guide to writing about nursing research.* Menlo Park, Addison-Wesley.

6
CHAPTER

Evidence-based nursing

Gavin Leslie and Judith Finn

LEARNING OUTCOMES

After reading this chapter the student should be able to:

- Outline what is meant by the term 'evidence-based nursing'.
- Identify the major criticisms of evidence-based nursing.
- Describe the five 'steps' involved in the practice of evidence-based nursing.
- Outline the role of the Cochrane Collaboration and the Joanna Briggs Centre for Evidence Based Nursing and Midwifery.
- Recommend internet websites that may provide useful evidence-based nursing resources.
- Discuss how evidence-based nursing might influence their own clinical nursing practice.
- Describe the relationship between evidence-based nursing and clinical nursing research.

Key terms

bibliographic database

critical appraisal

evidence-based nursing (EBN)

evidence-based practice (EBP)

levels of evidence

randomised controlled trial (RCT)

systematic review

INTRODUCTION

Evidence-based nursing (EBN) emerged from the evidence-based medicine movement in the last decade of the twentieth century to define a new driving force in the clinical practice of nurses. While this chapter will focus on evidence-based nursing, it is worthy of note that evidence-based practice (EBP) is not the prerogative or domain of any particular specialty, discipline or group in healthcare. Indeed, the principles of EBP can be applied across the full range of clinical contexts, within all healthcare professions.

The basic tenet underpinning EBN is to provide the most efficacious nursing interventions for patients, thus effecting a change in focus away from nursing care based on routine and ritual to that based on what works best to achieve the desired outcomes. Florence Nightingale herself espoused the virtues basing health policy and practice on systematically derived 'evidence', rather than conjecture (McDonald, 2001). And yet in the more recent history as a profession, nursing abounds with examples of practices that are based on anecdote and authority rather than on evidence. One example was the disconcerting array of potions and practices used over the years to promote 'healing' of decubitus ulcers (pressure sores), ranging from oxygen, honey, zinc paste, to mercurochrome or iodine-soaked dressings. Ironically, there was often a plausible biological rationale proffered for the therapy, as nursing moved into an era where being able to offer a logical explanation why something was done that way implicitly, if not explicitly, proffered sufficient justification for doing it.

However, few nurses at the time thought to suggest that perhaps it might be useful to actually find out if actual practices had ever been shown through research to be effective. For today's research-aware graduate nurse, this probably seems amazing, yet a large proportion of clinical practices in nursing (as with most other health professions, including medicine) remain based on tradition or professional opinion, rather than scientific evidence of what actually works. This 'evidence' may of course be the highest level available because of sound practical or ethical reasons. However, it was noted that it 'is generally accepted that contemporary nursing is often characterised by large variability in practice and a serious lack of research utilisation' (Joanna Briggs Institute for Evidence Based Nursing and Midwifery, 2000, 'About' section).

This chapter provides an introduction to the theory and practice of EBN, and identifies additional resources for further information. It seeks to put into context the relationship between EBN and clinical nursing research and to provide an awareness of the debate about what constitutes the appropriate evidence base for nursing. The chapter begins with a brief consideration of the history of EBN and progresses to the identification of the steps involved in the practice of EBN. As will become evident, the skills that are required of the physician to practice evidence-based medicine, namely, asking answerable questions and locating and critically appraising the literature, are equally relevant to the skills required by the professional nurse and EBN. What differs between the health professions are the questions asked, not necessarily the methods used to answer them.

BACKGROUND AND DEFINITION: WHAT IS EBN AND WHERE HAS IT COME FROM?

EBN has its roots in the evidence-based medicine movement that grew from concern by a group of clinicians about the proliferation of clinical trials without attempts to integrate research findings into medical practice. There was also recognition of the need to somehow bring together the ever-increasing volume of research literature, and to make the information accessible and meaningful to clinicians. In 1992, Guyatt and associates at McMaster University in Canada produced their landmark paper titled 'Evidence-based medicine—a new approach to teaching the practice of medicine' (Evidence Based Working Group, 1992), which called for a 'paradigm shift' towards greater integration of evidence from clinical research into medical practice. However, this was not to imply that EBM was simply the utilisation of research. The definition of EBM that has been most widely adopted is that by Sackett (also from McMaster University and previously Oxford University), thus: 'Evidence-based medicine is the conscientious, explicit, and judicious use of current best evidence in making decisions about the care of individual patients. The practice of evidence-based medicine means integrating individual clinical expertise with the best available external clinical evidence from systematic research' (Sackett et al., 1996, p. 71).

Similarly, definitions of EBN emphasise the principle of integration of the best available evidence with the nurse's clinical expertise, together with patient preferences within a context of limited resources, thus: 'evidence-based nursing is the process by which nurses make clinical decisions using the best available research evidence, their clinical expertise and patient preferences and values, in the context of available resources' (DiCenso, Cullum & Ciliska, 1998, p. 38).

Sackett and colleagues (1996) identified several factors that have fuelled the development of EBP, including:

- a growing recognition among clinicians of the daily need for research-based information to inform patient care decisions
- the inadequacy of traditional information sources such as textbooks
- the so-called experts
- didactic instructional techniques used to address the dynamic nature of clinical information.

Fortunately, the need to access a rapidly expanding volume of research literature has been accompanied by developments in strategies to locate relevant information (e.g. computer databases) and methods to synthesise information (e.g. systematic reviews) (Sackett et al., 2000).

Another impetus to the development of EBP, especially in the United Kingdom (UK), was concern over the standards of clinical care, exemplified by the now infamous case of the management of care of children receiving complex heart surgery at the Bristol Royal Infirmary prior to 1995 (Bristol Royal Infirmary, 2001). In 1997, the National Health Service (NHS) released a White Paper that described a new system of 'clinical governance' in NHS Trusts and primary care designed to 'ensure that clinical standards are met and there are processes to ensure continuous improvement, backed by a new statutory duty for quality in NHS Trusts' (National Health Service, 1997, 'newnhs' section). An essential component of clinical governance is clinical effectiveness, that is defined as a 'measure of the extent to which a particular intervention works' (Starey, 2001, p. 4), and relies heavily on EBP to discern practices that are or are not based on the best available evidence. The possible medico-legal implications of not following EBP are also alluded to (Starey, 2001).

HOW TO PRACTISE EVIDENCE-BASED NURSING

To effectively practise EBN requires a supportive institutional climate and active managerial leadership (see Chapter 7 for an example of this). This section discusses the steps involved, including asking answerable questions, and locating and appraising the evidence.

Steps in EBN

Several steps have been described in the practice of EBN, as shown in Table 6.1, beginning with the transformation of a clinical query or need for information into a structured answerable question which then forms the basis for the search for relevant evidence in the literature (see Chapter 3). The literature must then be critically appraised for its validity, size of effect and generalisability before being incorporated into clinical practice (if appropriate to the context and amenable to the patient) and the entire process evaluated (Flemming, 1998; Sackett et al., 2000).

TABLE 6.1 Five steps in the practice of evidence-based nursing

STEP	ACTIVITIES
1	Translate the clinical uncertainty into an answerable structured question.
2	Search for information that could be useful in answering the question developed in Step 1.
3	Critically appraise the information located in terms of validity, relevance and applicability.
4	Integrate the relevant information with own clinical expertise and context of care, together with patient preferences and clinical resources to plan and implement nursing care.
5	Assess the effectiveness of the process followed and the intervention in Step 4 and identify implications for future healthcare decisions.

Adapted from Flemming, 1998; Sackett et al., 2000.

Asking answerable questions

The variation in questions that nurses ask reflects the broad scope of current nursing practice as well as the differing priorities of concern for nurses working within different clinical contexts and with different patient groups (Flemming, 1998). Nurses are interested in the cause, clinical presentation and prognosis of disease as well as the experience and meaning of illness for their patients. However, nurses are also concerned about which nursing interventions do and do not 'work' (Finn, 2001), and it is questions about the efficacy and effectiveness of therapeutic interventions that form the basis of EBN.

Asking questions sounds a simple enough exercise, however, if the question is not well articulated, unnecessary time will be spent refining the literature searches and spurious information will initially be retrieved. It has been recommended that questions should consist of three to four parts, namely:

- Problem (either patient-related or another health issue)
- Intervention
- Comparison intervention (optional) or control
- Outcome (which can be measured).

These four parts form the acronym PICO.

An example would be, 'in adult patients who have had open heart surgery, should suction be applied to underwater seal drainage to encourage effective wound drainage?'. It should be clear that such a structured question would help to direct the searching of the literature much more efficiently than if one began the search with questions such as 'what is the best way to manage sternal wounds post-operatively?' or 'how should I care for a patient with an underwater seal drain in-situ?'. See Chapter 5 for further discussion of framing the question for systematic reviews.

Locating the evidence

Once the question is formulated, the search for information needs to be undertaken. Healthcare librarians are skilled in the process of information retrieval and can be of assistance in developing appropriate search strategies. Textbooks have traditionally been the written source of information for nurses and remain useful for the more 'stable' knowledge such as anatomy. However, within the more dynamic realm of clinical practice, the information presented in textbooks can become outdated soon after publication. This has led to some textbooks being made available online (e.g. books@ovid), thus enabling regular updates. See Chapters 1 and 3 for further discussion of online resources. Nonetheless, in most instances the most up-to-date clinical nursing information will come from journal articles, best located through the various bibliographic databases.

Bibliographic databases

There are a large number of databases available for searching (see the section on 'Electronic databases' in Chapter 3, pages 44–45, and Table 3.3 on page 43), however, the two most commonly searched databases by nurses are CINAHL (the Cumulative Index to Nursing and Allied Health Literature) and Medline. Most university and hospital libraries will subscribe to one or more of these databases, in addition to Medline and CINAHL (see Chapter 3).

Evidence-based databases and resources

Interest in EBP has given rise to the development of organisations that coordinate the conduct and dissemination of systematic reviews of clinical research (e.g. the Cochrane Collaboration and the Joanna Briggs Institute for Evidence Based Nursing and Midwifery).

The Cochrane Collaboration (www.cochrane.org), founded in 1993, aims to help people make well informed decisions about healthcare by 'preparing, maintaining and ensuring the accessibility of systematic reviews of the effects of health care interventions' (The Cochrane Collaboration website <www.cochrane.org>, 2001, para. 1). Cochrane systematic reviews and information about The Cochrane Collaboration are published electronically in The Cochrane Library, which also contains The Cochrane Controlled Trials

Register, a bibliographic database of around 300,000 controlled trials, and The Database of Abstracts of Reviews of Effectiveness (DARE), which includes structured abstracts of systematic reviews that have been critically appraised by reviewers at the NHS Centre for Reviews and Dissemination at York University and others (e.g. from the American College of Physicians' Journal Club and the journal *Evidence-Based Medicine*). Also included in The Cochrane Library is The Cochrane Methodology Register (a bibliography of articles on the science of research synthesis and a Reviewers' Handbook on the science of reviewing research), a glossary of methodological terms and Cochrane jargon, and contact details for review groups and other groupings in The Cochrane Collaboration. The Cochrane Library is published quarterly on CD-ROM and the internet and is distributed via subscription. Many university and hospital libraries subscribe to the Cochrane Library databases. Notwithstanding this, abstracts of Cochrane Systematic Reviews are available free of charge from the Cochrane Collaboration website.

The Joanna Briggs Institute for Evidence Based Nursing and Midwifery (JBIEBNM) (www.joannabriggs.edu.au) is an international research collaboration based at the Royal Adelaide Hospital and the Adelaide University with collaborating centres in Australia, New Zealand and Hong Kong, which was established in 1996 in recognition of the need for a collaborative approach to the evaluation of research and its integration into nursing and midwifery practice. As identified on its website, the JBIEBNM works with researchers, clinicians and managers to bring together a range of practice-oriented research activities to improve the effectiveness of nursing practice and healthcare outcomes by:

- conducting systematic reviews (SRs) and analyses of the research literature
- collaborating with expert researchers and clinicians to facilitate the development of practice information sheets based on an SR of research
- participating in the dissemination and implementation of Best Practice Information Sheets and evaluating their impact on nursing and midwifery practice
- designing, promoting and delivering short courses in EBN and midwifery for nursing clinicians, nursing researchers, nursing managers and nursing teachers
- offering direct fee-for-service consultancies to health server provider agencies to develop customised EBP training and EBP manuals
- initiating primary research when indicated by the findings of the SR
- contributing to cost effective healthcare through the promotion of EBN and midwifery practice
- planning and organising regular colloquia.

(Joanna Briggs Institute for Evidence Based Nursing and Midwifery, 2000).

As of January 2002 there were 16 full SRs listed on the JBIEBNM websites on a diverse range of topics, including falls in acute hospitals, nursing management of chest drains, music as an intervention for hospital patients, nursing management of fever in children, and post harvest management of split thickness skin graft donor sites (www.joannabriggs.edu.au/ sysmenu.html).

The University of York (UK) Department of Health Sciences also hosts a Centre for Evidence Based Nursing (CEBN) (www.york.ac.uk/healthsciences/). The CEBN seeks to produce reliable research evidence for clinical nursing through primary research and systematic review. Projects include: systematic reviews of wound care (through the Cochrane Wounds Group); a systematic review of the evidence relating to support for carers of people with Alzheimer's Disease (published in the Cochrane Library); and a multicentre randomised controlled trial (RCT) of compression bandages for people with leg ulcers. The CEBN is also researching factors that promote or impede the implementation of EBP.

A recent EBP initiative in Australia was the establishment of the National Institute of Clinical Studies (NICS) in December 2000 in Melbourne, as an initiative of the Commonwealth Department of Health and Aged Care. The NICS was established to act as a national focus for the collection and dissemination of strategies that achieve best practice clinical care (www.nicsl.com.au/index.asp) by:

- initiating and supporting activities that provide a better understanding of successful approaches to translate evidence into clinical practice
- integrating the routine uptake of evidence into systems established to improve quality and accountability
- facilitating cultural and attitudinal change in clinical practices.

Secondary journals

Increasing interest in EBP has also given rise to a series of 'evidence-based' journals, which, rather than publish original primary research, screen for the 'best' original articles and systematic reviews published in other journals and bring them together into a secondary journal that provides commentary on the original article by 'experts' in the particular field, who can place the new research in context. 'Secondary' journals have thus been promoted as a means of offering busy clinicians the evidence-based clinical information necessary to practice effectively (Cullum, DiCenso & Ciliska, 1998). Examples of such secondary journals include *Evidence-Based Nursing* (www.evidencebasednursing.com/), *Evidence Based Medicine* (www.evidence-basedmedicine.com/) and the *American College of Physicians (ACP) Journal Club* (www.acpjc.org).

Other internet resources

Over the last decade there has been exponential growth in the amount of information relevant to EBP that can be accessed via the internet. However, one does need to be cognisant of the fact that there is no inherent 'quality control' of what is posted on the internet, and as such, there is a need to be cautiously critical of some of the information found. Nonetheless, there is a wealth of information accessible via the world wide web, and extensive lists have been published in evidence-based medicine books and journal articles (McKibbon & Marks, 1998a; McKibbon & Marks, 1998b; Snowball, 1999). It would be impossible to list all useful sites here, however, one recommended strategy is to go to a site like the JBIEBNM Recommended Nursing Links site (www.joannabriggs.edu.au/links.html) and then browse through the multitude of links to other websites provided.

Another recommended means of locating EBP information is via the free-of-charge site called Netting the Evidence (www.nettingtheevidence.org.uk/), which is produced by the School of Health and Related Research (ScHARR) at the University of Scheffield (UK). It is intended to facilitate evidence-based healthcare by providing support and access to helpful organisations and useful learning resources, including an evidence-based virtual library, software and journals. The resources can be browsed alphabetically or by type and a search facility and self-assessment exercises are available.

In addition to EBP sites, there are other resources that are useful for accessing specific 'evidence' to answer clinical questions. For example, some full-text journals can be accessed free of charge via the internet, such as the *Medical Journal of Australia* (www.mja.com.au) and the *British Medical Journal* (http://bmj.com).

There are also various sites that publish evidence-based clinical practice guidelines, for example: the Australian National Health and Medical Research Council (NHMRC) Clinical Practice Guidelines (www.health.gov.au:80/hfs/nhmrc/publications/cphome.htm); New Zealand Guidelines Group (www.nzgg.org.nz/); and the US National Guideline Clearing House (www.guideline.gov/index.asp). Clinical practice guidelines are systematically developed statements to assist practitioner and patient decisions about appropriate healthcare for specific clinical circumstances (Cluzeau & Littlejohns, 1999), but as for all 'evidence' require critical appraisal rather than blind acceptance (Hayward, et al., 1995; Wilson, et al., 1995).

Also of use in searching for 'evidence' are specific sites, such as: the US Centers for Disease Control and Prevention (www.cdc.gov/) for information on infectious diseases; the Australian Institute of Health and Welfare (AIHW) (www.aihw.gov.au/) for Australian national health and welfare statistics; the World Health Organisation (www.who.int/home-page/) for information about worldwide public health issues; and the Australian Resuscitation Council (ARC) (www.resus.org.au) for resuscitation policy.

Other sources of 'evidence'

Unpublished theses and dissertations as well as government and private reports can also prove to be useful sources of clinical 'evidence', however they tend not to be widely available or are difficult to locate and, as such, are often termed 'grey' literature.

Levels of evidence

The type of research that constitutes the strongest evidence to answer a clinical question depends on the type of question being asked (Roberts & DiCenso, 1999). For a prognosis questions such as 'how likely is it that a child who has a febrile fit will fit again?', a cohort study often provides the best answers. For questions about cause/aetiology such as 'what are the risk factors for falls in hospitalised elderly people?', a case-control study may provide the best evidence. However, where the question involves efficacy of therapy, that is 'does this intervention achieve the desired clinical outcomes?', then RCTs do assume the greatest prominence. The best evidence for a therapy question will be provided by research that can demonstrate a difference in defined clinical outcomes in one group where the therapy was employed compared with another group(s) that did not receive the therapy; this 'evidence' is strengthened when systematic bias is minimised by the process of randomisation and blinding (Snowball, 1999).

All EBP organisations use a similar classification hierarchy to establish evidence for examining studies 'cause and effect' of therapeutic interventions. For example, the JBIEBNM publishes levels of evidence classification with each of their practice sheets. Table 6.2. outlines the classification hierarchy recommended by the NHMRC (1999).

TABLE 6.2 Hierarchy of evidence for cause and effect studies of therapeutic interventions

LEVELS OF EVIDENCE

All studies were categorised according to the strength of the evidence based on the following classification system.

Level I	Evidence obtained from a systematic review of all relevant randomised controlled trials.
Level II	Evidence obtained from at least one properly designed randomised controlled trial.
Level III.1	Evidence obtained from well designed control trials without randomisation.
Level III.2	Evidence obtained from comparative studies with concurrent controls and allocation not randomised (cohort studies), case-control studies, or interrupted time series with a control group.
Level III.3	Evidence obtained from comparative studies with historical control, two or more single-arm studies, or interrupted time series without a parallel control group.
Level IV	Evidence obtained from case series (post-test or pre-test/post-test).

National Health and Medical Research Council (NHMRC). (1999). A guide to the development, implementation and evaluation of clinical practice guidelines. Canberra, NHMRC. Copyright Commonwealth of Australia, reproduced with permission.

As noted above, the 'highest' level of evidence for a therapy question is a systematic review of all relevant randomised control trials, while the 'lowest' level of evidence is from the case series designs (post-test or pre-test/post-test). At this point in time, there is a dearth of RCTs of nursing interventions (Cullum, 1997), and as such, it is not uncommon for clinical practice to be based on lower levels of evidence.

Opinions of respected authorities based on clinical experience, descriptive studies, or reports of expert committees were designated Level IV evidence in previous classifications (e.g. Evans & Chang, 2000), but these forms of knowledge have now been questioned, as the findings do not arise directly from scientific investigation (NHMRC, 2000). However, when evidence from scientific investigation is lacking, then any recommendation must be acknowledged as being based on expert opinion, and should be reviewed as new evidence becomes available (NHMRC, 2000, p. 10).

It is relevant to note that even recommendations based on consensus of expert opinion is not equivalent to saying that nursing practice should be based on routine and ritual—or the personal opinion of the shift coordinator or team leader. In addition, the current classification does not value findings from research methods that are common in nursing (e.g. qualitative or descriptive observational designs). The section called 'Consideration of qualitative research' on page 102 provides further discussion of this issue.

CRITICAL APPRAISAL OF THE EVIDENCE

The aim of critical appraisal of the literature is to assess the quality of the research and to ascertain the applicability of findings to the clinical context where the question arose. The skill of critical appraisal has not necessarily been well developed for most clinicians (including nurses) (Meah, Luker & Cullum, 1996; Royle, et al., 1997), who traditionally have seen little clinical utility in research utilisation (Hunt, 1996). Nonetheless, like any 'skill', critical appraisal skills have the capacity to improve with practice and experience (Dawes, 1999).

Critical appraisal of the literature does require some understanding of research methods, statistical inference and effect measures (Ciliska, Cullum & DiCenso, 1999; Sheldon, 2000a; 2000b), but only to a level that enables the individual to be able to be a consumer of the research literature. There are a multitude of resources available, including this text and a series of Users' Guides published by the Evidence Based Medicine Working Group in the *Journal of the American Medical Association* (JAMA) and downloadable from the internet (www.phru.org.uk/~casp/index.htm or through Ovid full-text facilities). These Users' Guides include appraisal templates to assist with developing such critical appraisal skills. As of early 2002, 25 Users' Guides had been published, some in two parts (see the 'Additional resources' section on pages 106–07 for a selection of the Users' Guides).

Three key issues require consideration when appraising any paper, namely:

- Are the results of the study valid?
- What are the results?
- Are the results applicable to my patients?

Validity is concerned with the study being free from bias. The specific criteria to be addressed in the assessment of the validity will vary depending on the type of research method used in the study (Ciliska, Cullum & Marks, 2001; Cullum, 2000). For example, for RCTs, randomisation is a key issue impacting on the validity of the paper, whereas for epidemiologic studies such as case-control studies, identification of potential confounding factors is of importance (Mant, 1999).

In considering the results of the study, it is important to consider the clinical significance of the study as well as the statistical significance. It is possible for a study (especially if the sample size is large) to show a statistically significant result, even when the clinical effect is so small as to render it of little meaning to clinical practice (e.g. a reduction of mean blood pressure of 1mm Hg). The converse is also true, in that the results of a study may not reach statistical significance (often because of a small sample size not affording the study sufficient power) and yet a substantial difference is evident between the groups. It is for such reasons that the use of effect measures such as absolute risk reduction (ARR) and numbers needed to treat (the number of patients that need to be treated (NNT) with the experimental intervention for the duration of the trial to prevent one additional bad outcome), is replacing statistical inference in clinical research (DiCenso, 2001).

The question of applicability of the study to one's own clinical practice context relies on the experience and expertise of the clinician. Issues to consider include the generalisability of the study results to wider populations per se and to one's own patient group specifically. Specifically, the question that needs to be answered is 'Are my patients so different from those in the study that the results don't apply?' (Ciliska, Cullum & Marks, 2001).

INTEGRATION INTO CLINICAL PRACTICE

The process of asking clinical questions, finding and critically evaluating the evidence may result in the need to change some aspect of your clinical practice. If you are self-employed within your own private practice, then changing how you practice may not be so difficult. However, most nurses work within a multidisciplinary and often still hierarchical team structure. Changing one's own clinical practice without impacting on other members of the team is often not possible and therefore one is faced with tackling the time-honoured and valued practice traditions of other individuals or professions. As found by a team of UK researchers involved in a project to increase the use of research by hospital ward nurses, 'to some degree all nurses were resistant to change, but the topics about which they were resistant varied' (Newman, Papadopoulos & Melifonwu, 2000, p. 104).

A considerable volume of literature has been written about effecting organisational change within healthcare, a detailed consideration of which lies outside the scope of this chapter. It is worth noting that in a systematic review of 102 trials of interventions to improve professional practice, the authors concluded that 'there are no magic bullets', meaning no single activity or intervention clearly improves practice in healthcare (Oxman, Thomson, Davis & Haynes, 1995). While some interventions such as audit and feedback have tended to be inconsistent in efficacy across studies (Oxman et al., 1995; Thomson, 1998), those strategies that have been shown to be consistently effective include education outreach visits (one-on-one), reminders (prompts to professional practice), interactive educational meetings and multifaceted approaches (Thomson, 1998). Nonetheless, structural and organisational factors have been found to be major determinants of the successful implementation of change (Newman et al., 2000).

Evaluation and reflection

The fifth step in EBP is one of self-reflection and the evaluation of one's own performance in carrying out steps one to four (Sackett et al., 2000). It is a means of assessing the efficacy and effectiveness of personal EBP techniques. For example, it involves asking rhetorical questions such as 'Am I asking well formulated questions?', 'Are my searching strategies yielding appropriate results?', 'Are my critical appraisal skills improving?', and 'Am I successful in integrating the evidence into my practice?' (Sackett et al., 2000). However, perhaps even more fundamental questions to ask are 'Am I willing to accept that what I believe to be the "right" way of doing something may not be based on any evidence?', and moreover, 'Am I willing to change my perceptions of what is "best" practice if there is good evidence to do otherwise?'.

In addition to self-assessment, this step is also about evaluating the effect of any change in practice on patient outcomes, through an audit process (Dawes, 1999; Sackett et al., 2000). Nursing has enthusiastically embraced quality assurance and clinical audit, and now needs to extend these skills to the consideration of the processes and outcomes of care within a context of EBN. For example, based on the recommendations made in the respective JBIEBNM systematic reviews, 'has there been any change in the incidence of patient falls since our change in practices?' (Evans, Hodgkinson, Lambert, Wood & Kowanko, 1998) or 'are our patients on the oncology ward experiencing reduced problems with oral mucositis following recommended changes in practice?' (Kowanko, Long, Hodgkinson & Evans, 1998).

CONSIDERATION OF QUALITATIVE RESEARCH

Some nursing academics and practitioners have expressed concern that EBN devalues the qualitative approach to research and the holistic values that nurses aspire to in patient care (Closs & Cheater, 1999; McDonald & Smith, 2001), by placing emphasis on the randomised clinical trial (RCT). In referring to the definition of evidence-based medicine (EBM) previously cited (Sackett et al., 1999), it is worth noting that the term 'judicious use' refers to combining the evidence obtained through research and review with the contextual aspects of environment, resources, practitioner experience and patient desires, prior to implementation.

It is widely acknowledged that the RCT offers the best approach to testing the efficacy of a therapeutic intervention. However, to undertake an RCT, a clearly defined problem statement and research question must first be developed, and these are often drawn from preliminary research or previous findings. The basis of this work is often qualitative in nature and thus forms an important phase in research development. Nursing also has a clear interest in the contextual elements of healthcare, such as how a patient feels about an issue or the resourcing and processes associated with a procedure. Qualitative research approaches may better describe these issues and can co-exist and complement quantitative research (see section on 'Triangulation' on pages 31–34 of Chapter 2 for further discussion). The opposing schools of research thought are in fact an artificial divide, and often of little interest for the clinical nurse.

The value of any particular approach to research and subsequent evidence for practice lies in the question to be answered. If the issue is about experiences, feelings or attitudes, then qualitative research approaches will offer fertile ground for informing practice (Ploeg, 1999). When the clinical nurse seeks to determine which intervention is of greatest value in dealing with a particular problem, such as the most efficacious nursing interventions to prevent pressure areas, then quantitative research will be the most appropriate approach. If the nurse wishes to have a better understanding of why patients choose not to comply with treatment regimes, then qualitative research methods offer the most likelihood of providing the answer. Irrespective of the research approach used, it is important that the study has been conducted according to the standards set for that methodology, since its utility in answering the clinical question is dependent on the quality and rigour of the research (Giacomini & Cook, 2000).

FUTURE DEVELOPMENTS IN EVIDENCE-BASED NURSING

It appears clear that EBP will continue as a major driver of clinical practice development across all health disciplines for the foreseeable future. The ongoing commitment of resources by health departments and the development of major international organisations guarantees its existence. This section examines the major issues for the evolution of EBN in the future: at the clinical practice level; as a focus of nursing scholarship; and as a stimulus for clinical research.

EBN at the practice level

The original impetus for EBN came from a recognition of the importance of providing clinically effective nursing care and advice to our patients. Hence it is appropriate that EBN continues to be promoted within the clinical setting, be that in the community, clinic or hospital. However, the time required to sort through the vast amounts of information and resources available remains a limiting factor in the ability of clinical nurses to apply evidence-based principles to their clinical practice.

Organisations can assist in the practice of EBN by providing access to the resources needed to develop this approach. This is a clear imperative under any model of clinical governance. Therefore, access to the internet and search facilities is essential for all clinical nurses to practice EBN. There is little value in having access to expensive equipment and various search facilities to EBN reviews if they are only accessible in the hospital library or nurse educator's computer terminal at the community nursing base centre. To complement the available IT (information technology) facilities and resources, associated education and training for clinical nurses should include the search software as well as critical appraisal skills. As well, access to well prepared EBN reviews can substantially assist in providing easily useable information. This can be achieved by health services becoming members of organisations such as the JBIEBNM (described previously in this chapter).

Nurses need to understand the principles and steps of EBN so that they are able to seek out and critically appraise the 'evidence' to their own clinical questions. In addition, senior clinical and academic nurses need to promote the EBN process, rather than resort to routine and ritual when recommending care practices for patients on an individual or group basis.

Finally, it needs to be accepted that a lack of evidence to answer a question does not infer that an intervention is necessarily inappropriate. Moreover, there is a well worn adage that 'the absence of evidence is not evidence of absence'. Nursing, similar to most other healthcare professions, still lacks definitive research studies in many areas of practice, and thus we are required to resort to 'expert opinion' in many instances to guide nursing practice. However, where situations arise that reveal gaps in evidence to support practice, then clinical nurses should collaborate with researchers, educators, specialists and managers to highlight this as a research priority for a primary research study.

EBN and nursing scholarship

Both undergraduate and postgraduate clinical programs in nursing are ideal avenues to introduce the evidence-based approach to nurses (Wallace et al., 1999). The facilities that are essential to conducting EBN are basic to most university nursing schools, where access to the library and internet resources is well established in most academic programs. With these resources available, the option of producing evidence-based reviews and guidelines should assume the same level of recognition within honours and graduate programs as the traditional research thesis or academic project. In essence, the systematic review consists of a number of key elements that are regarded as essential for postgraduate projects, including academic writing, literature review and critique, and synthesis with clinical problem solving and interpretation to professional practice. Thus, university postgraduate courses provide an ideal forum for the development of evidence-based systematic reviews (SRs).

EBN as motivation for clinical research

As already acknowledged earlier, there is a dearth of nursing research that supports clinical practice, and so many clinical questions developed and subject to the EBN process will reveal either low levels of evidence, or no research support at all (Closs & Cheater, 1999). This situation has the chance of disenfranchising individuals from using this approach. However, these apparent dead ends in fact provide a rich resource for clinically derived research questions. If nurses are informed at an undergraduate level of the research process and academic nursing schools develop strong links at the practice level, then EBN has the opportunity to inform and prioritise future primary research. In this way, repetitious studies that add little to the nursing body of knowledge can be minimised, and areas where nurses require guidance and support in providing care to patients can be identified. This can include informing the academic approach and design of the primary study.

EBN, like so much in nursing, requires a team approach. Busy clinicians cannot be expected to design, carry out and analyse clinical studies every time that information is not found in respect to each clinical problem they encounter. It is even impractical to expect them to conduct lengthy literature reviews and searches when planning patient care. However, they must become consumers of healthcare information, using the evidence in a way that best suits their patients' individual needs and circumstances. An EBN team should include an expert resource in information access, an organisational group to incorporate reviews and guidelines into agency procedures and policies, educators to teach and promote the process of EBN, and researchers to take up the challenge where evidence is lacking. The team requires the tools of the information age—the computer, technical support, appropriate software and network facilities.

EBN practice provides an impetus for clinicians to look to clinical nursing research as a possible source of evidence on which to base their practice. For many, EBN has demonstrated a practical utility of clinical nursing research that was previously not evident.

To conclude, EBN is a powerful tool for clinicians to ensure that patients receive care that has demonstrated efficacy and that should deliver the best possible outcomes based on the best available evidence at the time. It is a dynamic process that provides direction to the development of clinical practice. Over time, EBN recommendations will change as new findings come to light. As has been stated, it is more than the application of research findings to clinical practice. When applied effectively and as defined by the proponents of EBN, the evidence must be contextualised by the nurse in negotiation with the individual patient, taking into account factors such as cultural and religious beliefs, relevant patient preferences, and economic and environmental issues. Chapter 7 provides an example of how research evidence changed clinical practice at an organisational level.

KEY POINTS

- EBN is about applying the most efficacious nursing interventions to address a particular patient problem/issue where it is congruent with the patient's personal preferences/values. The nurse's clinical expertise tells her that it is appropriate to do so within the specific clinical context.
- The five key steps in the evidence-based approach are: translating a clinical query into an answerable question; locating the evidence; critically appraising the evidence; applying the findings to clinical practice; and evaluating the efficacy of the process and clinical outcomes.
- Critical appraisal of the literature is a skill that will improve with practice.
- Questions relating to therapeutic efficacy are most reliably answered by RCTs and systematic reviews of RCTs, however, other 'types' of questions will afford greater prominence to other research designs.
- Systematic reviews will sometimes identify a lack of evidence relating to a particular nursing practice that in turn can serve as a stimulus and rationale for clinical nursing research.
- When a review of information about a subject reveals inadequate information to manage a patient problem, then 'usual' practice may be the best approach until more substantive evidence can be sourced or developed.

CRITICAL THINKING CHALLENGES

- Discuss the claim that there is a difference between research utilisation and EBP in nursing.
- What is the value of EBN for the patient, for the individual nurse, and for the discipline of nursing?
- A colleague suggests that to practise EBN just requires finding a few relevant journal articles to list at the end of each procedure in the ward procedure manual. What would be your response?
- A senior member of staff that you are working with is dismissive of EBN, claiming that it is just a passing fad. She claims that she has been nursing for 20 years and that she knows what works and what doesn't. Think about the strengths and limitations of basing clinical nursing practice on personal experience alone.
- Consider what strategies you might use within your own work environment to implement a change in one aspect of clinical practice. Conversely, think about what strategies might influence you to change your own practice.
- Identify one nursing practice from your own clinical experience where you are uncertain of the evidence that underpins it.

Additional resources

Billhult, A. & Dahlberg, K. (2001). A meaningful relief from suffering: experiences of massage in cancer care. *Cancer Nursing*, 24(3), 180–84.

Bondy, K., Jenkins, K., Seymour, L., Lancaster, B. & Ishee, J. (1997). The development and testing of a competency-focused psychiatric nursing clinical evaluation instrument. *Archive Psychiatric Nursing*, 11(2), 66–73.

Braunwald, E., Fauci, A.S., Isselbacher, K.J., Kasper, D.L., Hauser, S.I., Longo, D.L. & Jameson, J.L. eds. (2001). *Harrison's principles of internal medicine* (15th ed.). Colombus, McGraw Hill.

Caramanica, L., Maljanian, R., McDonald, D., Taylor, S., Kelly, A.S., McRae, J. & Beland, D. (2002). Evidence-based nursing practice, part 1: a hospital and university collaborative. *Journal of Nursing Administration*, 32(1), 27–30.

Centres for Health Evidence. (2002). Users' guides to evidence based practice. http://www.cche.net/usersguides

Dawson, S. (1997). Inhabiting different worlds: how can research relate to practice? *Quality in Health Care*, 6, 177–78.

Denwood, R. (1996). Data capture for quality management nursing opportunity. *Computers in Nursing*, 14(1), 39–44.

French, P. (2002). What is the evidence on evidence-based nursing? An epistemological concern. *Journal of Advanced Nursing*, 37, 250–57.

Greenhill, J. & Henderson, M. (1997). Report on the patient satisfaction survey: models of managing nursing care project. Unpublished work. Nursing Research Unit, Princess Alexandra Hospital, Brisbane, Queensland.

Guyatt, G.H. & Rennie, D. (1993). Users' guides to the medical literature [editorial]. *Journal of the American Medical Association*, 270(17), 2096–97.

Guyatt, G.H., Sackett, D.L. & Cook, D.J. (1993). Users' guides to the medical literature. II. How to use an article about therapy or prevention. A. Are the results of the study valid? Evidence-Based Medicine Working Group. *Journal of the American Medical Association*, 270(21), 2598–2601.

Guyatt, G. H., Sackett, D. L. & Cook, D. J. (1994). Users' guides to the medical literature. II. How to use an article about therapy or prevention. B. What were the results and will they help me in caring for my patients? Evidence-Based Medicine Working Group. *Journal of the American Medical Association*, 271(1), 59–63.

Huda, A. & Wise, L. (1998). Evolution of compliance within a fall prevention program. *Journal of Nursing Care Quality*, 12(3), 55–63.

Jaeschke, R., Guyatt, G. & Sackett, D.L. (1994). Users' guides to the medical literature. III. How to use an article about a diagnostic test. A. Are the results of the study valid? Evidence-Based Medicine Working Group. *Journal of the American Medical Association*, 271(5), 389–91.

Jaeschke, R., Guyatt, G.H. & Sackett, D.L. (1994). Users' guides to the medical literature. III. How to use an article about a diagnostic test. B. What are the results and will they help me in caring for my patients? The Evidence-Based Medicine Working Group. *Journal of the American Medical Association*, 271(9), 703–07.

Johnson, M. & Griffiths, R. (2001). Developing evidence-based clinicians. *International Journal of Nursing Practice*, 7, 109–18.

Ketefian, S., Redman, R., Nash, M.G. & Bogue, E.L. (1997). Inpatient and ambulatory patient satisfaction with nursing care. *Quality Management in Health Care*, 5(4), 66–75.

Kitson, A. (2001). Approaches used to implement research findings into nursing practice: report of a study tour to Australia and New Zealand. *International Journal of Nursing Practice*, 7(6), 392–405.

Laupacis, A., Wells, G., Richardson, W.S. & Tugwell, P. (1994). Users' guides to the medical literature. V. How to use an article about prognosis. Evidence-Based Medicine Working Group. *Journal of the American Medical Association*, 272(3), 234–37.

Lee, F-K., Chang, A.M. & Mackenzie, A.E. (2002). A pilot project to evaluate implementation of clinical guidelines. *Journal of Nursing Care Quality*, 16(2), 50–59.

Levine, M., Walter, S., Lee, H., Haines, T., Holbrook, A. & Moyer, V. (1994). Users' guides to the medical literature. IV. How to use an article about harm. *Journal of the American Medical Association*, 271(20), 1615–19.

Luther, K.M. (1996). Data-driven interventions to improve patient satisfaction. *Journal of Nursing Care Quality*, 10(4), 33–39.

Maljanian, R., Caramanica, L., Taylor, S., Kelly, A.S., McRae, J.B. & Beland, D. (2002). Evidence-based nursing practice, part 2: building skills through research roundtables. *Journal of Nursing Administration*, 32(2), 85–90.

Margarey, J. (2001). Elements of a systematic review. *International Journal of Nursing Practice*, 7(6), 376–82.

McKenna, H., Cutcliffe, J. & McKenna, P. (2000). Evidence-based practice: demolishing some myths. *Nursing Standard*, 14, 39–42.

Mitchell, A., Cummins, T., Spearing, N., Adams, J. & Gilroy, L. (2002). Nurses' experience with vancomycin resistant enterococci (VRE). *Journal of Clinical Nursing*, 11(1), 126–33.

Pearson, A. & Peels, S. (2001). A global view of nursing in the new millennium – 6: aspirations of nurses. *International Journal of Nursing Practice*, 7(6), S27–S30.

Thompson, C., McCaughan, D., Cullum, N., Sheldon, T., Mulhall, A. & Thompson, D. (2001). Research information in nurses' clinical decision-making: what is useful. *Journal of Advanced Nursing*, 36(3), 376–88.

Tronni, C. & Welebob, E. (1996). End-user satisfaction of a patient education tool: manual versus computer-generated tool. *Computers in Nursing*, 14(4), 235–38.

Watts, T., Jones, M., Wainwright, P. & Williams, A. (2001). Methodologies analysing individual practice in health care: a systematic review. *Journal of Advanced Nursing*, 35(2), 238–56.

7
CHAPTER

Implementing research into practice

Sanchia Aranda and Annabel Pollard

LEARNING OUTCOMES

After reading this chapter the student should be able to:

- Discuss three key factors influencing the implementation of research evidence in the clinical setting.
- Plan a project to implement an evidence-based practice change in their clinical setting.

Key terms

evidence-based practice

research utilisation

research-based practice

evidence-based guidelines

practice change

INTRODUCTION

As today's healthcare environment continues to undergo dramatic change, there is increasing emphasis on evidence-based practice (EBP). Improving healthcare outcomes requires a sustained effort to ensure that the findings of high quality research influence the daily practice of health professionals. Nurses can no longer rely on clinical experience, disease knowledge and expert opinion (Rosswurm & Larrabee, 1999) but must build their practice on an integration of best available evidence with clinical expertise (see Chapter 6 for further discussion of EBP). However, the important step of transferring research findings into practice has, until recently, received little attention in either nursing education or clinical practice.

Early efforts to understand the difficulties associated with implementing research findings into practice concentrated on identification of barriers. Four major categories of barrier were identified in recent Australian research: accessibility of research findings; anticipated outcomes of using research; organisational support to use research; and support from others to use research (Retsas, 2000).

While understanding the barriers to research use is critical in attempting to implement research in practice, factors that promote the use of research are now receiving attention (Kitson, Harvey & McCormack, 1998). Also important is consideration of how systematic (French, 1999) and organisational approaches (Gennaro, Hodnett & Kearney, 2001) can enhance nurses' use of evidence in practice. Building on these pro-active approaches this chapter aims to provide a framework for research implementation in the practice setting. The chapter draws on a local project to develop an evidence-based approach to the prevention of oral mucositis in people with cancer. The chapter first considers some of the key factors influencing practice change, and then moves to outline a ten-step process for change developed from existing literature and our experience with the mucositis project.

KEY FACTORS TO CONSIDER WHEN IMPLEMENTING EVIDENCE IN PRACTICE

Implementing evidence into the clinical setting requires health practitioners to systematically interconnect empirical knowledge with the tacit knowledge derived from practice experience (French, 1999). This is a deceptively complex and difficult task. Practitioners developing an evidence-based approach to health care delivery require a number of skills, including:

- An understanding of the concepts of effectiveness, safety and acceptability to ensure that the intervention being assessed achieves the desired patient outcomes.
- The ability to access and assess the quality and generalisability of the evidence presented. This includes access to resources such as databases and journals and the capacity to read and interpret published research.
- The ability to assess the applicability of the findings to the local population. Published research will have been undertaken in populations with varying degrees of similarity to the local population of interest. Assessing local applicability will help determine if the population and context are similar enough for immediate use or if further primary research in the target population is required.
- The capacity to effect practice change.

However, these skills alone do not ensure research findings will be adopted. A broader understanding of factors influencing practice change, beyond characteristics of the individual nurse, needs to be addressed. Kitson, Harvey and McCormack (1998) argue that practice change requires consideration of three key factors: evidence, context and facilitation. Sackett et al. (1996) define evidence as a combination of research, clinical expertise and patient choice, and thus each clinical decision relating to a patient intervention will reflect varying levels of influence in each of these areas. For example, there may be little primary research evidence to guide a clinical decision, and therefore clinicians predominantly use their clinical experience and feedback from past patients in determining how to care for the patient. Similarly, an intervention can be well supported by evidence as contributing to a particular patient outcome, but if it is unacceptable to the patient then it is unlikely to be adopted.

Context refers to the 'environment or setting in which the proposed change is to be implemented' (Kitson, Harvey & McCormack, 1998, p. 151) and consists of three components: culture, leadership and measurement. The culture of the organisation can be more or less patient-centred and can have varying approaches to involving staff in change processes, offering continuing education or valuing staff that challenge current approaches. Similarly, organisations will be more or less open to innovation (Rogers, 1993). Organisations with a questioning, learning culture and a commitment to staff empowerment are more likely to support evidence-based practice. The ideal environment for practice change is one where there are clear roles and responsibilities, effective teams, an organisational structure that facilitates change, and leadership that encourages innovation. In terms of measurement, organisations will have varying levels of commitment to processes such as audit, peer review and benchmarking. Organisations where there is a commitment to data collection on patient outcomes, along with processes to make this available to staff, will be more able to support practice change.

Kitson, Harvey and McCormack's emphasis on facilitation recognises that in order to change people may need help to 'understand what they have to change and how they change it to achieve the desired outcome' (1998, p. 152). Facilitation also takes account of the reality that most practitioners have heavy workloads and may find it difficult to keep the clinical change agenda at the forefront of their work commitments. Successful facilitators of practice change are supportive of others, approachable, reliable and confident, and have the ability to think innovatively and to listen to the perspectives of others.

A PROCESS FOR IMPLEMENTING PRACTICE CHANGE: THE PETER MACCALLUM CANCER INSTITUTE MUCOSITIS PROJECT

The mucositis project was the first project using an organisational approach to systematically build nursing practice interventions on an evidence-based approach. An evidence-based nursing group was established and given the responsibility of initiating the first project and of testing this as a model of implementing research-based practice.

The following ten-step process was developed from the experience of the group and adapted from a six-step process developed by Rosswurm and Larrabee, (1999):

1. identify the need for change
2. make current tacit knowledge explicit
3. identify and involve key stakeholders
4. develop an answerable question
5. gather, appraise and synthesise the evidence
6. compare the evidence to current practice and determine what, if anything, needs to change
7. plan for the practice change
8. implement and evaluate the change
9. sustain the change
10. share findings and what was learnt.

Structured approaches such as this consider evidence-based practice change as a research activity—albeit one derived from existing primary research and overlapping with other quality improvement activities. Essential to the process is an acknowledgement that evidence-based practice change is a rigorous, systematic and purpose driven activity that requires a clear audit trail to enable evaluation and replication of the process.

Step 1 Identify the need for change

The starting point for any practice-change endeavour is the identification of an issue or clinical problem where there is either controversy about practice or lack of clarity in how to provide clinical care for the patient. The stimuli for change might include 'awareness of patient preferences and dissatisfaction, quality improvement data, practitioner queries, evaluation data, or new research data' (Rosswurm & Larrabee, 1999, p. 3). The stimulus may also be internal (e.g. two nurses disagree about the clinical care of the patient), or external (e.g. a patient may question why something is done differently from their experience with another health service). In organisations where there is a questioning culture and willingness to explore new ideas, clinical change issues will be readily evident. In less questioning organisations, querying the current practice is likely to be met with responses such as 'We've always done it like this' or 'We tried that and it doesn't work here'. Initially, nurses with little experience in questioning practice may find it difficult to identify issues amendable to an evidence-based project. It is also important to recognise that there is unlikely to be consensus about the need for change. Rogers (1993) describes significant differences between innovators and those driving or open to change (early adoptors), and those who tend to require group pressure to change (late adoptors), or those who cling to the past (laggards).

When the project began, focus groups were initially conducted to determine suitable clinical issues for the first project, but had little success. The project group therefore selected mucositis because it was a common problem encountered by the patient population and there were variations in practice throughout the organisation, no assessment tool was in use, confusion centred on prevention versus treatment of mucositis, and significant costs were associated with the provision of oral care solutions.

Step 2 Make current tacit knowledge explicit

The next step to be considered was to what extent current care was evidence based, and to make explicit the tacit knowledge practitioners were using to guide their clinical care. The aim was to identify staff understanding of the rationale for what they do and to acknowledge that practitioners' knowledge and experience is important and relevant to determining best practice (French, 1999). This step can also help to identify potential points of resistance to practice change and will assist with assessment of the relevance of available research. In many areas of practice, the only available knowledge is the practitioner's clinical experience. For example, in a practice-change process on constipation in palliative care, there was no available evidence to guide practice in intervention decision-making when the patient was close to death (Bailey & Gephart, 1999).

In the mucositis project, clinical nurses demonstrated a clear understanding of the importance of oral care in the cancer context and considerable understanding of the specific needs of people with cancer. However, few were able to provide specific evidence supporting the interventions used. A number of ritualistic practices were identified including avoidance of brushing when experiencing low platelet counts, use of the institutional mouthwash, and prophylactic use of anti-fungal agents to prevent oral candidiasis. In addition, there was a perception that nurses could not change oral care as it was a medically controlled procedure. This was despite the reality that new doctors were generally told what to prescribe by experienced nurses.

Step 3 Identify and involve key stakeholders

Stakeholders are individuals within the organisation with a specific interest in the practice of the organisation (e.g. nurses, doctors, allied health practitioners, managers and patients). Approaches to stakeholder involvement will vary and may range from ongoing consultation, through advisory group membership to project leadership. Increasingly there is a commitment in government policy to involving consumers in service planning and delivery (Draper, 1997). The consumer perspective helps to ensure that any planned change is acceptable to consumers and may provide motivation to change, such as when practitioner resistance is encountered during implementation. As top-down approaches to change are likely to encounter more resistance than 'near-peer' approaches (Rogers, 1993), early involvement of practitioners of the level most affected by the change can be important to success.

Non-nurse stakeholders in the mucositis project included staff representing the dental clinic, pharmacy, radiation oncology, medical oncology and dieticians. The identification and involvement of stakeholders was not ideal, occurring as issues arose, with only the dentist being involved early in the project. Initially the project was conceptualised as principally a nursing activity. It was only later when considering ways to implement the change that other stakeholder involvement became critical, and involving these individuals at this later stage slowed progress.

Earlier involvement would have enhanced the speed of the project and may have helped to overcome critical problems in adapting the change to specific patient groups, particularly those receiving radiotherapy to the head or neck. Experience suggests that almost all projects involving a change to patient-related practice are best developed at the outset as multidisciplinary to ensure the best outcomes. This project was managed by a team, including a project coordinator, two experienced clinical nurses, one of whom acted as the project worker, a nurse manager, a dentist, a radiation oncologist, a pharmacist and a nurse academic researcher.

Step 4 Develop an answerable question

A clear question is required to determine the project's scope, to guide literature searching and to ensure that the project is manageable. Rosswurm and Larrabee (1999) suggest defining the problem in ways that link it to a focus on patient outcomes or interventions. This means defining the kinds of interventions or outcomes that are the focus of the project and refining these to ensure that the appropriate literature is selected.

In the mucositis project, the group began looking at oral care generally but narrowed the scope of initial work to prevention and early detection of oral mucositis in patients undergoing cancer treatment. The question became 'What is best available evidence in the prevention of oral mucositis?'. In the literature review this allowed a clear separation between research dealing with complications associated with oral mucositis, such as treatment of oral candidiasis or management of pain. Thus the focus included oral assessment for early detection of lesions, maintenance of oral hygiene, and consideration of factors increasing the risk of oral mucositis in this population, such as pre-existing dental or oral disease, smoking and poor nutrition.

Step 5 Gather, appraise and synthesise the evidence

Gathering the appropriate literature is a critical step in any implementation process. If the implementation project utilises an existing systematic review, then the review activities in this step will function only to update the current information. This is the ideal situation and a comprehensive search of databases housing systematic reviews is an essential part of preparation for change. If a systematic review is not available, significant resources would be needed to conduct one for the project. Thus it may be necessary to undertake a pragmatic review that gathers appropriate information and appraises and synthesises it to the level that is possible within available resources. If a systematic review is not used to guide the development of the practice change, this should be acknowledged as a limitation of the outcome and approaches should be made to organisations that conduct systematic reviews to initiate one on the topic.

In the mucositis project a pragmatic literature review was initially conducted, but during the course of the project a systematic review of mucositis management was published (Kowanko, Long, Hodgkinson & Evans, 1998) that reinforced both the need for practice change and the conclusions that the project team had drawn from their pragmatic review.

Despite the availability of a systematic review it is important that project team members appraise and assist to synthesise the literature (see Chapter 4). Appraisal of the evidence involves both an assessment of the quality of the research and an evaluation of its applicability to the current clinical problem, context and patient population. Stetler (1994) offers a useful model for assessing research applicability (see Box 7.1).

Project group appraisal and synthesis of the evidence assists in challenging pre-held assumptions about the rationale for current practice and increases facilitators' confidence when persuading others of the need for change. Involvement of project group members in critical appraisal of the literature can also enhance skill development if there is relative inexperience in this area.

BOX 7.1 Refinement of the 'Stetler/Marram tool for evaluation of applicability of research findings'

Phase I: preparation (purpose and context of research utilisation)

A What initiated review of this article/topic?

1 ______ general interest
2 ______ a problem
3 ______ task assignment
4 ______ knowledge update
5 ______ other

B If relevant, what is the desired *outcome* of this or multiple-related reviews? In particular, for option 2, how will you evaluate if the problem is 'solved' or, for option 3, if the task has been effectively completed?

C What intervening factors, if any (environmental/personal characteristics), might influence your decision-making?

______ tight deadline
______ need for consultation in the topical area
______ committee approval
______ other

Phase II: validation (scientific soundness and potential for application)

A What are the methodological strengths of this study?

B What are the major methodological weaknesses and the limitations of this study relative to acceptability for potential application?

C Given A and B above, rate scientific soundness in terms of the degree to which the findings are acceptable for *potential* application in practice:

Non-acceptable/low degree   High degree

______ ______ ______ ______ ______ ______

Applicable statement of findings

In your own words, write a brief statement specifying the findings of the study: use operational definitions; state results in day-to-day terms; indicate qualifiers and limiting conditions of application.

Phase III: comparative evaluation (criteria of applicability)

A Fit of setting:

1 How similar are the characteristics of the sample to those of the population with which you work?
STUDY SAMPLE =
YOUR CLIENTS =
Level of similarity: ______ acceptable ______ unacceptable

2 How similar is the study's environment to the one in which you work?
STUDY SETTING =
YOUR SETTING =
Level of similarity: ______ acceptable ______ unacceptable

B Current practice:
1 Do you have a theoretical/scientific basis for your current practice behaviour? ______ No ______ Yes (Describe)
Is it congruent with the basis for this study? ______ No ______ Yes
2 How *effective* is your current method of practice in this area?
Not at all effective _____ _____ _____ _____ _____ Highly effective
How do you know? What are your source/s of evaluative data?
Or: ______ don't know
Do you need evaluative data before proceeding?

C Feasibility (risk, resource and readiness):
1 What degree of potential risk could be associated with implementation of these findings? (Consider patients and staff)
No risk ______ ______ ______ ______ ______ High risk
2 Readiness:
a What level/s of the organisation would need to be involved in this change in practice? Check all that apply.
______ only you as an individual practitioner
______ other nurses on a single unit
______ inter-disciplinary healthcare team
______ collaborative management team
______ nurse managers
______ upper nursing administration
______ private attendings
______ other departments
______ others
b Given the level/s involved, what is the degree of readiness of each for such a change in practice?
Not at all ready _____ _____ _____ _____ _____ Highly ready
(Specify level ______)
Not at all ready ______ _____ _____ _____ _____ Highly ready
(Specify level ______)
Not at all ready ______ _____ _____ _____ _____ Highly ready
(Specify level ______)
Not at all ready ______ _____ _____ _____ _____ Highly ready
(Specify level ______)
3 What amount of resources would be needed to implement such a change?
No resources ______ ______ ______ ______ ______ Great resources
4 What is the risk/benefit ratio involved?

D Substantiating evidence (Is there an integrated review; should there be one?):
1 What other research has been conducted that examined a similar question/hypothesis?
2 Were the findings the same, similar or conflicting? (Specify)
3 What other non-research information/knowledge is available regarding this topic?
4 Overall, to what degree are the findings substantiated?
Low degree ______ ______ ______ ______ ______ High degree

Phase IV: decision-making (use or non-use; nature of use)

A Given all of the above factors, do you believe these research findings are:
____ Not applicable at this time (Reject)
____ May be used in the future in light of additional, scientific information (Delay)
____ Can be considered for use in light of additional, practical information (see B, below)
____ Can be used *now* to validate, discontinue or change practice (see C, below)

B Consider use: [Then return to start of Phase IV: decision-making]
1 How can such practical information be obtained?
______ through day-to-day observation
______ through routine evaluation
______ through discussion/input of others
______ through an action test or other formal pilot/evaluation of the innovation
______ other
2 Who would be involved?
______ self
______ peers/other professionals
______ committee/task force
______ experts/consultant
______ other

C Use now: [Then go to Phase V below]
1 What type(s) of use?
______ cognitive
______ instrumental
______ symbolic
2 What method?
______ informal
______ formal
3 What level?
______ by an individual
______ by a group
______ by an organisation
4 Potentially, how to use?
______ for validation
______ for discontinuation
______ modification/change

Phase V: translation/application (synthesis and specification)

A Organise and synthesise the separate findings and state results in terms of meaningful concepts and generalisation(s) about the identified issue/area.

B In practical terms, specify exactly how you will use these findings:
______ as orientation/background/reference information
______ as part of a set of principles or guiding framework
______ as part of routine nursing process or practice [specify]
______ for a policy/standard/critical path/etc. [specify]

______ for persuasive purposes [describe]
______ for identification of QM indicators
______ for routine measurement
______ others [describe]

C List any caveats/qualifiers/special circumstances of the above use.

D Have you 'applied' too far beyond the knowledge base?
______ No ______ Yes/Maybe [re-review or recognise that the application is *not* research-based]

E Will 'planned change' be required? If yes, proceed to related project management planning/dissemination/etc. Refer back to readiness assessment.

Phase VI: evaluation (results of utilisation)

A Reaffirm/state the outcomes you expected/needed to achieve; make sure they are measurable [refer back to Phase I].

B Given the type/method/level/nature of application, indicate exactly the how, what, who, where and when of evaluation.

Stetler, C. (1989). A strategy for teaching research utilisation. *Nursing Education*, 13, 17–20; modified by Stetler C. et al. (1995). Enhancing research utilisation by clinical specialists. *Nursing Clinics of North America*, 30(3), 457–73.

Practice in the prevention of mucositis at the institution was believed by many to be based on best available evidence (this evidence being a study of 36 patients undertaken more than 15 years ago). The study was influential because it was one of the first of its type and provided a safety net to practice that supported the rituals of not brushing teeth when platelet counts were low and appeared appropriate in advocating an anti-bacterial rinse solution. However, the systematic review highlighted more recent randomised controlled trials that disputed the findings of this early study. Project group members were often surprised by the extent to which their previous beliefs about best practice in mucositis prevention were challenged by the evidence. In addition, persuasion of others about the merits of change was greatly assisted by being able to refer to quality research findings in an articulate and authoritative way.

Step 6 Compare the evidence to current practice and determine what, if anything, needs to change

In step 1 the need for change was identified, however it is only at step 6 that the need for and extent of change can actually be determined. The question, 'To what extent does current practice concur with the evidence?' can help to guide this assessment. During this step, the care activities requiring change are described, usually as a practice guideline, a clinical protocol or a standard of care (Rosswurm & Larrabee, 1999) and clear recommendations for change are developed. The focus of the practice change should be aspects of clinical care covered by the evidence base assessed, and should ideally include the level of evidence for each aspect of care (see Chapter 6 for a further discussion of levels of evidence). Where no evidence is identified and clinical care is based on expert opinion, this should also be clearly indicated. Where evidence is absent, step 6 may involve identification of primary research questions aimed at providing the level of evidence needed to enhance practice. The complexity of the change should also be assessed at this point. Essentially, the more complex the change (i.e. difficult to understand or use or where new skills are needed), the more likely implementation will be difficult (Rogers, 1993).

The mucositis project identified that a significant issue in the approach to oral care was the lack of emphasis on good oral hygiene, a factor greatly contributing to the risk for developing oral mucositis. The previous approach centred on providing the patient with mouthwash solutions, and in some cases encouraging them to undertake a less rigorous oral hygiene regimen by removing tooth brushing and flossing from their daily oral care. The systematic review provided a high level of evidence for the aspects of clinical care identified for change. While the complexity of required change was not high, there was a context of highly routinised and ritualistic practice, which was likely to increase resistance to change. Change centred on the development of organisationally endorsed best practice guidelines in the prevention and early detection of oral mucositis, including:

- Introduction of an oral assessment tool to document oral status.
- Pre-treatment risk assessment to identify patients requiring early referral to the dental oncology department—including allowance for nurse initiated referral.
- Development of a self-care brochure for patients that emphasised a good oral hygiene approach to mucositis prevention.
- Cessation of practices using prescribed agents in the prevention of oral complications, except in situations where these are clinically indicated.

The project also identified a paucity of knowledge available to guide the management of oral complications and reinforced the chosen scope of the project to prevention alone. Best practice guidelines in the management of oral complications were identified as a future need for the organisation.

Step 7 Plan for the practice change

Planning for change is a critical step in the implementation process. This step should include discussion with all key stakeholders to help identify potential points of resistance to the change and to identify facilitators that may assist with implementation. Organisational requirements also need consideration, such as approvals from practice committees, documentation change requirements and funding requirements. The plan should include development of resource materials required for the change and processes for staff skill development, if required. A pilot study to test the implementation process can be a key strategy for success and should include piloting the evaluation framework, evaluation endpoints such as quality improvement instruments or surveys, and any changed documentation or educational resources before finalisation. The pilot may also indicate significant problems with implementation that may require further testing before implementation or a decision not to go ahead with the change at this point.

At this step in the mucositis project one member of the project team underwent extensive training in clinical assessment with the dental oncology service to ensure her ability to educate the nursing staff on oral assessment. Relevant committees approved the protocol as well as the developed documents, namely a patient self-care brochure and an oral assessment tool. In addition, the group planned a staged implementation across all wards and clinical departments of the hospital, spent considerable time informing relevant department heads of the change, and ensured that the organisation was ready for the change. The change was initially tested in one clinical area before a wider scale implementation commenced. In fact, selection of an appropriate pilot site was critical to the ongoing success of this project, as initial success instilled confidence in the project as a whole and facilitated problem solving at an early stage. In this project the pilot identified that practice change was acceptable to both patients and staff and the change implementation strategy was feasible.

Negotiating exceptions to the protocol was necessary to obtain buy-in from medical staff; for example, patients designated at high risk of developing oral mucositis continued to receive prophylactic treatment, but this was in addition to and not a substitute for attention to good oral hygiene.

Step 8 Implement and evaluate the change

Implementation consists of organisation-wide adoption of the practice change. This process requires full endorsement of key people in the organisation to ensure that staff members are aware of expectations to change. However, motivation to change must focus on benefits for patients and their families, with staff aware of the clinical rationale for the change. Implementation should include appropriate staff orientation to the change and provision of any necessary education or skills training. A pre-determined implementation timeframe should be set, allowing sufficient training time and a period of implementation, followed by a formal evaluation. The evaluation might include questions such as:

- Did the implementation go as planned? What went well? What might have been improved? Unintended outcomes can be an important part of learning how to successfully implement practice change.
- What is the current level of compliance with the change? Is the new protocol being fully implemented, partially implemented or strongly resisted? A poorly implemented change may have unintended negative outcomes, making it critical to assess the extent to which an initiative was adapted in practice. What was the effect of the change on patient outcomes?
- What are patients' and their families' perceptions of the change?

Evaluation of the mucositis prevention protocol included an audit of whether patients received appropriate oral care information and education, review of referral patterns to the dental clinic, and use of oral care agents. Findings suggested that the broad approach to patient education (content and format of information) was acceptable to patients. However, information dissemination, ensuring all patients received access to self-care information, was not as successful. Reasons for this included:

- difficulties in getting nurses to routinely disseminate information
- overcoming nurses' perception that the change implied criticism of their current practice, and
- ensuring nurses reinforced patient compliance in a more active self-care role.

Usage of prophylactic oral care agents decreased across the organisation, resulting in substantial cost savings. Lastly, some of the more helpful critical discussion came from stakeholders who were most resistant to the proposed changes, but who were willing to listen to the evidence and adapt their practice.

Step 9 Sustain the change

An important issue in any practice change is ensuring the change is maintained in the long term. Many of the steps taken thus far, including stakeholder involvement, clinician participation and piloting, all help to increase sustainability, although sustained change is not guaranteed. Including ongoing evaluation of the change into routine quality improvement processes, presenting the changed practice into orientation for new staff, and providing feedback on the evaluation cycles to clinical staff, can all help sustain the change. Offering rewards to units demonstrating quality performance can also increase sustainability (Greco & Eisenberg, 1993).

Sustainability efforts in the mucositis project continue. Uptake of the practice change remains mixed, and continued efforts are required to reinforce the need for change and to assess ongoing compliance. Attitudes of staff were a core component of the resistance experienced during the implementation process. In hindsight the approach did not fully acknowledge the need for nurses to move to a more pro-active prevention/education role in order to promote patient self-care. Future projects would emphasise the importance of self-care in the context of decreased inpatient stays. Also, the approach required a greater near-peer focus. Including a staff member from each unit as part of the project team with responsibility and authority for education and implementation process would have ensured local facilitation of the change process but would have needed additional funding.

Step 10 Share findings and what was learnt

Implementing evidence into practice is a relatively new aspect of nursing research and there is minimal guidance for practice change efforts. It is therefore imperative that implementation efforts are shared with colleagues through local meetings, conference presentations and journal publications. If organisations are open to sharing intellectual efforts, it might also be appropriate to place practice guidelines and evaluation outcomes on websites, making them readily available for others to utilise.

SOME REFLECTIONS ON THE PROCESS

Implementing practice change in the prevention and early detection of oral mucositis was both a rewarding and frustrating experience. Initially the project was undertaken within current resources and there was considerable difficulty in maintaining the effort required for practice change. The work rate increased considerably when a small grant was obtained that allowed a half-time project officer to implement the project. Other key success factors for work included access to a supportive library service to minimise effort in tracking and obtaining relevant literature, and supportive management. In future, projects would begin with more emphasis on a multidisciplinary approach and on communicating with clinicians about progress. A greater emphasis on near-peer facilitation would avoid resistance from a perceived top-down demand for practice change.

KEY POINTS

- Before beginning a practice-change initiative, it is important to have an understanding of the organisation in terms of level of openness to change, the culture of learning, and the availability of data to assess patient outcomes.
- Do not expect to gain group consensus for the need to change practice. More success will occur by working with a small group committed to a thorough investigation of the issue and who exhibit a willingness to change.
- Practitioners are more likely to collaborate with practice change initiatives when their expertise is acknowledged and overt criticism of their current practice is avoided.
- Approach a practice-change initiative like any other research process. A structured approach and meticulous planning will help ensure success.
- Project success will be enhanced if funding is available to support project work. Projects undertaken in addition to clinical responsibilities will take longer and may lose momentum.
- Identify and involve stakeholders early. This can be facilitated by mapping out the likely progress of the full project and considering who will need to be consulted at each step.
- Practice change must be clearly justifiable and confined to those aspects of care where evidence indicates a need for change.
- Select a pilot site and patient group where opportunities for success are high (local staff expertise, local staff commitment).
- Disseminate information about the project and its progress through targeted consultation, open forums and ongoing discussion that encourage expressions of resistance, identification of problems and alternative ideas.
- Involvement of unit-based staff as near-peer facilitators of the change may reduce local resistance and overcome feelings of being overburdened by change demands.

CRITICAL THINKING CHALLENGES

- Do you agree or disagree with the following statement: 'The findings of nursing research are largely irrelevant in my daily practice'. Support your position with examples from current literature.
- Consider the statement: 'Our unit is open and accepting of practice change'. Support your position with examples of innovative, evidence-based practice changes that have taken place in your unit.

Acknowledgements
The authors wish to acknowledge the contribution to this work of the mucositis project group, in particular Kate Wells.

Additional resources

Bassett, C. (1992). The integration of research in the clinical setting: obstacles and solutions. A review of the literature. *Nursing Practice*, 6(1), 4–8.

Clifford, C. & Murray, S. (2001). Pre- and post-test evaluation of a project to facilitate research development in practice in a hospital setting. *Journal of Advanced Nursing*, 36, 685–95.

Closs, G.J. & Cheater, F.H. (1994). Utilization of nursing research: culture, interest and support. *Journal of Advanced Nursing*, 19(4), 762–73.

Dawson, S. (1997). Inhabiting different worlds: how can research relate to practice? *Quality in Health Care*, 6, 177–78.

Department of Human Services and Health Victoria Australia. (2002). *Victorian public hospital web sites.* Retrieved 2 February 2002 from http:/www.health.gov.au/hospitals/pubwebs.htm

Donabedian, A. (1981). Criteria, norms, and standards of quality: what do they mean? *American Journal of Public Health*, 71(4), 409–12.

Donaldson, L.J. & Gray, J.A.M. (1998). Clinical governance: a quality duty for health organisations. *Quality in Health Care*, 7, S344.

English, S. (1994). Nursing as a research-based profession: 22 years after Briggs. *British Journal of Nursing*, 3(8), 402–40.

Gift, A. (1994). Nursing research utilisation. *Clinical Nurse Specialist*, 8(6), 306.

Huda, A. & Wise, L. (1998). Evolution of compliance within a fall prevention program. *Journal of Nursing Care Quality*, 12(3), 55–63.

Johnston, G., Crombie, I.K., Alder, E.M., Davies, H.T.O. & Millard, A. (2000). Reviewing audit: barriers and facilitating factors for effective clinical audit. *Quality in Health Care*, 9, 23–36.

Kitson, A. (2001). Approaches used to implement research findings into nursing practice: report of a study tour to Australia and New Zealand. *International Journal of Nursing Practice*, 7, 392–405.

Lepper, H. & Titler, M.G. (1997). Program evaluation. In Mateo, M. & Kirchhoff, K., eds, *Conducting and using nursing research in the clinical setting.* (2nd ed.). Baltimore, Williams & Wilkins.

Moss, F., Garside, P. & Dawson, S. (1998). Organisational change: the key to quality improvement. *Quality in Health Care*, 7, S1–2.

Peter MaCallum Cancer Institute (2001). Retrieved 2 February 2002 from http://petermac.Server101.com/

Rutledge, D.N. & Donaldson, N.E. (1995). Building organisational capacity to engage in research utilisation. *Journal of Nursing Administration*, 25(10), 12–16.

Stenger, K. (1994). Putting research to good use. *American Journal of Nursing Supplement*, 30–38.

Stetler, C. (1989). A strategy for teaching research utilisation. *Nurse Education*, 13, 17–20.

Titler, M.G. (1997). Research utilisation: necessity or luxury? In McCloskey, J.C. & Grace, H., eds, *Current issues in nursing.* (5th ed.). St Louis, Mosby.

Watts, T., Jones, M., Wainwright, P. & Williams, A. (2001). Methodologies analysing individual practice in health care: a systematic review. *Journal of Advanced Nursing*, 35(2), 238–56.

8

CHAPTER

Developing a research proposal

Zevia Schneider

LEARNING OUTCOMES

After reading this chapter the student should be able to:

- Describe the structure and content of a research proposal.
- Identify the statement of the problem in research studies.
- Identify the significance of the problem in research studies.
- Identify the aims and objectives in research studies.
- Describe the difference between aims (purpose), and objectives.
- Discuss some of the differences between quantitative and qualitative research proposals in terms of format and style.
- Discuss the criteria and rationale for examining ethical issues.
- Discuss ethical considerations.

Key terms

aims
anonymity
budget
confidentiality
ethical and legal considerations
human rights
informed consent
institutional ethics committee (IEC)
intellectual property
operational definition
pilot study
research proposal
research questions
significance of the problem
theoretical or conceptual framework
timeframe

INTRODUCTION

If, as Sir Arthur Quiller-Couch (1954) argues, the primary aim of speech is to be understood, it follows that the more clearly you write the more easily you will be understood. For students hoping to gain approval of a higher degrees committee or institutional ethics committee for their proposal, the essence of success is in their writing and their ability to make a clear, cogent argument about the need for the research they are proposing. In few cases is clarity of thought and word more necessary than in writing a proposal.

WHAT IS A RESEARCH PROPOSAL?

A proposal is a plan or blueprint for an investigation of some kind. A research proposal then is a plan that details a reasoned, rigorous and systematic enquiry into some topic in order to justify the need for the study and to gain a clearer understanding of the area. The format of the proposal is influenced by the specific purpose of the research and by the audience for whom it is intended. However, no matter who the audience is, the proposal must demonstrate the following:

- the investigator is competent to undertake the research
- the topic is worthwhile, that is, the findings will be of benefit to society
- the design, method and timeframe are feasible and appropriate
- the risk–benefit for participants is acceptable
- participant privacy and safety are protected
- if the proposal is submitted for the purposes of a higher degree, assurance from the head of department that the student will have appropriate supervision and access to the required facilities.

A research proposal may be written for any of the following reasons:

- the purpose of gaining the approval of a higher degrees committee in an academic institution to undertake a research project
- an ethics committees (human subjects or animal experimentation) requesting permission to conduct research using human subjects or animals
- the purpose of gaining approval of a relevant committee to undertake an academic activity not related to a research higher degree, e.g. a minor thesis that may require a literature review, or a meta-analysis of the literature
- funding agencies requesting financial assistance
- a pilot study.

WRITING A PROPOSAL

Writing a proposal involves good writing skills, clarity, logic, and commitment to whatever purpose for which the proposal is written. Putting pen to paper and talking about the proposed study will frequently highlight any potential problems and alert the researcher to any limitations or weaknesses in the plan. Nurses considering higher degrees should bear in mind that they are not expected to write a proposal without any assistance. Providing skilled guidance for students writing proposals is part of an academic's teaching role, and thus includes issues about interpersonal relationships between student and academic (Phillips & Pugh, 1994). This guidance becomes more obvious when one considers that it is the responsibility of the academic to inform the student about the feasibility, appropriateness, and potential value of the research, availability of resources in the department/university, and availability and appropriateness of adequate supervision should the proposal lead to a higher degree by research.

While academic staff are there to assist students, there are some strategies that may be helpful when considering a project. It may be useful to write a draft of the significance of the project (this may be in a particular discipline in nursing, e.g. palliative care, neonatal intensive care, the clinical area, community health or IT [information technology] programs). This activity may form part of the application process for higher degree candidature.

The structure and content of a research proposal is basically the same, although there may be some variations between the kinds of proposal being written (e.g. thesis or grant), and the universities and funding agencies. A good research proposal is evidence of the investigator's written skills, how the problems are conceptualised, the understanding of the literature, research design, data collection and data analysis. Success in writing a research proposal may be seen as an indication of how thoroughly the researcher has understood the information relating to research (as in Chapters 9 to 23 of this book). Generally, the following structure and content are required:

- the title of the research project
- the investigators
- an abstract or summary
- a statement of the problem being investigated
- the significance or importance of the project
- a literature review
- assumptions and definitions
- the aims and objectives of the project
- the research plan
- ethical issues (including the participant information sheet and informed consent form)
- dissemination of the findings
- the budget (including justifications for items).

Each component of the research proposal will now be discussed in more detail.

The title of the research project

Keep the title shorter rather than longer. The title of the project should not be too long as this may result in confusion about the question or issue one wants to research. It should be concise and clear as to the purpose of your research. It must also be explicit and unambiguous and say what the research project is about. Initially, the use of a subtitle may be useful, e.g. 'Health outcomes of patients undergoing cardiac surgery: level of agreement between index and proxy respondents using the SF-36 and 15D health status instruments'. During the course of writing a proposal, some ideas may change and it may be necessary to change the title as well. Therefore, a working title is acceptable; it is imprudent to cling to a title slavishly when your thinking about the research dictates otherwise.

The investigators

As noted earlier, proposal reviewers need to assess the ability of the investigators to undertake the research. Therefore, proposals require some information about the research team (e.g. name, qualifications, employment position) as a minimum. In some instances (e.g. NHMRC grants) a short biography (research track record) and publications list are necessary for each chief investigator.

All authors on the research team should provide intellectual capital to the research project. Following some unfortunate episodes of 'honorary authorship' to persons in authority who provided no academic input to research and related publications, there are now guidelines on the issue of authorship, sponsorship and accountability, issued by, among others, the International Committee of Medical Journal Editors (ICMJE) (see, for example, the *New England Journal of Medicine* http://www.nejm.org) and the Australian Vice-Chancellors' Committee (http://www.avcc.edu.au) websites.

An abstract or summary

It is often useful to begin the introductory paragraph with the original question. In this way the topic or key sentence provides the focus and alerts the reader from the outset to the point of the proposal. Having explained what the proposal is about, the next point is to describe how to address the issue and answer the research question. In some cases, keywords or disciplinary field codes may be required.

The statement of the problem and justification for the project

This section of the proposal informs the reviewer about the nature of the problem. The statement, sometimes called 'the plain language statement' or 'lay person description', should provide the rationale and justification for undertaking the project. The clarity required for the plain language statement will be the same for proposals that use a quantitative or qualitative research approach. The research question should be stated and an indication given of the pragmatic value of the findings and the implications of the knowledge gained for the field (e.g. theory building).

The literature review

A careful literature review is undertaken to discover what is known about the topic under consideration; it provides an indication of the current knowledge about the topic. Reviewing the literature will help in conceptualising the research project (see the section called 'Purposes of a literature review' on pages 74–76 of Chapter 5). The aims in this section are to summarise the previous research and provide a cogent argument as to why the proposed research is important. Reasons should be based on an analysis of the shortcomings of the reviewed literature (e.g. appropriateness of design and/or tests administered, gaps in knowledge, conflicting or inconclusive findings, problems with the samples such as numbers, selection or profile). The literature review also substantiates the case for the project. It is usual to cite studies less than five years old unless they are seminal works or, if little research has been conducted in the area.

The aims and objectives of the project

Aims are usually broad and are a statement of purpose. Objectives should be specific and describe the activities employed to achieve the aim(s). Both aims and objectives should be feasible and achievable. The purpose of the project should be very clear, that is, why the project is important in itself and what the benefits might be. There should be no room for misunderstanding or misinterpretation. In writing the proposal, the investigator must be ever-mindful of the congruency between the aims and objectives and the plan of the project.

When considering the aims and objectives of the project, it is important to remember that these aims constitute the boundaries of the research. The aims guide the ways in which data are collected and analysed. For example, if the aim is to find out whether nurses think as clearly immediately after coming from a night's work as they do after a night's sleep, an objective might be to administer some kind of cognitive test which will yield results that can be measured. These issues are important because other nurses may want to replicate or repeat the design and test(s) to see whether they obtain the same results. If, on the other hand, your aim is to find out how women cope with breast cancer, the design will probably include a face-to-face interview at different times (e.g. at diagnosis, following surgery and three months after surgery).

In some quantitative studies the aim may be to find out if there is a relationship between certain variables, and how they may be related. For example, the aim may be to know if there is a relationship between a group of nurses who have completed Year 12 mathematics and a group of nurses who have not completed Year 12 mathematics, in their accuracy of drug calculation. The question could be asked another way: 'Are nurses who have completed Year 12 mathematics more accurate in their drug calculations than those nurses who have not completed Year 12 mathematics?'.

Assumptions and definitions

Assumptions and definitions should be clearly stated to avoid any ambiguity or confusion, and variables should be operationally defined where appropriate. For example, if the plan is to administer a self-care program to a group of patients, an assumption may be that most people want to learn how to care for themselves. Humans may be further defined in terms of health status, education, age and cultural background. A definition of self-care refers to the acceptance of responsibility by individuals for their care in those activities of daily living considered appropriate for their particular health status. There may well be other definitions of self-care. However, an important point is that having given a particular definition considered appropriate for the project, the researcher can then decide how best to measure the success of the program in terms of paradigm and design.

The research plan

This section specifically details the paradigm (research approach), design, proposed mode of study, and exactly what is intended and how it will occur. The plan includes the method, design, sampling and sample profile, intervention (if appropriate), measuring instruments, procedure, data gathering and data analysis techniques/strategies, projected timeframe for the stages of the project, an acknowledgment of the limitations or weaknesses and sources of bias, and finally, recommendations for further investigation if this proposal forms part of a larger program of study.

Notwithstanding the importance of the literature review, the design section is probably the most important part of the proposal. As with other sections of the proposal, it is important to present the design in detail; this section can be refined and shortened later if necessary. The design must be carefully explained in order to convince reviewers that the research approach and methods entailed in the proposal are the most logical and appropriate for this particular research project. Be prepared to write several drafts of the proposal prior to submission.

Chapters 9 to 16 are devoted to qualitative research approaches: grounded theory, phenomenology, historical research, ethnography, evaluation research, action research, critical social theory and feminist methods. Each research approach has its own philosophy and theoretical or conceptual framework, and strategies for data collection and analysis. It would be wise to be familiar with the different approaches before committing to a particular one. The main consideration must always be to find the research design that will best answer the research question(s). A major difference between quantitative and qualitative approaches is what each seeks or claims to do. Quantitative approaches aim to test theory, establish cause and effect (if ... then) relationships, and test hypotheses and/or theory in a purportedly objective, scientific, systematic and rigorous manner.

The qualitative research approaches are discussed in terms of their theoretical or conceptual frameworks, questionnaires, interview techniques, data collection strategies, their credibility, auditability, fittingness, sampling, sample profile, data analysis, an acknowledgment of the weaknesses or limitations of the study, and finally, recommendations for further investigation. This is not to suggest that qualitative research approaches are less disciplined than quantitative methods. Hypotheses may also be generated in qualitative approaches but in this case the hypotheses are more intuitive. Qualitative approaches use questions that are wide-ranging and generally focus on personal narratives and social interactions in groups, organisations and society.

Chapters 17 to 23 are devoted to quantitative research approaches. Appropriate articles included in the chapters illustrate how the investigators have matched their research designs to their research questions. These chapters should be carefully read and understood prior to writing a proposal. Whether a qualitative approach or quantitative design is chosen, bear in mind the feasibility of the project in terms of access to the sample(s), ethical issues and financial restraints. The various stages of the research proposal are discussed in this and other chapters; namely, theoretical and conceptual frameworks, hypotheses, sampling and sample profile, intervention (test(s), questionnaires, procedures, programs), data collection techniques, reliability and validity, internal validity and external validity, data analysis, and an acknowledgment of the limitations of the project and recommendations for further investigation.

Ethical and legal considerations

Ethical and legal issues are concerned with the protection of human and animal subjects in research. The regulations aim to ensure the absence, or minimisation, of harm, trauma, anxiety and discomfort to participants, be they human or animal. Researchers must take every precaution to protect people being studied from physical or mental harm or discomfort. It is not always clear what constitutes harm or discomfort. Nurses should be aware of their role in the research process, whether functioning as researcher, caregiver (including patient advocate) or research consumer.

Ethical and legal considerations in research: an historical perspective

Ethical and legal considerations in research first received attention after World War II, when it was learned that the trials for war criminals would focus on justifying the atrocities committed by Nazi physicians on concentration camp prisoners as 'medical research'. As a consequence, the American Medical Association was asked to develop a code of ethics for research. The ten rules included in what was called the Nuremberg Code appear in Box 8.1.

BOX 8.1 Articles of the Nuremberg Code

1. The experimental subject should be of legal age to voluntarily consent to participate in the experiment. The subject must be given all the details of the experiment (nature, purpose, consequences on health) in order that an informed decision to participate can be made in an environment in which there is freedom of choice.
2. The results of the experiment should be of benefit to society and not be achievable by means other than human experimentation.
3. The experiment should be based on the scientific results of animal experimentation and an understanding of the disease process such that the results justify the conduct of the experiment.
4. Every endeavour should be made to avoid undue mental and physical suffering and injury.
5. Experiments that have a known injury to, or result in the death of a subject, should not be conducted. The exception is when investigating physicians are also participating as subjects in the experiment.
6. The importance of the experiment to humanity should be greater than the risk involved.
7. Every precaution should be taken in the experiment to prevent injury, disability or the death of a subject.
8. Only appropriately qualified investigators should conduct experiments.
9. The human subject must be free to withdraw from or discontinue the experiment.
10. The investigators conducting the experiment must be prepared to terminate the experiment at any stage, if there is reason to believe that continuation of the experiment will result in danger, disability or injury to, or the death of, the subject.

Adapted from http://www.raven1.net/nurm Permissible medical experiments. *Trials of war criminals before the Nuremberg Military Tribunals under Control Council Law No. 10. Nuremberg October 1946–April 1949.* (vol. 2, pp. 181–82). Washington, US Government Printing Office, (n.d.) Accessed online 30 June 2002.

The definitions of the terms 'voluntary', 'legal capacity', 'sufficient understanding' and 'enlightened decision' have been the subject of numerous court cases and commissions involved in setting ethical standards in research (Creighton, 1977). The code requires 'informed consent' in all cases but makes no provisions for any special treatment of children, the elderly or the mentally incompetent. Other international standards followed, including the Declaration of Helsinki, which was adopted in 1964 by the World Medical Assembly and later revised in 1975 (Levine, 1995) and 1989.

An example of unethical research occurred in New Zealand in the 1980s at the National Women's Hospital in Auckland. The researcher, gynaecologist Dr Herbert Green, aimed to prove that untreated carcinoma in situ would not progress to carcinoma of the cervix. One hundred and thirty-one women with this condition in the study were not treated. The study was unethical because the women were not informed of the true nature of the study and did not give their informed consent to withhold treatment. The mortality rate was four times that of the treatment group of 817 women. There was a known risk that the untreated women might die earlier, and the study was not subjected to adequate review of its scientific merit and ethics by peers and expert committees (Coney, 1988).

In Australia, guidelines for the ethical conduct of research involving humans or animals have been developed by the National Health and Medical Research Council (NHMRC). These guidelines build on the principles laid down by the Nuremberg Code and the Helsinki Declaration and provide a framework for the ethical conduct of research. All institutional ethics committees in Australia require research projects to adhere to these guidelines. A copy of the NHMRC Statement on Human Experimentation and all the supplementary notes can be found on the world wide web at URL <http://www.health.gov.au/nhmrc/ethics/humanexp/contents.htm>. In New Zealand, the Health Research Council of New Zealand is the equivalent body and their guidelines can be found at URL <http://www.hrc.govt.nz/ethigud3.htm>.

Currently in Australia, standards for nursing research are being developed by the Australian Nursing Federation. These standards will contain statements about the ethical conduct of research undertaken by Australian nurses. The role of both guidelines for the ethical conduct of research and the role of institutional research and ethics committees cannot be overstated. Both are vitally important for ensuring that the research we conduct is of high quality and acceptable to our communities. The concepts of 'human rights' and 'informed consent' require further explanation.

Protection of human rights

The term 'human rights' was outlined in the American Nurses Association (1985) guidelines as follows:

- right to self-determination
- right to privacy and dignity
- right to anonymity or confidentiality
- right to fair treatment
- right to protection from discomfort and harm.

These rights apply to everyone—participants and team members involved in a research project. Both researchers and consumers of research must realise that any issues highlighted in Box 8.1 should be identified and resolved before the research project is submitted for approval.

Informed consent

Informed consent is the legal principle that, at least in theory, governs the patient's ability to accept or reject individual medical interventions designed to diagnose or treat an illness. It is also a doctrine that determines and regulates participation in research (Katz, 1972; Pranulis, 1996; Silva, 1995). A useful definition of informed consent, quoted from the Code of Federal Regulations (USA) (1983) is:

> The knowing consent of an individual or his/her legally authorised representative, under circumstances that provide the prospective subject or representative sufficient opportunity to consider whether or not to participate without undue inducement of an element of force, fraud, deceit, duress or other forms of constraint or coercion.

The National Health and Medical Research Council (NHMRC) (1992) states that:

> the investigator is responsible for providing the subject at his or her level of comprehension with sufficient information about the purpose, methods, demands, risks, inconveniences and discomforts of the study. Consent should be obtained in writing unless there are good reasons to the contrary.

No investigator may involve a human being as a research subject before obtaining the legally effective informed consent of a participant or their legally authorised representative. The language of the consent form must be understandable and at a level of comprehension suitable for the individual or group concerned. Subjects must not be coerced into participating, nor may researchers collect data on participants who have explicitly refused to be involved in a study. An ethical violation of this principle occurred when an audit conducted in 1994 indicated that medical data on at least three dozen women were collected and analysed without authorisation, against the women's expressed wishes (Snowdon, 1994).

Careful consideration must be given to the following points when planning a research project:

- individuals should not be involved in research without asking them whether or not they wish to participate
- information should not be withheld from participants
- information provided should not be misleading
- participants should not be made to do or say things that violate their moral standards or expose participants to mental or physical stress
- anonymity or confidentiality of participants, organisations and institutions should be maintained
- privacy should not be invaded
- benefits should not be withheld from the control groups
- results should be made known to participants
- the informed consent of the participant should be gained—also consider the long-term effects of the study on the participants
- consider the welfare of laboratory animals or other animals participating in the project
- consider storage and safety of data.

It is advisable to review the NHMRC website (http://www.nhmrc.gov.au/issues/researchethics.htm) for numerous publications related to the ethical conduct of research.

Legal and ethical considerations in animal experimentation

In the 1970s, animal activists and anti-vivisectionist societies drew the public's attention to animal experimentation in research. Following World War II, there was an increase in the use of animals in research and a number of States passed legislation called 'pound seizure laws' that allowed, even mandated, the release of unclaimed animals from pounds to laboratories. The first pound seizure law was enacted in 1949 and repealed only in 1972. Regulations governing the welfare of animals in research can be found in the Australian Code of Practice for the Care and Use of Animals for Scientific Purposes (NHMRC, ARC, CSIRO, AVCC, ARMCANZ, 1997). The guidelines are summarised in the NHMRC Statement of Animal Experimentation and outline the principles for the care and use of experimental animals. They can be found on the world wide web at the URL http://www.ro.unsw/edu.au/animeth.htm

This section serves only as an introduction to the concept of legal/ethical issues related to animal experimentation. Principles of protection of animal rights in research have evolved over time, as has a growing body of literature in the area (Langley, 1989; Mackie, 1977; Singer, 1991). Animals, unlike humans, cannot give informed consent, but conditions safeguarding their welfare must not be ignored. Nurses who encounter the use of animals in research should be alert to the rights of all animals.

Dissemination of findings

If the research is worth doing, it is worth publishing the findings for the benefit of adding to the knowledge base of nursing. It is sometimes said that if findings are not published, it is as though the research has not been done—certainly the research process has not been completed. The proposal application form from funding agencies requires specific information as to the proposed dissemination of findings. Examples of sources for disseminating findings are conferences, lectures, and refereed journals of nursing, midwifery, public health and education.

The budget

A detailed itemised account of all expenditures (e.g. personnel, equipment, travel, accommodation, printing, telephone charges, photocopying, and stationery) is required by funding agencies and when applying for a grant from a nursing department or university. The university may charge a fee for managing a research account. Some funding agencies stipulate that the university must manage the account. In this event, it is important to add about 15% on-costs for this purpose. This figure should be discussed with the university research office.

References and appendices

References should be up-to-date and arranged in a standard format. This is most frequently the Harvard system (author–date system), or Vancouver system (numbered system); whichever format is used, consistency is the key element. This book uses the APA style of referencing, which is a variant of the author–date style. Increasingly, online resources will be used as references, and the reference format must also include the date the information was accessed, as well as the other bibliographic details, for example:

> Thede, L.Q. (2001). Incorporating evidence based practice into nursing practice: an introduction. *Online Journal of Knowledge Synthesis for Nursing*. Available at http://www.stti.iupui.edu/library/ojksn/e_jebpnp.html (June 11). Accessed 4 January 2002.

Appendices will include a participant information sheet and related informed consent form, as well as other documents such as questionnaires or an interview schedule that will be used in the research. Often the hospital/health service or university have a proforma or template to be used for submission of a proposal.

Inclusion of a theoretical or conceptual framework

An issue in writing a proposal is the question of a theoretical or conceptual framework. Finding an appropriate theoretical or conceptual framework for a study appears to cause many nurses and midwives some difficulty. Some research studies benefit from specific theoretical frameworks and some do not. Some research topics may be investigated or explored from a non-theoretical standpoint. Interest in a topic may arise from the clinical area, e.g. how proficient graduate nurses are in calculating drugs, or whether a labouring woman's anxiety levels are lower or higher when her partner is present. Similarly, interest in a topic may be because of its social or community importance, e.g. what factors influence the utilisation of the health system in 20- to 30-year-old men from a non-English speaking background. Generally, however, some kind of framework should be used to help clarify the concepts and their relationships. Students should discuss this issue with their lecturer or supervisor and be guided by their advice.

The importance of a conceptual framework is in linking the proposed or current study to the previous knowledge base on the concept of interest—this may be through examining relationships between concepts or building on known and established theories or models. As an applied discipline, nursing can legitimately use appropriate frameworks from the social or medical sciences as well as from within the discipline.

INTELLECTUAL PROPERTY

Another sometimes contentious issue for health professionals planning a research project is the question of intellectual property. The issue of what constitutes a student's rights regarding intellectual property is an important one. Meanings and interpretation of intellectual property can be found in a discussion paper written by the Australian Vice-Chancellors Committee (1995). See also the report 'National principles of intellectual property management for publicly funded research' (Australian Research Council et al., 2001). Most universities provide students with a copy of 'acceptance of conditions of offer of higher degree candidature' to read and sign. The paper sets out, inter alia, conditions regarding candidature, intellectual property and commercial agreements, and information about maintaining contact with your supervisor(s).

It is important for a student to understand his/her rights and obligations should their research have the potential to result in patentable inventions or any other discoveries that have potential commercial value. Such inventions or discoveries may be likely to arise out of research conducted by higher degree students in departments of biomedical science, toxicology and animal research (e.g. salmonella in pigs and chickens). Students engaged in research that may result in discoveries are usually included as one of a number of senior academic researchers undertaking funded research of a commercial nature. These students would be informed about the nature of the research project.

THE PILOT STUDY

A pilot study is a small-scale study undertaken to test the feasibility of conducting a larger study. A pilot study may be a requirement for a research unit and may be advised for students enrolled in a Doctor of Philosophy (PhD) program. In any event, it would be useful to administer any proposed instrument (questionnaire, test(s)) to a few interested colleagues or people to ensure that everyone is interpreting the questions in the same way. Funding agencies often ask applicants whether they have undertaken a pilot study.

Similarly, a pilot study could be done in the clinical area. For example, if new protocols or procedures were being introduced into the clinical area, it is important that the nurses or midwives are familiar with the new procedures and understand what is required of them. A pilot study would highlight any ambiguities or misunderstandings the staff may have. When new procedures are understood, their implementation in the clinical area is likely to result in less stress for the nurses and improve the conduct of the project.

THE PRE-PROPOSAL STAGE: CHOOSING A TOPIC

The structure and contents of the research proposal have been discussed in some detail. It is now timely to consider the activities leading up to the writing of the proposal. This preliminary stage is called the pre-proposal stage.

This stage involves identifying and clarifying a researchable topic and exploring the literature. Sometimes a student has a clear idea of what he/she wants to research, but equally, at times, there are students who are not sure what it is they want to research. There are many places where research ideas can be found: the clinical area in which you work; conference presentations; networking at conferences and elsewhere with people who have a similar interest; your reading; the internet; friends and other people you may meet. The clinical area, nursing management and nursing education provide unlimited opportunities for nurses to identify problems and challenges (e.g. nursing care, nursing rituals, communication with patients, family and colleagues, patients' understanding of their medical condition, reading habits of graduate nurses, the concerns of first-time mothers on leaving hospital).

When considering a topic for a research project, the nature of the proposal—that is, whether the proposal is for a higher degree, for the purpose of applying for a grant, or some other academic exercise—will be an important factor. Your supervisor will tell you what the research objectives and goals are in the faculty's strategic plan. Recognition of faculty goals is important, particularly if you are seeking funding from the department/faculty or university, or even from an external agency. It is unlikely that the head of department or dean will agree to spend money on research that is incongruent with faculty goals. The faculty in which you are enrolled may encourage research in a particular area, for example, two or three students may develop the same topic from different standpoints. If the proposal is directed to a funding agency, it may be that certain criteria have been stipulated and these criteria may impact on your choice of topic and design. It may also be that you have been given a certain amount of freedom in choosing the area you wish to research. These, and other factors, are important when thinking about a topic.

While your choice of a topic may or may not be limited by what the faculty considers important and worthwhile, faculty resources are important. These resources include appropriate supervision by academics who have the interest and knowledge to guide you. Your choice may also be restricted by the facilities (e.g. equipment, computers, space), apart from supervision, that the faculty can provide for you. Finally, your choice of topic may be limited by ethical considerations.

Most universities also offer postgraduate support grants. The amount of the grant may differ, but the purpose is generally to assist students with various costs related to the research being undertaken (e.g. conference attendance, use of photocopy machines, accommodation, special materials). Information about intellectual property may be obtained from your supervisor, head of school, the intellectual property office or the university solicitor. It is most important that the prospective student understands exactly what these conditions mean.

FORMAT REQUIREMENTS FOR THE PROPOSAL

Most academic institutions use a standard format for writing proposals. A separate standard form requiring different information may be required by a hospital human ethics committee. These forms may differ from those used by funding agencies who usually provide their own application forms. Also, the funding agency's criteria will certainly be different, as will the specific areas they are committed to funding. Most academic institutions also require a plain language statement about the research topic. This requirement is necessary for the review panel, which may include academics outside of the student's particular discipline, to understand clearly what the research is about. In addition, hospital ethics committees will have lay person members, as do animal experimentation ethics committees; this requirement is mandated by the NHMRC. These committees make decisions about proposals on the basis of their purpose, clarity, logic, standard and appropriateness.

KEY POINTS

- Identifying a feasible research question and finding the design that will best answer the question are key preliminary steps in writing a research proposal.
- The proposal must demonstrate the competency of the investigator to undertake the research.
- The topic must be worthwhile and relevant to the strategic research plan of the university, faculty, department or funding agency.
- The method, design and timeframe must be appropriate and feasible.
- Assumptions, definitions and operational definitions in the research proposal should be clearly stated and explained.
- A research proposal provides evidence of your written skills, how you conceptualise problems, and your understanding of the literature, research designs, data collection and analysis.

CRITICAL THINKING CHALLENGES

- Ethical considerations must be included in your proposal. Why is this so? Discuss.
- You have been asked by the faculty higher degrees committee or funding agency to justify the research design in your proposal. What factors would you consider in your answer?

- Your research class is debating the importance of aims and objectives in a research proposal. Are they important? Provide examples.
- Why do you think it is important to provide definitions in a research proposal? Give examples.

Additional resources

Aveyard, H. (2000). Is there a concept of autonomy that can usefully inform nursing practice? *Journal of Advanced Nursing*, 32(2), 352–58.

Ayer, S. (1994). Submitting a research proposal for ethical approval. *Professional Nurse*, 9(12), 805–06.

Bosek, M.S.D., Savage, T.A., Shaw, L.A. & Renella, C. (2001). When surrogate decision-making is not straightforward. *Journal of Nursing Administration* 3(2), 47–57.

Brink, P.J. & Wood, M.J. (1988). *Basic steps in planning nursing research: from question to proposal.* (3rd ed.). Boston, Jones and Bartlett Publishers.

Chenitz, W.V. & Swanson, J.M. (1985). *From practice to grounded theory. Qualitative research in nursing.* California, Addison-Wesley Publishing Co.

Cobb, A.K. & Hagemaster, J.N. (1987). Ten criteria for evaluating qualitative research proposals. *Journal of Nursing Education*, 26, 4.

Cohen, M.Z., Knafl, K. & Dzurec, L.C. (1993). Grant writing for qualitative research. *Image: Journal of Nursing Scholarship*, 25(2), 151.

Cormack, D.F.S. (1996). *The research process in nursing.* (3rd ed.). London, Hartnolls Ltd.

Hall, M. (1988). *Getting funded. a complete guide to proposal writing.* (3rd ed.). Portland, Oregon, Continuing Education Publications.

Haller, K.B. (1989). Preparing the research proposal: half science, half art. *Maternal Child Nursing*, 14, 230.

Marshall, C. & Rossman, G.B. (1989). *Designing qualitative research.* California, Sage.

Olsen, D.P. (2000). Equipoise: an appropriate standard for ethical review of nursing research? *Journal of Advanced Nursing*, 31(2), 267–73.

Orb, A., Eisenhauer, L. & Wynaden, D. (2001). Ethics in qualitative research. *Journal of Nursing Scholarship*, 33(1), 93–96.

Parahoo, K. & Reid, N. (1988). Research skills number 3. *Nursing Times*, 84(41), 49–52.

Pinch, W.J.E. & Graves, J.K. (2000). Using web-based discussion as a teaching strategy: bioethics as an exemplar. *Journal of Advanced Nursing*, 32(3), 704–12.

Sanchez-Sweatman, L.R. (2000). Reproductive cloning and human health: an ethical, international, and nursing perspective. *International Nursing Review*, 47, 28–37.

Sandelowski, M., Davis, D.H. & Harris, B.G. (1989). Artful research: writing the proposal for research in the naturalist paradigm. *Research in Nursing & Health*, 12(2), 77–84.

Tornquist, E.M. (1986). *From proposal to publication. An informal guide to writing about nursing research.* Wokingham, England, Addison-Wesley Publishers.

Watts, G.C.M. (1990). Development of health services research applications. *Health Bulletin*, 48(1), 41–49.

Wright, G. & Fowler, C. (1986). *Investigative design and statistics.* London, Penguin Books.

SECTION TWO

Qualitative research methods

9

CHAPTER

Approaches in qualitative research

Debra Jackson, John Daly and Esther Chang

LEARNING OUTCOMES

After reading this chapter the student should be able to:

- Identify nursing phenomena that lend themselves to using qualitative research methods.
- Discuss the terms 'ontology', 'epistemology' and 'methodology'.
- Discuss the characteristics of qualitative research methods.
- Understand the differences between the following research approaches: constructive-interpretive; post-positivist; feminist; post-structural; and critical.
- Appreciate the importance of qualitative research methods in understanding the experiential and contextual aspects of human existence.
- Discuss the relevance of conducting a literature review.

Key terms

constructivist–interpretive approach
critical approaches
epistemology
feminist approach
focus group
in-depth interview
methodology
naturalistic setting
observational methods
ontology
post-positivist approach
post-structural approach
sampling

INTRODUCTION

Qualitative methods of research provide a means to guide the study of everyday life, and because of this, many nurses are interested in using qualitative approaches to develop knowledge into aspects of human existence that, although prosaic, are poorly understood. Qualitative approaches can be used to wholly guide a study, or may be used with quantitative methods in a methodological triangulation type approach (see Chapter 2). Qualitative researchers use a range of research designs and methods, and many of these specific methods are addressed in depth in later chapters in this book. While there are important differences between the various qualitative approaches, all qualitative methods share some commonalities. It is these areas of commonality that are discussed in this chapter.

Nursing is a people-centred process concerned with health and healing, as well as with providing support and therapeutic care for people undergoing traumatic life events (such as illness or surgery) or major life transitions (such as the transition to parenthood that accompanies the birth of a baby). Nursing derives much of its knowledge from a range of biomedical sciences. However, biomedical knowledge does not supply all the knowledge that is required to adequately provide holistic care for clients. For example, biomedical perspectives do not necessarily explain or acknowledge the influences of factors such as gender, education, cultural issues, socio-economic status, previous experience and age, on an individual's health. Similarly, the biomedical model does not always take account of a client's expectations and perceptions of care, and their experience of recovery from illness or adaptation to changed life circumstances. Often in nursing it is the ordinary activities of everyday life that are the focus of nursing care and nursing problems. Therefore when investigating nursing, qualitative researchers use humanistic frameworks which are derived from the social sciences (e.g. sociology, anthropology) and philosophy as well as nursing knowledge to examine phenomena of interest.

WHAT IS QUALITATIVE RESEARCH?

Qualitative research is a broad term used to describe research that is focused on human experience, and represents a different philosophical view towards reality from the positivist or scientific approach. It is conducted in naturalistic settings and involves close, often sustained contact between the researcher and research participants (Oiler Boyd, 1993). Qualitative research does not focus on establishing cause and effect relationships, rather they allow exploration of a range of human experiences that are of interest to a discipline such as nursing, for example:

- What is the experience of suffering for people living with terminal cancer?
- What are the health beliefs pertaining to pregnancy and lactation of Arabic-speaking refugee women recently arrived in Australia?
- What is the meaning of comfort for recipients of nursing care?
- What is the meaning of 'quality of life' for wheelchair dependent brain-injured adults?
- What are the factors that influence students' beliefs about nursing?

Though it may be possible to study these types of phenomena using a quantitative approach, such an approach could be very limiting. The advantage of using a qualitative approach is that the phenomenon may be studied holistically and contextually. There is a focus on human experience, and it is possible to develop a rich description and deep understanding of the phenomena under investigation. Qualitative research involves:

> broadly stated questions about human experiences and realities, studied through sustained contact with persons in their natural environments producing rich, descriptive data that help us to understand those persons' experiences. The emphasis (here) is on achieving understanding that will in turn, open up new options for action and new perspectives that can change people's worlds (Oiler Boyd, 1993, pp. 69–70).

It is clear from the text above that qualitative writing is rich and descriptive. Methods used by qualitative researchers enable the collection of abundant, rich data, and it is important to carry that richness through to the 'write up' stage. The writing up stage is addressed comprehensively further in this chapter. Qualitative researchers operate under a set of beliefs and assumptions that differ from those held by quantitative researchers. These relate to ontology and epistemology, truth and objectivity, and researcher/participant relationships.

ONTOLOGY AND EPISTEMOLOGY

All research that is qualitative requires consideration of three philosophical concepts—ontology, epistemology and methodology (Denzin & Lincoln, 1994; Parse, 2001). These are highly philosophical areas, and qualitative researchers need to consider these concepts and develop a position in relation to them. Frameworks for qualitative researchers:

> combine beliefs about ontology (What kind of being is the human being? What is the nature of reality?), epistemology (What is the relationship between the inquirer and the known?), and methodology (How do we know the world, or gain knowledge of it?) (Denzin & Lincoln, 1994, p. 13).

Clearly, philosophical ideas such as these are based on values and beliefs, hence there is scope for contention and difference. However, internal consistency and logic are achieved in a qualitative study when the links between these three concepts are coherent (Parse, 2001, p. 15). Differing views exist regarding these concepts and the ways they interrelate. Key ideas from the literature regarding the interrelationship of these concepts suggest that:

- ontology provides the world view that guides a study
- epistemology provides focus for a study
- methodology provides a design for conducting a study.

These issues are discussed more fully in the following sections.

TRUTH AND OBJECTIVITY

Qualitative researchers reject the notion of a single, objective truth. Rather, they recognise the existence of multiple realities, in that there is acknowledgment that people's experiences of and perspectives on phenomena differ according to where they are positioned in relation to the phenomena. For example, the feelings and experiences associated with organ donation will be very different depending on a person's position as a family member of the donor, a family member of the recipient, or whether they are a nurse or doctor working in the intensive care unit or the operating theatre. The feelings and experiences of each of these people are likely to be different in some ways, even though they are all associated with the same phenomenon.

Qualitative researchers acknowledge that they are influenced by their own beliefs and feelings about a subject. This is quite unlike other methodological approaches in which researchers present themselves as neutral and objective. Qualitative researchers also acknowledge any subjective feelings they have about a phenomenon, and critically reflect and acknowledge their own assumptions and understandings about the phenomena under investigation. For example, in her study on withdrawal of life support in the intensive care unit, Watts (1998) made her assumptions about nursing and death clear, right at the beginning of the thesis.

RESEARCHER/PARTICIPANT RELATIONSHIPS

One of the characteristics of qualitative research is that it involves a close relationship between the researcher and participant. This is quite different from research conducted within the quantitative paradigm, where there is frequently no direct contact (i.e. as in return of mailed survey forms or receipt of test results). Research participants are viewed as 'knowers', that is, they are viewed as having the knowledge that the researcher seeks to gain. This is because they have lived through an experience, or they are part of the culture that the researcher is examining.

The relationships that develop between researchers and study participants may be short term or more sustained, depending on the research design. For example, in a grounded theory study that aimed to explore the professional identity of Japanese nurses, Gregg and Magilvy (2001) conducted in-depth qualitative interviews as well as observing participants in their natural settings. Subsequent to data collection the researchers then again interacted with research participants as they engaged in a process of member validation (Gregg & Magilvy, 2001). Clearly these researchers had an ongoing relationship with participants on at least three occasions. Ethnographic studies require researchers to enter the culture or sub-culture under investigation and so generally require a longer, more sustained relationship than some other approaches, which may require one contact only (i.e. one interview). The nature of the relationships means that there are specific ethical issues associated with qualitative research designs, and these are addressed later in this chapter.

Qualitative researchers have a range of research approaches available, depending on the nature of the study and the type of knowledge that the researcher wishes to develop. Broadly speaking, these are the constructivist–interpretive, post-positivist, feminist, post-structural and critical approaches (Denzin & Lincoln, 1994). Each of these approaches holds a set of ontological, epistemological and methodological beliefs that inform and shape research studies, and many of these are discussed in later sections of this book.

METHODOLOGICAL ISSUES WITHIN THE QUALITATIVE PARADIGM

The qualitative researcher can choose from a range of research approaches or methods. Each approach or method incorporates a way of structuring the study, selecting the research participants, and collecting and analysing the data. The aim for any researcher is that their work be accepted by the community of scholars and practitioners as rigorous and sound, and that it becomes a part of the knowledge base that underpins the discipline. As with all research, qualitative research needs to be well designed and rigorous. The conduct of research is a creative endeavour, and like other creative activities a plan or design is essential. There are several steps or stages that the researcher needs to move through in planning and conducting a qualitative project. The major steps are outlined below.

Identifying a research question or problem statement

The catalyst for undertaking research is usually a desire to know and understand something that is poorly understood in some way. A qualitative study is often borne of a need to understand the social, cultural and experiential aspects of a particular aspect of human existence. In the qualitative paradigm the focus of a research project is usually written as a problem statement or a research question, rather than hypothesised, as in quantitative research. The research issue may arise in a number of ways, including:

- Ideas arising from clinical practice often lead to research projects. Nursing seeks to improve and continue to develop clinical practice, and this requires that good quality research projects be undertaken and findings disseminated.
- Changes in treatments brought about by technological advances frequently raise ethical, experiential and other issues requiring research.
- Study of the literature can raise many questions, and frequently a gap in the literature is identified as the catalyst for commencing a research project.
- Recommendations of previous projects commonly call for further research.
- Brainstorming and discussion with clients, peers, teachers and colleagues can raise issues that are researchable.

It is evident from the list above that a substantial amount of preliminary work is required even before commencing a research study. Developing a research question or problem statement requires a sound knowledge of the particular area of interest.

Use of the existing literature

It is important to understand that no piece of research exists in isolation. Developing a research proposal requires that researchers draw on previous research. The literature represents what is known about a topic and also the attitudes and beliefs that are held about it by a discipline (Raftos, Mannix & Jackson, 1997). Because of this, the literature itself can be the subject of research and many published articles have used a selection of literature as data about which questions are raised and conclusions drawn. See, for example, Jackson, Raftos and Mannix (1996), who used a sample of the literature to look at trends in the nursing literature.

Though it is argued that some approaches call for the review of literature to be undertaken after data analysis (Streubert & Carpenter, 1995), most require a literature review very early in a project. All research requires a thorough examination of relevant literature (Daly, Elliott & Chang, 2000). Use of the literature is important for a range of reasons, including:

- the literature tells us what is already known about a topic
- the literature assists in identifying the gaps, shadows and what is not known
- study of the literature illuminates the problems and pitfalls that other researchers in the area may have come up against
- the literature can highlight ethical issues that may be of relevance when designing the study
- when the data are analysed and findings established, they are then discussed in relation to the literature, and in this way, new research findings are drawn into the existing body of knowledge.

When gathering literature for a proposal or a literature review it is important to search thoroughly. Use of databases such as CINAHL and Medline will help ensure that all current and relevant literature is identified. However, when reading the literature, it is not enough to be merely descriptive; it is important to read critically. Critical reading is a skill that takes time to develop. It is important to approach the task systematically, as it is also important to be able to clearly articulate the nature of your critique (see Chapter 4). Use of a tool or checklist can be very helpful, and there are many tools to assist readers develop the necessary skills and proficiency. The tools are generally presented as a series of subheadings, such as 'purpose', 'method' and 'sampling', and each subheading usually features a series of questions designed to trigger reflection and deliberation on different aspects of the paper (see the criteria used to critique studies used throughout this book and specifically in Chapter 4). Some tools are developed with a focus on quantitative reports and some focus on qualitative reports (e.g. Forchuk & Roberts, 1993; Streubert & Carpenter, 1995), but either approach is generally suitable as a guide to assist in developing skills for critically reading research papers.

CHOOSING A METHODOLOGICAL APPROACH

There are various approaches within the qualitative paradigm, and it is important to select a method that is appropriate for the research question or problem statement. For example, if the area of interest is a study of the lived experience, a researcher might choose a phenomenological approach, and this would guide the selection of participants and lead the researcher to ways of gathering and analysing data, as well as how to write the study report. Once the methodology has been selected, it is necessary to clearly demonstrate how the ideas, assumptions and principles underpinning the methodology are being used in the study. It is important that there is coherence between the research question or problem statement, the sample, methods used to collect data, analysis of data, write up and presentation of data.

Ethical implications of qualitative research

It is very important for qualitative researchers to be aware of and sensitive to ethics and ethical issues. Unlike quantitative research, the qualitative methods always involve a direct relationship with participants, and this raises ethical concerns. As with any research involving recruitment of human participants, approval from an institutional ethics committee (IEC) is essential prior to recruiting participants. IECs take guidance from, and are accountable to, the National Health and Medical Research Council (NHMRC). The IEC keeps records about the conduct of research carried out within the institution. Most institutions have their meeting dates, guidelines and application forms available on the internet (see, for example http://www.uws.edu.au/uws/uwsn/admin/research/ROethics/human/index.htm). It is an interesting exercise to browse through the documents on such sites. Researchers have to submit a detailed application to the IEC, including a complete project outline and various attachments. All researchers are responsible to the IEC. The IEC may call for additional information at any time and may suspend or withdraw approval for a project if they have any concerns (see Chapter 8 for further discussion of developing proposals for submission to ethics committees).

Special guidelines are available for researchers working with people who may have limited ability to give free consent, for example, young children, people with intellectual impairments, and people who are very ill, such as comatose people. People in dependent relationships are also recognised as a vulnerable group, and these include armed services personnel, prisoners, students and hospital staff and patients. It is also important to remember that some methods have particular ethical issues, for example, observational methods can lead to invasion of privacy (Adler & Adler, 1998).

Sampling

Sampling is the process of choosing suitable participants or text for inclusion in the study. It is a very important part of the research process because inappropriate sampling procedures will jeopardise the integrity, findings and outcomes of a project. There are a number of ways that sampling can be approached, and the choice of method will help guide the researcher through the process of sample selection. To be suitable for inclusion in a study, participants will need to have certain characteristics and meet certain requirements. The elements that need to be present are commonly referred to as the inclusion criteria (Crookes & Davies, 1998). For example, in a study of women's experiences of recovery from myocardial infarction, the stated inclusion criteria 'required that potential participants be female, recently discharged from hospital following a first-time MI, able to converse fluently in the English language, and be willing to participate in the study' (Jackson et al., 2000, p. 1406) (see Appendix A).

The three main types of sampling used in qualitative research are convenience sampling, purposive sampling and snowball sampling (Crookes & Davies, 1998). Convenience samples are those that recruit anyone who meets the inclusion criteria. Purposive or purposeful sampling provides information-rich cases for in-depth study (Coyne, 1997). Snowball sampling is especially useful where there is a marginalised or stigmatised group, who may be reluctant to come forward without the reassurance of knowing someone who has already participated in the study. A snowball sample is obtained through locating a participant who meets all criteria for inclusion, and using the networks and word-of-mouth of that initial participant to generate other participants. Sampling is discussed in more detail in Chapter 17.

Methods for collecting data

Qualitative research requires the collection of qualitative data and seeks to understand the 'emic' or insider view of a phenomenon, culture, social world or issue (Holloway & Wheeler, 1996). It is important to remember that qualitative methods require a direct relationship with research participants, and this is one of the major ways it differs from quantitative research, which does not require a direct relationship between researcher and subject.

Oral narrative is frequently the basis of much qualitative research and this narrative is most often gained through a direct encounter between researcher and participant, either in qualitative in-depth interviews (sometimes called qualitative conversations) or focus groups (Lane, McKenna, Ryan & Fleming, 2001). More recently use of computer-generated text such as email is becoming a source for qualitative studies, and this is likely to increase as use of the internet widens (Cooper, 2000). The way in which an in-depth interview or focus group is conducted is important, as a poor interview will yield poor quality narrative data. The participant needs to be made to feel as comfortable as possible. It is necessary to ensure adequate privacy, comfortable seating and that all items required for the encounter are available, for example, recording equipment, tapes, consent forms, participant information sheets, tissues and water or some other beverage. Researchers should take steps, such as posting 'do not disturb' signs and disabling telephone or pager devices, to ensure that interruptions are avoided. It is also important to pay proper attention to the structure and conduct of the interview, and a warm and non-judgemental demeanour towards the participant must be established and maintained.

There are many skills associated with qualitative interviewing. Minichiello, Sullivan Greenwood and Axford (1999, p. 399) propose that it is an art, and suggest three particular techniques:

- funnelling—beginning the interview with general and broad opening questions and then narrowing down
- story telling—asking questions in a manner which encourages story telling, for example, 'Tell me about ...'
- probing—eliciting further details or seeking clarification.

During the encounter it is important to be responsive to the participant, to concentrate on what is being said, as well as being alert to other, particularly non-verbal cues. It is also crucial to adopt an active listening stance, and to encourage the participant to be reflective (Holloway & Wheeler, 1996). Some researchers find it useful to keep a journal to record the non-verbal aspects of the encounters with participants, as well as their own thoughts and feelings about the qualitative interview and the issues raised in it, and this too can form part of the data set.

Observational methods are commonly used in qualitative research designs, and may vary between a range of modes: the complete participant; the participant-as-observer; the observer-as-participant; and the complete observer (Adler & Adler, 1998). The differences in these roles revolve around researcher involvement or detachment with participants. Though positivist researchers also use observation (see Chapter 16), observation which is qualitative in nature is:

> fundamentally naturalistic in essence; it occurs in the natural context of occurrence, among the actors who would naturally be participating in the interaction, and follows the natural stream of everyday life. As such, it enjoys the advantage of drawing the observer into the phenomenological complexity of the world, where connections, correlations, and causes can be witnessed as and how they unfold. Qualitative observers are not bound, thus, by predetermined categories of

measurement or response, but are free to search for concepts or categories that appear meaningful to subjects (Adler & Adler, 1998, p. 81).

Though qualitative observation may be unstructured as described above, it may also have some structure. For example, observers in a ward or clinic may focus their observations on certain phenomena of interest, such as episodes of violence, or acute hospital admissions. Though focused observations, they would still be holistic and contextual. Observational techniques are more than simply visual and Adler and Adler suggest that qualitative observation 'consists of gathering impressions of the surrounding world through all relevant human faculties' (1998, p. 80).

Not all qualitative studies involve oral interviews or observations of people or events. Much useful information can be gleaned from other sources. Insights which can help inform nursing knowledge and practice can be gleaned from a range of literary and artistic media, including photographs (Short, 1995), paintings (Darbyshire, 1994), literature (Begley, 1996; Darbyshire, 1995a; 1995b; De Vries, Dunlop, Goopy, Moyle & Sutherland-Lockhart, 1995; Jackson, 2000), and other art forms (Hess, 1995).

When is enough enough?

Unlike quantitative approaches that aim to establish statistical significance by sampling a predetermined number of subjects (Streubert & Carpenter, 1995), qualitative researchers do not usually begin a project with a fixed preset number of participants in mind. Rather, they continue collecting data until theoretical saturation or redundancy of data is achieved. Though there is some controversy as to whether it is really possible to achieve true saturation, its accepted meaning is 'repetition of data obtained during the course of a qualitative study [and] signifies completion of data collection on a particular culture or phenomena' (Streubert & Carpenter, 1995, p. 317). The point at which saturation will be achieved varies with each study and cannot be predicted (Holloway & Wheeler, 1996). Once the researcher is satisfied that saturation has been achieved, data collection can cease.

Analysis

Qualitative research yields quantities of rich data. The purpose of qualitative research is to gain insights and understandings into aspects of the human experience and the focus is on deep understanding. It is important that qualitative richness is not lost in the process of analysis, and the challenge for researchers is to put the data through a systematic and rigorous analysis that will not distort or reduce the richness of the data or fragment participants' stories and experiences.

The first step in analysing narrative data usually involves transcription of products from a verbal and personal encounter into a documented textual account. Sandelowski (1991, p. 163) states that 'any transcription is necessarily incomplete' because when transcribing there is necessarily a limitation to those aspects of an encounter that are able to be maintained in a textual form, and various non-verbal aspects of the encounter may be lost. One of the ways that this can be overcome at least in part is to listen to the tapes as well as read the text when analysing the narrative, and in this way it may be possible for the researcher to relocate and preserve as much as possible the context of the encounter.

There are several ways the text itself can be dealt with. These include thematic analysis and discourse analysis, among other approaches. The choice of method will help guide the researcher to an analytical path. Computer-assisted analysis is often used by qualitative researchers, however, as Grbich (1999, p. 239) suggests, 'computers are only aids for the management of qualitative data. They cannot analyse it. The process of interpretive analysis rests with the researcher'. Grbich (1999) also points out that learning to use some of the software may be difficult and time-consuming, and that proficiency in the use of the program may be the major outcome of software use, rather than knowledge of the data.

RIGOUR AND QUALITATIVE RESEARCH

In order to contribute to knowledge, research must be scholarly and rigorous, and therefore all research, regardless of design or approach, must address the issue of rigour. The need to establish and maintain rigour informs actions and decisions throughout a research project. Hitherto, the criteria for establishing rigour have been largely quantitative, however, as Koch and Harrington (1998) suggest, it is not reasonable to transfer criteria for credibility from one paradigm to another (similarly Hill Bailey, 1997). The ways of establishing rigour and how it can be conceptualised in the qualitative paradigm is very much a continuing conversation, and nurses have yet to reach agreement on how rigour can be achieved (Koch & Harrington, 1998). The challenge for qualitative researchers is to identify and institute strategies to establish rigour that are also compatible with the philosophical and methodological tenets of the study. One way to ensure that research findings are in fact a genuine and legitimate portrayal of the phenomenon under investigation is to utilise member validation procedures (Webb, 1992; Sandelowski, 1993). Member validation involves seeking feedback from study participants to ensure that findings are reflective of their experiences. However, in establishing rigour it is important not to jeopardise the focus of the project, as Sandelowski eloquently suggests:

> There is an inflexibility and an uncompromising harshness and rigidity implied in the term 'rigor' that threaten to take us too far from the artfulness, versatility, and sensitivity to meaning and context that mark qualitative works of distinction. It is as if ... we were more preoccupied with building fortifications against attack than with creating the evocative, true-to-life, and meaningful portraits, stories and landscapes of human experience that constitute the best test of rigor in qualitative work (Sandelowski, 1993, p. 1).

Like Sandelowski (1993), other scholars and researchers have sought to develop processes for establishing rigour in a qualitative paradigm. Strategies such as establishing an audit trail (Koch, 1994a), credibility, transferability, confirmability (Byrne, 2001), internal logic (Koch & Harrington, 1998), fittingness, and member checks or member validation (Sandelowski, 1993), have been proposed as demonstrating rigour in qualitative research (see Table 9.1).

TABLE 9.1 Criteria for judging scientific rigour: credibility, auditability, fittingness and confirmability

CRITERIA	CRITERIA CHARACTERISTIC
Credibility	Truth of findings as judged by participants and others within the discipline.
Auditability	Accountability as judged by the adequacy of information leading the reader from the research question and raw data through various steps of analysis to the interpretation of findings.
Fittingness	Faithfulness to everyday reality of the participants, described in enough detail so that others in the discipline can evaluate importance for their own practice, research and theory development.
Confirmability	Findings that reflect implementation of credibility, auditability and fittingness standards.

Examples of credibility

King and Wilson (1998) stated that a report of the analysis of their ethnographic study of diabetes education in the people of Nunkuwarrin Yunti, was provided to all participants so they could confirm that the findings were true to their experience. This is an example of a strategy aimed at ensuring that the findings are credible. In a study of the lived experience of men diagnosed with an AIDS-defining illness, Kermode (1995) interviewed each participant twice to provide them with an opportunity to clarify issues arising from the first interview and comment on the researcher's interpretation of their experiences. In her study of pregnant women's experiences of models of care in some hospitals in Victoria, Schneider (2002) posted a hard copy of the transcript to each woman, giving her the opportunity to read her transcript and comment on the accuracy of the researcher's interpretation.

Examples of auditability

Barclay, Donovan and Genovese (1996) provide the reader with some insight into the audit trail of their study into men's experiences of their partner's first pregnancy by illustrating how the conceptual categories were established and how they relate to the concepts identified in the data and the core category of 'confusion'. The reader's understanding of Barclay and colleagues' interpretation of the data is enhanced by being able to follow their analysis of the concepts and relating this to the words of the participants as presented in the study. Walters (1995a) explains the steps he used in analysing the data in a hermeneutic study of the experiences of relatives of critically ill patients. Walters details how he used Reinharz's method to transform the data to arrive at a hermeneutic interpretation of the meaning of the experience of the participants. By informing the reader of the process that he undertook, auditability of the study was enhanced. However, in many qualitative studies the audit trail of the researcher is not clearly explained. This omission makes the task of the reader of research reports difficult and invites questions about the validity of the findings.

Examples of fittingness

The use of the literature to support or refute the concepts emerging from the data provides another avenue for judging fittingness. Barclay et al., (1996) discussed their findings in the context of other research studies in the area. The authors argue that some of the conceptual categories emerging from this study are similar to those previously reported, adding support to the theories developed by the researchers. In a study of the delivery of nursing care in Western Australia (Williams, 1998), the researcher used a grounded theory approach that led to the development of a substantive theory of the delivery of quality nursing care from the nurses' perspective. Evidence of fittingness of the theory to the literature was proposed by the discussion of the theory in relation to recent research findings from other studies in the same area that focused on the patient's perspective. Williams (1998) considered that the match between the research and the literature confirmed the accuracy of data interpretation.

However, many of these approaches have ethical or practical problems. For example, Koch and Harrington (1998) describe practical problems in returning transcriptions to elderly research participants, and in trying to locate participants when a substantial amount of time has elapsed since initial recruitment. Rather, they draw on Marcus (1994), and argue for reflexivity to be woven through qualitative research designs, and suggest that its characteristics of self-critique and reflection establish the credibility and plausibility of qualitative research.

WRITING UP QUALITATIVE RESEARCH, INCLUDING QUALITATIVE APPROACHES AND LANGUAGE

Qualitative research is written up quite differently from positivist research. These paradigms are different in the ways that they construct written research reports. In seeking to demonstrate its supposed acontextuality, objectivity and neutrality, the traditional quantitative research report adopts a particular use of language (Hall & Stevens, 1991; Jackson, 1997; Webb, 1992). The voices that construct traditional research reports are passive. Careful to present themselves as neutral and impartial, they cloak themselves in the language of science and disguise themselves as invisible and anonymous (Hall & Stevens, 1991; Webb, 1992). Webb (1992) suggests that although the use of this language aims to convince the reader that the ideas being presented are proposed from a position of impartiality, this is in fact seldom the case. As discussed earlier in this chapter, qualitative researchers dispute the notion of true objectivity, and therefore do not need to limit themselves to neutral and impartial language. Study participants are not rendered invisible in the research reports and are often ascribed non-identifying biographic details and nom de plumes. Qualitative writers do not usually adopt a dispassionate stance, and use of the first person is not uncommon in written research reports. Writing has a particular function in the qualitative paradigm:

> Writing gives form to the researcher's clumps of carefully categorized and organized data. It links together thoughts that have been developing throughout the research process. The act of writing also stimulates new thoughts, new connections. Writing is rewarding in that it creates the product, the housing for the meaning that you and others have made of your research adventure. Writing is about creating a text. As a writer, you engage in a sustained act of construction,

which includes a particular 'story' to tell from the data you have analyzed, and creating the literary form that you believe best conveys your story (Glesne & Peshkin, 1992, p. 151).

It is evident from the text above that writing is more than the act of dissemination of findings for qualitative researchers; it is a crucial part of the research process itself. Writing involves reflection and the act of writing makes links and patterns explicit. Koch and Harrington (1998) use the metaphor of tapestry to convey the artistry and craft that goes into the completion of a qualitative research project.

In her examination of critical ethnography, Bruni (1994) presents the notion of 'authority', which questions the voices that construct research findings or text. If there is acceptance of the idea that qualitative research is concerned with hearing the voices and recognising the perspectives of participants, there must be recognition of the power researchers have to silence those voices. 'Gatekeeping' and the editorial process are factors that contribute to the silencing of participants' voices, therefore affecting research findings and ultimately the construction of knowledge (Bruni, 1994). As an issue, this is not confined to ethnography; it has relevance for all of the qualitative methodologies. In seeking to 'know' a phenomenon as it is experienced by others, it is not enough to merely gather data that are participant centred. There must be scrupulous adherence to accuracy in the presentation of findings.

HOW CAN QUALITATIVE RESEARCH FINDINGS INFORM NURSING PRACTICE?

Though it is important to remember that qualitative researchers do not claim generalisability, the findings from qualitative research can inform nursing practice by the contribution of new insights about the phenomena that concern them (e.g. grief or hope). Awareness of these insights can heighten nurses' sensitivity and understanding of the patients' experiences of such phenomena. This new understanding can enhance empathy. Qualitative findings can guide and enhance the quality of nursing practice and contribute to the development of theory for practice. There are many examples of good qualitative studies in the literature which have implications for nursing practice. These implications relate to the heightened awareness of the feelings and perceptions that can be associated with certain life events. For example, Jackson et al., (2000) conducted a study on women's recovery from first-time myocardial infarction (see Appendix A). Using a feminist qualitative approach, findings of the study illuminated the uncertainty, fear and emotional lability that characterised the early recovery period for the women in the study. Findings also revealed that the women had unmet needs for information, and raised questions about the timing and nature of information given to women recovering from myocardial infarction. Clearly these findings have implications for further research, nursing practice and healthcare service provision.

Another study found that nurses in acute care settings used a basic social process of 'enabling care', rather than the 'nursing process' because certain factors hindered work in that framework (O'Connell, 2000). Using a grounded theory approach, semi-structured interviews and field observations, O'Connell was able to examine the reality of practice for nurses, and the resulting conflicts between theory and practice (see Appendix B).

KEY POINTS

- The qualitative researcher in nursing can choose from a range of approaches and methods.
- The area to be investigated and the purpose of the study will influence choice of method.
- Qualitative methods allow for holistic exploration of the phenomenon of concern, and have a focus on meaning, interpretation and understanding.
- Qualitative research processes have contributed to the development of nursing as a discipline. Aspects of this include enhanced understanding of life processes, including individual and group experiences of health-related phenomena.
- The emphasis on meaning within this tradition calls for nurses to consider and seek to better understand human beings' lived experiences of health.
- Exploration of health and illness using qualitative approaches enables a broader understanding and deeper insight into complex human behaviours. This provides a basis for the development of sensitive, humanistic quality nursing care for patients and their families.

CRITICAL THINKING CHALLENGES

- Discuss the major differences between qualitative and quantitative research methods.
- Researchers using qualitative methods acknowledge that they are influenced by their own beliefs and feelings about a subject. Discuss.
- Discuss the ways in which quantitative and qualitative research approaches maintain rigour.
- No piece of research exists in isolation. Discuss.
- What are the features of a 'good' environment for the conduct of interviews in qualitative research?
- Data analysis for qualitative methods aims to make meaning from narrative data. How is this achieved?
- Ethical issues in qualitative research involve issues related to the naturalistic setting, emergent nature of the design, researcher–participant interaction and researcher as instrument. Think of examples of ethical issues relating to this statement.

Additional resources

Aldridge, D. & Stevenson, C. (2001). Social poetics as research and practice: living in and learning from the process of research. *Nursing Inquiry*, 8, 19–27.

Atkinson, P. (1995). Some perils of paradigms. *Qualitative Health Research*, 51(1), 117–24.

Baker, C., Wuest, J. & Stern, P.N. (1992). Method slurring: the grounded theory/phenomenology example. *Journal of Advanced Nursing*, 17, 1355–60.

Billhult, A. & Dahlberg, K. (2001). A meaningful relief from suffering: experiences of massage in cancer care. *Cancer Nursing*, 24(3), 180–84.

Cioffi, J. (2000). Recognition of patients who require emergency assistance: a descriptive study. *Heart & Lung: the Journal of Acute and Critical Care*, 29, 262–68.

Dunn, S.V. & Yates, P. (2000). The roles of Australian chairs in clinical nursing. *Journal of Advanced Nursing*, 31(1), 165–71.

X Happ, M.B. & Kagan, S.H. (2001). Methodological considerations for grounded theory research in critical care settings. *Nursing Research*, 50(3), 188–91.

Hewitt-Taylor, J. (2002). Case study: an approach to qualitative enquiry. *Nursing Standard*, 16, 33–37.

Kralik, D., Koch, R. & Brady, B. (2000). Pen pals: correspondence as a method for data generation in qualitative research. *Journal of Advanced Nursing*, 31(4), 909–17.

Kvale, S. (1996). *Interviews: an introduction to qualitative research interviewing.* Thousand Oaks, California, Sage.

Locsin, R. & Matua, A.G. (2002). The lived experience of waiting-to-know: ebola at Mbarara, Uganda—hoping for life, anticipating death. *Journal of Advanced Nursing*, 37(2), 173–81.

Maggs-Rapport, F. (2000). Combining methodological approaches in research: ethnography and interpretive phenomenology. *Journal of Advanced Nursing*, 31(1), 219–25.

Mason, L., Glenn, S., Walton, I. & Hughes, C. (2001). Women's reluctance to seek help for stress incontinence during pregnancy and following childbirth. *Midwifery*, 17, 212–21.

McCutcheon, H.H.I. & Pincombe, J. (2001). Intuition: an important tool in the practice of nursing. *Journal of Advanced Nursing*, 35(5), 342–48.

Melia, B. (2000). Conducting an interview. *Nurse Researcher*, 7(4), 75–89.

Minichiello, V., Aroni, R., Timewell, E. & Alexander, L. (1997). *In-depth interviewing.* (2nd ed.). Australia, Longman.

Offredy, M. (2000). Advanced nursing practice: the case of nurse practitioners in three Australian States. *Journal of Advanced Nursing*, 31(2), 274–81.

Orb, A., Eisenhauer, L. & Wynaden, D. (2000). Ethics in qualitative research. *Journal of Nursing Scholarship*, 33(1), 93–96.

Scott, D. (1997). The researcher's personal responses as a source of insight in the research process. *Nursing Inquiry*, 4, 130–34.

Street, A. (2001). The criteria for appropriateness and feasibility (editorial). *Nursing Inquiry*, 8, 1–2.

Taft, L.B. (1993). Computer-assisted qualitative research. *Research in Nursing & Health*, 16, 379–83.

Tetley, J. & Hanson, L. (2000). Participatory research. *Nurse Researcher*, 8(1), 69–88.

Wilton, T. & Kaufmann, T. (2001). Lesbian mothers' experiences of maternity care in the UK. *Midwifery*, 17, 203–11.

Yi, M. & Jezewski, M. A. (2000). Korean nurses' adjustment to hospitals in the United States of America. *Journal of Advanced Nursing*, 32(3), 721–29.

10

CHAPTER

Historical methods

Judith Godden and Sue Forsyth

LEARNING OUTCOMES

After reading this chapter the student should be able to:

- Understand the basic process involved in historical research.
- Define and identify primary and secondary sources in historical research.
- Recognise key questions to be asked when interpreting historical sources.
- Appreciate why historians value using different types of primary sources.
- Understand the purpose of footnotes and referencing in historical research.

Key terms

footnotes

historical research

primary sources

references

secondary sources

INTRODUCTION

Historical research is frequently likened to detective work: piecing together clues in order to arrive at the most probable solution to a question. It involves the collection, collation and critical analysis of surviving evidence which is interpreted in the context of its time and place. Historical research does not have a formula or a single historical method, just 'rules of evidence and guideposts to follow' (Lynaugh & Reverby, 1987, p. 4). As Cramer (1992, p. 5) stressed: 'Ultimately, writing history is an exercise of creative thought grounded in dimly perceived evidences of the past'. In this chapter the main rules of evidence and guideposts for imaginative, evidence-based nursing history are outlined.

There are many reasons for doing historical research, not the least because it can be an enjoyable and interesting hobby. Historical research is also an important means of understanding both the past and present. To ignore history is like gaining a new friend but refusing to hear anything about their life before you met them; subsequent knowing of your new friend would always be inadequate. As then Governor-General, Sir William Deane (1999, p. 47), explained paraphrasing the American author William Faulkner: 'The past is never fully gone. It is absorbed into the present and the future. It stays to shape what we are and what we do'. It would be difficult to understand today's nurses' roles, for example, without reference to an historically specific value system about sex roles (Versluysen, 1980).

Historical research should not be undertaken to confirm pre-existing convictions: 'You've got to keep the capacity to be surprised, to let the evidence change your mind' (Reynolds, 1992, p. 23). As indicated in the article associated with this chapter, for example, it has been (wrongly) assumed that Lucy Osburn as founder of Nightingale nursing in Australia, conformed to current ideas about the ideal Victorian-era nurse and lady (Godden & Forsyth, 2000). All good research must be open to the possibility that one's assumptions are wrong or inapplicable.

The best advice for researching history is to read good history. When reading, try to think what it is about the information that is interesting, attractive and worth pursuing. Good historical research depends on sound and intensive research, good writing skills and the writer's ability to appeal to one's historical imagination so that the differences and similarities about the past are understood. McCalman (1998, p. vii) does this in her foreword to a history of the Royal Women's Hospital in Melbourne:

> On 22 January 1866 at two o'clock in the morning, Miss Bridget Kelly, aged twenty-two and born in Ireland, delivered herself of a baby daughter in the Melbourne suburb of Prahran. She knew she needed help … We don't know how long it took her to walk the four miles … It was dark and the roads unlit … she found the Melbourne Hospital … But it was the wrong place … she needed the Lying-in Hospital, further up the hill … The hill became steeper … But this time she was taken in … and it was discovered that she 'had the infant in her arms with the *funis* and placenta attached'.

By this simple evocative story, constructed from the casebooks of the hospital, we learn the harsh realities of life for working class women in the mid-nineteenth century and how essential were the services offered by the hospital. It sets the scene and illustrates our shared humanity with the people we are studying.

Like other disciplines, historical research was influenced by positivism, including an optimistic belief that an objective truth not only existed but everyone reading an historical work could identify with its truth. The historian's task was to simply gather the facts of history which would then speak for themselves. More recently, post-modernism has challenged these beliefs, especially the belief that we could know and recognise an objective truth. Before the post-modernist debate, however, Carr (1961, pp. 26–27) pointed out that it does not follow that, because a mountain appears to take on different shapes from different angles of vision, it has objectively either no shape at all or an infinity of shapes. It does not follow that, because interpretation plays a necessary part in establishing the facts of history, and because no existing interpretation is wholly objective, one interpretation is as good as another.

One form of problematic interpretation is known as Whig history. Whig history emphasises progress in history through evolutionary advancement and assumes that the past inevitably leads to the present pinnacle of enlightenment. The problem with such histories is that the past is presented as ratifying, if not glorifying, the present (Davies, 1980). For example, the assumption that nursing training in hospitals was the result of strong matrons succeeding in imposing their will may be far from accurate (Godden & Forsyth, 2000). The opposite problem to Whig history is nostalgia, when the past is seen as a place of safety, certainty and purer values. The assumption that nurses should return to hospital training is frequently due to nostalgic memories of the past. When undertaking historical research, you view a mountain (of evidence) from certain perspectives. These perspectives need to be tempered with as much impartiality and rigour as possible.

SECONDARY SOURCES

Once an area of interest has been tentatively identified, the next step in historical research is to look at what evidence has already been uncovered and interpreted, that is, the secondary sources should be read. These are interpretations of the past produced after the period being researched. Most secondary sources are books, articles or theses but not all are written works. There are a number of useful films, for example, about nursing history.

Secondary sources are read for two main reasons. First, these sources provide important context. Nursing does not exist in isolation to surrounding social, economic and political events. If writing about the 1890s, for example, it is important to understand that Australia was in a major depression. A number of reputable general histories of Australia provide this essential context, such as the Oxford History of Australia series (e.g. Macintyre, 1986) and *The Macquarie Book of Events* (Fraser, 1983). Secondly, secondary sources are read to find specific information and to avoid undertaking research into a question that has already been well researched. Reading secondary sources and later researching the primary sources, enables a constant refining of the research question or area.

Like all sources, secondary sources need to be evaluated. More reliable sources include those with in-built quality checks (such as refereed journals) and whose authors provide checkable evidence for their claims, usually in footnotes. Historical knowledge, like all other sources of knowledge, dates. Many older secondary sources will still be valid; others will be hopelessly superseded by new evidence, new understandings such as those provided by feminism, and more rigorous standards of analysis.

A good place to start when researching a prominent nurse such as Lucy Osburn, for example, is the multi-volumed *Australian Dictionary of Biography* (Ritchie, 1996), which includes short articles on individuals by reputable researchers. Databases such as CINAHL are useful, albeit limited sources, as are bibliographies of healthcare (e.g. Department of Community Services and Health, 1988). If access to a large research library is available, useful references can be found by a keyword search of the catalogue and by browsing through selected journals. Refereed journals only publish articles well grounded in research. Relevant Australian journals include *Nursing Inquiry*, *Health and History*, *Australian Historical Studies* and *Labour History*. Conference proceedings, especially those that focus on the history of medicine (McCarthy, 1999), or edited collections (Rafferty, Robinson & Elkan, 1997), also provide good starting places for secondary sources in nursing history.

Many secondary sources about nursing are histories of a hospital or organisation. Particular care must be taken with works commissioned, funded or facilitated by organisations whose history it is: few organisations will employ or help fund an historian if they think the result will be critical of the organisation. Nevertheless, such books are valuable sources, especially for understanding general developments as they affected specific institutions. Others such as Strachan (1996) and Bessant and Bessant (1991) provide valuable information about State-based developments. (See Chapter 3 for information on online databases.)

PRIMARY SOURCES

Primary sources are the mainstay of historical research and its main source of enjoyment and fascination; they are original sources, produced at the time of the events/issues. Much of the skill of the historian lies in the ability to locate all available primary sources and to use unlikely sources to extrapolate otherwise unobtainable information (Tosh, 1999). Primary sources are mostly written documents, some in manuscript form such as letters, minutes and diaries, while others are in printed form such as examination papers, newspapers, books, journals, annual reports and government papers. Godden and Forsyth (2000) use a range of primary sources, including letters to Florence Nightingale and institutional records of Royal Prince Alfred Hospital.

Non-written sources of evidence should not be overlooked. Cartoons, photographs and advertisements in newspapers and journals can be as revealing as the accompanying text. For example, Russell (1990) uses cartoons to illustrate the problems of the nursing shortages in the 1970s, and there is the moving film of the Victorian nurses' strike (Everell & Brown, 1986). Paintings and photographs are more than a source of illustrations. Photographs, like other sources, reflect the viewpoint of the photographer: they are frequently staged and need to be interpreted. Artefacts such as uniforms and badges also provide evidence of conditions and attitudes. The uniforms of hospital-based nursing students with their aprons, caps and capes, have yielded a rich source of analysis about the domestic service, religious and middle class origins of nursing ideology. Such artefacts can be viewed in museums of nursing, health and medicine, many of which are associated with large teaching hospitals. Material evidence from the built environment, such as the architecture of nurses' homes and hospitals, is also a crucial source of evidence.

Oral history is an example of a source straddling the distinction between primary and secondary sources. Oral history refers to interviews with people, usually at a later date, about historical events. Despite being produced after the event, the information is generally counted as a primary source. Oral history is especially important because so much about nursing was not written down. Frequently the only way to learn about past nursing practice is to talk to older or retired nurses. The best oral history practitioners understand the importance of the present in shaping memories of the past and treat oral sources with the same combination of respect and scepticism as any other source of evidence. Thomson (1994) illustrates how private memories are shaped by public ideologies. Oral history is usually less reliable regarding precise details but can be highly reliable in understanding individual perspectives on past events. Like all types of evidence, oral history is best used in conjunction with other sources of information (e.g. Castle, 1984; Durdin, 1999). Similarly, reminiscences by individual nurses are also useful sources of evidence but must be used on the understanding that they represent just one person's view and are rarely based on thorough research (e.g. Hamilton, 1989).

An historical research project is not feasible without sufficient primary sources of evidence. Parts of the past which were unrecorded, or where primary source records have been destroyed, are lost forever. Sometimes primary sources are found serendipitously. For example, few primary sources about nursing practice in Australian hospitals in the 1820s remain. Other potential projects, such as the writings of Florence Nightingale, suffer from a surfeit of sources. In these cases, the project is normally limited so that mastery of the sources is possible for a researcher with limited time.

Analysing primary sources

Historical research using primary sources suffers from many disadvantages: knowledge about the past cannot be gained through direct observation or replicated in an experiment. Most historians are also eclectic in their approach to theory and rarely draw on any one definitive approach. Instead of certainty and well-defined method, historical research emphasises the art and technique of assessing evidence in all its forms.

The usual procedure is to 'amass as many pieces of evidence as possible from a wide range of sources—preferably from all the sources that have a bearing on the problem' (Tosh, 1999, p. 65). Baly (1996, p. 71) pointed out that histories 'written entirely from official papers are usually not only unbalanced but also dull'. Histories written almost entirely from a more interesting source, such as letters or oral history, may not be so dull but their viewpoint will be unbalanced. The ideal bibliography for an historical research project should include a variety of works such as private papers, institutional or government records, contemporary newspapers or journal articles.

Historical research is evidence based and it is important that the document used is genuinely what it purports to be. Authenticity is not usually a problem for historical researchers despite some well publicised cases of fraud. If in doubt, consult a reputable librarian, archivist or experienced historian. Claims must be based on evidence and, most importantly, no claims should be made that are known to be contrary to the evidence (Cramer, 1992). Perhaps the easiest way evidence can be misused is by selectively quoting, or paraphrasing, out of context. Claims must also be proportional to the reliability and representativeness of the source. A brilliantly evocative account of a nurse's life in the 1950s, for example, remains just one account unless other evidence indicates it is representative or typical.

Chronology has a particular role to play in constructing an historical argument. For example, the Nightingale Pledge, as repeated by generations of graduating nurses, cannot be used as an example of Florence Nightingale's (1820–1910) views, but only as a later interpretation of her views. The pledge was written in 1893 by an American nurse, Lystra Gretter (Seymer, 1954). To be used as an example of Nightingale's views, it would be necessary to uncover evidence that Nightingale knew and approved of the pledge.

The reliability of a source can only be judged through knowledge of the historical context and understanding of human motivations of the time. Basic questions to ask are 'How, when and why did that particular record come into existence?'. That is, we can only judge reliability by understanding 'the intention and prejudices of the writer' (Tosh, 1991, p. 61). Understanding the author's intentions is not to say that the information given is wrong, just highly shaped by particular needs and interests. Primary sources are generated for all sorts of purposes but rarely to provide an unbiased account for an historian. However, bias does not make an historical source invalid. Understanding the bias and the intentions of the writer can be of enormous help in understanding the context of the times and the motivations of the people studied (Tosh, 1999).

When critically examining a document for the author's intentions, it is useful to recall Rice-Davies' comment when giving evidence in 1963 about a spy and prostitution scandal. When told that Lord Astor denied her allegations about sex parties, her famous reply was: 'He would [say that], wouldn't he?' (*Oxford Dictionary of Quotations*, 1999, p. 626). Annual reports of institutions are usually produced to report successes or to raise money. As Rice-Davies said, they would say that, wouldn't they?

The importance of the intention of the author is also reflected in a major problem in nursing history: that the caricature of Sairey Gamp created by Charles Dickens was taken as a literal representation of pre-Nightingale nurses. More astute historians have pointed out that, while grounded in reality, nursing reformers used the image of Gamp to emphasise their difference and success (Dingwall, Rafferty & Webster, 1988). They would, wouldn't they?

Analysis of specialised types of documents generates additional questions. Newspaper sources need to be read understanding their editorial policies, their market and reader profile, their political bias and that of their owner (Baly, 1996). Similarly, much historical material was written to be prescriptive, not descriptive. Thus, textbooks and procedure manuals are very good sources for what nursing practices were prescribed and what was ideally meant to happen. They have less validity when used as evidence of what actually happened.

Generally, it is best if your purpose for using the documents does not coincide with the purpose of the writer. Godden and Forsyth (2000), for instance, quote a letter from Onslow to indicate how Osburn did not conform to the later stereotype of the Nightingale nurse, whereas the original writer was simply recording her impressions of Osburn. This example also indicates how documents meant to be private are normally much more revealing than documents written for an audience. Assumptions about the privacy of documents, however, must be questioned. Often, letters were written with the expectation that, as happened to Onslow's letter, they would be passed on to others to read. The source also tends to be more valid if, as in the above case, the author of the original document has first-hand experience of the events mentioned: hearsay was no more reliable a hundred years ago than it is now. For the same reason, it is best if authors write about something they have sufficient insight or expertise to understand and accurately describe.

An important aspect of interpreting primary sources of evidence is understanding that the 'past is a foreign country' (Lowenthal, 1985, p. xvii). In historical research, 'presentism' must be avoided by questioning every assumption. One common assumption is that words in the past have the same meaning as they have now (Lowenthal, 1985). The word 'nurse', for example, is highly problematic for nursing historians. However, as noted in Godden and Forsyth (2000), the distinction between a nurse and a doctor has not always been clear. Another common problem is to omit mental health nurses from an understanding of past nurses (Godden, Curry & Delacour, 1993).

Similar care must be taken in adopting the terminology of the past, with all its ideological baggage. For example, Australian nineteenth-century records will often record the names of men but not the names of women or non-Anglo-Saxon men. Other records refer to high-status women such as matrons as 'Miss' or 'Mrs', while lower status men and women were referred to using only a first name or surname. To reproduce this terminology without question is also to reproduce nineteenth-century notions of gendered class and status.

Silences, or what is not recorded, can be just as revealing as what is recorded: the silences reveal much about perceptions of what was important. In the case of women and nurses, the silences could also reveal notions that women were seen as belonging to the private sphere and that it was inappropriate for women to be named in a public document. Other notable silences can occur when documents repeatedly praise a member of staff, and then no longer do so. Such a change may mean a change in writer, or an indication of a major dispute within the institution.

At first sight, statistical compilations may seem to be free from bias. Rows of precise figures can be enticing, and certainly such sources as statistical registers and census returns are important. Like all sources of evidence, however, they must be used with caution. Deacon (1985) pointed out a major bias in census returns: whether or not a woman is counted in the workforce heavily depended on the statistician's ideology. Nurses working part-time and/or as married women before 1966 were more likely to be counted as dependents than in the workforce. The resulting estimated numbers of nurses are likely to be a significant under-estimation.

WRITING UP AND CONCLUSION

There are three main, and overlapping, stages of historical research: the search for sources of information; critical analysis of the material; and then synthesis and evaluation of the evidence collected. The later stage involves compiling all the evidence gathered and weighing it up in terms of comparative reliability and validity. The synthesised result is then usually written either chronologically and/or thematically. The use of footnotes or in-text references enables readers to locate and check for themselves the interpretation of the sources of evidence used.

The final result, whether a piece of written work, film or exhibition, should be a product which a reasonable person would want to read or view. The argument should be shaped by extensive and intensive sources of evidence, interpreted with logic and clarity of thought, but fired in the kiln of imagination and humanity.

KEY POINTS

- Historical research is the collection, collation and critical analysis of empirical evidence about the past that is interpreted in the context of its time and place.
- Historical methodology has three main, but overlapping, stages: searching for the sources; critical analysis of the material; and synthesis and evaluation of the evidence collected.
- Primary sources are the original sources produced at the time of an event; they provide the evidence of historical research and different perspectives on an issue.
- Secondary sources in history are interpretations of the past produced after the period being researched and provide context.
- Evidence needs to be analysed in terms of its inherent biases—understanding who produced it and how, when and why.
- Imagination grounded in extensive research and a sound understanding of context is essential.
- Footnotes/references provide sources of evidence so claims can be checked, and extended, by other researchers.

CRITICAL THINKING CHALLENGES

- Can historians ever be objective? Give reasons and examples to explain your answer.
- What sources would a future historian need to get an accurate picture of nursing/nursing education at your workplace/educational institution?
- Compare a current textbook in use to teach a nursing subject with one published decades ago. What do the main differences and similarities tell us?
- A nursing history research article you are reading is written primarily from secondary sources. How is this problematic?

Additional resources

Brush, B. & Stuart, M. (1994). Unity amidst difference: the ICN project and writing international nursing history. *Nursing History Review*, 2, 191–204.

Hisama, K. (2001). Patterns of Japanese clinical nursing: a historical analysis. *Journal of Clinical Nursing*, 10(4), 451–54.

Nelson, S. (1997). Reading nursing history. *Nursing Inquiry*, 4, 229–36.

Pickering, A. (1992). *Science as practice and culture*. Chicago, University of Chicago Press.

Rafferty, A. (1991). Historical knowledge. In Robinson, K.M. & Vaughn, B., eds, *Knowledge for practice.* London, Heinemann.

Strachan, G. (1995). 'A good nurse cannot be bought with money': the development of the professional and industrial roles of the nursing organisation in Queensland, Australia, 1904–1950. *Nursing History Review*, 3, 235–56.

Walker, K. (1994). Confronting 'reality': nursing science and the micropolitics of representation. *Nursing Inquiry*, 1(1), 46–56.

11

CHAPTER

Grounded theory

Merilyn Annells

LEARNING OUTCOMES

After reading this chapter the student should be able to:

- Identify the key purpose of grounded theory method.
- Explain how and why grounded theory can inform nursing practice.
- Identify and explain the key components of grounded theory method.
- Discuss how a grounded theory can be generated (or constructed).
- Recognise different versions of grounded theory method.
- Distinguish between grounded theory research and other types of research, including those that may use some research process elements and techniques traditional to grounded theory method.
- Evaluate, at a beginning level, the worthiness of grounded theory research results.
- At a beginning level, present ideas about the possible and/or desirable future of grounded theory research for informing nursing practice.

Key terms

axial coding

basic social process

coding framework

constant comparative analysis

core category

open coding

Paradigm Model

selective coding

theoretical coding

theoretical sampling

theoretical saturation

theoretical sensitivity

INTRODUCTION

Australians have not traditionally talked about someone or something being 'grounded', but the term 'down to earth' remains common, as does 'feet on the ground'. All these expressions metaphorically infer that there is an admirable, sensible and positive connection to what happens in actuality rather than being unconnected—'up in the air'.

Barney Glaser and the late Anselm Strauss, two non-nurse sociologists in a US-based department of nursing doctoral studies in the 1960s, formulated techniques for generating theory about social processes so that the theory is 'grounded', rather than the product of 'armchair' theorising. That is, instead of someone coming up with a theory from just sitting and thinking, the theory originates from analysing data collected from where human action and interaction occurs, from speaking with and listening to those who have been engaged in the action and interaction, and perhaps from documents pertaining to the action and interaction. Theory grounded in this manner was considered by them to produce more useful, pragmatic outcomes than what arises from pure theorising.

'Grounded theory' within research discourse refers to the method initially developed and introduced by Glaser and Strauss (1967) and as further discussed by them (Corbin & Strauss, 1990, 1996; Glaser, 1978, 1992, 1999; Strauss, 1987, 1993; Strauss & Corbin, 1990, 1994, 1997, 1998; see this chapter's 'Additional resources' on pages 177–78 for other readings), and others (e.g. Charmaz, 1994, 1995, 2000).

It is important to understand that although grounded theory research analyses mostly qualitative data, quantitative data can also be collected and analysed. Therefore, grounded theory is not essentially only a 'qualitative' research method.

PURPOSE OF GROUNDED THEORY

Grounded theory is popular among some nurse researchers, sociologists, and researchers in other healthcare professions, education, management and business studies. These days, grounded theory research is not necessarily just focused on social processes but has also evolved to explain human action and interaction in social, psycho-social or spiritual dimensions of life.

Nursing practice involves not only applying so-called factual knowledge about the physical body, but also knowledge about 'the person' regarding social, psychological and spiritual dimensions of being. Human action and interaction are intrinsic to how and why people approach and respond to health issues in their lives. Helping people deal with the impact of health issues multi-dimensionally upon their lives and quality of life may be the 'real stuff' of nursing care (Annells & Koch, 2001), and may be that which somewhat sets nursing apart from other healthcare professions. So, grounded theory nursing research provides understandings (Artinian, 1998) that can potentially be very useful for effective, best practice nursing care.

Grounded theory nursing research, according to the area of interest, tends to concentrate on either the patient primarily, the nurse involved in nurse–patient action and interaction, or both. Table 11.1 presents recent examples of Australian and New Zealand grounded theory nursing research and lists the research focuses, which encompass action and interaction in either the social, psycho-social or spiritual dimensions of people, or combinations thereof.

TABLE 11.1 Australian and New Zealand grounded theory research examples

RESEARCH PROJECT	FOCUS
Concentration on patients	
Holliday, Lowe & Outram, 2000	Women presenting for treatment after a myocardial infarction.
Higgins, Dunn & Theobald, 2000	Recovery after coronary angioplasty.
Irurita, 1999a, 1999b	Delivery of quality nursing care—patient's perspective.
Thomas & Retsas, 1999	Developing a spiritual perspective to strengthen approach to life and death when terminally ill.
Thornhill & Stevens, 1998	Cardiac rehabilitation.
Reaby, 1998	Breast restoration decision making.
Concentration on nurses	
Watters, 2000	Nurses teaching psychiatric patients about their medicines.
O'Connell, 2000	Nurses determining, delivering and communicating patient care in acute care hospitals.
St John, 1999	Role of the community health nurse in Australia.
Williams, 1998	Delivery of quality nursing care—nurse's perspective.
Pearson, 1998	Empowering nursing students in a clinical context.
Woods, 1997	Maintaining a nursing ethic.
Concentration on patients and nurses	
Henderson, 2000	Facilitating patient participation.
Seibold, Miller & Hall, 1999	Partnership between midwives and women.
Annells, 1997a	Nurse–patient interaction when a patient has a flatus problem.

Levels and types of grounded theory

Strauss and Corbin (1998, p. 25) define theorising as 'the act of constructing from data an explanatory scheme that systematically integrates various concepts through statements of relationship'. A grounded theory is most likely to be a middle-range theory, that is more than some working hypotheses used in everyday life but not an all-inclusive 'grand' theory beyond the context of human action and interaction (Glaser & Strauss, 1967). Grounded theory is usually context dependent. The resultant theory may be about a substantive area (e.g. seeking solutions to 'nits' in a child's hair) or is formal theory developed from data across various substantive areas about an abstract over-arching issue (e.g. regarding 'stigma' from researching actions and interactions of people feeling stigmatised for various reasons, including those impacted upon by 'nit' infestation).

Most grounded theories about nursing are substantive, though some formal theory development is occurring, such as theorising about the process of 'negotiating' in regard to women carers interacting with professionals in helping systems (Wuest, 2000). However, not all reported 'grounded theory research' has fully engaged in theorising. In grounded theory development, according to Strauss and Corbin (1998), there are three levels:

- Description—using language to convey ideas that purport to describe aspects of the action and interaction.
- Conceptual ordering—organising ideas into abstract concepts and grouping (classifying) these into like-groups (categories) and possibly sub-groups (sub-categories) in order to make sense of action and interaction.
- An explanatory scheme—offers plausible but contextualised explanatory relationships between the categories (and includes also the levels of description and conceptual ordering).

Some reports of grounded theory nursing research offer conceptual ordering rather than explanatory scheme grounded theories. Glaser (1999) says this type of research results in 'theory bits' that lead to 'story-talk' or an 'incident trip' rather than an integrated, multivariate theory. Conceptual ordering can, however, usefully inform nurses about human action and interaction; for instance to gain basic understanding that builds empathy or that assists in communicating meaningfully with patients.

It is increasingly being accepted that grounded theory does not offer prediction (i.e. if this happens, then that will occur), unlike theory developed in other sciences such as physics, chemistry or bio-science, where so-called factual laws or 'truths' can be 'found'. Human action and interaction is so subject to individual variation (even within similar cultures and with similar contextual factors), that there is no certainty able to be predicted. Rather, likely possibilities are presented according to a carefully and systematically researched explanatory scheme, where a contextualised 'plausible explanation of some phenomenon' (Miller & Fredericks, 1999, p. 543) is offered as well as 'an inductive argument for its plausibility' (Miller & Fredericks, 1999, p. 550).

FRAMEWORK

It is generally agreed that the framework of a grounded theory is that which is developed from data analysed to form and support the grounded theory developed through the research. That is, the theoretical framework 'evolves during the research itself' (Strauss & Corbin, 1990, p. 49). However, broad theoretical stances may in some way overall inform the theorising 'lens' of the researcher from the beginning. Therefore, grounded theorists may:

1. value a certain type of broad theoretical stance to look productively at data and do so deliberately
2. neither deliberately use a broad theoretical stance nor actively seek to not use it
3. actively seek to not use any broad theoretical stance.

Regarding the first option, the selected broad theoretical stance can vary, with some examples being:

- symbolic interactionism (underpinning the initial formulation of grounded theory method)
- continual permutations of action (Strauss, 1993)
- types of feminism (e.g. Keddy, Sims & Stern, 1996; Wuest, 1995, 2000).

Apart from a broad theoretical stance being a theorising 'lens' overall, it is also possible that more narrow theories may be selected to guide theorising at some point(s) during development. As Strauss and Corbin (1990, p. 50) state, 'you can incorporate seemingly relevant elements of previous theory, but only as they prove themselves to be pertinent to the data gathered in the study'.

The second option seems to be quite common for grounded theory nursing research, although some researchers realise the subconscious influence of a personal broad stance theory about human action and interaction formed by a collected store of integrated ideas from many sources (e.g. Annells, 1997a). Within this option, as also with the third option, there may also be some conscious, deliberate use of appropriate narrow theories at some points in theory development.

There is a debate among methodologists as to whether the third option can be totally achieved, and whether even striving for it is wise and justifiable. This debate relates to whether grounded theory is (or should be considered) objectivist or constructivist (Charmaz, 2000).

Objectivism and constructivism

Grounded theory research can be conducted according to a variety of perspectives about what can be known concerning human action and interaction, and how it can be known (Annells, 1996, 1997b; Benoliel, 1996). Objectivism considers that as in the natural sciences, there are realities/truths/facts (an object) to be revealed, albeit that in human 'social' science reality can only be incompletely revealed. Objectivist grounded theory aims to find and uncover what is believed to be 'there' (to be real) about human action and interaction, and to do so rigorously, seeking to limit 'bias' using specified technique. The theory is thought to purely 'emerge'. Data must not be 'fitted' specifically to previous ideas, notions and theories about the research focus (though a broad theoretical stance is acceptable, such as symbolic interactionism), and prescription may be possible.

In contrast, constructivism considers that in human 'social' science there are multiple, constructed realities, subject and relative to the opinion of the person experiencing and the person theorising. Constructivist grounded theorists view their research product (theory) as representing one of multiple, intangible realities about what may be happening regarding human action and interaction. Suitable research techniques are applied, realising that there can be flexibility in aspects of technique. The theory is 'constructed'. One's theorising 'lens' is shaped by factors such as culture, political ideology, moral stance, or discourse as either personally selected or inculcated, conscious or subconscious. However, rather than this resulting in damaging 'bias' in grounded theory research, it is believed that multiple factors inherent in personal meaning–making assist creativity, and are intrinsically tied to why there are multiple realities about what and why things happen in human action and interaction.

APPROACH

The classic grounded theory method, as formulated and published originally by Glaser and Strauss (1967), has been subject to modification until at present there are multiple approaches to, or versions of, the method (e.g. Strauss & Corbin, 1998; Charmaz, 1994, 1995, 2000). These versions primarily reflect different ideas about how data are analysed to the point that a theory results. However, some other ideas pertaining to the method differ. Researchers aligned with either classic grounded theory method or one of the newer versions may claim that their favoured version is 'correct' or 'more useful' (e.g. Chenitz & Swanson, 1986; Melia, 1996). Glaser, who champions the classic method (http://www.groundedtheory.com), has sometimes criticised modifications of the method, especially as delineated by Strauss and Corbin (1990, 1994, 1998).

Most commonly, either classic grounded theory or the more recent Strauss and Corbin (1990, 1994, 1998) version is used within grounded theory nursing research. It is generally accepted that classic grounded theory was developed from an objectivist perspective regarding human science. There are differing views about whether Strauss and Corbin's version is objectivist or leaning towards constructivism (Annells, 1996, 1997c; Charmaz, 2000; Hall & Callery, 2001), while Charmaz's (2000) version is ostensibly constructivist.

However, most importantly, a grounded theorist is not bound to approach their research focus in an objectivist or a constructivist manner by following either the classic or a more recent version of grounded theory method. There is freedom to design the project according to an objectivist or a constructivist perspective (usually, but not necessarily, to reflect one's own philosophical view about human 'social' science enquiry) and applying a suitable adaptation of either the classic or another version of grounded theory (Annells, 1997b).

While the variety of versions can be frustrating for someone planning a grounded theory research project, this situation provides choice and an enhanced possibility of also being able to justify analysis and theorisation steps that suit your own philosophical, cognitive and meaning–making processes, as appreciated by Annells (1997a), Charmaz (2000) and Eaves (2001). To adopt and adapt the method is common (Glaser, 1999).

Fundamental elements

Despite there being various versions of how to 'do' grounded theory research, the fundamental elements generally considered essential are:

- theoretical sampling
- constant comparative data analysis
- theoretical sensitivity
- memo writing
- identification of a core category
- a resultant explanatory theory.

One or some of these elements may also be included within research that is different in design and intent to grounded theory. For instance, constant comparative data analysis and open or axial coding have been applied to other methods. Sometimes research using one or several elements of grounded theory method, and/or use data coding techniques are presented as using a 'grounded theory approach'. This does not render the research less in status, just different in purpose and outcome. Therefore, grounded theory method development has introduced elements and techniques valuable to other methods of research.

SAMPLING

Grounded theory method focuses on samples of events and incidents pertaining to the research interest, rather than people (populations) per se (Strauss & Corbin, 1998), although people will be involved in the events and incidents. Statistical samples conforming to probability sampling rules are not applicable to grounded theory method. Initially, researchers will purposefully select a site where it is believed that there is the maximum possibility of data collection occurring related to the research interest (Glaser, 1978). Strauss and Corbin (1998) state that although maximising the potential to gain relevant data is most important, accompanying reasons for selecting the initial sample may include:

- deciding what type of data may first need to be acquired (e.g. interview data)
- accessibility, including the likelihood of gaining permission to enter a site from institutional ethics committees and management, and also accessibility of potential participants involved in relevant events and incidents
- available resources, including the researcher's time and budget.

Theoretical sampling

Once analysis commences (which starts as soon as initial data have been collected), sampling is directed and controlled by theory development that suggests the characteristics of incidents and events needing to next be accessed for further development of the theory. This is theoretical sampling, defined by Glaser (1978, p. 36) as 'the process of data collection for generating theory whereby the analyst jointly collects, codes, and analyses his data and decides which data to collect next and where to find them, in order to develop his theory as it emerges'. Thus the developing emergence (or construction) of theory controls the process of data collection.

Operational memos written during data analysis theorising can direct theoretical sampling. Theoretical sampling is a form of purposeful sampling (Coyne, 1997) with sampling becoming more purposeful and focused 'until all categories are saturated; that is, no new or significant data emerges, and categories are well developed ...' (Strauss & Corbin, 1998, p. 215). Sampling includes looking for negative cases, and may require multiple sites. The researcher may 'begin with a single site, develop initial theory; then utilising theoretical sampling move to the multiple sites' (Strauss, 1987, p. 275). O'Connell (2000), researching how and why nurses determine, deliver and communicate care in selected acute care settings, sampled incidents and events guided by theoretical sampling within five acute care settings.

All versions of grounded theory method stipulate theoretical sampling as an essential element of the research process, as outlined in Table 11.2. A difference exists in that Corbin and Strauss (1996) stipulate three forms of coding (open, axial and selective coding—to be discussed in the next section of this chapter), and direct that the focus of theoretical sampling changes according to the type of coding in which the researcher is primarily engaged at that time.

TABLE 11.2 Comparison of the procedural steps of two versions of grounded theory method

	CLASSIC GROUNDED THEORY METHOD	STRAUSS AND CORBIN'S GROUNDED THEORY METHOD
Sampling	Theoretical sampling directed by emerging codes until categories are saturated.	Theoretical sampling: open, relational/variational, and discriminative.
Sources of theoretical sensitivity	Knowledge of coding families, conceptual ability, and literature.	Professional and personal experience, literature, and the analytic process.
Constant comparative data analysis		
Coding:	Open and theoretical.	Open, axial and selective.
Coding framework:	Choice from multiple coding families depending on best 'fit' to data.	Specified coding framework named the 'Paradigm Model'.
Memos:	Primarily for sorting to form hypotheses.	Code, theoretical, and operational notes.
Focus on process:	Movement over time with at least two stages—a basic social process.	Linking of action/interaction sequences or non-progressive movement.
Category development:	Relevant categories and relevant properties emerge by comparing incident to incident and/or to concepts looking for the relevance, the fit, and emergent patterns until theoretical saturation occurs.	In terms of properties which are then dimensionalised and the categories grouped. Relationships validated against data. Gaps in categories are filled until theoretical saturation is reached.
Core category emergence:	The basic social process emerges and is the core category that accounts for most of the variation in the problematic pattern.	Explicating a story line about the central phenomenon around which other categories are integrated using the Paradigm Model.
Conditional/ consequential matrix:	Nil—micro levels of analysis only.	Specified—moves between micro and macro levels of analysis.

Reproduced from Annells, 1997c; used with permission.

DATA COLLECTION AND ANALYSIS

Benoliel (1996) opines that multiple types of data need to be collected for grounded theory research to be productive. However, the type and variety of data collected are determined by what events and incidents are pertinent to the human action and interaction being researched. Data are usually qualitative but may also be quantitative. Commonly, the types of data collected are:

- Interviewing—usually open-ended questions within a conversational semi-structured formal interview, although informal 'on-the-spot' interviews (chats) can also be used.

- Observation—either as a participant observer, an observer participant, or simply as an observer of pertinent events and incidents.
- Reading/studying documents that pertain to the events and incidents sampled.

For instance, O'Connell (2000) interviewed nurses, patients and patients' relatives, engaged in participant field observation, and studied patients' medical records. In addition, other ways of data collection relevant to the research focus can also be used, such as:

- 'Think-aloud sessions' where people record reflective thoughts and impressions into a hand-held audiotape recorder about events and incidents, e.g. patients when making self-management decisions about their diabetes (Thorne & Paterson, 2001).
- 'Focus groups' of people reflecting upon events and incidents experienced (e.g. St John, 1999, when using a focus group of community health nurses).

Aspects of data collection that may enhance (or restrict) grounded theory development need to be considered, such as the style of interviewing (Wimpenny & Gass, 2000) or the suitability of using focus groups (Webb & Kevern, 2001).

Ways of data collection are being debated as to whether (or to what degree) data are actually 'collected' or whether data are co-constructed by the researcher and the people communicating experiences about events and situations (Charmaz, 2000). Some constructivist grounded theorists prefer to use terms like 'generation of text' rather than 'data collection' (e.g. Annells, 1997a).

Constant comparative data analysis

According to Glaser and Strauss (1967), rather than a researcher going out and collecting a whole body of data, then fracturing data into abstract concepts, then later integrating concepts into categories, a grounded theorist collects some data then pauses to commence data analysis before collecting more data to pause again for analysis to occur. There is a 'continuously growing process' where the researcher:

- compares data about newly sampled incidents and situations to data about previously categorised incidents and situations
- integrates categories and properties (characteristics of a category)
- modifies and solidifies the integration (linking) of categories to form a theory
- and after a while, starts to write and re-write the theory.

It is, however, a 'back and forth' process with previously analysed data prone to being re-analysed in light of later analyses. As constant comparative data analysis occurs, decisions are being made as to what events and situations need next to be sampled. The intention is to develop a rich, dense, explanatory schema through a continual dialectic between constant comparative data analysis (text interpretation) and theoretical sampling.

Coding

Coding is the analytical process through which data are fractured (divided into abstract bits), conceptualised (abstracted grouping of fractured data) and integrated (linked) by the researcher. Classic grounded theory method talks primarily about just two forms of coding: open and theoretical coding (see Table 11.2). According to Glaser (1992), open coding is considered to be the looking for underlying meaning, uniformity or pattern in and across data with the researcher remaining 'open' to possibilities and not trying to fit data to preconceived notions and ideas. Theoretical coding involves the connecting of categories formed through open coding with connections 'emerging' as relationships between categories and their properties (Glaser, 1992). 'Selective' coding is seen to be a subset of theoretical coding and is the point at which open coding ceases and analysis is focused on delimiting and refining integrated categories along the dimensional level to form a theory with 'validated' relationships among concepts, including selection and refinement of a core category (Strauss & Corbin, 1998).

However, other types of coding are possible, as proposed to be beneficial by Strauss and Corbin (1990, 1994, 1998), who suggest axial coding should occur between open and selective coding (see Table 11.2). Axial coding is defined as 'relating categories to their subcategories, termed "axial" because coding occurs around the axis of a category, linking categories at the level of properties and dimensions (Strauss & Corbin, 1998, p. 123). Therefore, categories are dimensionalised (ranges along which properties of a category vary). The suggestion to use axial coding is debated among grounded theorists (see a critique by Glaser, 1992), with some deciding not to use it (e.g. O'Connell, 2000), some finding it useful for theory development (e.g. Thomas & Retsas, 1999; see Figure 11.1), some finding it not useful when tried (e.g. Kendall, 1999), while others developed their own synthesis of various coding types (e.g. Eaves, 2001).

Core category

Grounded theory has a core category. Classic grounded theory seeks to discover a basic social process as a core category that has at least two phases and which accounts for most of the variation in the problematic pattern being researched. For instance, O'Connell (2000) theorises that a two-phase basic social process of 'enabling care: working through obscurity and uncertainty' is how nurses in acute care settings in Australia deal with the problem of 'unknowing' in regard to structuring nursing care.

Not all grounded theorists purport to identify a 'basic social process'. For instance, Strauss and Corbin (1998) advocate for the core category to be an explicated story line about a central phenomenon around which other categories are integrated with linked action/interaction sequences. An example is the grounded theory of Thomas and Retsas (1999) (see Figure 11.1) where a story line is presented of spiritually 'transacting self-preservation' when terminally ill.

Coding framework

Classic grounded theory method proposes that the researcher has flexibility in what manner coded categories are relationally linked (in a pattern) to each other to form a theory. Glaser (1978) listed 18 possible 'coding families', noting that there may be others possible, that they are not mutually exclusive, and there can be overlap. The 'coding family' used may be prompted by how the theorist likes to make sense of human action and interaction events and situations but, according to Glaser (1978), should also consciously be selected from a repertoire of coding families as appropriate for an emerging theory—that is, theory development should not be limited to just one pattern of integrating categories.

FIGURE 11.1 **Core category diagram**

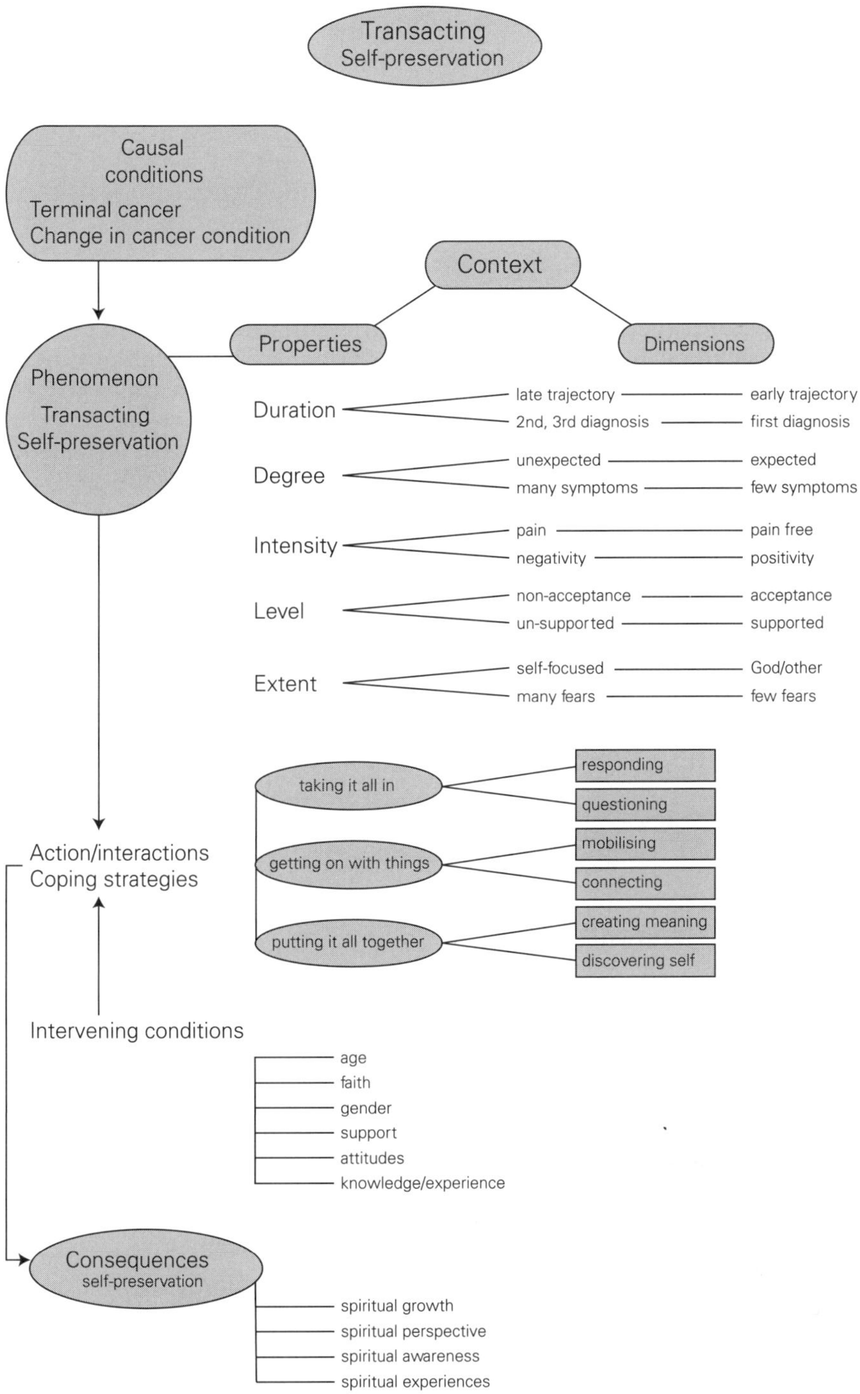

Reproduced from Thomas & Retsas, 1999; used with permission.

The Strauss and Corbin (1990, 1994, 1998) version of grounded theory method works with just one of these coding patterns (families) that they call the Paradigm Model, which provides understandings of causal, conditional and intervening factors related to context and with consequences (see Figure 11.1 as a result of using the Paradigm Model). This type of coding family uses a conditional/consequential matrix.

Therefore, grounded theorists have freedom about coding family (pattern) choice—one of the coding families listed by Glaser (1978), Strauss and Corbin's Paradigm Model in full or in part, or development of their own coding family (e.g. Eaves, 2001).

Memos

Constant comparative data analysis is facilitated by the writing of memos, which are notes written to yourself as researcher. Strauss and Corbin (1998, p. 110) define memos as a 'record of analysis, thoughts, interpretations, questions and directions ...' Memos can be different types, such as code, theoretical, and operational notes (directing modification of interview questions, theoretical sampling requirements, and possible literature to be read), and sub-varieties of these. Some computer software programs, such as NUD*IST, not only facilitate management of copious data but also the writing of memos (Bazeley, 1999; Morison & Moir, 1998).

Theoretical sensitivity

From an objectivist view, 'theoretical sensitivity' is being able to see what is supposedly present in the data, as explained by Glaser and Strauss (1967). Glaser (1978) has written a text on theoretical sensitivity where key sources are conceptual ability, knowledge of different coding families, and literature. Strauss and Corbin's (1990, p. 42) explanation of theoretical sensitivity is 'having insight, the ability to give meaning to data, the capacity to understand, and capability to separate the pertinent from that which isn't'. Professional experience, personal experience, certain techniques in analytical process, and literature, are proposed as key sources of theoretical sensitivity. When and why to use pertinent literature in grounded theory research is a debatable point (Cutcliffe, 2000) but the use of literature to enhance theoretical sensitivity is widely agreed.

Theoretical saturation

Theoretical sampling and constant comparative data analysis (with various forms of coding) continue until new data are either not adding to variations in major patterns theorised, or only providing additions in minor ways (Strauss & Corbin, 1998). The theory is said to be 'saturated'. However, the veracity of any such statement is open to debate and some grounded theorists avoid making this declaration (e.g. Charmaz, 2000).

CRITERIA FOR EVALUATING GROUNDED THEORY

There is also debate concerning how to judge or evaluate whether a grounded theory is worthy of application or not to nursing practice. Table 11.3 lists varying sets of evaluation criteria. Strauss and Corbin (1998) state that their suggested criteria are not absolute rules but guidelines, and that grounded theorists may compile their own criteria for quality in research process and product, but they should list those criteria when reporting the research. There are other suggested ways of judging grounded theory, including addressing post-modern concerns by using criteria evaluating reflexivity and contextualisation (Charmaz, 2000; Cutcliffe, 2000; Seale, 1999) with perhaps the inclusion of relationality criteria, which address power and trust relationships between participants and researchers (Hall & Callery, 2001).

TABLE 11.3 Comparison of the criteria for judging grounded theory according to two versions of the method

CLASSIC GROUNDED THEORY METHOD (1967)	STRAUSS AND CORBIN'S GROUNDED THEORY METHOD (1998)
Judgements about the theory itself	**Judgements about research process**
1. Fit	1. How and on what grounds was the original sample selected?
2. Work	2. What major categories emerged?
3. Relevance	3. What were some of the indicators (events, incidents or actions) that point to some of these major categories?
4. Modifiability	4. On the basis of what categories did theoretical sampling proceed, how did theoretical formulations guide data collection, and how representative of data are the categories?
5. Parsimony and scope in explanatory power	5. What were some of the hypotheses pertaining to conceptual relations among categories and how formulated/validated?
	6. Were there incidences in which hypotheses did not explain data, were discrepancies accounted for, and hypotheses modified?
	7. How and why was the core category selected, was data collection gradual or sudden, difficult or easy, and on what grounds were final analytical decisions made?
	Judgements about empirical grounding
	1. Are concepts generated?
	2. Are concepts systematically related?
	3. Are there many conceptual linkages with categories well developed and having conceptual density?
	4. Is variation built into the theory?
	5. Are the conditions under which variation can be found built into the study and explained?
	6. Has process been taken into account?
	7. Do the theoretical findings seem significant and to what extent?
	8. Does the theory stand the test of time and become part of discussions and ideas exchanged among relevant social and professional groups?

Modified from Annells, M, 1997c; used with permission.

For nurses, the most stringent and vital of criteria and the ultimate test is whether the grounded theory informs nursing practice in a productive, useful manner so that ultimately there are positive gains for the patient. The usefulness of grounded theories when applied to nursing practice is rarely reported in the literature though, which is a deficit that needs to be addressed in the future. The future will, however, no doubt, bring a burgeoning of grounded theory nursing research, as it is realised that there is no one precise way of doing grounded theory, that the focus is not limited to studying just social interaction, that post-modern concerns can somewhat be addressed, and that there is freedom to select:

- an objectivist or a constructivist (or other) approach
- either a suitable or preferred broad theoretical stance, or have no ostensible broad theoretical stance
- techniques from a variety of grounded theory research process versions
- from among a variety of coding patterns (families), including what may arise from one's own cognitive reasoning.

Creativity is encouraged within parameters of certain elements as being part of the research process. There is, therefore, much potential for grounded theory research, in evolving forms, to increasingly inform multidimensional nursing practice.

KEY POINTS

- Grounded theory nursing research ideally offers constructed explanatory schemes (either as substantive or formal theory) about social, psycho-social, or spiritual dimensions of human action and interaction process, and can therefore inform and guide the practice of nursing.
- A grounded theory is constructed through data–theory interplay by constant comparative analysis of relevant data gained through theoretical sampling.
- Some grounded theory nursing research may not fully construct a theory (as explanatory theme) but may offer conceptual ordering about human action and interaction process.
- Grounded theory research is not essentially qualitative as quantitative data can also inform theorising.
- For a research project to be classified as grounded theory research, the present consensus is that certain fundamental elements of the research process should be applied.
- Although there are some generally specified essential elements of the research process, there are varying versions/modes of grounded theory method.
- The versions/modes offer varying suggestions about steps within the research process, such as how to proceed with coding and conceptualising data.
- Some steps of the research process and some qualitative data analysis techniques developed initially for grounded theory method may be used in other forms of research.

- Grounded theory research can be conducted according to a variety of philosophical perspectives about what can be known concerning human action and interaction, and how it can be known.
- Although the framework of a grounded theory is that which is constructed from data analysed, broad theoretical frameworks (e.g. symbolic interactionism or feminism) may inform theorising.
- There are a variety of criteria from which to select to evaluate the credibility and trustworthiness of grounded theory.
- Grounded theory method is evolving and responding to various contemporary concerns and debates about research methodology appropriate for human science, but continues to offer a product very useful to inform nursing practice.

CRITICAL THINKING CHALLENGES

- To what extent do you think it is possible to predict what may happen when an older person needs to find solutions to self-manage a health problem (e.g. constipation)? How could a grounded theory developed about action and interaction pertaining to this situation in one Australian State inform community nurses wanting to assist older people with this problem in that State and elsewhere—and in what contexts would it be potentially useful?
- From your experience and observation of nursing in acute care settings, how 'grounded' does the theory seem as proposed by O'Connell (2000)? Does this theory seem credible, and if so, why? Does your answer to these questions assist you in deciding how you would like (at least in part) to evaluate the quality of a grounded theory? If so, why? If not, why not?
- Study the recommendations suggested by O'Connell (2000) arising from her grounded theory research about ways to improve nursing care for patients in acute care settings. Discuss whether you think the research was worth doing, with reasons stated.
- Do you think that grounded theory nursing research should ideally be primarily concerned about patients, or nurses, or both patients and nurses, or are all required equally? Why?
- Think of specific human action and interaction relating to nursing practice about which you would like to see grounded theory developed relating to each of the social, psycho-social, or spiritual dimensions of people. Which would you personally prefer to develop, and why?

Additional resources

Glaser, B. (1991). In honour of Anselm Strauss: collaboration. In Maines, D., ed., *Social organisation and social process: essays in honour of Anselm Strauss*. New York, Aldine De Gruyter.

Glaser, B., ed. (1994). *Examples of grounded theory: a reader*. Mill Valley, Sociology Press.

Glaser, B. (1994). Introduction. In Glaser B., ed., *More grounded theory methodology: a reader*. Mill Valley, Sociology Press.

Glaser, B., ed. (1995). *Grounded theory, 1984–1994* (vols 1–2). Mill Valley, Sociology Press.

Glaser, B. (1998). *Doing grounded theory: issues and discussions.* Mill Valley, Sociology Press.

Glaser, B. (1999). The future of grounded theory. *Qualitative Health Research*, 9, 836–45.

Happ, M.B. & Kagan, S.H. (2001). Methodological considerations for grounded theory in critical care settings. *Nursing Research*, 50, 188–92.

Morgan, A.K. (2001). A grounded theory of nurse–client interactions in palliative care nursing. *Journal of Clinical Nursing*, 10, 583–84.

Strauss, A. (1994). Awareness contexts and grounded formal theory. In Glaser, B., ed., *More grounded theory methodology: a reader*. Mill Valley, Sociology Press.

Strauss, A. (1995). Notes on the nature and development of general theories. *Qualitative Inquiry*, 1, 7–18.

12
CHAPTER

Ethnography

Grace Tham

LEARNING OUTCOMES

After reading this chapter the student should be able to:

- Explain the relevance of ethnography in the study of cultures and sub-cultures.
- Describe the relationship between access, and covert and overt research.
- Identify the different types of sampling used.
- Explain the terms 'gatekeeping', 'reciprocity' and 'reflexivity'.
- List the different triangulation methods used to validate data.
- Compare the four types of participant observation.
- Explain the term 'informants'.
- Describe the different types of data that may be collected in ethnographic research.
- Describe how data can be managed during field work.
- Describe the steps in data analysis.
- List different ways to report ethnographic findings.
- Discuss the ethical issues confronting an ethnographer.

Key terms

access
anonymity
anthropology
culture
disengagement
emic/etic perspectives
ethnography
field work
gatekeepers
informants
participant observation
reciprocity
sampling
triangulation

INTRODUCTION

Ethnography is a qualitative research approach that is considered a 'naturalistic methodology'. In naturalistic research, the social world is observed in its 'natural' state, not manipulated and controlled, but respected and appreciated (Hammersley & Atkinson, 1983), to gain insights into the subjective experiences and actions of the people being observed so as to develop, test and refine theories. This chapter takes the reader through the processes of conducting and reviewing ethnographic research.

WHAT IS ETHNOGRAPHY?

The term 'ethnography' originates from the Greek word 'ethnos' and the Latin word 'graphia' (*Websters Dictionary*, 1972, p. 628). 'Ethnos' means character, customs, race or group (*Websters Dictionary*, 1972, p. 628); and 'graphia' means drawing, writing or description (*Websters Dictionary*, 1972, p. 795). Combining the terms therefore means writing about or the description of a custom, group or culture. Ethnography is considered synonymous with anthropology (the study of humankind), as ethnography is a category of anthropological research devoted to the descriptive study of cultures (Seymour-Smith, 1986, pp. 98–99). Brewer (2000) explains that ethnography is not a particular data collection method but a style of research with the objective to understand the activities and meanings of a social group. An ethnographic approach to research is now seen in the fields of anthropology of nursing, medicine, education, feminism and linguistics, to name a few.

Inherent in ethnography is the concept of culture. According to Spradley and McCurdy (1972, pp. 7–9) culture is the emotions, childbearing practices, art, law, institutions of society, as well as all the man-made artefacts, such as spears, cars and buildings, made by members of the group. Culture is knowledge learned, shared and understood by each member of the group so that their interactions and behaviours can be interpreted and understood by its members.

Ethnography is considered holistic as it aims to understand the behaviour of a group of people within the context of its culture. This is achieved by long periods of observation, the gathering of many kinds of data, and employing multiple methods and hypotheses to cover all aspects to form a picture of the social whole (Fetterman, 2000). This is to say that behaviours and events are studied in relation to other factors that may influence or generate the events and behaviours. Hanna (2001), in her ethnographic study of teenagers coping with motherhood, observed how teenagers coped with a six-month-old child and dependency on government supports and healthcare professionals. To gain a better understanding of the plight of the teenagers, she also studied their backgrounds, their family circumstances and their reasons for leaving home. What Hanna had done was to understand two different realities that impact on their behaviours: the realities from the viewpoint of the teenagers, or the emic (insider) perspective; and realities from the perspective of the social scientist, or the etic (outsider) perspective. Fetterman (2000) explains that an emic perspective is the reality shared and perceived by the people being studied and considered to be the insider's reality. There could also be multiple realities within the group as different individuals in the group could each have his/her own subjective version and understanding. Etic, in contrast, is the outsiders' version, understanding or interpretation of the reality, derived from the theoretical underpinnings of the study.

FIELD WORK

All ethnographers have to enter a research site, be it a community setting or a hospital ward, to conduct their studies. The research setting is the conceptual 'field' and the conduct of their research in the field is known as 'field work'. The selection of the field depends on the research topic. It is always ideal for a researcher to locate the study in an exemplary site. However, in practice, Burgess (1984, p. 59) noted that sometimes a researcher does not always select a 'typical' or 'representative' site for the study but rather the site is chosen because of the cooperation of individuals or convenience.

The study by Manias and Street (2001) was a typical example of convenience affecting the selection of a research site. Their research on nurse–doctor interactions during ward rounds occurred in a critical care unit because one of the researchers was a staff member of the unit. While some studies require one site for research, there are studies that may require multiple sites. Hanna's (2001) study on teenage motherhood required observations at different sites because the five teenage mothers she studied were each living on their own. Even in an institution, multiple sites may also be involved. While selection of research sites may be made by cooperation of colleagues or convenience, Glesne and Peshkin (1992) caution that sometimes, these 'backyard' studies may be problematic, as work may take precedence and opportunities for observations may be lost. In addition, being an insider can also create ethical and political dilemmas for the researcher. It may become difficult to conduct research at the place of work because the researcher may uncover, what Glesne and Peshkin (1992, p. 23) call, 'dangerous knowledge' that could be risky for an insider. An insider conducting research may also be criticised for being unethical because staff may participate in the study under duress, especially when the researcher is in a more influential position than those being studied. Selection of research sites is not simple and it is suggested that a site be selected that allows the researcher to have a certain level of freedom, accessibility and participation to carry out the research (Spradley, 1980).

SAMPLING

In the field, the researcher observes and records the events and behaviours of the people and this can become overwhelming as to what and where to begin. Burgess (1984) acknowledges that it is impossible for the researcher to study every event and behaviour in a social situation. It is necessary, therefore, for the researcher to select situations, events and people to observe and to reject others in the field. These decisions are guided by the researcher's theoretical and substantive interests. Often, the researcher has to engage in sampling time, people and context (Brewer, 2000; Hammersley & Atkinson, 1983).

Time sampling

Attitudes and activities vary over time and any systematic study will reveal different patterns of work, activity and interactions according to the time of day, night or week (Hammersly & Atkinson, 1983). Burgess (1984) noted that every organisation has its own social rhythm. Therefore, certain routines and interactions take place at certain times of the day. Depending on the study, certain times have to be selected for observations. For example, in the study by Manias and Street (2001) on doctor–nurse interactions during ward rounds, the researchers selected times when ward rounds were being conducted for observations. Similarly, in their study on the handover practices of the nurses they had to observe the times when handovers were given (Manias & Street, 2000b).

Sampling people

Sampling people requires adequate representation, and depending on the study, gender, race, age, occupation, qualifications, status and memberships must be considered, as these variables influence behaviours (Hammersley & Atkinson, 1983). In ethnographic studies, non-probability sampling is more often used (Brewer, 2000). Because there is no way of estimating that every element has a chance of being studied, Burgess (1984) suggests the following sampling strategies:

- Judgement sampling—occurs when the researcher selects people who have the required status or experience or are endowed with special knowledge to provide the researcher with the vital information.
- Opportunistic sampling—occurs when the researcher selects people who are willing to cooperate by supplying the necessary information.
- Snowball sampling—occurs when the researcher starts with gathering information from a few people and then relies on these people to put the researcher in touch with others who may be friends, relatives, colleagues or other significant contacts. This method of sampling is also referred to as networking.
- Theoretical sampling—occurs after the initial data have already been analysed and a decision is made as to what data need to be collected next and where to find the additional data. Theoretical sampling is most useful when theory has begun to emerge and more data are necessary to test the emerging theory.

Selection of events

Behaviours always occur within contexts, and observation of different events is important (Hammersley & Atkinson, 1983). This was well illustrated by Manias and Street (2000b) when they found that the behaviour of nurses changed from being docile, passive and uncritical during global handover (that is, from one shift to another) to anxious and fearful during bedside handover.

When considering events, Burgess (1984) identifies three types of events to observe:

- Routine events that are part of daily activities.
- Cyclical events that repeat over a period, such as festivities, births, deaths and marriages.
- Untoward events, such as emergencies, dramatic situations and crises. These events present some of the best opportunities to observe and to understand human behaviours.

Time, people and events are the threads woven into the tapestry of individuals' lives. In conducting ethnography, these three dimensions cannot always be clearly separated and have to be observed in their entirety.

ACCESS

When a researcher has selected a topic and a field, the next step to consider is how to gain access into the field. This is an exercise in field relations for the researcher. Entry to the field and access to participants are never always straightforward and there are levels of entry that have to be negotiated and renegotiated (Burgess, 1984). Glesne and Peshkin (1992) consider access a process to acquire consent to settings and to conduct observations, to interview people, and to obtain necessary documents to meet the needs of the research.

The usual way for a researcher to gain entry is by obtaining permission from power holders within the organisation, such as the heads of departments, management committees or ethics committees. Sometimes, access can be obtained with the assistance of an intermediary (Brewer, 2000). Fetterman (2000) mentions that the intermediary may be a teacher, gang member, or director, who has an association with the group or has credibility within the group. In the event that an intermediary is not available, the researcher may have to join an appropriate group or volunteer time to build relationships with the group members to earn their trust and respect. Whyte (1955), who conducted the classic study on street gang societies at Conerville, had to speak initially to many social workers at Norton Street House. One of the social workers understood what he needed and introduced him to 'Doc' (who used to be active at Norton Street House). Doc, in turn, introduced him to the gang members.

It is relatively easy for the researcher if all personnel agree to participate in the study. However, it is possible that some staff may wish to be observed but not to be interviewed and vice versa. Some may not wish to participate and may view the researcher with suspicion, while others may believe that their performance is being evaluated. While participation is the prerogative of the individual, sometimes power holders and different levels of staff may not grant the researcher access to certain people, situations or documents necessary for the research. This is when the researcher has to be aware of 'gatekeepers' in ethnographic study.

Gatekeepers

Gatekeepers are individuals who have the power to withhold from the researcher access to people, situations and/or documents necessary for the purpose of research (Burgess, 1984). Gatekeepers may exercise some control and surveillance to block off certain lines of enquiry and to direct the researcher in certain directions. This is because gatekeepers are concerned with the way the ethnographer might present the organisation, and they regard it as their role to ensure that they and their colleagues are presented in a favourable light (Hammersley & Atkinson, 1983). Gatekeepers can be at any level in an organisation and not confined only to those in authority positions. Sometimes, the clerk who has access to documents may effectively frustrate the research by not providing the researcher with the required documents or archival material.

An example of gatekeepers at work can be seen in the study attempted by Greenwood, Holmes and Bidewell (2001). The authors submitted a research proposal to the local institutional ethics committee (IEC) to investigate the policies and practices of health service ethics committees in the greater Sydney area. The local IEC refused to approve the study. One of the reasons given to the authors for the rejection of their proposal was that the local ethics committee was reluctant to expose its operations to external scrutiny.

Ethical issues regarding access

The main ethical question regarding ethnography is the process of access and the openness of the research. This has to do with whether the research is conducted covertly or overtly. Research conducted by nurses is generally 'overt', meaning that the study is known to the participants concerned; as opposed to 'covert', when the people involved are not aware that they are being observed. However, there is also a grey area: if, for example, the head of an organisation knows about research taking place but the rest of the staff are not informed that a researcher is in their midst (Burgess, 1983; Whyte, 1955). In ethnographic studies, there are many arguments for and against both types of research and the relevance of each has to be evaluated against the purpose and context of the study (Glesne & Peshkin, 1992; Fetterman, 1989; Burgess, 1984; Hammersley & Atkinson, 1983). It is a requirement that research is approved by the relevant IEC of an organisation (see Chapter 8).

DATA GATHERING STRATEGIES

In ethnographic research, participant observation is one of the most important data gathering methods and the researcher is the main instrument of social research. However, the researcher cannot rely on himself or herself as the sole instrument of data collection by conducting observations only. Depending on the kinds of data needed for the study, methods such as interviews, photography and videotaping are used to collect data, as well as materials such as archives, records and documents.

Participant observation

Participant observation is a central data collection technique in ethnographic research (Punch, 1998). It involves participation in the daily life of the people in their natural setting to discover their interpretations, social meanings and activities (Brewer, 2000, p. 59). Participant observation ranges across a continuum from participation to observation, and the researcher could be at any point on this continuum during different times of the research (Glesne & Peshkin, 1992). Along this continuum, four distinct roles of participation and observation can be distinguished: complete participant; participant as observer; observer as participant; and complete observer (Burgess, 1984; Hammersley & Atkinson, 1983).

Complete participant

The complete participant is a functioning member of the community under observation as well as a researcher (Glesne & Peshkin, 1992). Complete participation gives the researcher the best opportunity to observe peoples' behaviours as this role is usually associated with covert research. Burgess (1984) and Hammersley and Atkinson (1983) warn of several pitfalls when taking on this role:

- The researcher may alter the behaviour of the group.
- The researcher may identify with the community (by 'going native') to the extent that it interferes with the objectivity of the research.
- By living out the lives of the people, the researcher is expected to fulfil the roles and expectations of a community member to the extent that there is no time for observations and documentation.
- If the people find out that they are being observed, the project is jeopardised. The uncovering of a researcher can also destroy the trust the community has of outsiders. To overcome these problems, the researcher has to take frequent breaks to record, analyse and reflect on the data collected (Burgess, 1984).

Participant as observer

The participant observer does not conceal the research in acting as both participant and observer. This openness allows the researcher to develop relationships with the informants, to observe what is considered important, and to come and go as he or she pleases (Burgess, 1984). Although there is considerable freedom as a participant observer, it does not allow the researcher to participate to the extent that is possible as a complete participant (Denzin, 1978).

Observer as participant

As an observer as participant, the role of the researcher is made public. The researcher is first an observer, and participation is secondary. Burgess (1984) noted that in this situation, contact with informants is brief and formal, and only observations can be carried out. This form of data gathering does not allow the researcher to fully understand the behaviours of the people. Denzin (1978) noted that, in this role, there is no attempt to establish any sense of an enduring relationship with the people.

Complete observer

This role removes the researcher entirely from interaction (Denzin, 1978) and is confined to observations only. A complete observer faces the risk of failing to understand the perspectives of the participants, which could lead to serious misunderstanding of the behaviour of those being observed (Hammersley & Atkinson, 1983).

With regard to how much a researcher should participate, Bogdan and Taylor (1975, pp. 51, 53) advise that the researcher must remember that the primary purpose of participation is to collect data and any participation that interferes with data collection should be avoided. They also remind the researcher not to lose sight of ethical issues raised by the researcher's participation. Sometimes, those observed might try to involve a researcher in activities that violate the researcher's sense of ethics; and sometimes, the researcher feels ethically bound to participate or intervene in the activities of those observed. Their advice is that the researcher must participate only to the extent required to establish rapport, unless ethics demand more participation.

Informants

When in the field, the researcher has to make sense of the setting, the events, the people and their roles. Hence, the researcher needs an 'informant', who is an 'insider to the group', knows the 'language' and is a source of information. Some of the roles of the informant are to assist the researcher with access to the group, to teach the researcher how to fit into the group, and to direct the researcher to the events for observation and to the important people to interview.

McNeill (1985, p. 68) notes that the informant is one with whom the researcher develops a close relationship, and the key informant is 'almost a partner in research'. Given the roles of the informant, Van Maanen (1988) suggests that the researcher needs to establish relationships with several informants because it is not possible for one informant to know about all aspects of the group's culture.

Conversations and interviews

Central to ethnography are conversations that the researcher has with the people in the setting. These daily conversations occur naturally while interacting with the people being observed, and they are also data gathering opportunities. Often, valuable information can be gathered even during a coffee break or a ten-minute 'chat' with someone in a corridor. Data gathering needs to be more focused and this is when the researcher has to decide whether to conduct unstructured or structured interviews.

Burgess (1984) considers interviews as conversations and prefers unstructured interviews in ethnographic research. They complement participant observation in different ways (p. 106) and help the researcher to:

- gain access to situations that, through time, place or situation, are 'closed'
- obtain details of situations that are not witnessed by the researcher
- gain access to information regarding situations that the researcher may not be privy to.

Hammersley and Atkinson (1983) state that ethnographers do not have predetermined questions; rather, they conduct unstructured interviews with a list of issues to be covered. In these interviews, the questions are non-directive, open-ended, and are designed to be triggers to stimulate the participant to talk about a broad topic. These interviews rely on the social interaction between the researcher and informant to elicit information (Minichiello, Aroni, Timewell & Alexander, 1995). While events allow the researcher to observe behaviours, interviews allow the researcher to understand how the participant would behave if the circumstances were different (Hammersley & Atkinson, 1983).

Besides unstructured interviews, semi-structured or focused interviews and group interviews are also used to gather information. The questions in semi-structured interviews or focused interviews are more unstructured than structured, in that a particular topic guides the questions but the interview is conducted following the unstructured interview process (Minichiello et al., 1995). In group interviews, the researcher gathers the informants together to engage in dialogue with each other. This allows the researcher to examine the relationship between the participants and their perspectives (Burgess, 1984). Group interviews have the advantage of being more economical to conduct than individual interviews.

Other types of data

There are many different types of data a researcher could gather depending on the study, including filming, audiotaping and videotaping events. They have an advantage over handwritten notes because it is sometimes impossible to record everything one observes, or even to observe everything that occurs in an event.

These forms of documentation are useful for detailed analysis and for comparison of changes to the circumstances of people over time, such as observations of cultural groups, organisational behaviour or nurse–patient interactions.

Other forms of data include historical records, archival material, minutes of meetings, biographies, personal and organisational diaries, letters and personal documents. Documents provide historical and contextual dimensions to observations and interviews, as well as supporting, challenging and expanding the perceptions of the researcher (Glesne & Peshkin, 1992).

Triangulation

One of the concerns of ethnographers is that people can act in ways and provide information that they think the researcher wants to observe or to hear. The researcher also needs to know that the informant is not giving his or her own perspective but the perspective of the group. Many researchers use multiple strategies, commonly referred to as 'triangulation', to address the issue of validity. The researcher uses different research methods, forms of data and theories, to validate (or corroborate) the observations and data gathered. In research, triangulation provides not only a validity check, but also gives depth to the description of the social meanings within the setting (Hammersley & Atkinson, 1983, p. 198). (See Chapter 2 for different approaches to triangulation.)

REFLEXIVITY

When conducting research, the researcher must be mindful of the fact that he or she is also part of the social scene which inevitably affects the phenomena being observed. As a product of society, the researcher also has their own personal beliefs, biases and individual tastes (Fetterman, 2000), which may colour the observations and interpretations of the behaviours of others. Hammersley and Atkinson (1983) state that it is impossible for the researcher to escape the social world to study it or to eliminate the researcher effect. And as 'participants in the social world, we (researchers) are still able, at least in anticipation or retrospect, to observe our activities "from the outside" as objects in the world' (Hammersley & Atkinson, 1983, pp. 16–17). The effect of the researcher on the people is best illustrated in Whyte's (1955) Street Corner Society, when Doc (Whyte's informant) admitted that since he had known Whyte, he had slowed down and had also started to think about his actions rather than acting upon instinct.

RECIPROCITY

The researcher in ethnographic research is obligated to the people who participate in the research. This obligation comes with the privilege of being given the opportunity to participate in the life of the group. Glesne and Peshkin (1992) observe that the degree of indebtedness varies according to the length of study, the topic of the study, and the relationships that have been developed. For these reasons, the researcher is obligated to return certain favours. Fetterman (2000) suggests that while payment is not usually recommended, the researcher may offer time and expertise or a sympathetic ear as bartering tools. His final advice is that some form of reciprocity is essential during field work, but it should not become obtrusive, contaminating or be an unethical activity.

DISENGAGEMENT FROM THE FIELD

It is not always easy to leave the research setting after investing much time and energy into developing relationships. There might be an exchange of gifts or sentiments, and some relationships may outlast the field work. The researcher may either never return to the field again or it may become a long lasting relationship with the agency for future collaborations. Whatever the relationship, the researcher is expected to leave the field in such a manner that future researchers would be afforded a similar opportunity to conduct their projects.

MANAGING DATA

When conducting field work, the researcher very quickly accumulates a large amount of notes taken from observations, conversations and interviews. As these data do not come in a neat and tidy form like those in a questionnaire, they have to be managed. The following section discusses the organisation and analysis of the data.

Organising data

Ethnographic research involves the simultaneous collection and analysis of data (Brewer, 2000, p. 107). It is a normal practice for ethnographers to review their data at the end of the day so that they can decide who and what to observe and what theory to test during the next visit at the site. As a result, data are not confined to just field notes, but are also made up of analytic notes of different kinds. Burgess (1984) suggests that the data be grouped into substantive field notes, analytic notes and methodological notes.

Substantive field notes are records of situations, events, interviews and conversations that the researcher has participated in or observed (Burgess, 1984). These notes can also include diagrams of a room setting, positions of participants in a meeting, and other sketches and drawings. Substantive field notes are also referred to as descriptive notes (Glesne & Peshkin, 1992) and observational notes (Hammersley & Atkinson, 1983).

Analytic notes are generated after the material gathered for the day has been read and new questions and theoretical ideas begin to emerge (Burgess, 1984; Hammersley & Atkinson, 1983).

Methodological notes consist of impressions, reflections, hunches and processes, and procedures associated with field work (Burgess, 1984). Burgess (1984) emphasises that these notes are reflections of the researcher and they assist the researcher to speculate on ways to adopt, adapt and develop methods for use in particular settings. The different types of notes are interrelated: substantive field notes lead to the development of analytical and methodological notes; analytical and methodological notes then guide and refine the direction of the research.

Given the complexity of the notes, the researcher has to find some ways of managing the data. Burgess (1984) suggests that field notes may be recorded in different columns on cards, and that the notes be subdivided according to paragraphs for easy identification. Field notes can also be indexed according to themes or categories, with several copies made so that the same set of notes can be placed in different files. Hammersley and Atkinson (1983) suggest that initially, field notes can be organised chronologically, but later, they still have to be organised and indexed according to themes, codes or categories.

Making sense of the data: analysis

When analysing the observational, interview or documentary data, the researcher can do so manually or use computer software to assist in the process. This software stores data in orderly clusters, under the concepts or codes developed by the researcher, which can be retrieved efficiently and which aids analysis and interpretation (see, for example, http://www.qsrinternational.com). The advantages and disadvantages of this software are discussed by Glesne and Peshkin (1992, pp. 141–45). The analytic process the researcher engages in depends on the research question and the theory that guides the study (Brewer, 2000). Forms of analysis range from thematic analysis to theoretical analysis. For more general analysis, the following methods are suggested.

When analysing the data, the researcher initially reads through the material carefully to note interesting or emerging patterns or themes. These patterns will give ideas for the development of broad categories, themes, concepts and hypotheses, under which data could be grouped. Hammersley and Atkinson (1983) suggest that when the initial analytic categories are identified, the next step is to develop these into theoretical themes, to find links between the concepts and to add new ones. This process of sifting and comparing will eventually produce a clear picture of the phenomena. Strauss and Corbin (1990) suggest a different way of analysing the data, using open, axial and selective coding processes. Analysis begins with open coding, which identifies categories of concepts. This process 'fractures' the data and allows categories to be identified. Axial coding follows, allowing data to be re-constructed by making connections between a category and its sub-categories. This places the categories within contexts. In the next step, selective coding is used to integrate categories to form the total picture. The reader is directed to other chapters in Section 2 and other sources (e.g. Punch, 1998; Strauss, 1987; Strauss & Corbin, 1990) for further discussion of qualitative data analysis.

TELLING THE STORY

At the end of the research, the story must be told. When telling the story, there are two factors to consider: the audience and the presentation of the story. Fetterman (1989) notes that the format, language and level of abstraction used will be different depending on the audience. On the one hand, if the project is sponsored by an agency, the report may have to be brief and direct. On the other hand, if the report is written for a particular academic journal, a certain level of analysis and abstraction will be necessary.

An ethnographic study can be presented in different ways, with the final product providing a descriptive account (telling the story) of a group, a culture or a unit. Hammersley and Atkinson (1983) liken it to a narrative laden with theme and argument. Fetterman (1989) calls it thick description, where the cultural meaning and the ethnographer's analysis are included in the variety of cultural scenes and episodes. Verbatim quotations are often used to convey the different thoughts and emotions that give meaning to human existence, as well as to give a sense of immediacy to the reader. Presentations could also be in the form of case studies (see Chapter 2). Examples of ethnographic studies, where stories are told with meaningful interpretive analysis and verbatim accounts, can be found in Joan Cassell's (1991) *Expected Miracles*, on the professional life of surgeons; and Marcia Inhorn's (1994) *Question for Conception*, on the impact of in vitro fertilisation technology on Egyptian women.

When presenting the accounts, the researcher must ensure the anonymity of the people concerned. It is not always sufficient to use pseudonyms to maintain anonymity, as the events, time and place where the research was carried out may give clues to identify the person(s). Sometimes, the researcher may need to alter certain details to prevent the person or organisation being identified. The researcher also has to exercise discretion in the publication of information given in confidence by a person (or persons) or certain pieces of information that might happen to be 'discovered' during the course of the study. This is to protect the person(s) or the organisation from being exposed, as well as to protect the researcher from libel action. When a person or an organisation opens up for scrutiny by a researcher, the parties have entered into a contract of trust that must be honoured.

KEY POINTS

- Ethnography allows in-depth enquiry of a phenomenon within its cultural context. This perspective is congruent with the concept of holism in nursing.
- The strength of ethnographic research is in the emic and etic interpretations of phenomenon.
- When attempting to access a research site and its participants, the researcher must be mindful of the ethical issues governing informed consent.
- Substantial field work is crucial for adequate sampling of people and events over time.
- The different types of data gathered in ethnographic research provide the richness in description and interpretation.
- When conducting ethnographic research, the researcher must be theoretically informed, either to be able to guide the study or to recognise emerging theories for testing, as well as to be able to build on existing theories.
- Triangulation is important in ethnography for validation of data.
- The pillar of ethnographic research is the relationships developed between the researcher and the participants. The researcher must uphold the ethical and moral obligations, such as respect, trust, confidentiality, anonymity and reciprocity.

CRITICAL THINKING CHALLENGES

- What are the elements in ethnography that make it a powerful tool for the development, testing and building of theory for nursing practice?
- How can ethnography as a research methodology assist in the advancement of nursing as a profession?
- In what ways can nurses employ ethnography to promote relationships, understanding and collaboration with other healthcare professions to enhance teamwork for the benefit of the patient?

Additional resources

Agee, E. (2000). Menopause and the transmission of women's knowledge: African American and White women's perspectives. *Medical Anthropology Quarterly*, 14(1), 73–95.

Brink, P.J. (1998). The Fattening Room among the Annang of Nigeria. In Morse, J.M., ed., *Cross-cultural nursing*. (pp. 131–43). Philadelphia, Gordeon and Breach Science Publishers.

Burgess, R.G., ed. (1986). *Key variables in social investigation*. London, Routledge & Kegan Paul.

Byrne, M. (2001). Ethnography as a qualitative research method. *Association of Operating Room Nurses Journal*, 74(1), 82, 84.

Ford, K. & Turner, D. (2001). Stories seldom told: paediatric nurses' experiences of caring for hospitalized children with special needs and their families. *Journal of Advanced Nursing*, 33(3), 288–95.

Gilbert, N. (1993). *Researching social life*. London, Sage Publications.

Hammersley, M. & Atkinson, P. (1983). *Ethnography: principles in practice*. London, Tavistock.

Jordan, B. (1993). *Birth in four cultures*. (4th ed.). Illinois, Waveland Press.

Kvale, S. (1996). *Interviews: an introduction to qualitative research interviewing*. Thousand Oaks, California, Sage.

Leininger, M.M. (1985). Ethnography and ethnonursing models and modes of qualitative data analysis. In Leininger, M.M., ed., *Qualitative research methods in nursing*. Orlando, Grune & Stratton.

Lipson, J.G. & Meleis, A.I. (1989). Methodological issues in research with immigrants. In Morse, J.M., ed., *Cross-cultural nursing*. (pp. 103–15). Philadelphia, Gordon and Breach Science Publishers.

MacCormack, C.P., ed. (1994). *Ethnography of fertility and birth*. (2nd ed.). Illinois, Waveland Press.

Manias, E. & Street, A. (2000). Legitimation of nurses' knowledge through policies and protocols in clinical practice. *Journal of Advanced Nursing*, 32, 1467–75.

Manias, E. & Street, A. (2001). Rethinking ethnography: reconstructing nursing relationships. *Journal of Advanced Nursing*, 33(2), 234–42.
Mardiros, M. (1989). Conception of childhood disability among Mexican–American parents. In Morse, J.M., ed., *Cross-cultural nursing*. (pp. 55–68). Philadelphia, Gordon and Breach Science Publishers.
Martens, K.H. (1998). An ethnographic study of the process of medication discharge education (MDE). *Journal of Advanced Nursing*, 27, 341–48.
Maslin-Prothers, S. (2001). Gender issues in ethnography. *Journal of Advanced Nursing*, 35(3), 468–69.
Melia, B. (2000). Conducting an interview. *Nurse Researcher*, 7(4), 75–89.
Peacock, J.L. (1986). *The anthropological lens: harsh light, soft focus*. New York, Cambridge University Press.
Sanday, P.R. (1989). The ethnographic paradigm(s). In Van Maanen, J., ed., *Qualitative methodology*. Newbury Park, California, Sage.
Sanjek, R., ed. (1990). *Fieldnotes: the makings of anthropology*. New York, Cornell University Press.
Shomaker, D.J. (1989). Age disorientation, liminality and reality: the case of the Alzheimer's patient. In Morse, J.M., ed., *Cross-cultural nursing*. (pp. 91–101). Philadelphia, Gordon and Breach Science Publishers.

13
CHAPTER

Phenomenology

Louise O'Brien

LEARNING OUTCOMES

After reading this chapter the student should be able to:

- Describe the basic frameworks for conducting phenomenological research.
- Discuss the appropriateness of phenomenological frameworks for nursing research.
- Describe the value of the knowledge gained from phenomenological research for nursing.
- Identify the types of questions that could be best answered by the use of a phenomenological framework in research.

Key terms

being
Dasein
epistemology
hermeneutics
interpretative
interview
lived experience
ontology
participants
phenomena
phenomenon
phenomenology
qualitative research
temporality
themes

INTRODUCTION

Phenomenology as a framework for research enquiry has been embraced by nursing researchers as a way of understanding phenomena that occur within the domain of nursing. Nurse researchers have found phenomenology particularly useful for the study of those phenomena that do not lend themselves readily to the processes of quantification, control or comparison. A phenomenon is defined as 'something that is shown, or revealed, or manifest in experience' (Blackburn, 1994, p. 285).

Phenomenology was first a philosophy and subsequently has been utilised as an approach to research enquiry. While phenomenology as a philosophical movement has provided nursing with incredible riches in terms of understanding human existence and experience, it also provides considerable challenge to the nurse researcher. The nurse researcher needs to have a good understanding of the underlying assumptions about the philosophical framework in order to produce research that is true to this framework.

This chapter provides an overview of the history, philosophical concepts and assumptions of phenomenology that provide parameters for the conduct of nursing research within a phenomenological framework. Nursing research using a phenomenological framework is discussed and suggestions for further reading are provided.

HISTORICAL PERSPECTIVE

Phenomenology as a philosophical movement has its origins in Greek philosophy. The German philosopher, Husserl (1859–1938) is credited with being the founder of the 20th century phenomenological movement. Husserl moved philosophical discussion from the question of whether or not objects in our conscious awareness had a separate existence, to the systematic analysis of consciousness and its objects. For Husserl, human beings were subjects in a world of objects and it was the study of consciousness of those objects that he called phenomenology. Husserl's phenomenology is epistemological in that it is concerned with asking questions of knowledge about objects gained through conscious awareness. He aimed to separate out (bracket) mood, thoughts, memories and emotions to focus on conscious awareness of objects (McGee, 1987).

Heidegger, a pupil and colleague of Husserl, questioned the relationship between consciousness and objects and thus diverged significantly from Husserl's project. Heidegger argued that people do not relate to their worlds in a theoretical way, but as concerned human beings, historically situated with many more ways of relating to their worlds than 'knowing' (Inwood, 1997). For Heidegger the practical situatedness of human experience takes precedence over scientific theorising or cognition about objects (Fell, 1992). It was to the study of that practical situatedness of human experience, of understanding the necessary conditions for people being in their worlds, that Heidegger focused his efforts. Thus Heideggerian phenomenology is ontological in that it seeks to understand the conditions whereby human beings can understand their existence and thus the nature and the meaning of being.

The differences between a Husserlian epistemological tradition and a Heideggerian ontological tradition are important because they impact on the questions that can be asked, and the kinds of answers that can be sought. Several Australian nurse phenomenologists have explicated the importance of these differences (Koch, 1995; Walters, 1994). Questions that can utilise a Husserlian approach to research are epistemological questions of knowing 'How is this phenomenon known?'. Studies using this approach utilise bracketing of both the researcher's and the participant's prior knowledge of the phenomenon. Questions that can utilise a Heideggerian approach to research are ontological questions of experience: 'How is this phenomenon understood through experience of the phenomenon?'. Heideggerian phenomenology thus lends itself to a research framework that addresses questions concerning meaning in the practical everyday life of people and seeks to provide an interpretation of the practical understanding of human actions and experiences.

KEY CONCEPTS OF HEIDEGGERIAN PHENOMENOLOGY

This section provides a basic overview of some key concepts that need to be considered when undertaking phenomenological research. These key concepts have implications for how research studies using this approach are conducted.

Being

The mode of being belonging to a person as described by Heidegger is 'Dasein' (Heidegger, 1962, p. 67). The German verb 'dasein' means 'to exist', 'to be there', 'to be here' and refers to both the human being and to 'the type of being that humans have' (Inwood, 1997, p. 22). The nature of human being is described by Heidegger (1962, p. 33) as having four *a-priori* structures of existence:

- Dasein's ability to be aware of its own being
- Dasein's ability to exist in such a way as to belong to the world
- Dasein's capacity for relationships
- Dasein's ability to use the world and for the world to be available to Dasein.

The implication of these structures of existence is that people live in their worlds in contextualised ways. People are aware of their own existence and question what it means to be. They question the meaning of their experience of being and can thus interpret their worlds. The world is not made up of objects but of a context with meaning. People can reflect on the meaning of their experience, and can look forward to possibilities of being. People have the capacity for relationships with others; others are of concern. People can use their world in a constant and uncritical way but can also stand back and critically reflect on the objects in the world and their use with meaning and understanding. Guignon (1983, p. 19) suggests that 'self is not distinct from the roles through which we participate in the world. Self is inextricably woven into the wider context of the community and a cosmos'.

Temporality

For Heidegger (1962, p. 386), being in the world is always understood in terms of temporality. Life as lived now cannot be divorced from the historical experience of living a life and the potential for that life in the future. Temporality is thus intrinsically involved in the meaning of life experience.

Meaning, understanding, language and the hermeneutic circle

Heidegger described Dasein as being in the midst of a world that is familiar and that is understood. This 'hermeneutic circle' (Heidegger, 1962, p. 119) describes the historical, cultural and personal preconceptions from which understanding is developed. However, the hermeneutic circle is not a static entity; it is dynamic. The preconceptions contained in understanding are challenged by new understandings. It is by making the background preconceptions explicit in language that the testing of assumptions is possible. The process is kaleidoscopic as different patterns emerge in the process of the illumination of taken-for-granted understandings. People come to an encounter with a history of culture and experience that is bound in language. The process of understanding is bringing together perspectives influenced by pasts and articulated in shared language.

Hermeneutic phenomenology thus provides a framework that defines a view of persons and their being-in-the-world. It also defines how meaning and language are understood and thus how knowledge about human beings and their world is subjective, temporal and historical. These concepts provide a framework that has implications for the process of research and it is adherence to these implications that affects the coherence of the phenomenological study.

PHENOMENOLOGY AND NURSING KNOWLEDGE

Phenomenology can illuminate phenomena and disclose hitherto unnoticed or overlooked aspects through exploring the experience of phenomena. Phenomenology provides descriptions rich in detail and exemplars that open the possibilities of understanding. Phenomenology reveals meanings embedded in the situation rather than makes inferences, or identifies causes. The result of such knowledge is that nurses may better understand the possibilities embedded in the experience of phenomena.

Phenomenology has found appeal in nursing research because it reflects values and beliefs that are coherent with nursing and allows questions to be explored that are important to nursing. The kinds of questions that nurses ask often focus on understanding experiences of phenomena related to health and illness, treatment and care, from the perspective of both those cared for and those providing care.

Phenomenology and nursing share basic premises related to beliefs about individuals and their relationship to the environment. Phenomenology offers a methodology that intrinsically values an holistic perspective of experience and the individual's ability to make sense of, and reflect on, those experiences.

Phenomenology also has the potential to raise awareness of the need for change when situations are critically examined in light of phenomenological findings. It can provide a way of critically evaluating health and nursing care in light of the participants' experience of phenomena related to such care (Benner, 1994). Chesla (1994) used hermeneutic phenomenology to explore the caregiving practices of parents of offspring with schizophrenia. This study widened the understanding of this experience, usually accepted as a 'burden' and provided a means for understanding the families' perceptions beyond that concept. This study provided understanding that could inform interventions that were more coherent with the possible ways that these families understood their experience. Harvey (1993) used phenomenology to uncover the experiences of women in the perinatal period, nursed in hospital, and considered 'at risk'. The understandings of the experience generated by the study led to changes to the mode of nursing care towards listening to the narratives of the women and responding in ways that were individual, holistic, and responsive to change.

USING A PHENOMENOLOGICAL FRAMEWORK FOR RESEARCH

The goal of phenomenology is to develop an understanding of a phenomenon through the specific human experience of the phenomenon, in order to better understand that experience of being in that life-world. The process of phenomenological research therefore, does not fragment the experience that is being studied but provides descriptions that are rich and full and interpretations that illuminate what it means to be a person in that life-world. The research approach is one of sensitive awareness to the participants' descriptions of their experiences, while maintaining a questioning, reflective stance about the particular phenomenon and its context.

The role of the researcher

The researcher comes to the study with an attitude of care. It is because of the researcher's interest in the question that the study is undertaken. The researcher has a preliminary understanding of what is going on, knows that the question is a legitimate one and can envisage possibilities that may emerge from the study. In phenomenological research it is important that this position of pre-understanding is made explicit. By making the background assumptions explicit, the researcher can test assumptions and new knowledge. This historical background of experience, knowledge and assumptions needs to be made explicit in a first-person account.

The selection of participants

Persons are viewed as self-interpreting beings able to reflect upon and articulate their experience. They are seen as amidst their world and caring about their world. Phenomenological research is an interactive involvement of both the person who researches and the participants in research. The participants of phenomenological studies are chosen because of their experience of the phenomena being studied and because of their ability to articulate that experience. The number of participants involved in a phenomenological research study is usually based on a combination of pragmatic acceptance of the restrictions imposed by the research process and of the acceptance of the infinite nature of experience of phenomena. The richness of the data collected is more important than the number of participants in the study.

The data collection process

Phenomenology is based on acceptance of language as the only tool with which to develop a shared world of meaning. Phenomenological studies use the language of the participants in the study to reflect as accurately as possible the meanings embedded in the experience. The collection of data usually involves tape recorded interviews.

Phenomenological interviews

The phenomenological research interview serves as an arena in which the researcher can establish a relationship with a partner (interviewee), focused on the meaning of the experience. The conversation that emanates from the focused relationship provides a means of collecting descriptive material that can be used to understand and interpret the experience of the phenomenon (van Manen, 1990).

The task of the researcher is to understand what it is that the participant is saying about their experience and to engage the participant in such a way that rich descriptions of the participant's experience are gained. The interview material needs to be specific to the phenomena being studied and to contain sufficient material in stories, anecdotes and examples to provide the reader with an understanding of the experience as lived (Kvale, 1996; van Manen, 1990).

Transcription of recorded material

The taped interviews are transcribed into printed form. The art of transcription includes being able to overcome the limitations of language, and to do this, transcripts need to be created that reflect as closely as possible the experience of the conversation. Notes taken during or following the interview are useful to provide comment on feeling–tone, body language, and the researcher's experience of the interview.

Analysis of data

The aim of data analysis is to provide an understanding of the experience through the identification of themes. The analysis of data is often the most difficult area of the phenomenological research process for the novice researcher to grasp. A number of authors have provided processes that may assist the analysis of data (Kvale, 1996; van Manen, 1990), however, there is no standard method of text analysis. A number of processes are undertaken in the analysis and construction of meaning. Analysis of the data is commonly achieved by reading, and rereading in whole and in parts, identifying themes that illuminate the meaning of the experience, and writing narrative interpretations of the text. Parts of the experience are examined in light of the whole experience. The focus of analysis moves from part to whole and whole to part, identifying structures of meaning and themes as they emerge from the text, considering the pre-understanding of the researcher and moving back to the text for verification of the emergent meanings. Themes are defined as essential aspects of the experience that provide illumination and meaning. The emerging narrative needs to reflect the context and time frame of the experiences, the understandings of the researcher, and the context of meanings contained in other sources. It is necessarily a writing and re-writing process. The descriptions are not judged according to the exact replication of incident but of the intertwining of understanding of the researcher and the participant. The interpretation of data and how it illuminates a particular phenomenon needs to be shown in the pattern of meaning in which it exists. It is insufficient for phenomenological studies to claim a particular interpretation of a human phenomenon. The consequences of the interpretation and the suppositions that it challenges within the circle of understanding need to be made clear.

RIGOUR AND PHENOMENOLOGICAL RESEARCH

The challenge of conducting phenomenological research that is rigorous is similar to the process of achieving rigour in all qualitative studies (see Chapters 9–16). The following points, however, are particularly important to phenomenological research. What can be judged as rigorous in phenomenological studies is influenced by:

- the acceptance of the validity of the participants' descriptions of the experience and the understanding that the stories emerge out of the unique context of their conversations
- the use of the researcher's perspective of the experience of the phenomenon
- the use of other sources of understanding and contextualising the phenomenon
- the bringing together of participant, researcher and other sources in the interpretation
- the provision of an interpretive narrative illustrated by concrete examples in anecdotal form
- a recognition that the experience being described resonates with the reader's understanding of what it is, or what it might be, to experience a life in that context.

ETHICAL ISSUES RELATED TO PHENOMENOLOGICAL RESEARCH

While ethical issues related to qualitative research are applicable to phenomenological studies, there are some specific concerns that need to be considered. Often the phenomena that nurses explore are sensitive human experiences. The timeliness of the research for the researcher needs to be considered. Researchers who undertake phenomenological studies are concerned about the research question. However, while immersed in the study, they need to be able to stand back enough to allow new perspectives to emerge. Researchers also need to consider the appropriate time for participants to be invited. The participant's sensitivity related to the experience of the phenomena needs to be considered.

The process of interviewing may be emotive for both the researcher and the participant. Participants in phenomenological research often identify that the process is therapeutic, however, the researcher needs to consider how they will handle emotional distress if it arises. Phenomenological nursing studies have been undertaken in areas as sensitive as incest, family breakdown, pain, and life-threatening and chronic illness (e.g. Gullickson, 1993; Kondora, 1994; Krasner, 1996; Saunders, 1994; Shin, 1999; Wray, 1995).

SKILLS REQUIRED FOR PHENOMENOLOGICAL RESEARCH

Many skills are required in the conduct of phenomenological research, including philosophical understanding, attention to the details relating to the study, interviewing skills, interpretative skills, and the ability to write descriptively.

Philosophical understanding

Undertaking phenomenological research requires a commitment to philosophical understanding. Researchers need to be able to:

- reflect on what it means to be a person in the world
- reflect on one's own experience and explore one's own understandings of a phenomenon
- think beyond the 'proving of facts' to a desire to explore the experiences of self and others, of a phenomenon, in a particular context
- have sufficient understanding of the phenomenological framework in order to explicate how it informs the method of the study and the findings of the study.

Attention to detail

Phenomenological research requires the meticulous recording of details related to the study, such as thoughts and decisions about the research question, the sources that are used to provide a background context, the researcher's own perspective, the selection of participants, the data collection process, and the interpretative process.

Interviewing skills

Researchers need to have skills in interviewing. The researcher enters into a partnership with participants to explore the phenomenon within that person's experience. The researcher needs to keep the interview focused on the phenomenon while allowing the participant to explore what may be important to them about the phenomenon. The researcher needs to be able to encourage exploration of the meaning of the experience of the phenomenon for the person and to ask for concrete examples that can help illuminate the meaning.

Interpretative skills

Phenomenological studies are interpretative from beginning to end. The researcher first of all identifies the phenomenon and asks the question, and in so doing, interprets it as an important question to ask. The exploration of a range of sources related to the phenomenon is an interpretative process that refines the phenomenon and the experience through which it can be revealed. The process of interviewing is an interpretative process that brings together the researcher's perspective and that of the participants. It is because of the researcher's perspective that they can ask the questions that allow the experience of the phenomena to be explored. The researcher interprets the transcribed interviews in light of their own understandings and that provided from other sources. The researcher uses the interpretative process to identify the implications of this new understanding of the phenomenon.

Writing skills

Phenomenological research is a writing project. The product of the research is the final written interpretation of the experience of the phenomena. Researchers need to be able to write descriptively, and have a strong affinity for the imaginative use of language in order to illuminate the phenomenon in such a way as to provide a new way of seeing this phenomenon.

EXAMPLES OF PHENOMENOLOGICAL NURSING RESEARCH

The following are examples of Australian phenomenological nursing research studies. This is not an exhaustive list but provides an indication of some of the phenomena that have been explored in the Australian context.

Walters (1995b) focused on the role of critical care nursing practice. Walters interviewed eight critical care nurses to elicit the meaning of caring in the critical care unit. The themes 'being busy', and 'balancing', were identified. 'Being busy' was related to the 'ability of the nurses to manage technology skilfully and to perform technical tasks competently' (p. 494). Alongside this busy-ness was the closeness that the nurse develops to the patient from being in close proximity for extended periods of time. The paradox between the technological control in the intensive care unit and the human connectedness of the patient and the nurse was expressed in the theme of 'balancing'. The process of tidying the bed area and reducing the visibility of the technology helped to make the patient more visible. Critical care nursing emerged as a balancing and integration of these apparent polarities. This study offered nurses new ways of understanding nursing care in the critical care environment that acknowledged technical competence and skill while maintaining the centrality of the patient's humanity.

Kralik, Koch and Wotton (1997) undertook a study of post-operative patients' perceptions of what was important about nursing care in an acute hospital context. Their aim was to gain understanding of what it is like to be nursed in order to inform nursing of what matters to patients. The authors interviewed nine women recovering from total hip replacement surgery. Two major themes of 'engagement' and 'detachment' were identified from the interview data. The participants described the engaged nurse as having such attributes as showing consideration and care, consulting, being gentle, using humour and being compassionate. The detached nurse was busy and efficient, sharp and cold, rough with physical care and giving little information. The literature related to these themes was explored to further illuminate the findings. The authors concluded that the engagement between the patient and the nurse is important to the patient's perception of receiving quality care.

Walsh (1999) studied the nurse–patient encounter in order to 'uncover meaning and generate understanding of the psychiatric nurse' (p. 2). Walsh interviewed seven nurses and asked them to relate significant encounters exemplifying being a psychiatric nurse. The study revealed three elements of the encounter, 'being-with as understanding', 'being-with as possibility', and 'being-with as careful concern' (p. 2). 'Being-with as understanding' was related to the nurses' ability to grasp the patients' plight in its complexity and entirety; to be able to give meaning to the story. In 'being-with as possibility' the nurse projected towards the future with hope. The activity of the nurse was towards the manifestation of that possibility. 'Being-with as careful concern' exemplified the multitude of ways that the nurses were there for patients. The study revealed a unifying theme of 'shared humanity' (p. 7) that made possible the genuine being-to-being encounter and provided a matrix for the use of self. This study provides a way of articulating the nurse–patient relationship and making sense of the complex interaction in that encounter.

O'Brien (2000; 2001) also studied nurse–client relationships, bringing together the perspective of community psychiatric nurses and clients with a mental illness. The nurses identified 'being-there', 'being concerned', 'establishing trust' and 'facilitating transition' as central to their experience of the relationship (2000, p. 9). The clients identified 'having someone looking out for me, working in collaboration, and being understood and gaining understanding' as central to the relationship (2001, p. 10). O'Brien interviewed five experienced community psychiatric nurses and five clients with long-term mental illness. In bringing the themes from the nurses and the clients together the relationship was revealed as an arena in which the clients could 'be' and in which they could explore the 'possibilities of being' (2000, p. 191). There were distinct similarities in what was important to clients about the relationship and what was important to nurses. This study provided confirmation that the issues that nurses see as important in their work with clients are also important to the clients. The knowledge that nurses bring about mental illness, mental health, responses to illness and health, community responses to mental illness, and a range of treatments for mental illness, was revealed as important. However, this knowledge needed to be utilised within the artistry of the relationship with the client.

The above studies focus on aspects of nursing that cannot be accessed by observation alone. What are revealed are the complex and intricate interactions that occur in nurse–patient encounters. The studies provide a way of articulating the purpose and value of those interactions. These studies have implications for understanding and teaching nursing practice, for nursing services and for further nursing research.

CRITICAL REVIEW OF PHENOMENOLOGICAL NURSING RESEARCH

The framework used to critique phenomenological nursing research overlaps with that of other qualitative methodologies (see Chapters 10–14). There are, however, specific issues that need to be addressed when critically analysing phenomenological studies. Attention to the following issues helps ensure that the methodology that is described is consistent with the phenomenological philosophy identified:

- Does this study reflect a phenomenological view of persons and their worlds? Are the participants seen as able to reflect on their experience of the phenomenon and to develop shared meaning with another?
- Does the researcher describe their own experience and perspective of the phenomenon?
- Is the context of the phenomenon and of the participants described in sufficient detail so that the reader can identify similarities and uniqueness in how the phenomenon might be experienced?
- Are the process and the content of the interview described in narrative?
- Does the analysis of the data focus on the meaning of the experience of the phenomena?
- Does the researcher bring together the background understanding of the phenomenon from multiple sources, their own understandings and that of the participants?
- Do the identified themes provide a way of understanding the meaning of the experience for the participants?
- Are the findings discussed in light of their implications?
- Are the findings discussed in light of phenomenological understandings of what it means to be a person in the world?

KEY POINTS

- Phenomena can be understood through the experiences people have of them.
- Phenomenology provides an understanding of persons and their relationships with their worlds.
- Phenomena are always viewed in their complete concrete context.
- Language is accepted as a means for understanding others' experience of phenomena.
- The researcher is committed to understanding the experience of the phenomena holistically.
- The participants are considered able to reflect upon and articulate their experience of the phenomenon.
- The phenomenological interview is a conversational process between the researcher and the participant(s) that provides an arena where shared meaning can be established.
- The transcriptions attempt to reflect as nearly as possible the experience of the conversations.
- The process of interpretation involves both an awareness of the pre-understandings that the researcher brings to the study and close reading of the text.
- The pre-understandings of the researcher need to be explicated as part of the research data.
- Phenomenological writing is a creative process that reaches beyond narrative description to reveal meaning and understanding.
- The meaning of the experience of the phenomenon needs to be illuminated with its concrete context in order to question beliefs and assumptions.

CRITICAL THINKING CHALLENGES

- Identify phenomena that can be explored within the nursing domain.
- Identify the basic assumptions about persons in Heideggerian phenomenology.
- Consider how the basic assumptions affect the conduct of phenomenological research studies.
- Consider how knowledge gained through phenomenological studies can contribute to the development of clinical practice in nursing.

Additional resources

Atkinson, P. (1995). Some perils of paradigms. *Qualitative Health Research*, 5(1), 117–24.

Baker, C., Wuest, J. & Stern, P.N. (1992). Method slurring: the grounded theory/phenomenology example. *Journal of Advanced Nursing*, 17, 1355–60.

Barkway, P. (2001). Michael Crotty and nursing phenomenology: criticism or critique? *Nursing Inquiry*, 8, 191–95.

Beck, C.T. (1991) How students perceive faculty caring: a phenomenological study. *Nurse Educator*, 16(5), 18–22.

Beck, C.T. (1992). The lived experience of postpartum depression: a phenomenological study. *Nursing Research*, 41(3), 166–70.
Beck, C.T. (1994). Phenomenology: its use in nursing research. *International Journal of Nursing Studies*, 31(6), 449–512.
Gelvin, M. (1989). *A commentary of Heidegger's being and time*. (rev. ed.). Illinois, Northern Illinois University Press.
Koch, T. (1996). Implementation of a hermeneutic enquiry in nursing: philosophy, rigour and representation. *Journal of Advanced Nursing*, 24, 174–84.
Lawler, J. (1998). Phenomenologies as research methodologies: from philosophy to researching practice. *Nursing Inquiry*, 5, 104–11.
Orb, A., Eisenhauer, L. & Wynaden, D. (2001). Ethics in qualitative research. *Journal of Nursing Scholarship*, 33(1), 93–96.
Rather, M.L. (1992). 'Nursing as a way of thinking': Heideggerian hermeneutical analysis of the lived experience of the returning RN. *Research in Nursing and Health*, 15(1), 47–55.
Scott, D. (1997). The researcher's personal responses as a source of insight in the research process. *Nursing Inquiry*, 4, 130–34.
Smith, B.A. (1999). Ethical and methodological benefits of using a reflexive journal in hermeneutic-phenomenological research. *Image: Journal of Nursing Scholarship*, 31, 359–63.
Taylor, B.J. (1992). 'Ordinariness' in nursing: a study (part 2). *Nursing Standard*, 7, 37–40.
Taylor, B.J. (1992). Relieving pain through ordinariness in nursing: a phenomenological account of a comforting nurse–patient encounter. *Advances in Nursing Science*, 15(1), 33–43.
Todres, L. & Wheeler, S. (2001). The complementarity of phenomenology, hermeneutics and existentialism as a philosophical perspective for nursing research. *International Journal of Nursing Studies*, 38, 1–8.
van Manen, M. (1984). Practicing phenomenological writing. *Phenomenology & Pedagogy*, 2(1), 36–69.

14

CHAPTER

Feminist and critical approaches

Debra Jackson, Judith Clare and Judy Mannix

LEARNING OUTCOMES

After reading this chapter the student should be able to:

- Discuss the basic belief systems underpinning critical research approaches.
- Identify the central tenets of feminism and how they relate to research practice.
- Explain how feminist and critical approaches may be linked in research practice.

Key terms

feminism

critical theory

emancipation

hegemony

power

research ethics

INTRODUCTION

What counts as knowledge and who defines it have long been central to social enquiry and as such, have become primary concerns in the scholarly nursing literature. These are issues that unsettle traditional theorists and researchers who have long taken for granted that there is only one way of 'doing' science, and that is through scientific method. However, for the last 50 years there has been an ongoing debate in the literature and in practice about the nature of knowledge, how knowledge is generated and transmitted, and how nurses might legitimately take part in knowledge making. While some authors have described various paradigms of scientific enquiry (such as positivist, interpretative, critical and post-modern) and others maintain the quantitative versus qualitative dichotomy, we contend that it is more useful to describe the underlying beliefs and assumptions about knowledge. The particular theoretical and methodological approaches used in a study or to underpin practice are drawn from a set of personal and professional beliefs and understandings about people and how we come to know and understand our social worlds.

For the purposes of this chapter we will demonstrate how critical and feminist approaches to knowledge generation provide both researcher and participant with the opportunities to explore together the nature of knowledge. The relationship between the knower and the known, the nature of understanding and the nature of reality can be revealed for critique and understanding to make sense of the social world. Both critical and feminist approaches to research use many of the methods and tests for rigour inherent within interpretative, critical and postmodern paradigms. Statistical (quantitative) methods sometimes may be used in critical and feminist research but data will always be interpreted from a critical or feminist perspective. This chapter introduces the reader to critical and feminist approaches to research. We outline the major beliefs and tenets of critical and feminist thought, and link them to the research and its outcomes. Practical issues associated with research using these approaches are discussed and links are drawn between critical theory and feminism.

FEMINIST PERSPECTIVES AND THEIR USE IN RESEARCH

Feminism is both philosophy and practice. That is, feminism is a broad term that represents a complex array of views, beliefs, activism, and political movements and, even as we write this chapter, the boundaries of feminist thinking and scholarship are growing and changing, ebbing and flowing (Barrett & Phillips, 1992; Oleson, 1994; Weedon, 1999). However, from a philosophical perspective, feminism has a central concern with recognising the inherent value of women's ways of being, thinking and doing (Tong, 1995). Feminist theory recognises the centrality of women's experience, and women's concerns and experiences are viewed as legitimate sources of knowledge (Olesen, 1994). Though traditional research approaches position objectivity as analogous to truth, Cook and Fonow (1986) suggest these traditional approaches frequently adopt research methods that are liable to distort the experiences of women. Indeed some of the so-called validated tools that are used in the conduct of research may be based on the belief that knowledge generated from research with men can be generalised to women, or simply biased against women research participants, or founded on unsupported gender-based assumptions.

WHY FEMINIST RESEARCH?

Health discourses have predominantly adopted quite reductionist and fragmented approaches to women, and frequently do not adequately reflect the experiences of women and/or the contexts in which many women live. Nursing has had an uneasy relationship with feminism (Cheek & Rudge, 1995), partly because of the uncritical way in which some early feminists accepted and reinforced sexist stereotypes about nurses (Vance, Talbott, McBride & Mason, 1985). However, feminist theory is compatible with and complementary to nursing, and more nursing researchers are now bringing a feminist consciousness to their work (e.g. Carryer, 1995; Jackson, 2000; Lumby, 1995a, 1997; Parker & McFarlane, 1991; Raftos et al., 1997, 1998; Speedy, 1997).

Feminist perspectives contribute insights important to the conduct of research and the subsequent production of knowledge, including:

- attention to the rights of research participants, and the responsibilities of researchers (Tong, 1995)
- sensitivity to relationships and collaborative endeavour (Lumby, 1995b)
- recognition of the tyranny of language, and its centrality in shaping the world (Spender, 1985)
- an awareness of power and oppression in the social world (Jackson, 1997)
- an understanding of research as an inherently hierarchical (and therefore potentially oppressive) process (Jackson, 1997)
- recognition of the potential for oppression and women's invisibility in the generation of knowledge (Horsfall, 1997; Jackson, 1997; Webb, 1992)
- a valuing of women and an interest in making the experiences and perspectives of women central (rather than marginal) to the process of knowledge production (Cheek & Rudge, 1995)
- a commitment to accessibility of research findings (Campbell & Bunting, 1991; Jackson, 1997; Webb, 1993), and
- transformative potential (Carryer, 1995; Parker & McFarlane, 1993; Speedy, 1991), which is especially relevant to a practice discipline such as nursing (Jackson, 1997).

WHAT IS FEMINIST RESEARCH?

Means of clearly identifying research that may be described as 'feminist research' has been the subject of consideration and controversy. However, despite this controversy, it is generally accepted that feminist research is, by definition, that which is undertaken to benefit women, and focuses on the concerns and experiences of women. Research may be considered to be 'feminist' if it is informed by feminist principles and ideals, and if these principles and ideals are visible in the research design. Stanley and Wise (1993, p. 61) propose that 'feminist research ought to be concerned with the implications of feminism itself'. This may be achieved by positioning women and women's experience as central to the production of knowledge (Cheek & Rudge, 1995), scrutinising feminist tenets and assumptions, and developing an understanding of how these may inform research practice (Stanley & Wise, 1993). Cook and Fonow (1986) identify several principles associated with feminist research and these provide a framework for researchers (see, for example, Jackson, 2000). These incorporate:

- the need for continuous recognition of gender as basic to all social life (including the conduct of research)

- recognition of consciousness raising as an integral aspect of methodology
- acceptance of intersubjectivity and personal knowing as legitimate sources of knowledge
- acknowledgement of ethical responsibilities in research, and
- understanding of the transformative and empowering aspects of feminist research (Cook & Fonow, 1986).

In addition, Reinharz (1992) adopts three criteria for distinguishing feminist research from research undertaken within other philosophical frameworks. These identify feminist research as that which:

- is undertaken by people who declare themselves to be feminist
- appears in feminist publications, or
- has received feminist honour or recognition (Reinharz, 1992).

Feminist literary criticism is an inter-disciplinary mode of enquiry, and has been instrumental in raising awareness of the androcentric influences that are represented in and through language (Ruthven, 1984). It presents a significant challenge to mainstream literature (Humm, 1989), and takes the view that from within a feminist world view, there are no neutral approaches to literature, rather 'all interpretation is political' (Belsey & Moore, 1997, p. 1). The possibilities that literary critiques bring to a practice-based discipline like nursing are captured by Chinn, who argues for the benefits of a scholarly 'shift embracing the humanities' (Chinn, 1995, p. ix), and contends that use of such approaches enhances understanding and facilitates the growth and development of insights for further study and research. Feminist literary critics may apply methods grounded in various forms of textual analysis, or they may aim to establish 'traditions in women's writing which are neither heterosexual, white nor Western' (Belsey & Moore, 1997, p. 11). Within feminist literary criticism, gender is accepted and understood as a basic experiential category.

TENETS OF FEMINISM AND HOW THEY MAY BE APPLIED TO RESEARCH

As acknowledged earlier, feminisms encompass various ideological perspectives and these different, but sometimes overlapping, perspectives each provide distinct approaches to feminist philosophy. However, despite the differences in feminist approaches, they share several common underlying understandings. The most central of these include the assertion that as a group, women are oppressed; the idea that the personal is political; and the concept of consciousness raising, which reflects the awareness raising the potential of feminism (Carryer, 1995; Stanley & Wise, 1993).

The personal is political

Feminist authors have noted that women do not tend to differentiate between their work and personal values, or between theory and practice (e.g. Campbell & Bunting, 1991; Lumby, 1995b). Though a generalisation, this statement highlights the fact that powerful political forces influence women's everyday private lives, and captures the idea that, for many women, their private lives cannot be separated from public existence (Stanley & Wise, 1993). Gatens (1991) suggests that males can achieve what she terms public disembodiment, and thus realise a public and private divide. However, this is only attainable because of the gendered nature of social life that permits men to bypass or transcend certain 'natural functions, childrearing, sensuality and so on' (Gatens, 1991, p. 6). These areas, she argues, have become women's domain, and are relegated to the realm of 'private life'. Thus, 'the conflicts and compromises involved for women who "choose" to be both wives and mothers and paid workers in the public sphere have no parallel in men's lives' (Gatens, 1991, p. 6). Hughes (1997, p. 26) makes a similar point in her discussion of what she terms 'the public/private divide', and Lumby (1995b, p. 197) states that feminist research 'brings the personal into the public arena for debate and scrutiny'.

Starting from the politics of the personal, in which women's subjectivities and experiences of everyday life become the site for the redefinition of patriarchal meanings and values and of resistance to them, feminism generates new theoretical perspectives from which the dominant can be criticised and new possibilities envisaged (Weedon, 1987). This is not to say that the 'political is limited to the personal' (Mohanty, 1992, p. 82), but rather, that personal, individual experiences are the beginning point from which feminists facilitate women's ways of knowing and being visible, and thereby challenge dominant structures oppressive to women (Tong, 1995; Weedon, 1987).

Raising awareness: feminist consciousness raising

In order to develop the understanding necessary to provide relevant and women-centred care, it is essential to have an awareness of issues of concern to women. Consciousness raising is a means through which an increased awareness of the gender asymmetry in the social world may be generated. It has been argued that consciousness raising is a uniquely feminist method (Reinharz, 1992), although feminists see it as rather more than a methodological concept. Reinharz (1992, p. 221) describes consciousness raising as 'a political, therapeutic, or educational activity. Its product is usually not a publication but a new way of thinking, relating, naming or acting'. Several key aspects of feminist theory are derived from consciousness raising, and these include understanding the value of women's experience as authoritative sources of knowledge; and recognition that the experience of being oppressed permeates all aspects of life (Humm, 1989). Consciousness raising is a means of raising awareness, and exploring previously unchallenged aspects of life through a feminist lens, and may result in understandings of gender asymmetry and oppression in the social world. This process of understanding is an important step in developing a feminist consciousness (Stanley & Wise, 1993).

Subjectivity and knowledge

Like other qualitative and critical approaches, feminists do not accept the notion of objective knowledge and a single truth, rather knowledges and truths are seen as constructed (Jackson, 1997; Tong, 1995). The personal perspectives and understandings that people bring to their work, and the futility of researchers attempting to suppress their subjective selves, are acknowledged and accepted (Jackson, 1997; Speedy, 1991). Within feminist thought, subjectivity and knowledge are also raised in relation to the issue of who can be a knower (Lumby, 1995a; Olesen, 1994).

Like everyone else, researchers bring their own culture and sets of values to their work and it is partly because of the centrality of intersubjectivity that many feminist researchers practice reflective techniques, so as to develop insights into their own prejudices and preferences (De Marco, Campbell & Wuest, 1993; Horsfall, 1997; King, 1994). It is only through knowing and understanding one's own experiences and biases that knowledges and insights into the realities of others are developed (King, 1994).

Acknowledging commonality and diversity

Though women have many areas of commonality and shared experience, women are not a homogenous group—'there is no universal "women's experience", because women's lives have never been shaped exclusively by gender' (Hall & Stevens, 1991, p. 17; see also, for example, Weedon, 1999). Coming from an Australian context, Gatens (1991, p. 78) suggests that while 'women may interpret, perceive or experience the same event in ways that differ radically from men', these differences may also be experienced among women of different sociocultural, economic, religious or political backgrounds. These types of contextual issues are becoming increasingly recognised and viewed as crucial to ensuring adequacy and credibility of research findings. Feminist researchers and scholars are continually developing ways to make women's experiences and concerns visible, and to represent the diversity as well as commonality of women and women's experiences.

PRACTICAL ISSUES FOR FEMINIST RESEARCHERS

Now that we have presented some of the ideas behind feminist thinking and feminist research, the next section describes ways in which these ideas transform research, particularly in terms of focus, design, collecting and analysing data, reporting findings, ethics, and achieving adequacy and credibility.

Identifying the focus of the research

The broad aims of feminist research are to illuminate, explicate and validate women's experiences, concerns and ways of being, and to challenge structures that marginalise and oppress women. Feminist researchers have a commitment to ensuring that their work does not contribute to the oppression or mistreatment of women. This may occur indirectly and feminist researchers are careful to consider the ramifications of their projects and to anticipate the possible uses to which findings may be put (Hall & Stevens, 1991).

Designing the study

When conducting research within a feminist framework, researchers need not follow any particular research design. Rather, they may choose methods most fitting to the topic at hand (Webb, 1993). Within feminist scholarship, the idea of taking insights from several (seemingly disparate) methodologies and disciplines and applying them to gain new understandings is acceptable. Indeed, feminist scholars have called for an end to 'methodolatry' (Ruthven, 1984, p. 25) and even urge feminist scholars to 'methodicide' (Daly, 1978, p. 23). Ruthven (1984, p. 25) makes the point that 'a dispersed field demands diverse methods', and argues that 'methodological tidiness leads to reductionism and oversimplification'. In the end, what is important is that the methods applied in the practice of feminist research be compatible with and reflective of the underlying principles of feminism (Cook & Fonow, 1986; Jackson, 1997; Reinharz, 1992; Sigsworth, 1995; Speedy, 1991; Webb, 1993).

Attention to issues of power relationships and equity are fundamental to feminist research. Feminism recognises the nature of power and oppression and therefore research conducted using a feminist approach should not contribute to the exploitation or oppression of any group (Jackson, 1997). The power inequity between researcher and research participant is also acknowledged (Patai, 1991). Reflexivity is a common approach in feminist research, where researchers raise their consciousness concerning their own beliefs and attitudes, and how these beliefs and attitudes influence the interpretation of findings and the construction of knowledge (Hall & Stevens, 1991). Reflexivity may be facilitated in several ways, including use of reflective journals, participation in discussions with supervisors, other students, and other feminist researchers.

Collecting data

The same fundamental data collecting procedures used in established social science investigations are used in feminist research (Hall & Stevens, 1991), including oral and life histories, story telling, in-depth interviewing and participatory action research. For feminist researchers, the collection of research data usually involves direct contact with research participants, and it is therefore important to carefully consider the nature and structure of the contact. As with all research encounters, care must be taken to ensure participant comfort and privacy. When considering interviews, Minister (1991) invites feminist researchers to be mindful of potential differences in communication styles between men and women. This reinforces the idea that a study designed for men may not be suitable for use with women participants. Attention to verbal and non-verbal cues and responses is essential when planning the structure of interviews and other information gaining encounters (Minister, 1991).

Feminist approaches recognise that the thoughts and responses of researchers are a crucial aspect of the research process and indeed are fundamental to the generation of knowledge. Intersubjectivity is embraced, and the researcher is viewed as an active participant in the process (Anderson & Jack, 1991). When considering data collection, researcher input such as memos, entries in reflective journals, thematic ideas, and notes are recognised as secondary sources of data (Thompson & Barrett, 1997).

Analysis of data

Feminist research aims to interpret, explain and validate women's experiences, concerns, and approaches to their world. It is important therefore that analysis of data does not diminish the very thing it is seeking to expound. Listening is the first step in the analysis of narrative data, and needs to occur in certain ways. Anderson and Jack (1991) caution against listening superficially, because doing so diminishes the possibility of seeing things in new ways, and limits the interpretative possibilities. Rather, they suggest three ways of listening that help to understand the narrator's interpretations of their own experiences, and can guide the analytical process:

- attention to moral self-evaluative statements, which make visible relationships between self-concept and accepted cultural norms
- attention to meta-statements, or points in the interview where the narrator stops of their own volition and makes some sort of reflective statement
- attention to the logic of the narrative, which refers to the internal consistency and the inter-relationship of themes in the narrative (Anderson & Jack, 1991).

In addition to listening, questioning the text is also useful to guide analysis (Jackson, 2000). Summary oral reflective analysis is another example of methodological development by feminist researchers that preserves the richness and contextuality of narrative data, and is responsive to the complexity of language used in the oral narrative (Thompson & Barrett, 1997).

Reporting the findings

Language is one of the key areas responsible for the oppression of women, and it is a way that women may be marginalised or excluded (Spender, 1985). Feminist researchers have an ethical commitment to avoiding language that is oppressive or denigrating either to women (Cook & Fonow, 1986) or any other oppressed group (Jackson, 1997). When conducting research or writing research reports, language should be used in a way that is sensitive and respectful, and which gives recognition to the intrinsic worth of women's ways of being and knowing.

Feminist research ethics

Feminist research theories demand a commitment to ethical research practices, as this is one of the key epistemological principles characterising feminist research (Cook & Fonow, 1986). In addition, feminist researchers are frequently interested in exploring issues relating to marginalisation and oppression, and this necessarily raises ethical issues relating to unequal power relationships, as well as possibilities of researcher exploitation (Patai, 1991). Within a feminist framework, ethics is considered to be 'grounded in caring', rather than justice, and this requires that the emphasis be on 'responsibilities and relationships rather than rights and rules' (Tong, 1995, p. 263; similarly Vance et al., 1985). This means that the relationships that develop between researcher and participants are pivotal to the practice of feminist research (Jackson, 1997), and there is recognition that these relationships, like all others, are affected by power and privilege (Patai, 1991).

Achieving adequacy and credibility

According to Olesen (1994) and Jackson (1997), the need to demonstrate credibility is one of the major challenges facing researchers who operate within a feminist framework. However, the criteria for establishing rigour in research have been largely quantitative, and are not able to be reasonably transferred from one paradigm to another (Koch & Harrington, 1998). Despite this concern, all research needs some sort of evaluative criteria for rigour, and feminist scholars (along with other qualitative researchers) have reconceptualised the concept of rigour, so as to make it compatible with feminist research designs. Much of what is written on rigour in qualitative and feminist research focuses on the relationships between the researcher and participants, and propose measures such as 'member checks' (Sigsworth, 1995, pp. 896–99; Webb 1993, p. 420), reflexivity, rapport, coherence, complexity, relevance, honesty and auditability (Hall & Stevens, 1991).

Coherence is established by carefully selecting research methodology and methods appropriate to the aims of the project, and through appropriate analytical and 'writing up' procedures. Hall and Stevens (1991, pp. 24–25) suggest that relevance can be achieved where the research 'questions address women's concerns and … the answers to these questions can serve women's interests and improve the conditions of women's lives'.

CRITICAL APPROACHES TO SOCIAL ENQUIRY

Critical approaches to research, with much of their theoretical foundations in critical theory, attempt to generate knowledge and understanding that is liberating. Proponents of critical social enquiry argue that conventional research from the positivist and interpretative paradigms maintain the status quo in a world that is fundamentally unjust and unfair, and these approaches contribute to this inequity by failing to be sufficiently critical of existing situations (Clare, 1993a, 1993b; Grundy, 1987; Smith, 1993). Critical social science challenges the status quo and offers an approach to change the inequitable state of affairs existing in the social world. To gain a greater understanding of the social world, researchers in the critical paradigm operate from a set of beliefs and assumptions that have the capacity to emancipate people from the constraints under which they are existing and operating.

Beliefs and assumptions in the critical paradigm

A fundamental belief of the critical paradigm is that no aspect of social phenomena can be fully understood exclusive of the historical, cultural, economic and political context in which it is situated (Habermas, 1972; Held, 1980). Further, in the critical paradigm:

- knowledge is believed to have a social dimension and is a product of human activity within a particular historical/economic/sociopolitical context
- the relationship between what is known and the knower does not occur in isolation from the wider societal context, and is not quarantined from society and its associated problems (McCutcheon & Jung, 1990)
- the nature of reality is regarded as being socially and economically based, existing within problems of hegemony (McCutcheon & Jung, 1990). Hegemony, first articulated by Gramsci (cited in Lawner, 1975), describes how the domination of one group (class, state or gender) over others occurs through a combination of political will (coercion) and, more importantly, ideological agencies (e.g. church, trade unions) in society which procure the consent of the dominated groups to be ruled by hegemonic classes/groups
- there is recognition of the existence of inequality between individuals and groups and beliefs that inequality is not a naturally occurring phenomena; it is constructed and maintained through the actions of humankind (Smith, 1993). The construction of inequality is generally undertaken by those in power at the expense of those who are in a much less powerful and more vulnerable position, and is invariably to the advantage of the former.

The nature of critical theory

As noted above, critical theories have their foundations in social change and hinge on notions of oppression and power (Hall, 1999). However, critical theory does not constitute a single entity and 'does not mean the same thing to all its adherents' (Held, 1980, p. 14). This is evident through the work of the theorists of the Frankfurt School, the contemporary work of Jürgen Habermas, and more recently, some forms of post-modernity. Nevertheless, inherent in critical theory are basic notions with a commonality of purpose, including:

- A focus on human activity and the way in which this activity both impacts on broader social structures and is affected by these social structures in the shaping of the social world (Ritzer, 1992).
- An acceptance that values can never be disregarded when considering facts (Kincheloe & McLaren, 1994).
- The recognition that human actors are not passive entities shaped by 'natural forces' but are subjective beings, able to be self-critical, self-reflective and have the capacity to act rationally.
- An acknowledgment that in the formation of subjectivity, 'language is central' (Kincheloe & McLaren, 1994, p. 140).
- The debunking of ideologies of male hegemony, capitalism, racism, heterosexism and classism through the process of rational critique. This critique offers more than negative judgements, taking a positive role in exposing 'existing forms of belief' in order to facilitate the emancipation of people in society (Abercrombie, Hill & Turner, 1984, p. 57). Through this emancipation, people are free to make rational choices in their own best interests of autonomy and with a sense of justice.
- An assumption that no individual wants to be oppressed (Hall, 1999, p. 90).
- A goal to create social conditions facilitating 'open, unconstrained communication' by means of uncovering hidden imbalances of power that 'inhibit free discourse' (Allen, 1985, p. 61).
- An assertion that there is an interconnectedness of theory and practice (Boutain, 1999; Perry & Moss, 1989). In other words, critical theories offer a process of critique comprising a cognitive component as a form of knowledge as well as providing a guide for human actions.

Although critical theorists recognise the impact of the historical influences on knowledge formation, they also acknowledge the possibility existing for truth claims to be determined rationally, independent of the immediate ideological constraints of a wider social context. However, for this to occur, certain conditions need to be present. For one critical theorist, Habermas, these conditions arise in an ideal speech situation, a central concept of his *Theory of Communication Action* (1984; 1987). Habermas (1984) argues each communicative act aimed at understanding is presupposed on a background consensus comprising a set of four universal 'validity claims':

- what is said is comprehensible
- the content is true
- what is spoken is right; and
- sincerity is embodied in what is spoken (Outhwaite, 1994, p. 40).

An ideal speech situation exists when these validity claims are satisfied, based on reciprocity and devoid of domination through force or power that, in turn allows the strength of the better argument to win out. The concept put forward by Habermas provides a useful framework for interviewing in nursing research because of the way equity is advocated between researcher and participant.

RESEARCHING USING CRITICAL APPROACHES

Conducting credible research depends on a researcher having a sound understanding of the theoretical underpinnings, concepts and language associated with a particular approach, irrespective of the paradigm. Therefore, when researching in the critical paradigm it is important to have an understanding of the nature of critical theory, particularly the notions of critique and critique of ideologies. It is also essential that any research conducted using a critical approach has an emancipatory intent aimed at uncovering oppressive ideologies in society, taking account of the sociopolitical, cultural and economic contexts of the research. Given these imperatives, those considering research in the critical paradigm need to be aware that a range of methodological approaches are available to conduct critical research. For example, a research project may be best suited to an action research methodology while another may be better suited to a critical hermeneutic approach or to critical case studies. In this section of the chapter, strategies for conducting credible research using a critical approach are discussed.

Focus of the research

In nursing, the obvious focus of research is the broad area of health and as such, it makes sense that the focus of critical research be aimed at uncovering oppressive aspects in the social world that can affect the health of individuals and groups, as well as the way health care is delivered. Oppressive features in society that may affect health include the position individuals find themselves in based on gender, race, class or economic status. Establishing links between oppression and health occur when critique is used to uncover ideologies that are rarely challenged (Boutain, 1999). The focus of research is not just to establish links and expose unequal power relationships, but also to provide insights into how to promote social change for a more just social world, where the health of all individuals is not impeded by oppressive practices based on particular ideologies.

Designing the study

The design of a study using a critical approach requires careful consideration to:

- The centrality of language, either written or spoken. Words and their meanings are 'symbolic and value-laden' (Campbell & Bunting, 1991, p. 5), and therefore the study needs to ensure a sufficient level of understanding of language.
- The connection between theory and practice, thought and action (Perry & Moss, 1989).
- Incorporating opportunities for self-reflection throughout the study—the process that enables one to look at oneself and the role one is playing in a given situation (Ray, 1992) needs to be incorporated into the research process for both researcher and all participants.
- Recognising that critical theory provides a theoretical framework or orientation for critical research—it is not something that can be tested or applied in a research project. For example, in Sigurdsson's (2001) study that explored what it means to be a perioperative nurse, notions related to language and communication contained in Habermas' theory of communicative action guided the study. At no stage was the theory tested or applied.
- Acknowledging that advocacy for those who are oppressed or marginalised is a central ethical concern in critical research. As Smith (1993, p. 242) points out, the conduct of critical research needs to be guided by 'the critical moral imperative of human emancipation and social justice'.

In the design stage a researcher may find it necessary to 'problematise' a situation or issue in order to ensure it is critical. For example, in Fulton's (1997) study of nurses' views on empowerment, the impetus for the study was the wide use of the concept of empowerment in the nursing world, largely without substantive evidence about what nurses thought of the concept. In designing the study, Fulton problematised the situation into research questions that sought to facilitate self-reflection and uncover unequal power relationships that would lead to change.

Collecting the data

As with feminist research, observation, interviews and examination of text as data are also available to the critical researcher, using similar skills and processes. Importantly though, it is the types of questions asked that shape a critical or feminist study. The processes of data collection in critical research may also be enhanced through other reflexive practices, for example, reflective journalling by the researcher and participants, and returning interview transcripts to participants for review and clarification. The use of such sources as data will largely depend on the nature of the study. For example, a reflective journal may be kept by the researcher during data collection as a way of tracking the project, or a study may use written texts as the only source of data.

Analysis of the data

Analysing data in critical research requires researchers to critically question the data, particularly in relation to sociopolitical, cultural and economic contexts, and in doing so, 'expose hidden power imbalances' (Campbell & Bunting, 1991, p. 5) that are oppressive. Questions asked during data analysis may include:

- whose interests are being served?
- whose reality is being privileged?
- whose voices are being excluded?, and
- who is gaining from the situation?

Analysis may be undertaken solely or collaboratively, and in some types of critical research, analysis may involve researchers and participants in the research collectively working together to 'co-identify the quality of the patterns of communicative interaction' (Ray, 1992, p. 100). Irrespective of the approach, a researcher needs to ensure adequate depth in the interpretation and analysis of the data, a process that will usually involve multiple readings of the data and associated note-taking so as to reflect the centrality of language.

Reporting the findings

Credible and ethical research requires reporting of the study to reflect the central tenets of the critical paradigm; critique of ideology and an emancipatory intent are evident. As Smith (1993, p. 243) comments, the research report should be 'empowering rather than victimising in its style and actions'. In reporting the findings of critical research, some broad similarities exist with other types of qualitative research, especially around presentation and format (e.g. including excerpts from the textual data to illustrate a point).

LINKS BETWEEN CRITICAL THEORY AND FEMINISM

When considering which research approach to use for a particular project there may be occasion to consider a combination of two or more approaches. Before considering this, a researcher needs to ensure sufficient compatibility between the approaches in terms of theoretical underpinnings, philosophical orientations and understandings. In the case of critical and feminist approaches to research, there exists a number of commonalities that enables critical–feminist research to be pursued, including:

- A strong sense of idealism in seeking a social world characterised by equality for all individuals, and a belief this equality can only be achieved through change that will transform society as it currently exists (Campbell & Bunting, 1991). This shared idealism is derived in part from the Marxist critique of positivism and the associated critique of the ideology of objectivity (Westkott, 1990).
- An emphasis on the importance of subjectivity and the experiences of the individual in making sense of the social world.
- A belief that the ability of the individual to be self-reflective and self-critical are intrinsically important to the process of understanding and knowledge production.
- The need for a strong interconnectedness between theory and practice so that 'what is known' is the same as 'what is done' by individuals in society. Both theoretical perspectives take the view that if this occurs, then all of society will benefit as the status quo is challenged and subsequent changes will result in a more egalitarian social world for all individuals regardless of class, race or gender.
- An acknowledgment of the influence of historical factors in the context of knowledge production. Feminists, however, tend to hold the view that historical influences have been detrimental to women and their position in the social world. As Marshall (1988, p. 222) notes, feminism views women's oppression as 'part of an historically situated totality' needing to be transformed
- The recognition that the act of communication is fundamentally important in society. Rational communication, particularly verbal communication, is regarded as the vehicle by which a new and transformed social world can be attained by providing new knowledge and understanding, with unequal power relationships and inequality being exposed.

KEY POINTS

- Nursing knowledge needs to keep pace with increasingly complex health problems and meet the health needs of increasingly diverse societies.
- Nurses are challenged to generate and transmit new knowledge using methods that have the capacity to uncover and critique unequal power relationships. Acknowledging the impact of gender and other socially constructed differences on people's health and ways of being will begin to transform oppressive practices.
- Critical and feminist methods have an emancipatory intent and transformative potential for nurses and other health workers, enabling the development of solutions for complex problems.

CRITICAL THINKING CHALLENGES

- Using an electronic database, search for two feminist research journal articles and two research articles using a critical approach. Discuss how the participants were selected and what methods were used for collecting data.
- Choose a clinical topic, such as recovery from an acute illness or pregnancy and childbirth. Using a database search, collect one published research report in the area that is quantitative and one that is informed by feminist or critical theory. In a small group, compare the reports in relation to the language used in the report, the way the participants are represented, the nature of the findings, and the implications of the research.

Additional resources

Denzin, N. & Lincoln, Y., eds. (1994). *Handbook of qualitative research.* Thousand Oaks, Sage.

Lane, V. & Lawler, J. (1997). Pap smear brochures, misogyny and language: a discourse analysis and feminist critique. *Nursing Inquiry*, 4, 262–267.

Street, A.F. & Kissane, D.W. (2001). Discourses of the body in euthanasia: symptomatic, dependent, shameful and temporal. *Nursing Inquiry*, 8, 162–72.

15

CHAPTER

Action research

Annette Street

LEARNING OUTCOMES

After reading this chapter the student should be able to:

- Understand the basic premise of action research and be able to decide when it is appropriate to use action research in nursing.
- Identify and describe the key values and significant differences between action research and other research methods.
- Describe the key stages of the action research process.
- Describe democratic enquiry.
- Understand the ethical concerns in action research.
- Identify the data collection and analysis methods most commonly used.
- Describe the limitations of the method.
- Understand how the process of reflection is used in action research.

Key terms

action research
catalytic validity
collaborative action
construct validity
democratic enquiry
ethical issues
facilitation
pluralism
preliminary investigation
reference group
reflection
spirals
stakeholders
sustainability
transferability
triangulation

INTRODUCTION

Professional nurses are expected to be advocates and change agents, capable of understanding and improving the health of those in their care through their knowledge and actions. They are also expected to be consumers of and participants in research. This chapter explores the action research process to demonstrate its value to nurses interested in not only understanding a healthcare situation but also being able to work with others to improve it. This connection between collecting evidence to understand a situation and collaborative action is the hallmark of an action research approach. Action research addresses three concerns raised by clinical nurses (Greenwood, 1994). Action research studies are:

- situational; that is, they address the specific needs in context
- participatory and so involve all those who are interested in, or will be affected by, the outcome
- self-evaluative, enabling individuals and groups to assess their own contribution to, and the functioning of, the research activity.

Action research is the method of choice when people want to join together to understand, critique and improve their situation.

THE HISTORY AND BASIC PREMISES OF ACTION RESEARCH

The term 'action research' was coined in 1946 by social psychologist, Kurt Lewin, to describe the research program he developed in response to serious post–World War II social problems in America (Lewin, 1946). Lewin's interest was in narrowing the gap between research recommendations and implementation so that democratic enquiry could lead the way to group decisions and a commitment to improvement (Lewin, 1951). He wanted to develop a concrete procedure for translating evidence into action. His research experiences led him to recognise that change introduced from outside was rarely effective because it is difficult to anticipate all the possible consequences of action in the real world (McTaggart, 1991). To deal with this Lewin argued for a cyclical research process that enabled action to be carefully monitored, analysed and evaluated as the basis for reflection on the success of the plan and the possibility for modifying it and starting another cycle of planning, action, data collection, analysis, evaluation and reflection. This cyclical process would continue until the situation had improved.

This early form of action research has generated many variations and related methods that are generally collected under the umbrella term of action research and are committed to the notion of emergent shared goals to close the theory–practice gap (Reason & Bradbury, 2001). Action research is more a style of research than a specific method (Dick, 1999). Research processes that cluster under the action research umbrella include action science, action enquiry, action learning, participatory research, cooperative enquiry, soft systems methodology, transparent research, and community development research.

There have been a number of attempts to classify these forms of action research depending on their interests and whether they take a 'bottom-up' approach (Holter & Schwartz-Barcott, 1993). Hart and Bond (1995) promote four basic kinds of action research:

- experimental
- organisational
- professional
- empowering.

Each of these methods has a different emphasis but they share common premises about the interrelationship between theory and practice, research and action. In the experimental model the researcher conducts the action research in a socially scientific manner that is focused on an experimental intervention to provide a controlled outcome with causal processes that can be generalised. The organisational model is managerial or client-focused, with the most powerful group defining the problem for others providing for a top-down directed approach to achieve tangible outcomes. The professionalising model has a reflective practice perspective and is practitioner focused. Professional problems arise from practice or experience and the group is professionally led with a dynamic style aimed at improvement in practice and on behalf of others affected by the changes. Finally, the empowering approach involves a consciousness raising bottom-up approach designed to allow the problem definition to develop and be addressed as awareness grows. As there are a number of vested interests involved in this form of research, there is also an allowance for pluralism in outcomes.

It is helpful to be able to categorise nursing research into these formats in order to see where the focus of the study is situated. Neither type is better than another, with each type being the most applicable in certain situations. Sturt (1999) and Meyer (2000) make the important point that most projects move between these typologies. For example, they may begin as professional action research that is initiated by a professional interest, and become empowering action research, where the stakeholders take over the shaping of the project and carry it on into the future. The kinds of topics that nurses have investigated can be loosely classified as organisational, professional or emancipatory approaches, as evident in Table 15.1.

TABLE 15.1 Types of nursing action research

TYPE	AUTHORS	FOCUS
Emancipatory	Selim, P., Bashford, C. & Grossman, C. (2001).	Tap water cleansing of leg ulcers in the community
	Walters, S. & East, L. (2001).	Homelessness in young mothers
	Koch, T. & Kelly, S. (1999).	Urinary incontinence in women with MS
	Blackford, J., Street, A. & Parsons, C. (1997).	Communicating with people from non-English speaking backgrounds
Professional	Webster, J. (1999).	Evaluation of implementation of bedside handover
	Rose, K., Waterman, H., McLeod, D. & Tullo, A. (1999).	Managing day surgery for cataract
	Street, A. F. & Robinson, A. (1995).	Advanced clinical roles

	Lindsey, E., Sheilds, L. & Stajduhar, K. (1999).	Effective nursing partnerships
	Street, A., Cuddihy, L., Wilks, D., Geladas, D., Chew, S. & Best, D. (1997).	Rostering practices
	Manley, K. (1997).	Advanced practice role
	Suderman, E. M., Johnson, L. S., Deatrich, J. V. & Sawatzky-Dickson, D. M. (2000).	Discharge preparation
	Balfour, M. & Clarke, C. (2001).	Self-administrative and medication
	Heslop, L., Elsom, S. & Parker, N. (2000).	Managing psychiatric crisis in emergency
	Bennett, B. (1998).	Increasing collaboration within a multidisciplinary research project
	Moyer, A., Coristine, M., Jamault, M., Roberge, G. & O'Hagan, M. (1999).	Identifying older people in need
	Kelly, D & Simpson, S. (2001).	Clinical practice facilitators in an acute setting
Organisational	Baillie, L. (1999).	Preparation for management roles
	Cowley, S. & Billings, J. R. (1999).	Implementing health visiting services
	Lauri, S. & Sainio, C. (1998).	Nursing care of breast cancer patients
	McElroy, A. & Sheppard, G. (1999).	Assessment and management of self-harming patients in A & E

Although there is some use of the organisational model, most nurses engaging in action research work within the professionalising and empowering modes that are in sympathy with the words of Wadsworth (1993).

Participatory action research is not just research which we hope will be followed by action! It is action which is researched, changed and re-researched within the research process. Nor is it simply an exotic variation of consultation. Instead, it is active co-research, by and for those who are to be helped. Nor can it be used by one group of people to get another group of people to do what is thought best for them—whether that is to implement a central policy or an organisational or service change. Instead, it is a genuinely democratic process whereby those to be helped determine the purposes and outcomes of their own enquiry. Paradoxically, it is quite close to a common sense way of going about 'learning by doing'. But at the same time it is very hard to achieve the ideal conditions for putting it fully into practice.

Likewise, McNiff and Whitehead (1996, p. 14) summarise the distinct features of action research as:

- it requires action as an integral part of the research process itself
- it is focused by the researcher's professional values rather than methodological considerations
- it is necessarily insider research, in the sense of practitioners researching their own professional actions.

THE ACTION RESEARCH SPIRAL

Most forms of research are constructed in a series of linear steps from hypothesis/question to recommendations for action; but action research is usually depicted as some variation of a spiral design. The spiral design used in this chapter is not dissimilar to Lewin's (1946) original design and was formed out of my research work with nurses over the last 20 years (Street, 1995). It is simple to understand and has worked well in many nursing projects.

FIGURE 15.1 Action research spiral

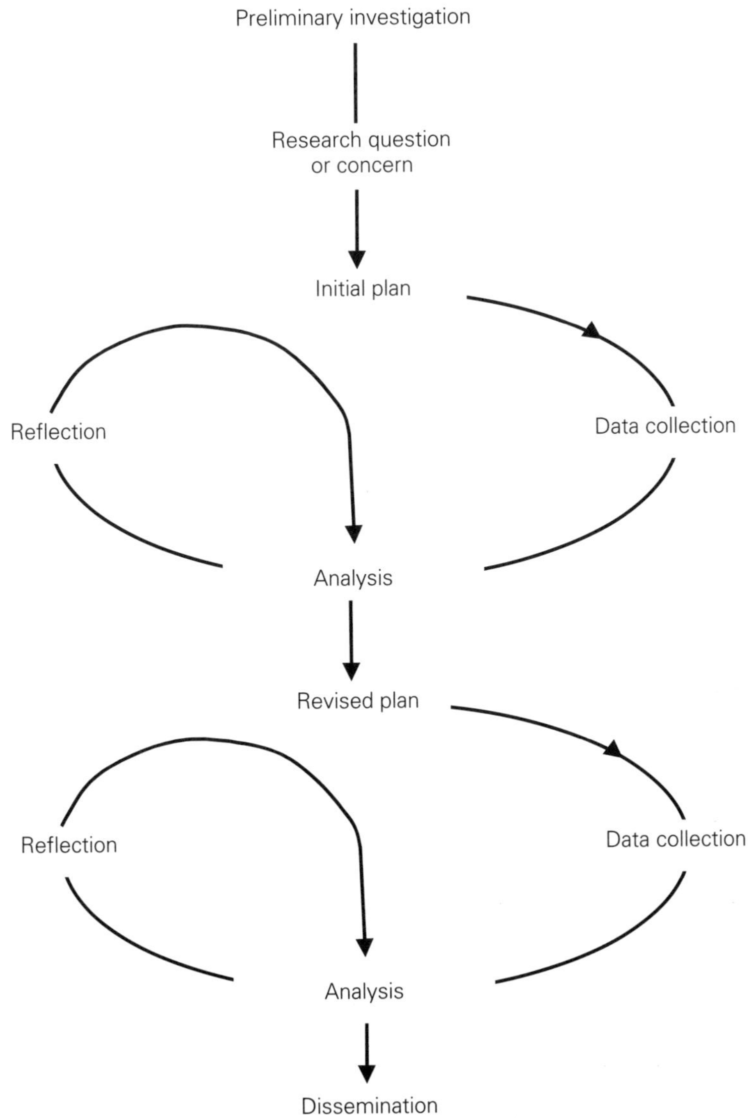

The spiral consists of a number of stages, some of which are repeated until the situation improves.

Preliminary investigation

A thorough investigation enables the research team to capture some information in order to understand the current situation and the evidence of the problem. This process generally involves:

- a literature review of the literature on the topic including government or hospital reports
- an analysis of the history to the problem that might include the healthcare context, the organisational procedures and practices, the rationale for the previous solutions to the problem, and issues relevant to personnel in the situation
- an analysis of solutions tried by others
- an identification of all those who are interested in this situation (stakeholders)
- the collection of baseline statistics about the situation that might be used to measure any improvement.

The preliminary investigation demonstrates the extent of the problems in the situation under consideration and assists the research team to develop a specific research question.

Research concern and objectives

The research concern might be quite broad as it relates to the whole situation. It is commonly followed by a number of objectives that define the key research questions that enable the research team to clarify the concern under investigation and keep focused. Engaging in action research is like opening a can of worms. New possibilities wriggle off in different directions and it is easy to get sidetracked following them. Reflecting on the main concern at various cycles in the project can re-orient the team.

The question needs to be asked in such a way that it is possible to know if it has been answered. For example, an Australian study directed at the management of urinary incontinence in women with multiple sclerosis (MS) arose because continence nurses had found that 80 of their referrals were from women with MS (Koch & Kelly, 1999). The study had four clear objectives:

- to identify ways in which women with MS self-manage their urinary incontinence
- to identify current nursing practice in relation to the management of urinary incontinence with women with MS
- to combine the information from women with MS and nurses to identify the best possible management of urinary incontinence among women with MS
- to disseminate the information to improve the management of urinary incontinence among women with MS.

These objectives contained a number of key elements of action research—collaborative investigation, strategies, education and dissemination.

Planning action

Planning action needs to be done systematically. McNiff and Whitehead (1996) remind us that research is systematic enquiry made public. As this is action *research* and not just action it is important to be very clear about the first action plan and how it is to be monitored and evaluated. It is best if the team agrees on one strategic action to be implemented and monitored. If more than one action is planned at the same time, it is not possible to discern whether the effect was caused by the combination of actions or just the result of one action. The planning stage takes account of the *objective* conditions or the physical and material conditions and constraints, along with the *subjective* conditions for action, that is, the patterns of formal and informal relationships, the competing values held by people and the expectations they hold (Kemmis & McTaggart, 1988). The action plan is prospective or future-oriented: it includes what will be done; what the expected outcomes are; and the means by which these outcomes will be assessed.

Implementation

Implementing action means sticking to the action plan for as long as has been agreed upon, unless there is evidence of serious harm—very uncommon in this form of research. Nurses are educated to react quickly and to deal with constantly changing situations. Sometimes nurses are tempted to treat action research as normal practice and want to change or add actions before sufficient evidence has been gathered to fully understand the alterations occasioned by the action plan. It is vital to be able not only to explain the effects of the action, but also able to account for the unintended circumstances and constraints that become evident. The constant changes in the healthcare situation mean that there are a number of unforeseeable circumstances that may affect the implementation of action. For example, nurses conducting action research in aged care facilities at the time of a change of government policy found that nurses became caught up in a need to rapidly prepare documentation for new accreditation procedures and abandoned their action plan and data collection strategies. They had to be reformulated and renegotiated after major accreditation activities were completed.

Data collection

There are a number of different ways that action researchers collect data about the effects of an action plan. Common methods are surveys, interviews, observation, audits and various forms of charting. These methods have been described in detail in other chapters in this book and so will not be repeated here.

An additional method that is very common to action research and has been adopted more widely in other methods is the use of a personal/professional journal where researchers document their ideas and local theories about the research and their role in it as it evolves. The use of a journal provides the individual with access to a rich resource of raw data about their professional lives for analysis and action. Through this process the nurse recognises the limitations of the solutions of the 'experts' and begins to pose appropriate new problems that contain the potential to transform their own professional nursing practice and the healthcare context in which it is practised.

Analysis

When the data collection strategy is put in place, then there needs to be a clear understanding of how the data will be analysed. The forms of analysis are consistent with those described in this book, especially in Chapter 23 and the relevant sections of Chapters 9 through 14. Decisions need to be made about the extent to which the research team will be involved in the analysis. This will differ depending on the skills required and the time available.

Computer packages are available to assist quantitative and qualitative researchers code, manage and analyse their data. Statistics packages like SYSTAT or SPSS have the capacity to analyse the data but qualitative packages like NUD*IST or ETHNOGRAPH require the researcher to do the analysis. The conceptual mapping, data integration and linking capacities of NVivo (Bazeley & Richards, 2000) are particularly helpful to manage complex action research projects.

Reflection

As descriptive data are collected and analysed, the values, theories, attitudes and assumptions in use in professional practice are exposed through a process of reflection (Street, 1991). This process needs to be systematic as it is the basis for developing or testing theories. This capacity to generate 'theories-in-use' and build them into theories or conceptual models is a distinguishing trademark of action research, separating it from continuous quality improvement (Waterman, 1996). Reflection can occur in two ways.

First, individuals who are keeping journals engage in a process of assessing their own taken-for-granted assumptions and habitual practices, along with the way their growing understanding of the social conditions assist or hinder the change process (Sturt, 1999).

Second, individuals share their reflective accounts and understandings with group members. This sets up a retrospective group assessment of the progress that has been made in light of the wider research question and the values, theories and assumptions that inform the current and desired situation. This group reflection has an evaluative component as the researchers judge the progress in preparation for the next planning stage. It also has a responsive component. During reflection, researchers not only examine the analysed data but also the research processes and the roles of all involved. So the interest is not only in *what* was discovered but *how* it was discovered, under what conditions, and how this relates to the wider concern. This is the 'lessons learnt so far' stage that provides a rationale to underpin the next action plan (Lindsey, Sheilds & Stajduhar, 1999). At this stage the group decides if the previous action plan needs to proceed with modifications or whether a new but related plan can be introduced to address the research question.

Revised plan

The revised plan needs to be clearly documented. Sometimes the previous plan will continue with a different form of data collection; at other times a related plan will be developed using all the steps taken in the initial plan.

Spirals upon spirals

It is worth noting that many projects develop mini sub-projects with their own spirals that are attached to the main spiral. These branch spirals reflect the different interests of group members in pursuing specific objections related to the main question. For example, in Robinson's study with an aged care assessment team, the team developed two related spirals depicting networking projects that developed out of an initial pilot networking project. One project was directed at establishing more effective networks with general practitioners in the community, whereas the second spiral was directed at improving networks with nurses in the acute sector. Each sub-project was part of the overall research intention to understand and improve the networking skills and capacity of the members of the aged care assessment team.

Dissemination

A common feature of the final stages of action research is the process of feedback to all the stakeholders in appropriate formats. These might take the form of forums, conference presentations, media releases, newsletters and reports. Interactive feedback methods such as focus groups and seminars can provide valuable information to fine-tune the intervention.

Research is not completed until it is published. All researchers who receive funds or institutional support for their research owe it to their colleagues, supporters and the wider nursing community to publish the results of their research. Publishing a paper on action research is a challenge because the spiral shape of the process is difficult to readily depict in the linear forms of papers. Whereas a thesis or large report has the capacity to allow the action researcher to demonstrate the various action cycles, articles for publication or conference presentations require the researchers to organise their work into sections. Thus the action plans may be listed together even though they happened over time. Likewise the various data collection and analysis strategies are often conflated into one section rather than being associated directly with the action plan. Alongside a section on limitations, a common feature of action research papers is a section on 'lessons learnt' as an aid to other nurses interested in a similar endeavour.

COLLABORATIVE RESEARCH PARTNERSHIPS AND INVOLVEMENT

In most chapters in this book the section following the framework is directed at explaining sampling. Although some sampling may occur in the implementation stages of the process, the focus of action research is on partnerships and involvement. As action research aims to be democratic and inclusive of those the research outcomes are expected to affect, there are a number of strategies that are used to facilitate the widest involvement possible.

The research relationships can be organised so that nurses and other stakeholders participate in one or more levels of involvement. These levels of involvement can be illustrated through an action research project that was designed to develop, trial and evaluate flexible rosters able to meet the demands of the nursing service as well as the needs of the individual nurses (Street et al., 1997). As this had implications for wages and conditions, there were many interested parties involved.

The first layer was the unit-based action research groups who were the people most affected by the outcomes of the research (Street, 1998). These were small unit-based teams of nurses and nurse managers, who met regularly with their colleagues to plan, implement and collect data on the project. The next layer consisted of the project research team. This team was a collection of elected or designated people who were given time release from their clinical, management or union roles to participate in the day-to-day running of the project. This time release was managed so that each day one person from the team was available to troubleshoot issues for the unit research groups or to participate in the wide variety of research activities used in this study. The third layer was the stakeholder project management group which met less frequently and acted more as a watchdog committee to ensure that their vested interests were being addressed in the group. This committee was called the reference group and involved state nursing union representatives, personnel, hospital management and government nursing advisors. Regular and structured input was sought from a fourth layer of other stakeholders involved with occupational health and safety, a brain research institute, other hospitals and health agencies. The following list in Box 15.1 depicts a plan of how these various stakeholder groups could interact with the action research process.

BOX 15.1 Action research project structure

- Identify a nursing situation that needs improvement.
- Establish a collaborative research group concerned with addressing the situation.
- Establish a reference group composed of all key stakeholders.
- Conduct training workshops for participating nurses in action research.
- Conduct a preliminary investigation to develop baseline data and understand the scope of the concern.
- Meet with the reference group to examine the data and assess the proposed plans.
- Implement the first action plan, collect and analyse data.
- Group reflection and re-planning through the spiral.
- Meet with the reference group to discuss project results.
- Disseminate the findings in accessible formats to all stakeholders.

Action research is necessarily insider research, in the sense of practitioners researching their own professional actions.

ETHICAL ISSUES

Although action researchers need to be mindful of all the ethical considerations outlined in Chapter 8, there are specific considerations to keep in mind. When the project begins it is not always possible to predict the data collection strategies that may be adopted in later planning stages. It may be necessary to gain provisional ethics support with an agreement that if there are changes in data collection that might necessitate further ethics approval, then this will be sought. Likewise, the number of participating researchers and stakeholders means that access to and storage of confidential material must be carefully addressed.

FUNDING

Action research projects that are funded are required to specify a timetable. It is usually the end of the funding period that marks the end of the project. This is often a difficult matter to predict. Many action research projects gain their own impetus and researchers want to keep working through more cycles to achieve a better outcome. If too little time is allocated then it is unlikely that sustainable change will occur. Widespread participation, time, effort and enthusiasm are necessary for effective action research (Karim, 2001).

VALIDITY AND RIGOUR

The dynamic and fluid aspect of action research and the involvement of stakeholders as novice researchers may mean that there are difficulties maintaining research rigour. The emphasis on finding concrete and practical solutions may become the focus of the research to the detriment of systematic recording, that is, the researchers may be more focused on *action* than on *research*. Time pressure can also affect rigour.

One of the key arguments for rigour in action research was the proposition advanced in the mid-1970s by influential methodologists concerning the use of triangulation, as described in Chapters 2 and 12. The argument for triangulation of methods assumed that the weaknesses in one method would be counter-balanced by the strengths in another. These arguments have challenged action researchers to develop conceptual triangulation. Each research approach that is incorporated into the design, whether it is in the form of surveys, interviews or document analysis, needs to be evaluated separately in accordance with its own methodological criteria. In this way each part can stand alone, while also being linked conceptually to other parts.

Many action researchers adopt the criteria of credibility, auditability and fittingness as already discussed in Chapter 9. Lather (1991) has argued that action researchers can also use catalytic validity to determine if the research was systematic and valid. Because action research is change-oriented with a focus on changing knowledge, language, practices and the situation, its outcomes need to be evaluated against these criteria. Catalytic validity is evident when the research provides the catalyst that produces a desired systematic change in most or all these areas (Balfour & Clarke, 2001).

LIMITATIONS OF THE METHOD

Like all research methods, action research has a number of limitations that need to be considered before engaging in an action research project: time, the involvement of many people, and the context-specific nature of the research design.

Novice researchers and the organisations supporting them can be influenced by the desire to solve problems swiftly. This may affect the quality of the analysis, and in many cases, time pressure truncates or eliminates the reflection process central to thoughtful research and the capacity to test theories and build theoretical models. Rigorous action research is a time-consuming process, as sustainable change takes time to accomplish.

The need for many stakeholders to be involved at different levels can also provide organisational difficulties and may affect the capacity of some people to be involved.

The findings of action research are context specific and therefore not generalisable from one setting to another. In response to this critique, action researchers argue for the transferability and sustainability of their work. Transferability refers to the capacity of the theories and techniques to be useful in another setting while sustainability relates to the capacity of the research changes to continue after the official life of the research.

In conclusion, action research has great value for clinical nurses. It involves and educates individuals as members of wider nursing groups, it is context specific and issue focused, it fosters change, it links action and analysis through a cyclical process, and it is relevant and inclusive of stakeholders.

KEY POINTS

- Action research is a useful method for nurses to use when they want to understand and improve a situation.
- Action research is action focused and context specific so can address problems of practical concern.
- Action research uses a cyclical process in which the research, implementation, evaluation and theorising are linked to reduce the theory practice gap.
- Triangulation of methods and data sources enable a broader picture to emerge.
- The involvement of all stakeholders means that those who will be affected by the research results are involved all through the process.
- The intention of action research is to produce systematic and sustainable change that can be widely disseminated and used in other settings that share the same concerns.

CRITICAL THINKING CHALLENGES

- Identify an issue that concerned you from your clinical experience and create an action research question. How can you justify that this is an action research question?
- How would you conduct a preliminary investigation on this topic? What might be an initial plan and what kind of data would you collect?
- What do you consider would be the limitations in conducting this project? How might you overcome them?
- Identify all the stakeholders who would be affected in a study on improving the sexual and reproductive health information available for Muslim teenagers.

Additional resources

Baillie, L. (1999). Preparing adult branch students for their management role as staff nurses: an action research project. *Journal of Nursing Management*, 7(4), 225–34.

Bennett, B. (1998). Increasing collaboration within a multidisciplinary neurorehabilitation team: the early stages of a small action research project. *Journal of Clinical Nursing*, 7(3), 227–31.

Blackford, J., Street, A. & Parsons, C. (1997). Breaking down language barriers in clinical practice. *Contemporary Nurse*, 6(1), 15–21.

Cowley, S. & Billings, J. R. (1999). Implementing new health visiting services through action research: an analysis of process. *Journal of Advanced Nursing*, 30(4), 965–74.

Heslop, L., Elsom, S. & Parker, N. (2000). Improving continuity of care across psychiatric and emergency services: combining patient data within a participatory action research framework. *Journal of Advanced Nursing*, 31(1), 135–43.

Kelly, D. & Simpson, S. (2001). Action research in action: reflections on a project to introduce Clinical Practice Facilitators to an acute hospital setting. *Journal of Advanced Nursing*, 33(5), 652–59.

Koch, T., Kralik, D. & Taylor, J. (2000). Men living with diabetes: minimizing the intrusiveness of the disease. *Journal of Clinical Nursing*, 9(2), 247–54.

Lauri, S. & Sainio, C. (1998). Developing the nursing care of breast cancer patients: an action research approach. *Journal of Clinical Nursing*, 7(5), 424–32.

Manley, K. (1997). A conceptual framework for advanced practice: an action research project operationalizing an advanced practitioner/consultant nurse role. *Journal of Clinical Nursing*, 6, 179–90.

McElroy, A. & Sheppard, G. (1999). The assessment and management of self-harming patients in an Accident and Emergency department: an action research project. *Journal of Clinical Nursing*, 8(1), 66–72.

Moyer, A., Coristine, M., Jamault, M., Roberge, G. & O'Hagan, M. (1999). Identifying older people in need using action research. *Journal of Clinical Nursing*, 8(1), 103–11.

Retsas, A. (1994). Problematic telephone orders: empowering nurses through action research. *Australian Journal of Advanced Nursing*, 11(2), 19–27.

Rose, K., Waterman, H., McLeod, D. & Tullo, A. (1999). Planning and managing research into day-surgery for cataract. *Journal of Advanced Nursing*, 29(6), 1514–19.

Selim, P., Bashford, C. & Grossman, C. (2001). Evidence-based practice: tap water cleansing of leg ulcers in the community. *Journal of Clinical Nursing*, 10(3), 372–79.

Street, A.F. & Robinson, A. (1995). Advanced clinical roles: investigating dilemmas and changing practice through action research. *Journal of Clinical Nursing*, 1995(4), 349–57.

Suderman, E.M., Johnson, L.S., Deatrich, J.V. & Sawatzky-Dickson, D.M. (2000). Action research sets the stage to improve discharge preparation. *Paediatric Nursing*, 26(6), 571–84.

Walters, S. & East, L. (2001). The cycle of homelessness in the lives of young mothers: the diagnostic phase of an action research project. *Journal of Clinical Nursing*, 10(2), 171–79.

Webster, J. (1999). Practitioner-centred research: an evaluation of the implementation of the bedside hand-over. *Journal of Advanced Nursing*, 30(6), 1375–82.

16
CHAPTER

Collaborative evaluation research

Tina Koch

LEARNING OUTCOMES

After reading this chapter the student should be able to:

- State the purpose(s) of evaluation research.
- Define impact, outcome, process and collaborative evaluation research.
- Describe the dominant approaches in evaluation in terms of generations.
- Understand why a review of the literature is important.
- Identify the research process in 'qualitative' evaluation.
- Appreciate ethical issues in collaborative enquiries.
- Identify evaluative criteria that may indicate rigour of the enquiry.
- Describe the likely nature of the outcomes using fourth generation evaluation.

Key terms

action
agenda
change
collaborative evaluation
concurrent analysis
construction
facilitation
feedback
formative evaluation
impact evaluation
negotiation
participation
process evaluation
responsive focusing
stakeholders

INTRODUCTION

Evaluation research in health has emerged as one of the most important activities in recent decades. Evaluation activities include assessing needs, passing laws, delivering health programs, health education and promotion, formulating policies, managing people and resources, nursing interventions, restructuring, changing organisational culture, educating students, intervening in conflicts and solving problems.

In nursing contexts, it can be argued that the goals of evaluation research are to provide evidence about our practice, service or programs. This evidence is necessary for decision-making by those who provide the funding as well as demonstrating accountability for our work. Evidence procured in this way provides assurances of quality in our practices. Those who fund health services and programs want to be reassured that health outcomes are achieved and that interventions we provide make a difference in the lives of clients and in the wider community. Indeed, evidence provided by evaluation can be used to convince funding agencies, clients and the community that our services, programs and projects are necessary and viable. Evaluations can work in our interest and protect our jobs (Koch, Marks & Tooke, 2001). If we are astute and generate evaluation data from everyday nursing practice, evidence so obtained can provide a persuasive argument for the maintenance of our roles. As Wass (2000, p. 121) writes, 'the daily practice of an individual health worker, the overall work of an agency or team, and specific health promotion activities or projects will all benefit from regular evaluation'. Although outsider consultants conduct evaluations, the argument presented here is that it is both impractical and costly for nurses not to do in-house evaluations. Not only should we take charge of our own evaluations, evaluating *with* stakeholders will provide evidence that our programs, services and practices are relevant for clients and the wider community. In this chapter, the focus will be on taking responsibility for evaluations that affect our lives, our services, our programs and our professions.

EVALUATION RESEARCH

Evaluation is applied research for the purpose of informing action, enhancing decisions and making and applying knowledge to solve problems identified in practice. The central evaluation question is, 'are people accomplishing what they want to accomplish?'. The term 'evaluation research' includes 'any effort to increase human effectiveness through systematic data based enquiry. Here it is assumed that human beings are engaged in all kinds of efforts to make the world a better place' (Patton, 1900, p. 11). A simple definition of evaluation is 'the systematic application of research procedures for assessing the conceptualisation, design, implementation and utility of services, programs or practice' (adapted from Rossi & Freeman, 1993, p. 5). Being *systematic* is the operating word. It is not useful entering the debates surrounding quantitative and qualitative evaluation research, but rather we should ask, 'what is the most appropriate methodology to answer the questions posed?'.

MEASUREMENT DRIVEN EVALUATION

Nevertheless, it is important to understand that the dominant approach in evaluation is driven by measurement, so before collaborative approaches are discussed, an overview of quantitative strategies is provided in the section to follow.

Indeed the term, evaluation research, has been applied to a wide spectrum of investigative activities. The most common evaluation method is to monitor or measure against predetermined objectives and indicators using a range of methods. The type of evaluation that we are most familiar with is derived from the experimental and testing traditions in sciences. In measurement traditions, evaluation is carried out so that judgements can be made about a practice, program, project or service. Two of the most basic questions asked are: Is this practice, program, service or project meeting its targets? Is it worth funding? The features of measurement driven strategies are:

- measuring effectiveness by examining whether or not a service has reached required standards on pre-specified criteria
- seeking objective numerical data
- use of parameters e.g. randomised use of large samples
- use of a control group
- findings are able to be generalised.

Evaluations are usually identified with measurement, and the results are used by managers to control and predict aspects of the health service, its staff and clients/patients. As such, evaluations appear as something done 'to', 'at' or 'on' us (Wadsworth, 1997). This chapter is about other kinds of evaluation tentatively known as qualitative evaluation, but before proceeding, some definitions are examined.

Impact, outcome and process evaluation

Consistent with evaluations based on measurement, the terms 'impact evaluation' and 'outcome evaluation' are often used. Impact evaluation refers to testing the performance of the program, project or service once it has been implemented and as soon as it has been completed. It is concerned with the immediate effects of the program, project or service. Evaluation is a political activity, and it is important to gain consensus on the program's objectives before the evaluation plan is established. When the program's objectives are clearly stated and verified, there can be no doubt what is to be tracked, measured and why. When the evaluation is driven by objectives (as the most common evaluation strategy), impact corresponds to achieving the objectives, recording both intended and unintended effects. In other words, outcome evaluation questions if the program, project or service has met its goals. Often this assessment includes the cost, and is concerned with longer term effects than those addressed in impact evaluation.

In contrast to impact evaluations and outcome evaluations, during 'process evaluation' or 'formative evaluation', the evaluator examines what happens while evaluating. 'The term *formative evaluation* refers to the provision of short loop diagnostic feedback about the quality and implementation of—and immediate responses to—methods, activities and programs' (Green & Lewis, 1986, p. 27). A broad view of this type of evaluation may include forming focus groups as well as seeking the immediate response of onsite people. Short loop feedback is required so that problems and issues identified during the implementation of the program can be communicated quickly to administrators, so that refinements and improvements can be planned and implemented.

Process evaluation is particularly valuable in practice when you want feedback on program implementation, site response, client response, practitioner response and the competencies of personnel. A focus on process is on how something happens rather than on the outcomes of the results obtained. Process implementation documents the extent to which a program is delivered as planned. As noted earlier, evaluation research is not conducted in an apolitical context; others may have vested interests in delaying the implementation or are capable of obstructing or subverting the program. Therefore, it is important to assess and monitor the site's political context. In the course of process evaluation, the satisfaction of those involved in the program, project or services, are recorded. This refers in particular to clients or beneficiaries of the service. Incorporating the insights and feedback of those practitioners implementing the program is essential for process evaluation. Implying that consultation takes place, practitioners can offer their interpretation of the situation and offer improvements. Feedback on the level of knowledge, skill and performance of the various healthcare professionals who deliver the program can be ascertained. Most agencies have established competencies for practice, with competencies being assessed through informal interviews, brief case analyses, short quizzes and self-evaluation and appraisal. Onsite observation of staff performance may also be indicated.

SELECTING AN EVALUATIVE STRATEGY

Selection of a strategy is based on the evaluation question(s). Whether you are conducting quantitative or qualitative research, and as discussed, the most common evaluation method is to monitor against predetermined objectives and indicators. So what is the service, program or project objective(s)?

There are many qualitative evaluation models. Illuminative evaluation (Green & Lewis, 1986) provides an intensive study of the whole program, with the model using three steps: observation, enquiry and explanation. Data are collected through observation, and accompanied by semi-structured interviews and/or open-ended questionnaires. Stake's model (1973) relies on historical records, questionnaires, interviews, standardised tests and instruments, thus combining quantitative and qualitative data generation strategies for describing a program. Scriven (1972) argues for a Goal-Free evaluation. The important difference here is that ideally the evaluator does not know the program's objectives. The main purpose is to investigate and judge if the program is meeting the needs of the target group. Data are generated as for Stake's model. The CIPP model (Stufflebeam, 1973) requires information for decision-making via description and analysis of components: Context, Input, Process and Product.

This has been a useful strategy for a number of recent evaluations, including the Collaborative Action Program (CAP) project, in which a new model of service is designed to meet the complex needs of older persons with mental health problems (challenging behaviours). This project is discussed further in the 'Literature review' section on pages 45–46. Context evaluation provides a basis for the program's objectives and it describes the environmental conditions in which the program is to operate. Data are generated through observation, interviews and analysis of archival material. Context and Input evaluations usually occur before a program begins. The latter component identifies and assesses relevant capabilities of the agencies involved with the program, and consultation of the literature (as is shown below) and/or other expert sources is undertaken. Product evaluation, the last component of CIPP, interprets program attainments during and on completion of the program. If the first three steps are completed successfully, program effectiveness and efficiency will be ascertained. In the CAP evaluation, which included an economic assessment, the information secured continued funding for the program. It is noted that a qualitative evaluation is primarily a process or formative strategy, allowing the use of collaborative enquiries to expand on process activity.

COLLABORATIVE EVALUATION

Collaborative evaluation moves beyond process evaluation strategies to include stakeholders in the evaluation. In other words, it is *with* people. A central notion driving this type of evaluation is negotiation. Collaborative evaluation:

- involves all participants affected by the evaluation
- enables participants to research alongside the evaluator
- integrates program development and implementation from the very beginning
- incorporates evaluation data throughout the life of a project so that actions become more congruent with evolving goals
- identifies views that may be in conflict and creates a safe place for their engagement
- integrates a new thinking process into an organisation's culture.

Regardless of the type of evaluation strategy, the phases outlined below are usually followed for a collaborative enquiry:

- evaluation questions
- literature review
- context in which the evaluation is carried out
- identifying key people with whom to collaborate
- identifying principles to guide the enquiry, including ethical considerations
- designing the research plan
- interview guided by concerns, claims and issues (CC&Is)
- recording the process
- data generation
  - observation
  - individual interviews
  - group work—negotiation
  - journal accounts as data
- rigour
- outcomes.

Evaluation questions

Before even thinking about particular methodologies, the evaluator needs to be clear on the purpose of the study and the topic to be investigated. The questions of 'why' and 'what' need to be answered before the question of 'how' can be answered. Is it to provide evidence for the funding continuation of a position(s)? Is it about articulating a practice, service, project or program so that decisions can be made about its viability? Is it to evaluate an alternative health service delivery model? Is an evaluation necessary for apprehending and describing program processes? Or is it to discover the success indicators of a dynamic program and to describe the program so that it can be replicated elsewhere? Is it for understanding the meaning of a program to its participants? Or is it to describe variations in program implementation at different sites? All investigations begin with evaluation questions.

Literature review

Following the research process, it is equally important for evaluation research to be informed by the literature. The objective of a review is to find if similar services, programs or projects exist, explore the way they have been evaluated and observe decisions made regarding their outcome. It may be useful to show the kinds of literatures reviewed before discussing evaluation of the CAP project (Koch, Marks, & Moss, 1999). It involves a systematic unpacking of issues and constructs surrounding these keywords. In fact the literature for each word in the project title is researched.

The first literature search was to locate the categorisation of mental health problems. It was found that the term 'mental illness' has its conceptual base within the dominant medical discourse and relies on the *Diagnostic and Statistical Manual of Mental Disorders* (DSM-4) (2000) developed by the American Psychiatric Association. The next stage of the review was to describe these categories. The narrow medical focus of this literature required consideration of the sociological literature. Utilising the database Sociofile, readings were consulted for a wider appreciation of the situation. Noted in the literature was that mental illness has two focuses: social construction of mental illness and a critique of the medical conceptualisation of a psychiatric illness. The setting in which mental healthcare is delivered was also pertinent to this review. It is recognised that the most significant change in mental healthcare policy has been the de-institutionalisation of people with a psychiatric disability into community-based care. Tracking its development from institutions into the community became part of the review. Recently, a number of Australian national and State government enquiries and reports have drawn attention to people with a mental illness and their need for community care. So the review turned to government reports for further clarification of issues.

Further, an extensive search of the major, relevant databases (Sociofile, CINAHL, PsycLIT, Australian Health Journals and Medline) was conducted from 1997 through to 1999 seeking literature which described and evaluated other service delivery models for people with challenging behaviours residing in the community. The review then turned to the way alternative service models were justified. In so doing, gaps in service delivery for this specific group were identified. Readings revealed that mainstream services were reluctant to include people with a serious mental illness in their programs. Next it was important to describe what constitutes challenging behaviour. After this was defined for the purpose of this evaluation, the literature around service delivery models in mental health, and in particular case management, was assessed. Five components of case management were described and these components were not unlike the CAP model envisaged, hence providing potential indicators of the evaluation.

In summary, these literatures were linked to provide a concise background and helped to shape the evaluation. This meant taking care to define constructs as it moved from categorisation, sociological constructs, de-institutionalisation, government reports and direction, other service delivery models and their justification, to what constitutes challenging behaviours and towards case management and identifiable criteria useful for evaluation.

Context in which the evaluation is carried out

Collaborative evaluations take account of wider contexts and are primarily concerned with description and interpretation. The first task of the evaluator is to become familiar with the day-to-day reality of the settings to be encountered and to unravel the social and political situation. Use is made of documents, often for historical data and to gain an insight into local politics. As for CIPP evaluations, the context is described and is included in the final report.

Identifying key people with whom to collaborate

Collaborative enquiries rely on participation of stakeholders (those who have a stake in the outcome of the evaluation) and the agenda for evaluation is devised by the participants. Stakeholders are defined as those who have a direct involvement with the group or setting that is to be evaluated. Deciding who can participate is the evaluator's second task. In addition, the evaluator has to be mindful that the enquiry is both feasible and manageable. The following examples illustrate the scope and feasibility of completed evaluations. In a nursing home study (Mitchell & Koch, 1997) all people employed (nurses, managers, cooks and gardeners) by this organisation (n = 50) were interviewed. Most importantly, residents and significant others were invited to 'have a say' (Koch, 2000). In a study exploring career options for district nurses at clinical nurse consultant level, 30 consultants participated in individual interviews. In addition, representatives from management, unions, and nurses working at clinical nurse or registered nurse levels provided additional interview data (Koch, Zadoroznji, Hudson, et al., 1999; Koch, 2000). In total, 80 people were interviewed and a group of 20 people (representatives) met around the negotiating table. In a Master of Nursing project evaluating a nursing unit (a nurse led ward), the student interviewed all healthcare professionals, and client opinion about CC&Is was sought (n = 40). Another Master of Nursing student chose all clients attending nursing clinics as the first stage in gaining an understanding of the concerns of this group (n = 30). Based on these experiences, stakeholders should not exceed 80, given that it is useful to complete individual interviews before groups are convened. Nevertheless, a ward or a small nursing centre is the ideal size for a collaborative evaluation and this strategy is manageable for insider or in-house evaluations.

Identifying principles to guide the enquiry, including ethical considerations

Evaluation research usually has to be approved by a legally established ethics committee. Institutional ethics committees are interested in ways participants are recruited, their self-determination and protection from harm. There are a few ethical principles worth considering. Evaluators ask stakeholders if they want to be involved in research and if they will give up time for interviews and similar activities. Individual interviews of staff are better organised outside working time, hence the stakeholders must be prepared to commit their own time and energy to ensuing group work. The evaluation study requirements must be discussed before informed consent can be given.

What are the benefits? What do interview participants get in return for sharing their time and insights with the evaluator? Will they or their communities benefit in some way from the results of the study? If promises are made (such as copies of reports or monetary payments), those promises should always be kept.

Of course it is not possible to promise confidentiality when people work in groups, however, it is possible that names of people and places will be fictionalised unless otherwise negotiated and agreed. Before commencement of the observation period allowing exploration of contextual issues, permission needs to be obtained from the organisation to read its data and files, correspondence or other documentation.

In collaborative enquiries, participants involved in the research have an equal right to be informed, and to engage in any decision-making affecting them. Participants have the right to say 'no' to an interview request, the right of reply, and the right to have a voice in the affairs of an evaluation that affects them; in fact, their participation is central. Evaluation in healthcare settings can be abused and to that end, coercion, overt or covert, is not tolerated. Questions to be answered are, 'What will happen to the data generated?' and 'What rights do participants have in relation to such data files?'.

Openness underlies all collaborative transactions, particularly in discussions between stakeholders (Koch, 1994a). If an interview is given, steps should be taken to ensure that the account reflects the concerns raised by the participant. The evaluator will almost certainly find that different individuals and groups will 'see' the same situation in different ways and that there are multiple realities according to the values people hold. Bringing common concerns and/or issues together is the task of the evaluator, and obviously this requires effective facilitation skills. It is not unusual to find that nurses working at senior levels (and these nurses are most likely to undertake evaluation research) have highly developed facilitative skills. So it is possible to organise an in-house evaluation utilising existing skills. Group dynamics are infinitely engaging, with each group having its particular needs and setting its own norms. Despite group diversity, the principles of respect, equity and ability to be heard make the process possible in any environment. It is important that any recommendations flowing from the report will be implemented, hence management is not only one of many stakeholders, but its commitment to see it through is central.

Designing the research plan

Fourth generation evaluation (FGE) as proposed by Guba and Lincoln (1989) is one possible collaborative research plan. To summarise, first generation evaluation relies on *measurement*, the second generation is driven by *measurable objectives*, and third generation is based on the *judgement* of the evaluators. In healthcare settings, most evaluations are derived from these generations. An evaluator external to the organisation is contracted to conduct the research. A report arising from the evaluation is owned by the organisation funding the study. Often, the evaluator has no independence and no control over the use made of evaluation findings. The evaluator is expected to provide an unconditional service to the organisations and policy makers who employ the evaluator. Often the evaluator is asked to accept the values of those who hold office. The evaluator's role is seen as a management consultant whose role is to offer information that will help the organisation to accomplish their policy objectives. Notions of service, utility and efficiency direct this type of evaluation.

Note that quantitative research represents first generation evaluation; the models of Stake (1973) and Stufflebeam (1973) fit into the second and third generations of evaluation; whereas FGE, as the fourth type of evaluation, is contingent upon *negotiation*. The appeal of a negotiation process is that the evaluation strives to give its participants (stakeholders) a voice or opportunity to have a say about things that affect them. It is an evaluation strategy that can be incorporated into daily practice and with some additional resources (e.g. time and expert guidance), it can be completed as an insider's evaluation project.

Interview guided by concerns, claims and issues (CC&Is)

Evaluation is a joint collaborative process and aims at the evolution of consensual constructions about what is being evaluated. FGE argues for all stakeholders to have a right to place their concerns, claims and issues (CC&Is) on the negotiating table. *Claims* are defined as 'favourable assertions', *concerns* are 'unfavourable assertions', and *issues* relate to situations where 'reasonable persons may disagree' (Koch, 1994b). This process is not unlike participatory action research, however this agenda is shaped by the CC&Is identified.

Recording the process

The evaluator is involved in individual interviews, and once an agenda has been formulated, group discussions take place. Decisions are made about recording the individual and group conversations, and as the evaluator is concerned with great detail, it is usual to find the use of audiotapes for at least some interviews. Verbatim transcription is very useful to capture language conventions and metaphors that characterise conversations. The analysis of these conversations can reveal tacit assumptions, interpersonal relationships and status differentials. Interviews and their transcripts produce a large volume of material that must be condensed, categorised or otherwise interpreted and made meaningful. It is ideal if a research support person is able to word-process the group conversation concurrently. It may seem resource intensive, but there is no doubt that an instant record obtained through having a support person to type the conversations as they evolve means analysis can proceed immediately.

Data generation

There are a number of ways in which data may be generated, including observation, interviews and reflective journals.

Observation

Observation is one of the main methods of generating data and is especially useful during the early 'immersion' period. The evaluator builds up a continuous record of events that might be considered on the fringe of the study, e.g. ward/community centre meetings, committee meetings and management meetings. Prolonged engagement in order to establish rapport and build trust is necessary if the evaluator is to uncover constructions and to become immersed in understanding the culture's context. This means being in the field for an extended time. If already working in the research setting, adequate time in the field is not an issue except that the evaluator may need to view the situation with 'new' eyes. Persistent observation means that the evaluator can identify those characteristics that are most relevant to the issues being pursued. Systematic recording and analysis of observational data are brought to the evaluation as another approach to tease out the relevant issues.

Individual interviews

Interviewees are asked to tell the evaluator their construction of concerns, claims and issues as they apply to the situation being evaluated. These focuses or reference points are the CC&Is, and form the basis of what must be asked of all stakeholders, namely, 'What are your concerns?'. In addition, this question gives shape to the analysis and the agenda for negotiation.

Stories told to the evaluator are taken to represent meaningful constructions that stakeholders form to make 'sense' of the situations in which they find themselves. Interviewing aims to uncover as much as possible of the participant's construction, understandings, reasoning and biographical perspective. As discussed, in FGE, the evaluator is more likely to use semi-structured interviewing (responsive focusing) so that CC&Is can be ascertained. The major advantage is that the data generated are systematic and comprehensive, while the tone of the interview still remains fairly conversational and informal. Teasing out the constructions that participants hold is the evaluator's main task.

Skill is required for the interviewer to be sensitive to non-verbal messages, effects of the setting on the interview, and nuances of relationships. These observations can be captured in a daily journal. Maintaining a daily reflective journal provides evidence about what is going on while researching. For instance, if the interviewer is fatigued, impatient or irritable, these influences are recorded and brought into the analysis.

While much of the value of qualitative interviewing lies in its flexibility and openness, it remains extremely important for the evaluator to think through the process and provide the basic structure and framework for analysis. In the case of FGE it is somewhat easier because questions are guided by CC&Is. However, in an FGE study involving residents of a nursing home (Michell & Koch, 1997), many participants could not relate to FGEs guiding CC&I questions, so a conversational style was developed instead—for example, participants were asked 'Tell me about your day', 'What do you like/do not like about this nursing home', and 'What do you feel strongly about?'. Here the skilled interviewer can use flexibility and insight to ensure an in-depth, detailed understanding of the participant's experience.

Group work—negotiation

Negotiation must be carried out under circumstances where all parties are in possession of the same level of information. This may mean that stakeholders require assistance in understanding what information means for their interests. The idea of 'hermeneutic' accepts that participants in the evaluation are self-interpreting and bring their constructions to the negotiating table. Views may be in conflict, however, emphasis is placed on creating a safe place for their engagement. The evaluator acts as broker and facilitator in exchanges of information between groups who want knowledge about each other.

As discussed, the negotiation process begins with open-ended interviews with stakeholders. Once all interviews have taken place and individual feedback has been offered, decisions are made about who is represented around the negotiating table. The agenda listing common CC&Is are presented at the first group meeting (Koch, 1994b; Koch, 2000), and is followed by prolonged and persistent engagement with stakeholders, with sometimes eight to ten group meetings. When group meetings are at regular intervals (say weekly, every fortnight, or monthly), concurrent analysis is essential. As information is collected, it is analysed immediately, and fed back for comment, correction and revision at subsequent meetings. Stakeholders at subsequent group meetings can view the analysis of issues emerging from previous conversations and renegotiate common issues. The process is a continuous, dialectic chain of questioning, answering, analysing and requisitioning.

Although the evaluator brings the agenda for negotiation to a representative group, this does not mean that the evaluation will end in consensus. However, it will be possible to create an agenda where CC&Is are clearly identified, even if only some items are acted upon. Social change is seen to take place when stakeholders themselves create their own solutions based on their understanding of the problem.

When common CC&Is are agreed upon and negotiated, there is a moral imperative that this form of evaluation will lead to action. Common CC&Is can direct negotiation in the process of action planning, action taking, and back into iterative cycles of evaluation. Once an agenda listing common issues is agreed, some items are usually identified for action. Participants decide which of the CC&Is they wish to act on and who is volunteering to follow it through. Facilitating action, participants can be asked to identify:

- objectives
- the tasks
- steps to be taken for each task
- the people involved
- the place where the activity will occur
- the timelines
- duration of the activity
- the resources required.

Evaluation data are incorporated throughout the life of the evaluation so that actions become more congruent with evolving goals. These are monitored and reported as part of the FGE process.

Journal accounts as data

If the evaluator is an insider, maintaining reflective notes is essential. A reflective journal or field diary is one way that a researcher can achieve insights and clarity of their project experiences. Reflective notes can provide valuable stimuli for the formation of ideas on the process and progress of the evaluation, responses to interactions with participants and a daily recording of events. Analysis of reflective notes can be incorporated into the final report.

Rigour

Clearly FGE cannot be evaluated with criteria from quantitative evaluation research, however it is important to ask if the account presented is believable. Guba and Lincoln (1989) discuss criteria for assessing the quality of FGE evaluation. As discussed, peer debriefing is cyclic and ongoing. Member checks are the essence of the negotiation process. The final construction (the report) is the summary of all recorded negotiations (even those not agreed upon) as feedback is given to stakeholders. In effect, the report is written concurrently. An audit should be able to be carried out as all journal accounts, actions and transactions of the evaluation process are recorded (Koch, 1994a; Koch & Harrington, 1998).

One of the appealing aspects of FGE is that the final report is written collaboratively. The onus is to write a report in a language that is not only accessible to all stakeholders but also for decision-makers who determine whether a service, program or practice is viable. If the evaluation report is to effectively communicate findings, it must meet ethical standards such as confidentiality and respect, be readable and be usable for its intended audiences. In some cases, different reports may be needed for different audiences.

Outcomes

Collaborative evaluation is a local process. Its outcomes depend on local contexts, local stakeholders and local values that cannot be generalised to other settings. Experience suggests that FGE is not always a neat, orderly activity that proceeds step-by-step through the process. The research relationship described here is dynamic and evaluation is a process with 'unpredictable outcomes' (Guba & Lincoln, 1989, p. 255).

On the other hand, FGE involves all participants affected by the evaluation, thus there is a stronger sense of ownership of the actions and outcomes. FGE is a process for sharing accountability. Equally important is the conviction or assumption that the engagement of practitioners in researching their own practice will prompt action. Value is attached to human decision-making and control of action lies with the stakeholders. The aim of an activist ideology is that action is taken by the participants to advance or improve the situation at hand. Outcomes of the evaluation process are considered successful when change prompted by the FGE has occurred. Whatever the outcomes, a transparent culture is created with FGE process in which stakeholders and funds providers will have greater clarity about the way the service, program or practice operates. Making the world a better place is the ultimate outcome.

KEY POINTS

- One of the goals of evaluation research is to provide evidence about practice, service or programs.
- Evaluating *with* stakeholders will provide evidence that programs, services and practices are relevant for clients and the wider community.
- The most common evaluation method is to monitor/measure against predetermined objectives and indicators, however, a range of methods can be used.
- Selection of an evaluation strategy is based on the evaluation question(s).
- Quantitative evaluations appear as something done 'to', 'at' or 'on' us.
- There are many qualitative evaluation models.
- Impact evaluation refers to testing the performance of the program, project or service once it has been implemented and as soon as it has been completed.
- Outcome evaluation questions if the program, project or service has met its goals.
- During process evaluation or formative evaluation the evaluator examines what happens while evaluating.
- Process evaluation is particularly valuable in practice for feedback on program implementation, site response, client response, practitioner response and the competencies of personnel.

- Collaborative evaluation (e.g. fourth generation evaluation or FGE) moves beyond process evaluation strategies to include stakeholders in the evaluation, in other words, it is *with* people.
- A central notion driving this type of FGE evaluation is negotiation.
- The objective of a literature review is to find if similar services programs or projects exist, explore the way they have been evaluated, and observe decisions made regarding their outcome.
- Collaborative evaluations take account of wider contexts and are primarily concerned with description and interpretation.
- Collaborative enquiries rely on participation of stakeholders (those who have a stake in the outcome of the evaluation) and the agenda for evaluation is devised by the participants.
- FGE is a joint collaborative process and aims at the evolution of consensual constructions about what is being evaluated.
- FGE argues for all stakeholders to have a right to place their concerns, claims and issues (CC&Is) on the negotiating table.
- The negotiation process begins with open-ended interviews with stakeholders.
- Social change is seen to take place when stakeholders themselves create their own solutions based on their understanding of the problem.
- When common CC&Is are agreed upon and negotiated, there is a moral imperative that this form of evaluation will lead to action.
- An audit should be able to be carried out as all journal accounts, actions and transactions of the evaluation process are recorded. As the final document is produced collaboratively the account is likely to be believable.
- Collaborative evaluation is a local process.
- FGE evaluation is a process for sharing accountability.
- The aim of an activist ideology is that action is taken by the participants to advance or improve the situation at hand. Outcomes of the evaluation process are considered successful when change prompted by the FGE evaluation has occurred.

CRITICAL THINKING CHALLENGES

- Why should we take responsibility for our evaluations?
- Can you say why some evaluations appear as something done 'to', 'at' or 'on' us?
- Is it important to be inclusive in evaluation? What are the benefits of inclusivity?
- Why is it important to articulate an evaluation question before you decide on the methodology?
- What are some reasons for conducting an evaluation?
- What is meant by the term 'context'? Why is it important to describe the context in which an evaluation takes place?
- How would you ensure that everyone around the negotiating table has a voice?
- Why is FGE an ideal model for insider evaluation research?
- What are the ethical considerations when conducting collaborative enquiries?

- What are the resources implications for tape recording the interviews and conversations? What are the alternatives to tape recording?
- What are the benefits of verbatim transcription?
- Can you list some activities that may enhance the rigour of the evaluation process?

Additional resources

Arts, S.E.J., Francke, A.L. & Hutton, J.B.F. (2000). Liaison nursing for stroke patients: results of a Dutch evaluation study. *Journal of Advanced Nursing*, 32(2), 292–300.

Baum, F. (1999). Public health issues for the 21st century. *Australian and New Zealand Journal of Public Health*, 23(2), 115–16.

Eriksen, L.R. (1995). Patient satisfaction with nursing care: concept clarification. *Journal of Nursing Measurement*, 3(1), 59–76.

Gerdtz, M. & Bucknall, T. (2000). Australian triage nurses' decision-making and scope of practice. *Australian Journal of Advanced Nursing*, 18(1), 24–32.

Greeneich, D.S., Long, C.O. & Miller, B.K. (1992). Patient satisfaction update: research applied to practice. *Applied Nursing Research*, 5(1), 43–48.

Ketefian, S., Redman, R., Nash, M.G. & Bogue, E.L. (1997). Inpatient and ambulatory patient satisfaction with nursing care. *Quality Management in Health Care*, 5(4), 66–75.

Koch, T., Kralik, D. & Taylor, J. (2000). Men living with diabetes: minimising the intrusiveness of the disease. *Journal of Clinical Nursing*, 9(2), 247–54.

Lindop, E. & Cannon, S. (2001). Evaluating the self-assessed support needs of women with breast cancer. *Journal of Advanced Nursing*, 34(6), 760–71.

Luther, K.M. (1996). Data-driven interventions to improve patient satisfaction. *Journal of Nursing Care Quality*, 10(4), 33–39.

Mahon, P.Y. (1996). An analysis of the concept 'patient satisfaction' as it relates to contemporary nursing care. *Journal of Advanced Nursing*, 24(6), 1241–48.

Megivern, K., Halm, M.A. & Jones, G. (1992). Measuring patient satisfaction as an outcome of nursing care. *Journal of Nursing Care Quality*, 6(4), 9–24.

Melia, B. (2000). Conducting an interview. *Nurse Researcher*, 7(4), 75–89.

Nehls, N., Owen, B., Tipple, S. & vanderMause, R. (2001). Lessons learned from developing, implementing and evaluating a model of community-driven nursing. *Nursing & Health Care Perspectives*, 22(6), 304–07.

Taft, L.B. (1993). Computer-assisted qualitative research. *Research in Nursing & Health*, 16, 379–83.

Wellard, S. & Palaster, L. (1996). An evaluation of two methods of pre-cannulation skin infection. *Australian Journal of Advanced Nursing*, 14(1), 3–7.

Wu, M., Courtney, M. & Berger, G. (2000). Models of nursing care: a comparative study of patient satisfaction on two orthopaedic wards in Brisbane. *Australian Journal of Advanced Nursing*, 17(4), 29–34.

SECTION THREE

Quantitative research methods

17
CHAPTER

Approaches in quantitative research

Zevia Schneider

LEARNING OUTCOMES

After reading this chapter the student should be able to:

- Discuss the aims and objectives of quantitative approaches.
- Discuss the approaches, outcomes and values of quantitative designs.
- Define 'population', 'sample', and 'sampling'.
- Discuss the purpose of sampling.
- Discuss the advantages and disadvantages of commonly used sampling strategies.
- Explain the difference between sampling size and sampling error.
- Discuss the eligibility criteria for sample selection.
- Define non-probability and probability sampling.
- Discuss the procedure for drawing a sample.
- Discuss the factors that influence determination of sample size.
- Discuss internal and external validity.

Key terms

data saturation
delimitations
directional hypothesis
external validity
hypothesis testing
inclusion criteria
internal validity
non-directional hypothesis
population
random selection
representative sample
sample
sampling
study validity
systematic sampling

INTRODUCTION

The paradigmatic and methodological differences between qualitative and quantitative approaches were discussed in Chapter 2. Quantitative research refers to those studies whose findings are quantified and reported as summary statistics and analysis (Cohen, 1988). Quantitative research approaches are often referred to as scientific or empirical methods that depict reality as something that is objective and external to the researcher. In contrast, qualitative or humanistic approaches provide emphasis on the personal and subjective nature of an enquiry with findings reported in a narrative form.

The word 'design' implies the organisation of research elements into a masterful work of art and represents the major distinctive research approach that has been chosen for the specific purpose of answering a specific question. The research question and the aims and objectives influence and guide the choice of design. In order to make an informed choice about which design will best answer the research question, and for the consumer to understand the implications and the use of research, a clear understanding of designs is important. This chapter provides an overview of the meaning, purpose and issues related to quantitative research design, and presents a variety of approaches used in quantitative research. The following chapters provide more detailed discussion on data collection (Chapter 18), and observational (Chapter 19) and interventional (Chapter 20) designs and related methods. Common to these approaches are issues of study validity and sampling, which are discussed later in this chapter.

The design must be able to answer the question posed by the researcher. On this basis alone nurses can begin to determine whether a paper describing a research study could be of value in informing their practice (Greenhalgh, 1997). A variety of considerations, including the type of approach chosen, affect the value of the study. For example, in quantitative research these considerations include objectivity in the conceptualisation of the problem, operational definition, accuracy, feasibility, control of the experiment, hypothesis testing, replication, internal validity and external validity. Of these, the most important concepts are control, operational definition, hypothesis testing and replication.

CONTROL

In quantitative research the researcher's main aim is to use a design to maximise the degree of control over the variables tested. A research variable is a defined concept that varies and has two or more properties (e.g. age, height). Control involves holding the conditions of the study constant, that is, allowing for variation, specifying the variation permitted, or distributing the variation equally. Included is the need to establish specific sampling criteria or subject inclusion criteria, which enable a representative sample to be drawn from a larger population. There are statistical principles behind the many forms of control, but a clear conceptual understanding is of greater importance for the research consumer. Basic to the concept of control is internal and external validity: internal validity refers to the degree to which it can be inferred that the experimental treatment, rather than an uncontrolled condition, resulted in the observed effects; while external validity refers to the degree to which the findings of a study can be generalised to other populations or environments.

OPERATIONAL DEFINITION

An operational definition refers to measurements used to observe or measure a variable and to the delineation of the procedures or operations required to measure or evaluate a concept. This procedure is necessary to avoid confusion or misunderstanding. Recall in Chapter 8 the definition of self-care (see page 127). It is possible that another researcher may provide a more restricted or broader definition. What is important is that by stating a particular operational definition, the researcher has identified the empirical referents, enabling the research consumer to judge the results of the study accordingly.

HYPOTHESIS TESTING

In quantitative studies, hypotheses are not always stated explicitly in a research article. Hypotheses flow from the problem statement, literature review and theoretical framework. An hypothesis is an assumptive statement about a relationship between two or more variables that suggests an answer to the research question. Hypothesis testing is the most commonly used purpose of inferential statistics, and answers such questions as 'Is there a difference between the two groups?' or 'What is the relationship between the two variables?' or 'What are the changes over time?'.

Regardless of the specific format used to state the hypothesis, the statement should be worded in clear, simple and concise terms. The three important points are:

- the variables of the hypothesis
- the population being studied
- the predicted outcome of the hypothesis.

Directional versus non-directional hypotheses

Hypotheses can be formulated directionally or non-directionally. A directional hypothesis is one that specifies the expected direction of the relationship between the independent and dependent variables. In this case the existence of a relationship is proposed as well as the nature or direction of that relationship. An example of a directional hypothesis is: 'Patients who report less support in the marital relationship also report more problems with emotional and physical adjustment to breast cancer than do patients who report more support' (Hoskins et al., 1996). Examples of directional hypotheses can also be found in Table 17.1, in examples 2–5, 7 and 8.

A non-directional hypothesis indicates the existence of a relationship between the variables, but does not specify the anticipated direction of the relationship. An example of a non-directional hypothesis is 'There will be a difference in competency in drug calculation among third-year Bachelor of Nursing students at hospital A and hospital B'. Examples of non-directional hypotheses can be found in Table 17.1 in examples 1 and 6.

In addition to directional and non-directional hypotheses, there is a causal hypothesis. As the name implies, a causal hypothesis postulates a cause for any change and is frequently used in the evaluation of interventions and new drugs. In a study evaluating clinical guidelines in nursing, midwifery and the therapies (Thomas et al., 1999), the causal hypothesis was 'The use of clinical practice guidelines leads to improvements in practice'. The independent variable (the

TABLE 17.1 Examples of wording of hypotheses

HYPOTHESIS	VARIABLES*	TYPE OF HYPOTHESIS	TYPE OF DESIGN SUGGESTED
1 There will be a relationship between self-concept and suicidal behaviour.	IV: Self-concept DV: Suicidal behaviour	Non-directional research	Non-experimental
2 Synchrony of maternal and newborn sleep rhythms will be negatively related to postpartum blues.	IV: Synchrony of maternal and newborn sleep rhythms DV: Postpartum blues	Directional research	Non-experimental
3 Structured preoperative education is more effective than structured post-operative education in reducing the patient's perception of pain.	IV: Preoperative education IV: Post-operative education DV: Perception of pain	Directional research	Experimental
4 The incidence and degree of severity of subject discomfort will be less after administration of medications by the **Z**-track intramuscular injection technique than after administration of medications by the standard intramuscular injection technique.	IV: **Z**-track intramuscular injection technique IV: Standard intramuscular injection technique DV: Subject discomfort	Directional research	Experimental
5 Progressive relaxation will be more effective in reducing indices of physiological arousal than hypnotic relaxation or self-relaxation in patients undergoing cardiac rehabilitation.	IV: Progressive relaxation IV: Hypnotic relaxation IV: Self-relaxation DV: Physiological arousal indices	Directional research	Experimental
6 There will be a relationship between years of nursing experience and attitude towards patients with human immunodeficiency virus (HIV) disease.	IV: Years of experience DV: Attitude towards HIV patients	Non-directional research	Non-experimental
7 There will be a positive relationship between trust and self-disclosure in marital relationships.	IV: Trust DV: Self-disclosure	Directional research	Non-experimental
8 There will be a greater decrease in post-test state anxiety scores in subjects treated with non-contact therapeutic touch than in subjects treated with contact therapeutic touch.	IV: Non-contact therapeutic touch IV: Contact therapeutic touch DV: State anxiety	Directional research	Experimental

*IV, Independent variable; DV, dependent variable.

dissemination of clinical practice guidelines to a variety of health professionals), was deliberately manipulated in order to assess its effects on the dependent variable (improvements in practice). The researchers claimed that the guidelines caused the improved practice.

Statistical versus research hypotheses

Readers of research reports may observe that an hypothesis is further categorised as either a research hypothesis or a statistical hypothesis. A research hypothesis, also known as a scientific hypothesis, consists of a statement about the expected relationship between the variables. A research hypothesis indicates what the outcome of the study is expected to be. A research hypothesis is also either directional or non-directional. If the researcher obtains statistically significant findings for a research hypothesis, the hypothesis is supported. For example, in a study exploring the relative effectiveness of one intervention—the side-lying position during breastfeeding to minimise fatigue—Milligan, Flenniken and Pugh (1996) hypothesised that 'postpartum women [who] delivered vaginally and who breast fed in the side-lying position would report less fatigue symptoms than women who breast fed in the sitting position'. The authors reported a statistically significant difference in the average number of fatigue symptoms between the two breastfeeding positions in subjects who had vaginal deliveries. As such, the hypothesis is supported, that is, the predicted outcome was supported by the study findings. The examples in Table 17.2 represent research hypotheses.

TABLE 17.2 Examples of statistical hypotheses

HYPOTHESIS	VARIABLES*	TYPE OF HYPOTHESIS	TYPE OF DESIGN SUGGESTED
Oxygen inhalation by nasal cannula of up to 6 L/min does not affect oral temperature measurement taken with an electronic thermometer.	IV: Oxygen inhalation by nasal cannula DV: Oral temperature	Statistical	Experimental
The incidence of pregnancy in adolescent girls attending birth control education classes will not differ from that of girls who do not attend birth control education classes.	IV: Birth control education classes DV: Adolescent pregnancy	Statistical	Experimental

*IV, Independent variable; DV, dependent variable.

A statistical hypothesis (also known as a null hypothesis) states that there is no relationship between the independent and dependent variables. The examples in Table 17.2 illustrate statistical hypotheses. If, in the data analysis, a statistically significant relationship emerges between the variables, the null hypothesis is rejected. Rejection of the statistical hypothesis is equivalent to acceptance of the research hypothesis. For example, in the study by Rudy et al. (1995), which compared the effects of a low-technology environment of care and a nurse case management delivery system (special care unit [SCU]) with the traditional high-technology ICU environment and a primary nursing care delivery system, null or statistical hypotheses were implied. One example of an implied null hypothesis is 'there is no difference in mortality, length of stay, infections, respiratory complications or life-threatening complications for chronically critically ill patients receiving care in the SCU versus the ICU environment'. Rudy et al., (1995) reported that there were no significant differences in patient outcomes in relation to these variables. Because the difference in outcomes was not greater than expected by chance, the null hypothesis was accepted (see Chapter 21).

Some researchers refer to the null hypothesis as a statistical contrivance that obscures a straightforward prediction of the outcome. Others state that it is more exact and conservative statistically and that failure to reject the null hypothesis implies that there is insufficient evidence to support the idea of a real difference. Readers of research reports will note that, in general, when hypotheses are stated, research hypotheses are more commonly used than statistical hypotheses. In any study that involves statistical analysis, the underlying null hypothesis is usually assumed without being explicitly stated.

Relationship between the hypothesis and the research design

Regardless of whether the researcher uses a statistical hypothesis or a research hypothesis, there is a suggested relationship between the hypothesis and the research design of the study. For example, when an experimental design is utilised, the research consumer would expect to see hypotheses that reflect relationship statements, such as the following:

- X_1 is more effective than X_2 on Y.
- The effect of X_1 on Y is greater than that of X_2 on Y.
- The incidence of Y will not differ in subjects receiving X_1 and X_2 treatments.
- The incidence of Y will be greater in subjects after X_1 than after X_2.

Such hypotheses indicate that an experimental treatment will be used and that two groups of subjects—experimental and control groups—are being used to test whether the difference predicted by the hypothesis actually exists.

In contrast, hypotheses related to non-experimental designs reflect associative relationship statements, such as the following:

- X will be negatively related to Y.
- There will be a positive relationship between X and Y.

Null hypothesis and alternative hypothesis

Prior to an experiment, the researcher sets up two mutually exclusive hypotheses:

1. The null hypothesis, which specifies hypothesised values for one or more of the population parameters, commonly involves the statement of 'no difference'.
2. The alternative hypothesis assumes the population parameter is other than the one hypothesised:
   i. The alternative hypothesis may be directional or non-directional. When the alternative hypothesis asserts only that the population parameter is different from the one hypothesised, it is said to be non-directional.

ii. When the alternative hypothesis states not only that the population parameter differs from the one hypothesised, but also the direction of that difference, for example, greater or less than that hypothesised (Runyon & Haber, 1980).

Figure 17.1 illustrates the decision path for determining the type of hypothesis presented in a study, as well as the study's readiness for a hypothesis testing design.

FIGURE 17.1 Hypothesis testing decision path

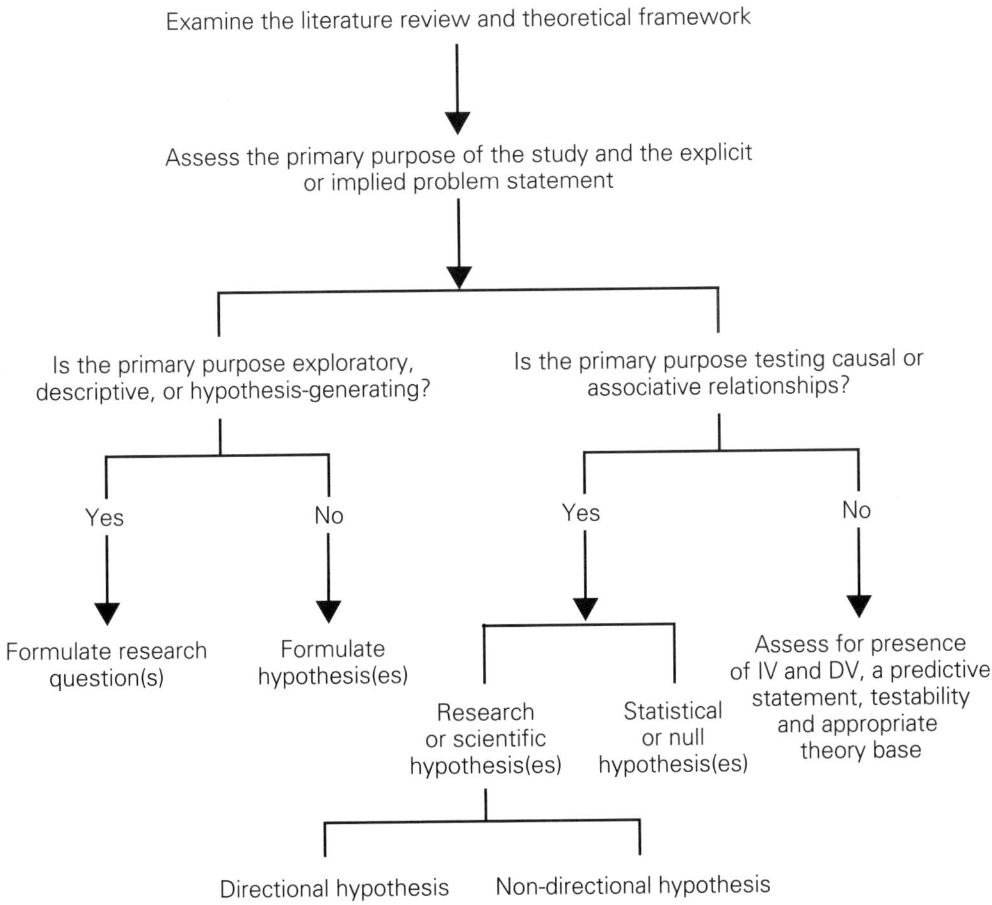

SAMPLING

Sampling is the process of selecting units of a population for study in a research investigation. For reasons of expediency, cost and feasibility, data are collected from a sample of cases, rather than the whole population. Sampling is a familiar process. For example, nursing students may make generalisations about the quality of nursing in a general hospital as a result of a single clinical placement in the medical ward. Patients may also make generalisations about a hospital's food during a three-day hospital stay.

Scientists also derive knowledge from samples. Many problems cannot be solved without employing sampling procedures. For example, when testing the effectiveness of a medication for patients with cancer, the drug is administered to a sample of the population for whom the drug is potentially useful. The scientist must come to some conclusions without administering the drug to every known patient with cancer or every laboratory animal in the world. But because human lives are at stake, the scientist cannot afford to arrive casually at conclusions that are based on the first dozen patients available for study. The consequences of arriving at erroneous conclusions or making inaccurate generalisations from a small, non-representative sample are much more harmful in scientific investigations than in everyday life. Consequently, research methodologies have expended considerable effort to develop sampling theories and procedures that produce accurate and meaningful information.

Sampling concepts

A population is a well defined set that has certain specified properties. A population can be composed of people, animals, objects or events. For example, if a researcher is studying third-year nursing students, the type of educational preparation of the population must be specified. In this instance the population consists of students enrolled in a Bachelor of Nursing program in, say, Victoria, or one may wish to sample a group of students from each Australian State. Examples of other possible populations might be: all patients admitted to hospital X for renal dialysis during 1999 and 2000; or all independent midwife practitioners in New Zealand. These examples show that a population may be broadly defined and potentially involve millions of people, or narrowly specified to include only several hundred people. It is important to remember that the basic unit of the population must be clearly defined, because the generalisability of the findings will be a function of the population criteria.

The reader of a research report should consider whether the researcher has identified the population descriptors precisely. Consider the student nurses enrolled in a Bachelor of Nursing program. Would this population include both part-time and full-time students? Would it include students who had previously attended another nursing program? Would it include year 1, 2 and 3 students? What about international students? Would nurses from an English-speaking background and those whose main language is a language other than English (LOTE) be included? In so far as it is possible, the researcher must demonstrate that the exact criteria used to decide whether an individual would be classified as a member of a given population have been specifically delineated. The population descriptors that provide the basis for eligibility criteria should be evident in the sample, that is, the characteristics of the population and the sample should be congruent. For example, if a population were defined as full-time, Australian-born, third-year nursing students enrolled in a Bachelor of Nursing program, the sample would be expected to reflect these characteristics.

Sample size and power analysis

Power analysis is a mathematical strategy used to determine the size of a sample. Stated simply, power refers to the ability of a statistical test to reject a null hypothesis that is false (Cohen, 1988). That is, a study with appropriate power provides more confidence in predicting that any differences found in the study reflect the true situation. See Chapter 23 for a more detailed discussion of power analysis.

Inclusion and exclusion criteria

The population criteria establish the target population, that is, the entire set of cases about whom the researcher would like to make generalisations. A target population might include all registered nurses in Australia. It is often not feasible, because of time, money and personnel, to pursue the entire target population. An accessible population—one that meets the population criteria and is available—is used instead. For example, in a study commissioned by the Australian Nursing Council (ANC), on nurses' views of indicators for continuing competence in nursing (Pearson & FitzGerald, 2001), the authors decided to accept a random sample of 2% of registered nurses in each State and Territory (except the Australian Capital Territory). Working in the ACT was an exclusion criterion because legislation in the ACT does not permit the nursing regulatory authority to release names and addresses of nurses on their register. The researchers sampled 2% (n = 4133) of the nurses, but only 1005 nurses responded, resulting in a final sample of less than 0.5%. Clearly, this was a study limitation, which questions any attempt at generalisability to the study population.

Think about the concept of eligibility criteria applied to a research study where the subjects are patients. For example, participants in a study investigating inpatient self-management of bipolar disorder (Pollack, 1996) had to meet the following eligibility criteria:

- age—between 18 and 65 years of age
- medication—receiving lithium carbonate, carbamazapine and/or valproic acid for treatment of their bipolar disorder
- status—sufficiently stable to be interviewed
- treatments—not receiving electro-convulsive treatment
- activity level—ambulatory
- language competence—English speaking
- physician endorsement—permitting participation in study protocol
- awareness of diagnosis—have been told their diagnosis
- co-morbid conditions—no evidence of organic brain disorder or known terminal illness.

Eligibility criteria may also be viewed as delimitations or those characteristics that restrict the population to a homogeneous group of subjects. Examples of delimitations include the following: gender, age, marital status, socio-economic status, religion, ethnicity, level of education, age of children, health status and diagnosis. In a study on Australian triage nurses' decision-making and scope of practice (Gerdtz & Bucknell, 2000), all Emergency Nurses Association of Victoria Incorporated (ENA Vic Inc.) members (n = 285) were invited to participate in the study. In this study, membership of ENA was the only criterion. However, emergency nurses working in Victoria who were not members of the ENA were not sampled, creating the possibility of bias. In a study about nurse–environment misfit and nursing practice (Takase, Kershaw & Burt, 2001), the sample consisted of registered nursing students currently undertaking either the post-registration conversion course or postgraduate courses in the School of Nursing at a university in Western Australia. These examples demonstrate the potential differences between the sample actually selected and a larger population.

The research consumer should remember that criteria for inclusion/exclusion in a study are not established in a casual or meaningless way, but are designed to control for extraneous variability or bias. Each criterion should have a rationale, presumably related to a potential confounding effect on the dependent variable. A confounding (confusing) or spurious (false, misleading) relationship exists when the findings falsely show that two or more variables are associated. An example will illustrate this concept. Suppose one domiciliary visit was made routinely to every woman who had radiation therapy prior to discharge from hospital X. And suppose too, that a questionnaire administered to this sample of women reflected physical and mental well-being and comfort. In the absence of knowing that the women belonged to a very effective self-help support group, the health professionals visiting the women might feel justified in assuming that their visit had made the difference. The association between the visit and the women's well-being and comfort may be a misleading or spurious association because it may well disappear when the other variable (self-help support group) is taken into account. A statistical association appears between the visit and the women's well-being because both variables are affected by a third variable—the self-help support group. Adequate design and statistical control should prevent such a problem from occurring.

Samples and sampling

Sampling is a process of selecting a representative portion of the designated population. The most common element in nursing research is individuals, but other elements, such as places or objects, can form the basis of a sample or population. A sampling unit is the element or set of elements used for selecting the sample. Sometimes the sampling unit and the element represent the same thing, and at other times it is more efficient to use a unit larger than the element for sampling purposes. For example, a researcher planned a study that compared the effectiveness of different nursing interventions on the healing rate of decubitus ulcers. Four hospitals, each using a different treatment protocol, were identified as the sampling units rather than the nurses themselves or the treatment alone.

The purpose of sampling is to increase the efficiency of a research study. Samples should be drawn in such a stringent way as to ensure that valid generalisations can be made from the sample to the population. The foremost criterion in evaluating a sample is its representativeness. A representative sample is one whose key characteristics closely approximate those of the population. If 70% of the population in a study of child-rearing practices consisted of women and 40% of them were full-time employees, a representative sample should reflect these characteristics in the same proportions. There is no easy way to guarantee that a sample is representative without obtaining a database about the entire population. Because it is difficult and inefficient to access a population, the researcher must employ sampling strategies that minimise or control for sample bias.

TYPES OF SAMPLES

Sampling strategies are generally grouped into two categories: non-probability sampling and probability sampling. In non-probability sampling, elements are chosen by non-random methods. The drawback of this strategy is that there is no way of estimating the probability that each element has of being included in the sample. Probability sampling uses some form of random selection when choosing the sample units. This type of sampling enables the researcher to estimate the probability that each element of the population will be included in the sample. Probability sampling is the more rigorous type of sampling strategy and it is more likely to result in a representative sample. A summary of sampling strategies appears in Table 17.3 for convenient reference.

TABLE 17.3 Summary of sampling strategies

SAMPLING STRATEGY	EASE OF DRAWING SAMPLE	RISK OF BIAS	REPRESENTATIVENESS OF SAMPLE
Non-probability			
Convenience	Very easy	Greater than any other sampling strategy	Because samples tend to be self-selecting, representativeness is questionable
Quota	Relatively easy	Contains unknown source of bias that affects external validity	Builds in some representativeness by using knowledge about the population of interest
Purposive	Relatively easy	Bias increases with greater heterogeneity of the population; conscious bias is also a danger	Very limited ability to generalise because sample is handpicked
Probability			
Simple random	Laborious	Low	Maximised; probability of non-representativeness decreases with increased sample size
Stratified random	Time consuming	Low	Enhanced
Cluster	Less time consuming than simple or stratified	Subject to more sampling errors than simple or stratified	Less representative than simple or stratified
Systematic	More convenient and efficient than simple, stratified or cluster sampling	Bias in the form of non-randomness can be inadvertently introduced	Less representative if bias occurs as a result of coincidental non-randomness

Non-probability sampling

The non-probability sampling strategy is less rigorous than the probability sampling strategy and tends to produce less accurate and less representative samples, thus limiting the ability of the researcher to make generalisations at a population level about the findings. When planning a research study the researcher must question how important it is that the results of this study be generalisable to a broader population. Non-probability samples are useful when the total population is unknown or unavailable. The three major types of non-probability sampling are: convenience sampling, quota sampling and purposive sampling strategies.

Convenience sampling

Convenience sampling (also called incidental sampling or accidental sampling) is the use of the most readily accessible persons or objects as subjects in a study. The subjects may include volunteers, such as the first 25 patients admitted to hospital X with a particular diagnosis, or everyone who enrolled in program Y during the month of September. For example, Bucknell and Thomas (1997) studied decision-making in critical care settings and selected a convenience sample of nurses who were members of the Confederation of Australian Critical Care Nurses (Victorian Branch) to participate in the study. Similarly, researchers who were investigating the reasons women attend childbirth education classes approached all women booked into four metropolitan hospitals in Victoria between the months of February and June 1996 (Dawson & Beanland, 1997).

A snowball sampling approach (also an effective convenience sampling method), was used to provide an insight into the work of nurse practitioners in three Australian States (Offredy, 2000). Snowballing (network sampling) is a strategy used for accessing samples difficult to locate. It uses social networks and the fact that friends or colleagues tend to have characteristics in common. Individuals who meet the eligibility criteria are asked to assist in getting in touch with others whom they know meet the inclusion criteria.

The advantage of a convenience sample is that it may be easier for the researcher to obtain subjects. The only concern is obtaining a sufficient number of subjects who meet the criteria dictated by the study. The major disadvantage of a convenience sample is that the risk of bias is greater than in any other type of sample. The problem of bias exists because convenience samples tend to be self-selecting, that is, the researcher ends up obtaining information only from the people who volunteer to participate, for example those who chose to return questionnaires sent to them. In this case the following questions must be raised: 'What motivated some of the people to participate and others not to participate?' or 'What kind of data would have been obtained if non-participants had also responded?', and 'How representative of the population are the people who did participate?'.

While recruiting research subjects is a problem for many nurse researchers, a variety of recruitment strategies may be used. For example, a study seeking to identify sources of stress and job satisfaction in the nursing environment (Healy & McKay, 1999), invited nurses to participate by using poster information placed on notice boards in ward areas. Other nurses, from different institutions, were recruited individually by the investigators. A researcher may even offer to pay the participants for their time, although subject motivation and the potential for bias should be considered. Another method of subject recruitment is the use of online networks (Cooper, 2000; Wilmoth, 1995).

However, convenience sampling is the weakest form of sampling with regard to generalisability and should be avoided whenever possible. When critically analysing a research study that has employed this sampling strategy, the external validity of the findings should be considered.

Quota sampling

Quota sampling refers to a form of non-probability sampling in which knowledge about the population of interest is used to build some representativeness into the sample. A quota sample identifies the strata of the population and proportionally represents the strata in the sample. The characteristics chosen to form the strata are selected according to a researcher's judgment based on knowledge of the population and the literature. The criterion for selection should be a variable that reflects important differences in the dependent variables under investigation. Age, gender, religion, ethnicity, medical diagnosis, socio-economic status, level of completed education and occupational rank are among those variables that are likely to be important stratifying variables in nursing research investigations. For example, the data in Table 17.4 reveal that 20% of the 5000 nurses in city X are diploma graduates, 40% are certificate qualified and 40% are bachelor degree graduates.

TABLE 17.4 Numbers and percentages of students in strata of a quota sample of 5000 graduates of nursing programs in city X

	DIPLOMA GRADUATES	CERTIFIED QUALIFIED GRADUATES	BACHELOR DEGREE GRADUATES
Population	1000 (20%)	2000 (40%)	2000 (40%)
Strata	100	200	200

Each stratum of the population should be proportionately represented in the sample. In this case, the researcher used a proportional quota sampling strategy and decided to sample 10% (500 nurses) of a population of 5000. Based on the proportion of each stratum in the population—100 diploma graduates, 200 certificate qualified graduates and 200 bachelor degree graduates—the quotas were established for the three strata. Subjects who met the eligibility criteria of the study were recruited until the quota for each stratum was filled. A quota sampling strategy addresses the issue of appropriate representation for each segment of a population.

The reader of a research study seeks to determine whether the sample strata appropriately reflect the population under consideration and whether the stratifying variables are sufficiently homogeneous to ensure a meaningful comparison of differences among strata. Even when these factors have been addressed, the reader must remember that, as a non-probability sample, the quota strategy contains an unknown source of bias that affects external validity.

The problem is that those who choose to participate may not be typical of the population with regard to the variables being measured. There is no way to assess the biases that may be operating. In cases where the phenomena under investigation are relatively homogeneous within the population, the risk of bias may be minimal. However, in heterogeneous populations the risk of bias is great.

Purposive sampling

In purposive sampling the researcher's knowledge of the population and its elements is used to handpick the cases to be included in the sample; those cases considered to be typical of the population. For example, in a qualitative research study investigating how Korean nurses adjust to hospital settings in the USA (Yi & Jezewski, 2000), a purposive sample of 12 Korean nurses provided the data for the study. Grounded theory was used to develop a substantive theory that explained their process of adjustment.

A purposive sample is also used when a highly unusual group is being studied, such as a population with a rare genetic disease such as Tay-Sachs disease. In this case the researcher would describe the sample characteristics precisely to ensure that the reader will have an accurate picture of the subjects in the sample. In another situation the researcher may wish to interview individuals who reflect different ends of the range of a particular characteristic. For example, the psycho-social needs of individuals who are sero-positive for the hepatitis C virus but have no symptoms, compared with individuals who have active hepatitis C.

As noted previously, online services can be of great value in helping researchers access and recruit subjects for purposive samples. When using a purposive sample in a quantitative research study, the researcher assumes that errors of judgment in over-representing and under-representing elements of the population in the sample will tend to balance out. However, there is no objective method for determining the validity of this assumption. The reader must be aware of the fact that the more heterogeneous the population, the greater the chance of bias being introduced in the selection of a purposive sample. As indicated in Table 17.4, conscious bias in the selection of subjects remains a constant concern for a researcher. As with any non-probability sample, the ability to generalise is very limited. The following are instances of when a purposive sample may be appropriate:

- the effective pretesting of newly developed instruments with a purposive sample of divergent types of people
- the validation of a scale or test with a known-groups technique
- the collection of exploratory data in relation to an unusual or highly specific population, particularly when the total target population remains an unknown to the researcher.

The limitations of using a purposive sample in quantitative studies should be remembered, particularly since generalisability of findings is important.

Probability sampling

The primary characteristic of probability sampling is the random selection of elements from the population. In other words, random selection occurs when each element (i.e. subject or participant) in the population has an equal and independent chance or probability of being selected in the sample. Four commonly used probability sampling strategies are simple random sampling, stratified random sampling, cluster sampling and systematic sampling.

Random selection of sample subjects should not be confused with random assignment or allocation to different groups. The latter refers to the assignment of subjects to either an experimental or a control group on a purely random basis, after the subjects have been selected for inclusion in the study.

Simple random sampling

Simple random sampling is the basic technique of probability sampling. It is a laborious and carefully controlled process with the more complex probability designs incorporating the principles of simple random sampling in their procedures. The researcher defines the population (a set), lists all of the units of the population (a sampling frame) and selects a sample of units (a sub-set) from which the sample will be chosen. For example, units specialising in respiratory problems are the sampling unit, and a list of all hospitals with such units would be the sampling frame. If certified clinical nurses constituted the accessible population, a list of those nurses would be the sampling frame.

Once a list of the population elements has been developed, the best method of selecting a sample is to employ a table of random numbers containing columns of digits, such as the one shown in Figure 17.2. Such tables can be generated by computer programs. After assigning consecutive numbers to units of the population, the researcher starts at any point on the table of random numbers and

FIGURE 17.2 A table of random numbers

1000 random integers between 0 and 99																			
40	23	0	29	10	94	17	58	12	85	13	25	80	84	72	74	54	63	55	31
32	98	49	23	74	97	51	42	21	87	48	64	54	38	84	68	14	17	35	48
84	34	84	14	53	65	67	37	2	45	84	21	71	34	10	80	72	27	11	13
86	37	24	89	23	4	44	40	72	81	44	69	25	44	34	34	34	75	50	50
50	58	85	8	22	24	73	20	63	35	60	87	91	92	96	80	19	22	87	24
1	87	43	82	9	31	40	88	33	28	82	73	18	6	48	64	59	45	34	3
21	19	42	76	84	67	29	68	8	66	93	89	96	28	12	14	38	47	52	65
32	66	33	21	81	97	39	76	67	27	97	22	76	89	41	11	91	29	6	66
16	82	42	75	35	42	92	90	77	24	21	8	36	16	5	54	89	51	57	85
74	32	63	65	93	96	18	36	82	72	39	69	37	97	51	17	36	71	38	30
50	94	4	66	17	37	10	53	8	29	67	74	88	38	11	59	60	91	56	17
71	47	81	18	53	98	7	87	29	37	22	93	13	6	95	7	95	71	14	6
71	93	48	16	33	19	46	21	60	44	52	91	52	58	10	9	41	31	35	18
20	94	13	99	45	6	53	54	1	25	79	28	1	48	36	26	68	37	59	7
75	22	69	56	62	40	64	45	40	99	94	14	98	84	22	38	24	87	43	71
16	87	41	0	88	83	11	37	71	78	22	39	43	37	75	84	84	11	55	58
92	90	80	2	30	37	85	55	56	50	3	71	24	13	62	74	82	44	90	32
96	89	31	32	37	45	70	67	80	55	58	9	55	60	61	55	86	44	27	77
38	29	36	94	65	39	56	29	29	65	88	13	71	38	71	8	81	66	31	44
20	6	61	66	90	13	70	60	92	53	87	49	34	42	14	47	75	33	26	9
63	44	94	21	14	13	41	80	39	72	29	3	25	89	44	88	13	49	18	58
13	32	93	90	31	75	86	95	18	51	61	59	84	95	67	54	40	30	29	63
26	35	48	81	19	24	36	36	76	16	46	5	93	41	97	46	79	54	95	49
89	74	96	95	94	69	31	60	16	69	76	42	28	71	69	34	46	55	20	42
50	39	28	64	20	68	60	33	92	82	61	70	5	68	95	88	12	85	18	94
55	86	5	96	87	69	75	93	54	79	0	57	45	8	86	59	25	21	9	29
75	35	1	2	86	62	70	83	85	13	97	37	13	73	16	38	36	23	54	11
74	50	1	77	87	92	68	87	57	36	17	47	0	97	78	72	72	45	54	51
34	24	35	13	26	42	22	75	47	2	34	87	15	50	65	27	5	72	28	68
73	33	42	65	91	24	44	84	71	55	70	1	27	30	8	61	65	61	18	92
7	55	12	6	61	17	23	95	91	58	60	30	35	61	34	27	75	44	35	64
10	94	18	4	3	19	21	37	28	55	76	25	10	29	80	64	8	81	20	32
20	48	92	87	95	58	57	73	42	1	12	81	94	85	63	97	24	19	93	51
81	10	92	49	70	15	76	4	36	92	62	99	78	32	86	74	43	22	98	46
66	67	82	94	67	75	16	88	84	98	0	52	37	0	43	9	0	51	2	62
64	92	36	11	3	52	44	65	45	67	97	86	92	2	50	5	93	66	73	40
36	29	98	46	88	23	28	44	8	71	69	43	53	16	87	21	56	23	37	24
15	11	82	30	59	94	23	30	40	25	87	26	24	30	44	53	33	65	72	55
89	57	49	79	83	88	42	45	41	93	38	24	15	80	97	18	61	12	13	42
23	36	65	9	64	26	93	37	26	44	42	17	45	68	27	77	74	56	49	34
9	93	90	61	45	40	75	85	64	66	36	89	72	43	99	90	92	10	10	85
53	94	30	31	62	92	82	30	94	56	40	4	50	53	9	74	87	2	36	36
18	69	77	38	89	78	30	68	71	92	22	93	91	74	52	1	97	69	71	42
50	20	76	36	6	20	75	56	36	5	14	70	9	78	23	33	91	33	25	72
30	46	1	10	16	72	69	26	94	39	80	36	36	68	92	74	22	74	41	42
59	47	7	92	77	55	2	12	5	24	0	30	25	62	83	36	92	96	36	75
93	22	3	20	82	44	16	69	98	72	30	57	77	15	90	29	32	38	3	48
9	55	27	41	40	94	77	14	54	10	25	75	1	74	72	15	69	80	33	58
70	8	3	5	46	89	28	86	40	6	25	40	81	26	63	97	87	48	26	41
19	6	89	31	80	60	13	89	17	69	38	93	58	55	54	69	74	33	8	55

reads consecutive numbers in any direction (horizontally, vertically or diagonally). The numbers corresponding with the sampling frame indicate units to be chosen for the sample. This process continues until a sample of the desired size is drawn. In the example above, a list of all eligible clinical nurses would be numbered. If the numbers 76, 16, 46, 5, 93, 41 ... were randomly selected, then the nurses corresponding with those numbers would form the sample.

The advantages of simple random sampling are:

- the sample selection is not subject to the conscious biases of the researcher
- the representativeness of the sample in relation to the population characteristics is maximised
- the differences in the characteristics of the sample and the population are purely a function of chance
- the probability of choosing a non-representative sample decreases as the size of the sample increases.

Simple random sampling may be used in a study examining the relationship between nursing care requirements and nursing resource consumption in home healthcare using both an intensity index and client needs. Using a table of random numbers, a random sample of, for example, 300 patient records could be drawn from patients discharged during a six-month period who received at least three nursing visits at home from a community nursing service.

Despite using a carefully controlled sampling procedure that minimises error, there is still no guarantee that the sample will be representative. Factors such as sample heterogeneity and subject dropout may yet jeopardise the representativeness of the sample. The major disadvantage of simple random sampling is that it is a time-consuming and inefficient method for obtaining a random sample. Consider the task of listing all of the Bachelor of Nursing students in Australia. It may be impossible to obtain an accurate or complete listing of every element in the population. Or imagine trying to obtain a list of all drownings in New South Wales for the year 2000? It may be the case that although drowning may have been the cause of death, another cause, such as cardiac arrest or respiratory failure, appears on the death certificate. It would be difficult to estimate how many elements of the target population would be eliminated from consideration. The issue of bias would definitely enter the picture. Thus, one must be cautious about generalising from reported findings, even when random sampling is the stated strategy, if the target population has been difficult or impossible to list completely.

Stratified random sampling

Stratified random sampling requires that the population be divided into strata or sub-groups. The sub-groups or sub-sets that the population is divided into are homogeneous, that is, they are composed of similar or identical elements. An appropriate number of elements from each sub-set are randomly selected on the basis of their proportion in the population. The goal is to achieve a greater degree of representativeness. Stratified random sampling is similar to the proportional stratified quota sampling strategy discussed earlier in the chapter. The major difference is that stratified random sampling uses a random selection procedure for obtaining sample subjects. Figure 17.3 provides an example that illustrates the use of stratified random sampling.

The population is stratified according to any number of attributes, such as age, gender, ethnicity, religion, socio-economic status or level of completed

FIGURE 17.3 Subject selection using a proportional stratified random sampling strategy

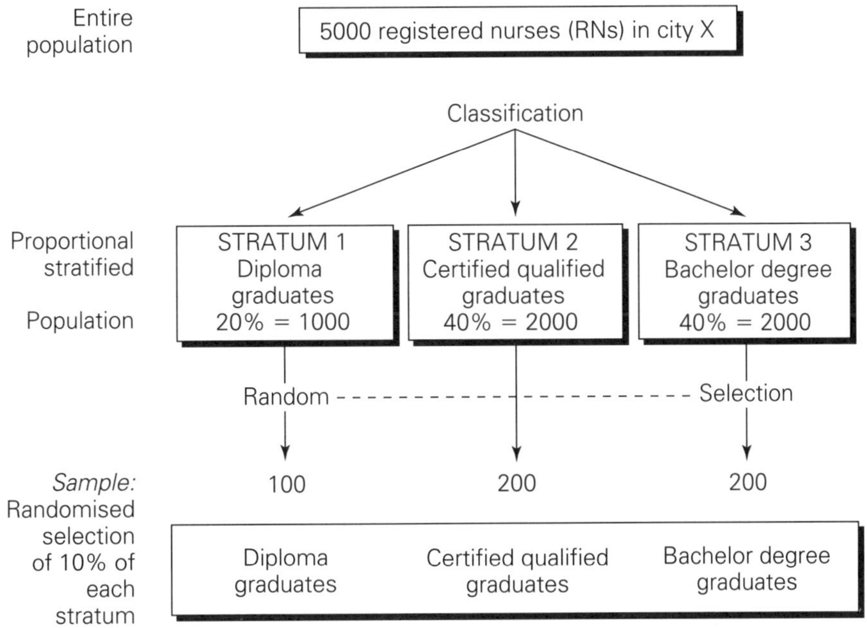

education. The variables selected to make up the strata should be adaptable to homogeneous sub-sets for the attributes being studied. The following criteria can be used for decision-making in the selection of a stratified sample:

- Is there a critical variable or attribute that provides a logical basis for stratifying the sample?
- Does the population list contain sufficient information about the attributes that will be used to divide the sample into sub-sets?
- Is it appropriate for each sub-set to be equal in size or is it more appropriate for each sub-set to be proportionally stratified based on the proportion of each sub-set in the population?
- If proportional sampling is being used, is there a sufficient number of subjects in each sub-set for basing meaningful comparisons?
- Once the sub-set comparison has been determined, are random procedures used for selection of the sample?

There are several advantages to a stratified sampling strategy:

- the representativeness of the sample is enhanced
- there is a valid basis for making comparisons among sub-sets if information on the critical variables has been available
- one can over-sample a disproportionately small stratum to adjust for their under-representation, statistically weigh the data accordingly and continue to be able to make legitimate comparisons.

The obstacles encountered when using this strategy include:

- the difficulty of obtaining a population list containing complete critical variable information

- the time-consuming effort of obtaining multiple enumerated lists
- the time and money involved in carrying out a large-scale study.

The reader should question the appropriateness of this sampling strategy for the problem under investigation. For example, in a post-hospitalisation telephone survey evaluating patient-centred care outcomes, 17 mid-western USA hospitals were selected from a pool of 69 acute care institutions in a single metropolitan area using a stratified random sampling strategy. The stratification was based on location (inner-city, urban and suburban) and the annual number of adult non-psychiatric, non-obstetric admissions (Minnick et al., 1995). It is appropriate for the researcher to strive to represent all strata proportionately in the study sample. In a previous example illustrated in Figure 17.3, the sample consisted of a representative proportion (in this case 10%) from each stratum of the population of registered nurses in city X.

Cluster sampling (multi-stage sampling)

Cluster sampling involves a successive random sampling of units (clusters) that progress from large to small and meet sample eligibility criteria. The first stage sampling unit consists of large units or clusters. The second stage sampling unit consists of smaller units or clusters and so on. For example, if a sample of clinical nurse specialists (CNSs) is wanted, the first sampling unit would be a random sample of hospitals obtained from a Commonwealth Department of Health and Human Services list, which meet the eligibility criteria (for example, size, type). The second stage sampling unit would consist of a list of CNSs practising at each hospital selected in the first stage: the list would be obtained from the director of nursing at each hospital. The criteria for inclusion in the list of CNSs were:

1. at least two years experience as a CNS
2. at least 50% of the CNS's time must be spent in providing direct patient care, and
3. full-time employment at the hospital. The second stage sampling strategy would be the random selection of two CNSs from each hospital who met the inclusion criteria.

When multi-stage sampling is used for large national surveys, such as those carried out by the Australian Bureau of Statistics, States are used as the first stage sampling unit, cities, suburbs and street blocks are used as the second stage sampling unit, and then households are used as the third stage sampling unit.

Sampling units or clusters can be selected by simple random or stratified random sampling methods. Suppose that the hospitals described in the example above were grouped into four strata according to size (number of beds): (1) 200 to 299; (2) 300–399; (3) 400–499; and (4) 500 or more. Stratum 1 comprised 25% of the population; stratum 2 comprised 30% of the population; stratum 3 comprised 20% of the population; and stratum 4 comprised 25% of the population. This means that either a simple random strategy or a proportional stratified sampling strategy is used to randomly select hospitals that would proportionately represent the population of hospitals in Australia. The main advantage of cluster sampling as illustrated in Table 17.3, is that it is considerably more economical in terms of time and money than other types of probability sampling, particularly when the population is large and geographically dispersed, or when a sampling frame of the elements is not available. Two major disadvantages are:

- more sampling errors tend to occur than with simple random or stratified random sampling
- the appropriate handling of the statistical data from cluster samples is very complex.

Systematic sampling
Systematic sampling refers to a sampling strategy that involves the selection of every '*k*th' case drawn from a population list at fixed intervals, such as every tenth member listed in the directory of the Royal College of Nursing Australia's Nursing Research Network. Systematic sampling might be used to sample every '*k*th' person presenting to the emergency department (ED) during the winter months or to be hospitalised with a diagnosis of AIDS in 2000. When systematic sampling is used, the population must be narrowly defined as consisting, for example, of all those people presenting to the ED for the sample to be considered a probability sample. If senior citizens were sampled systematically on entering the ED, the resulting sample would not be called a probability sample because not every senior citizen would have a chance of being selected (only those who were acutely ill). As such, systematic sampling can sometimes represent a non-probability sampling strategy.

Systematic sampling strategies can be designed to fulfil the requirements of a probability sample. First, the listing of the population (sampling frame) must be random in relation to the variable of interest. Suppose subjects were selected from every tenth hospital bed for a study on patient satisfaction with nursing care. Every tenth bed happens to be a single room in the hospital where the study is being conducted. It is possible that the responses of patients in single rooms with regard to satisfaction might be different from those of patients in shared rooms. Because of the non-random arrangement of the rooms, bias may have been introduced.

Second, the first element or member of the sample must be selected randomly. In this case the researcher, who has a population list or sampling frame, first divides the population (N) by the size of the desired sample (n) to obtain the sampling interval width (k). The sampling interval is the standard distance between the elements chosen for the sample. To select a sample of 50 nurse managers from a population of 500, the sampling interval would be as follows:

$$k = \frac{500}{50} = 10$$

Essentially, every tenth case on the nurse manager list would be sampled. Once the sampling interval has been determined, the researcher uses a table of random numbers (e.g. Figure 17.2) to obtain a starting point for the selection of the 50 subjects. If the population size is 500 and a sample size of 50 is desired, a number between 1 and 500 is randomly selected as the starting point. In this instance, if the first number is 51, the nurse manager corresponding to numbers 51, 61, 71 and so forth would be included in the sample of 50. Another procedure recommended is to randomly select the first element from within the first sampling interval. If the sampling interval is 5, a number between 1 and 5 would be selected as the random starting point. For example, if the number 3 is randomly chosen, and keeping in mind the sampling interval of 5, the next elements selected would correspond to the numbers 8, 13, 18 and so on until the sample was obtained.

Systematic and simple random sampling are essentially the same type of procedure. The advantage of systematic sampling is that the results are obtained in a more convenient and efficient manner (see Table 17.3). The disadvantage is that bias in the form of non-randomness can inadvertently be introduced into the procedure. This problem may occur if the population list is arranged so that a certain type of element is listed at intervals that coincide with the sampling interval. For example, if every tenth nursing student on a population list of all types of nursing students in Queensland was a Graduate Diploma of Nursing student and the sampling interval was 10, Graduate Diploma of Nursing students would be over-represented in the sample. Cyclical fluctuations are also a factor. Consider a list of nursing students using the university library each day. A biased sample will probably result if every seventh day is chosen as the sampling interval, because perhaps fewer and different nursing students study in the library on Sundays.

It is important to know whether a satisfactory random selection procedure was carried out. If randomisation was not used, the systematic sampling may have become a non-probability quota sample. In this case the implications related to interpretation and generalisability are drastically altered. Two other important issues when considering quantitative research designs relate to internal and external validity.

INTERNAL AND EXTERNAL VALIDITY

When reading research one needs to feel that the results of a study are valid, based on precision, and faithful to what the researcher wanted to measure. For a study to form the basis of further research, practice and theory development, the findings must be believable and dependable. There are two important criteria for evaluating the credibility and dependability of the results: internal validity and external validity. Threats to validity are listed in Table 17.5 and discussed below.

TABLE 17.5 Threats to validity

INTERNAL VALIDITY	EXTERNAL VALIDITY
■ history	■ effects of selection
■ maturation	■ reactive effects
■ testing	■ effects of testing
■ instrumentation	
■ study mortality	
■ selection bias	

Internal validity

Internal validity asks whether the independent variable really made the difference. This requires the researcher to rule out other factors or threats as rival explanations of the relationship between the variables. There are a number of threats to internal validity and six of the major threats to internal validity are defined by Campbell and Stanley (1963). These should be considered by the researcher in planning the design and by the consumer before implementing results in practice. The research consumer should note that the threats to internal validity are most clearly applicable to experimental designs, but attention to those factors that can compromise outcomes should be considered to some degree in all quantitative designs. If these threats are not considered, they could negate the results of the research. Threats to internal validity include history, maturation, testing, instrumentation, mortality and selection bias.

History

In addition to the independent variable, another specific event that may have an effect on the dependent variable may occur either inside or outside the experimental setting; this is referred to as history. For example, in a study of the effects of a breastfeeding teaching program on the length of time of breastfeeding, an event such as government-sponsored advertisements on the importance of breastfeeding featured on television and in newspapers may be a threat of history. The researcher would be in some doubt as to which event had a greater influence on the women.

Another example may be that of an investigator testing the effects of a breast self-examination teaching program on the incidence of monthly breast self-examination. Concurrently, a famous movie star may be diagnosed as having breast cancer—as happened in the case of Shirley Black (former child star Shirley Temple). The occurrence of this diagnosis in a public figure engenders a great deal of media and press attention. In the course of the media attention, medical experts are interviewed widely and the importance of breast self-examination is supported. If the researcher finds that breast self-examination behaviour has improved, the researcher may not be able to conclude that the change in behaviour was the result of the teaching program; it may well be the result of the diagnosis given to the well known figure and the resultant media coverage.

Maturation

Maturation refers to the developmental, biological or psychological processes that operate within an individual as a function of time and are external to the events of the investigation. For example, suppose one wishes to evaluate the effect of a specific teaching method on Bachelor of Nursing students' performance in giving intramuscular injections. The investigator would record the students' abilities before and after the teaching method. Between the pretest and post-test the students have had practice and experience in the nursing laboratory and hospital environment. This growth or change is unrelated to the investigation and may explain differences between the two testing periods rather than the experimental treatment.

Maturation could also occur in a study focused on investigating the relationship between two methods of teaching on children's knowledge of self-care measures. Post-tests of student learning would need to be conducted in a relatively short time period after the teaching sessions were completed. A relatively short interval would allow the investigator to conclude that the results were because of the design of the study and not maturation in a population of children who are learning new skills rapidly.

Testing

Testing is defined as the effect of taking a pretest on the score of a post-test. On certain tests, students taking the same or a similar test, usually do better than those students taking the test for the first time (Campbell & Stanley, 1963). Therefore, the effect of taking a pretest may sensitise an individual and improve the score of the post-test. Individuals generally score higher when they take a test a second time regardless of the treatment. The differences between post-test and pretest scores may not be a result of the independent variable but rather of the experience gained through testing.

Instrumentation

Instrumentation threats are changes in the measurement of the variables or observational techniques that may account for changes in the obtained measurement. Daniels, Poroch and De Roach (1995) compared several different glucometers to determine their accuracy when the timing and site of blood letting were varied. To prevent instrumentation risk, the researchers checked the calibration on each glucometer according to the manufacturer's specifications before and after data collection.

Techniques of observation are also important. If an investigator has several research assistants collecting observational data, all must be trained in a similar manner. If they are not similarly trained, a lack of consistency may occur in their ratings and therefore a major threat to internal validity will occur. The study by Botti et al., (1998) is an example of a study that trained observers to use the same methods of measurement and recording of data for each subject, thereby reducing the risk of instrumentation. At times, even though the researcher takes steps to prevent problems of instrumentation, this threat may still occur.

In a study by Lipson (1992) that was designed to explore the health and adjustment processes of Iranian migrants, the investigator who was an American, and two highly qualified research assistants who were Iranian and spoke Persian, conducted semi-structured interviews with the study's participants. The researcher noted that when the interviewer was an Iranian, the subjects described the political nature of their migration responses to the Iranian interviewers, but when the interviewer was an American, they did not. This is a problem that would be difficult to prevent because of the delicate political circumstances of the immigrants. When an evaluator finds such a threat, it needs to be assessed within the total context of the study as the researcher did in this study.

Mortality

Study mortality or dropout is the loss of study subjects from the first data collection point (pretest) to the second data collection point (post-test). If the subjects who remain in the study are not similar to those who dropped out, the results could be affected. If most dropouts were non-breastfeeding women in a study of the ways a media campaign affects the incidence of breastfeeding, the perception given could be that exposure to the media campaign increased the number of breastfeeding women, whereas it was the effect of experimental mortality that led to the observed results. A study in which mortality may have influenced the results was conducted by Ziemer, Cooper and Pigeon (1995). The study evaluated a dressing to reduce nipple pain and improve skin condition in breastfeeding women. The investigators reported a high dropout rate and noted several reasons for this, such as the timing of data collection (all were new mothers), and discomfort of the dressing (discomfort of dressing removal). Even though the dropout rate was high, the results do provide valuable information on the problem area, the possible use of the dressing and the continued need for more research in the area.

Selection bias

If precautions are not used to gain a representative sample, a bias of subjects could result from the way the subjects were chosen. Selection effects are a problem in studies in which the individuals themselves decide whether to participate in a study. In Waldenström and Nilsson's (1994) study, the researchers investigated the effects of birth centre care on a number of outcomes. To draw conclusions of cause and effect with confidence, women participating in the study were randomly allocated to the intervention group (birth centre care) or the control group (standard obstetric care). It would not be ethically acceptable to allocate women to a model of care they did not want and the study would be biased if women, allocated to a model of care they did not want, dropped out to receive care elsewhere, thus creating a design dilemma for the researchers. The researchers were able to solve this problem because, when the study was conducted, it was the only program offering birth centre care in Sweden. All women interested in birth centre care were invited to participate in the study knowing that they had a 50% chance of being allocated to the group that would receive birth centre care. Women randomly allocated to the control group received the same standard of care that they would have had if they had not participated in the study. This strategy was feasible, ethical and prevented selection bias due to women dropping out because of allocation to a model of care they did not choose.

The list of internal validity threats is not exhaustive. More than one threat can be found in a study depending on the type of study design. Finding a threat to internal validity in a study does not invalidate the results and is usually acknowledged by the investigator in the results or discussion section of the study.

External validity

External validity deals with possible problems of generalisability of the investigation's findings to additional populations and to other environmental conditions. External validity questions under what conditions and with what types of subjects the same results can be expected to occur. The goal of the researcher is to select a design that maximises both internal and external validity.

The factors that may affect external validity are related to selection of subjects, study conditions and types of observations. These factors are termed effects of selection, reactive effects and effects of testing. The reader will notice the similarity in names of the factors of selection and testing and those of threats to internal validity. When considering them as internal threats the research consumer assesses them as they relate to the independent and dependent variables within the study, and when assessing them as external threats the research consumer considers them in terms of the generalisability or applicability outside the study to other populations and settings. Figure 17.4 illustrates the way threats to internal and external validity can interact with each other. It is important to remember that this path is not exhaustive in describing the types of threats and their interactions. Problems of internal validity are generally easier to control. Generalisability issues are more difficult to deal with because it means that the researcher is assuming that other populations are similar to the one being tested. As noted in Table 17.5, external validity factors include effects of selection, reactive effects and effects of testing.

FIGURE 17.4 **Interacting threats to study validity**

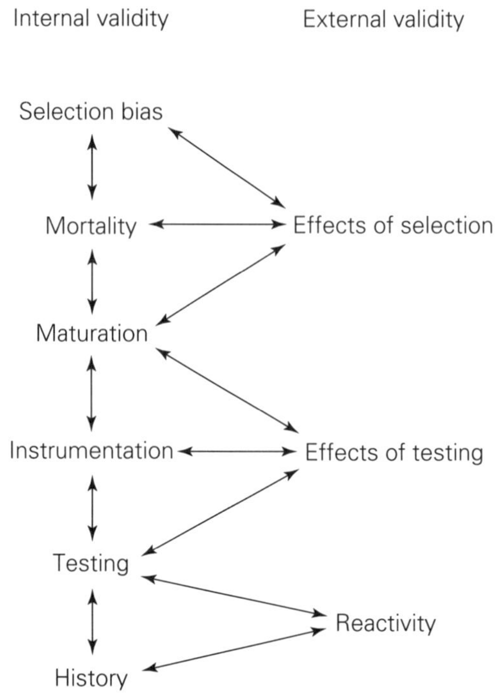

Effect of selection

Selection refers to the generalisability of the results to other populations. An example of the effect of selection occurs when the researcher is not able to attain the ideal sample population. At times, numbers of available subjects may be low or not accessible to the researcher; the researcher may then need to choose a non-probability method of sampling over a probability method. Therefore the type of sampling method utilised and how subjects are assigned to research conditions affect the generalisability to other groups or the external validity.

The effect of selection is highlighted in the following example. Koniak-Griffin and Brecht (1995) studied the relationship of sexual risk-taking to substance use and acquired immunodeficiency syndrome (AIDS) knowledge in pregnant adolescents and non-pregnant young mothers. The sample consisted of 58 pregnant adolescents and 93 non-pregnant young mothers. The researchers cautioned that the findings should be interpreted in light of the study limitations. A convenience sample of moderate size was used and the possibility of self-selection bias influencing the findings must be considered. The investigators also commented on the comparability of their sample to other urban samples in general and on the steps they took to ensure complete anonymity of data collection. These remarks caution the reader but also point out the usefulness of the findings for practice and future research aimed at generating knowledge in this area.

Reactive effects

Reactivity is defined as the subjects' responses to being studied. Subjects may respond to the investigator not because of the study procedures but merely as an independent response to being studied. This is also known as the Hawthorne effect, named after Western Electric Corporation's Hawthorne plant, where a study of working conditions was conducted. The researchers developed several different working conditions (that is, turning up the lights, piping in music loudly or softly and changing work hours). They found that no matter what was done, the workers' productivity increased. They concluded that production increased as a result of the workers knowing that they were being studied rather than because of the experimental conditions.

A threat to internal validity can also be a threat to external validity. In the study with Iranian migrants, the reaction to the interviewer in this study was a threat to instrumentation and reactivity and therefore a threat to the generalisability of the findings (Lipson, 1992). It should be noted that even though this is a problem in the study, the study is important because it points out the many needs of migrants in the area of healthcare and healthcare providers. Chrisman (1992), a reviewer, noted that the migrants demonstrated concerns related to language and different ways of expression and explanation of their illnesses. Chrisman noted also that more research in this area is needed so that nurses can better assess and intervene with migrants. This study is a good example of how a researcher took an interest in a relevant nursing care issue, developed a study to explore the issue, dealt with the real problems of research in the area and is also developing an area of specialty that will ultimately improve patient care.

Effect of testing

Administration of a pretest in an experimental situation affects the generalisability of the findings to other populations. Just as pretesting affects the post-test results within a study, pretesting affects the post-test results and generalisability outside the study. For example, suppose a researcher wants to conduct a study with the aim of changing attitudes towards people with mental illness. To accomplish this, an education program on mental illness is incorporated. To test whether the education program changes attitudes towards mental illness, tests are given before and after the intervention. The pretest on attitudes allows the subjects to examine their attitudes regarding mental illness. The subjects' responses on follow-up testing may be different from those of individuals who were given the education program and who did not see the pretest. Therefore, when a study is conducted and a pretest is given, it may prime the subjects and affect the ability to generalise the findings of the study to other situations or populations.

When reviewing a study, be aware of the internal and external threats to validity. These threats do not make a study useless but are actually useful to readers. Recognition of the threats allows researchers to build on data, and consumers to think through what part of the study can be applied to practice. Specific threats to validity depend on the type of design and the type of generalisations the researcher hopes to make.

There are other threats to external validity that depend on the type of design and methods of sampling utilised by the researcher, but these are beyond the scope of this text. The most detailed coverage of the issues related to internal and external validity is offered by Campbell and Stanley (1963).

STRENGTHS AND LIMITATIONS OF QUANTITATIVE APPROACHES

Three main strengths of the quantitative approaches are in the objectivity, precision and control afforded through design, sampling strategies, and analytical tests. Since hypotheses are generally tested in quantitative approaches, the researcher can make statements about causation. In addition, quantitative data can be analysed using inferential statistical analysis to establish generalisability of the findings from a representative sample.

A criticism of the scientific/quantitative approach when the sample is made up of people, (as opposed, for example, to evaluating treatments used in wound care), is that it is reductionist: that is, it attempts to describe human behaviour in terms of chemical and electrical events and to find neurological correlates for all kinds of human behaviour (i.e. perceiving, thinking, acting). By showing physical relationships between a behaviour and its neurological correlate, that is, between behaviour and the central nervous system, it offers neat causal explanations for behaviour. The limitation of the reductionist viewpoint is that it does not take account of a person's individuality or subjective human experience within a cultural or situational framework (Peele, 1981).

There are clearly situations where a quantitative approach is appropriate, and there is a tendency now for some researchers to use triangulation of both quantitative and qualitative approaches in the same study (see Chapter 3). An initial qualitative approach may also be used to question individuals or group/s and provide the basis for the research question, design and analysis for a quantitative study.

KEY POINTS

- The purpose of the design is to provide the format for a creative piece of research.
- There are many types of designs. No matter which type of design the researcher uses, the rationale for its selection is to credibly answer the research question.
- The research consumer should be able to locate within the study design a sense of the question that the researcher wished to answer. The question should be proposed with a plan or scheme for the accomplishment of the investigation. Depending on the question, the consumer should be able to recognise the steps taken by the investigator to ensure control.
- Control affects not only the outcome of a study but also its future use. The design should reflect how the investigator attempted to control threats to both internal and external validity.
- Internal validity and external validity must be considered within the sampling design.
- Sampling is a process that selects representative units of a population for study. Researchers sample representative segments of the population because it is rarely feasible or necessary to sample entire populations of interest to obtain accurate and meaningful information.
- Criteria for drawing a sample vary according to the sampling strategy. Systematic organisation of the sampling procedure minimises bias.
- An appropriate systematic sampling plan will maximise the efficiency of a research study. It will increase the accuracy and meaningfulness of the findings and enhance the generalisability of the findings from the sample to the population.

CRITICAL THINKING CHALLENGES

- It has been suggested that the drawback of using non-probability sampling limits the generalisability of the findings. Why?
- A final-year Bachelor of Nursing student wants to send a questionnaire to every final-year Bachelor of Nursing student in Australia. What sampling strategies could she use?
- You are interested in finding out about the eating habits of student nurses on night duty in hospital X. It was suggested that you use purposive sampling. Discuss.
- Discuss the research situations in which you may want to use stratified sampling.
- List the six major threats to the internal validity of an experimental study. Prioritise them and defend the one that you have made the essential or the number one threat to address in a quantitative study.

Additional resources

Byrnes, M. & West, S. (2000). Registered nurses' clinical reasoning abilities: a study of self perception. *Australian Journal of Advanced Nursing*, 17(3), 18–23.

Dunn, S.V., Lawson, D., Robertson, S., Underwood, M., Clark, R., Valentine, T., Walker, N., Wilson-Row, C., Crowder, K. & Herewane, D. (2000). The development of competency standards for specialist critical care nurses. *Journal of Advanced Nursing*, 31(2), 339–46.

Dunning, T. & Martin, M. (1996). Developing a questionnaire: some methodological issues. *Australian Journal of Advanced Nursing*, 14(2), 31–38.

Gattuso, S. (1996). The meaning of home for older women in rural Australia. *Australian Journal on Ageing*, 15(4), 172–76.

Hicks, C. (1995). The shortfall in published research: a study of nurses' research and publication activities. *Journal of Advanced Nursing*, 21, 594–604.

Jackson, M.S., Schmierer, C.L. & Schneider, Z. (1996). Development, refinement and future usage of the scale: attitudes toward learning in pregnancy. *International Journal of Nursing Studies*, 33(1), 37–46.

Lyneham, J. (2000). Violence in News South Wales emergency departments. *Australian Journal of Advanced Nursing*, 18(2), 8–17.

Patterson, E., Del Mar, C. & Najman, J. (1999). A descriptive study of nurses employed by general practitioners in South-east Queensland. *Australian Journal of Advanced Nursing*, 17(2), 13–20.

Timmerman, G.M. (1996). The art of advertising for research subjects. *Nursing Research*, 45(6), 339–40.

Wassertheil-Smoller, S. (1990) *Biostatistics and epidemiology: a primer for health professionals*. New York, Edwards Brothers, Inc.

Williams, K.S., Crichton, N. & Roe, B. (1997). Disseminating research evidence. A controlled trial in continence care. *Journal of Advanced Nursing*, 25, 691–98.

Wu, M-L. & Courtney, M. (2000). Models of nursing care: a comparative study of patient satisfaction on two orthopaedic wards in Brisbane. *Australian Journal of Advanced Nursing*, 17(4), 29–34.

Yarandi, H.N. (1991). Planning sample sizes: comparison of factor level means. *Nursing Research*, 40(1), 57–58.

18

CHAPTER

Quantitative data collection

Doug Elliott

LEARNING OUTCOMES

After reading this chapter the student should be able to:

- Define the types of data collection methods used in quantitative nursing research.
- List the advantages and disadvantages of each of these methods.
- Critically evaluate the data collection methods used in published research studies.

Key terms

bias
close-ended item
concealment
consistency
intervention
interviews
Likert Scales
objective
open-ended item
operational definition
physiological measurement
questionnaires
reactivity
scale

INTRODUCTION

Nurses use all of their senses when collecting data from the patients for whom they provide care. Nurse researchers also have many available ways to collect information about their research subjects. As noted earlier, data collection for qualitative research includes in-depth interviews, observation, written journals, photographs and other media. Data collection methods in quantitative research include the use of questionnaires, observation and physiological measurement. When collecting this data, the methods need to be objective and systematic—the aims are for the data to not be influenced by the observer or person who collects the information, and to be collected in the same way for each subject.

The methods and procedure that researchers use to collect information about subjects are identifiable and repeatable operations that enable the major variables to be studied in a systematic and rigorous manner. The process of identifying the concepts of interest and defining how they will be actually measured by the researcher is termed the procedure, or 'operationalisation', of the research. There are often a number of ways to define the same concept, and therefore, operationalise the concept to collect the relevant data. For example, researchers interested in measuring anxiety in patients with acute coronary syndrome admitted to a coronary care unit, could take physiological measures such as blood pressure or heart rate, or administer an anxiety questionnaire such as the State-Trait Anxiety Scale (STAI) (Spielberger, 1973) or the Depression Anxiety and Stress Scales (DASS) (Lovibond & Lovibond, 1995). Researchers could also directly observe patients to see whether they displayed any signs of anxious behaviour. These types of measures all reflect different ways of deriving an operational definition for the concept of anxiety. The method chosen by a researcher would depend on their definition of the concept being studied, the research question and method selected to answer the research question, the nature of the subjects, and the relative costs and benefits of each method.

MEASURING VARIABLES OF INTEREST

To a large extent the success of a study depends on the quality of the data collection methods chosen and employed. Determining what measurement to use in a particular investigation can be a difficult and time-consuming period in study design, requiring substantial review of the background literature. In addition, as nursing research continues to evolve, for researchers there is an increasing array of instruments with proven reliability and validity from which to choose. The process of evaluating and selecting the available tools to measure variables of interest is of critical importance to the potential success of the study. In this section the selection of measures and the implementation of the data collection process are discussed. An algorithm to assist researchers in their choice of data collection methods is illustrated in Figure 18.1.

Researchers use many different ways to collect information about concepts or phenomena of interest to nurses. Nurses are interested in biological and physical indicators of health, such as blood pressure and heart rates, as well as complex psycho-social questions. Psycho-social variables—such as anxiety, hope, social support, self-concept or health-related quality of life—can be measured in several different ways, including observation of behaviour, self-reports of feelings or attitudes and by means of interviews or questionnaires. Researchers may also use

FIGURE 18.1 Data collection methods decision path

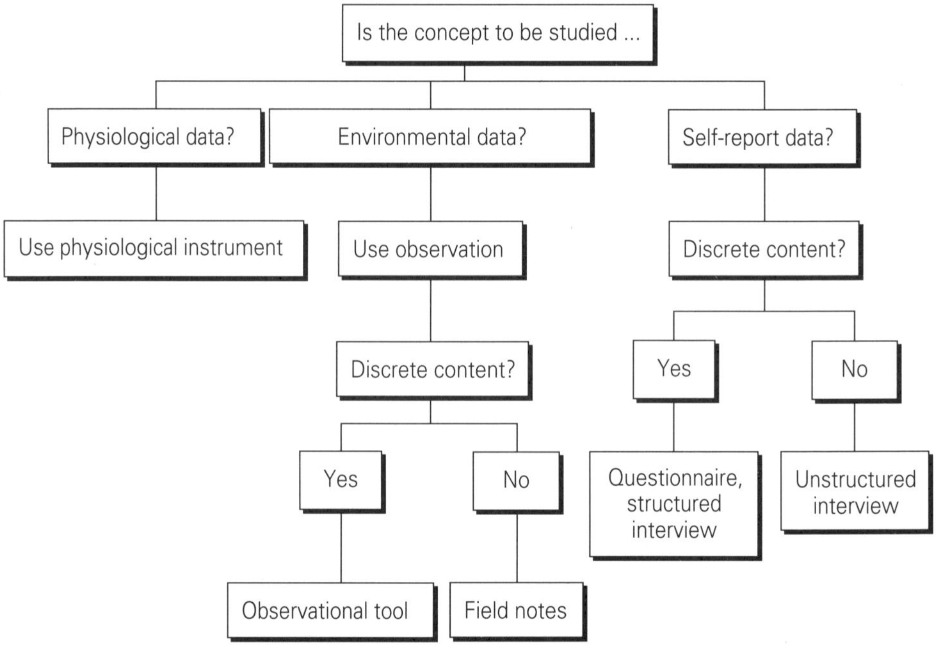

data that have already been collected for another purpose, such as records, diaries or other media. Choosing the most appropriate method and instrument requires careful consideration. The method must be appropriate to the problem, the hypothesis, the setting and the sample. For example, if a researcher is interested in studying the behaviour of three-year-old children in day care, it would not be sensible to give the children some kind of paper-and-pencil tool. Although the children might be able to draw on the paper, they would not be able to answer written questions appropriately.

Conceptual and operational definitions

As noted above, selection of the data collection method begins during the literature review. One purpose of the review is to provide clues on how best to measure a concept. As the literature review is conducted, the researcher begins to explore how previous investigators defined and operationalised variables similar to those of interest in the proposed study. The researcher uses this information to formulate a conceptual definition of the variables to be studied. Once a variable has been defined conceptually, the researcher returns to the literature to define the variable operationally. This operational definition translates the conceptual definition into a form that can be measured for the study. The researcher may then search for instruments that measure the concept of interest as operationally defined.

Elaboration of the previous example of anxiety may clarify the relationship of the conceptual and operational definitions. A conceptual definition of anxiety might be 'a subjective feeling of apprehension and tension, manifested by physiological arousal and varying patterns of behaviour'. While this definition enables a reader to understand the concept, clearly in this form of definition anxiety cannot be measured in an operational sense. However, the use of an operational definition does allow the concept to be measured. For example, an operational definition for anxiety of 'a subject feeling of apprehension and tension, as measured by the State-Trait Anxiety Inventory (STAI) (Spielberger, 1973)' can be studied. As noted, the operational definition provides a statement that enables measurement of the concept of interest. There are various levels of measurement possible (see Chapter 17), each with specific statistical analyses approaches (see Chapters 22 and 23).

Measuring instruments

Instruments found during a literature search may be used in original form or adapted for use in a new study (although any modification may alter its accuracy and validity). If instruments are available, the researcher needs to obtain permission for their use from the original author or copyright holder (often the publisher of the journal where the instrument or article was first published). Examples of instruments that examine quality of life issues are provided by the MAPI Research Institute's Quality of Life Instruments Database (QOLID) (http://qolid.org); this site lists over 800 instruments with information and contact details. Many other resources of measuring instruments are also available (e.g. Frank-Stromberg, 1992; Waltz, Strickland & Lenz, 1991).

It is sometimes the case that no suitable measuring tool exists, so the researcher needs to decide whether the variable is important to the study and whether a new tool should be constructed. This is often a challenge in nursing research, because many variables of interest have not been adequately studied. In constructing new instruments for data collection, reasonable reliability and validity must be ensured (see Chapter 21). Sometimes researchers decide not to study a variable if no suitable measuring tool exists; at other times the researcher may decide to invest time and energy in tool development, or consider exploratory research aimed at identifying and clarifying the concept.

However, instrument development is a complex and time-consuming process, often requiring many years of developmental work. For example, the Medical Outcomes Study Short-Form 36-item (SF-36) originated from a larger battery of 149-items (Functioning and Well-Being Profile) developed from questionnaires in the 1970s to 1980s. The SF-36 examines eight concepts reflecting self-evaluation of physical and mental functions (physical functioning, physical role, bodily pain, general health, vitality, social functioning, emotional role and mental health) (Ware, 2000). The instrument was presented in developmental form in 1988 and standard form in 1990. Continued psychometric testing in international and a variety of clinical cohorts enabled development of version 2, as well as a related instrument (SF-12), which was designed for population surveys. The revised SF-36 has improved layout and item wording, and increased precision for role functioning, as well as population norm-based transformed scores for easier interpretation and comparison to the general population. Unfortunately, there are currently no Australian population-based data for the revised instrument to allow score transformation, and so its utility is limited.

Whether the researcher uses available methods or creates new ones, once the variables have been operationally defined in a manner consistent with the aims of the study, the population to be studied and the setting, the researcher will determine how the data collection phase of the study will be implemented. This decision deals with how the instruments for data collection will be administered to the subjects. Consistent implementation of the study procedure and data collection is the most important issue for this phase in quantitative research. Consistency means that the data are collected from each subject in the study in exactly the same way or as close to the same way as possible. Consistency can minimise the bias introduced when more than one person collects the data.

The researcher must also consider ways to maintain subject motivation to complete the data collection process (Bariball & While, 1999), and data collectors must be carefully trained and supervised to ensure consistency in collection; that is, researchers must rehearse with data collectors in the methods to be used in the study so that each person collects the information in the same way. Information about how to observe and collect data is often included in a kind of 'cookbook' protocol for the research project. A researcher may spend several months developing the protocol and training research assistants to collect data systematically and reliably. If data collectors are used, the reader should expect to see some comment about their training and the consistency with which they collected the data for the study.

For example, Alsop-Shields and Alexander (1997) studied the errors that can occur when weighing infants, exploring the factors that influenced measurements of infant weight at child health clinics. Four potential sources of error were identified:

1. instrument error (related to calibration and use of the scales)
2. intra-observer error (inconsistency in measurement of weight by the same operator)
3. test–retest stability (changes in the weight of the baby over short time periods due to biological factors)
4. inter-observer error (errors in measurement due to different operators weighing the same baby on the same scales).

The latter issue is also called inter-rater reliability, and is discussed in Chapter 21.

DATA COLLECTION METHODS

In general, data collection methods can be divided into the following five types:

- physiological
- observational
- interviews
- questionnaires
- records or other documentation.

Each of these methods has a specific purpose, as well as certain advantages and disadvantages inherent in its use. These methods and their respective uses and limitations are discussed below.

Physiological or biological measurements

In everyday practice, nurses collect physiological data about patients, such as their temperature, pulse rate and blood pressure. Physiological and biological measurements involve the use of specialised equipment to determine the physical and biological status of the subject. Physiological measures can be: physical, such as weight or temperature; chemical, such as blood glucose level; microbiological, as with cultures; or anatomical, as in radiological examinations. What separates these measurements from others used in research is that they require the use of special equipment to make the observation.

A study by Caudell and Gallucci (1995) provides an example of the use of physiological data collection methods, where the purpose was to measure neuroendocrine, immunological and psycho-social variables before and after the application of a particular stressor. To study this problem, it was important for the researchers to provide the stressful stimulus in the same manner to all subjects and then measure the physiological and psycho-social variables at similar intervals for all subjects. The study used both psycho-social instruments (mood, stress appraisal, stress symptoms) and physiological measurements (urine catecholamines, plasma catecholamines, cortisol, autonomic nervous system activity) to study responses to the stimulus.

Another study determined the appropriate site and timing of blood collection for accurate measurement of blood sugar levels (BSL) using a number of glucometers (Daniels, Poroch & De Roach, 1995). The study required careful standardisation of the procedures so that blood samples were all collected in the same way. This included formulating a written protocol for sample collection that specified procedures and conditions for participants' hand washing, skin temperature, and activity level prior to sample collection. Written protocols were developed for researchers in relation to the consistent use of one type of lancet for blood collection, randomisation of selection of specific sites for blood sample collection on both hands, and recording of the puncture sites used for blood sample collection.

Physiological or biological measurement is particularly suited to the study of several types of nursing problems. The latter example given above is typical of studies designed to determine the effectiveness of certain nursing actions. In another example, an experimental study compared the effects of pressure bandaging on complications and comfort in patients undergoing coronary angiography (Botti et al., 1998). One of the variables measured was haematoma (bruise) size, measured in square centimetres. The researchers used a standard measurement protocol and measures of inter-rater reliability to ensure that all data collectors were rating or measuring haematoma size in the same way for all participants in the study. To increase reliability of data collected, information sessions for data collectors were conducted throughout the study period. The results of the study showed that there was no difference in bruise size between the bandage and no bandage groups, but that participants who were not bandaged expressed greater comfort than those who were.

The advantages of using physiological data collection methods include their objectivity, precision and sensitivity, assuming that calibration and instrument error have been addressed. Such methods are generally objective because unless there is a technical malfunction, two readings of the same instrument taken at the same time by two different nurses are likely to yield similar results. Such instruments are intended to be sufficiently precise and sensitive to pick up subtle variations in the variable they are designed to measure. However, physiological measurements are not without inherent limitations, including the expense of obtaining the specialised knowledge and training to collect the data reliably, or the effect of instrumentation and testing (see Chapter 17 for threats to internal validity). For example, the presence of a heart rate monitoring device may elicit a stress response and make some patients anxious and increase their heart rate, unless suitable information is provided to allay concerns.

Observational methods

Sometimes nurse researchers are interested in determining how subjects behave under certain conditions. Depending on the aims and questions of the study, a researcher may opt for a qualitative or quantitative observational approach. For example, a researcher may be interested in how children respond to painful situations. Children could be asked how painful an experience was, but they may not be able to answer the question or quantify the amount of pain, or they may distort their responses to please the researcher. Observing the subject may give a more accurate picture of the behaviour in question than directly asking the patient.

Although observing the environment is a normal component of nursing care, observation using a quantitative approach places emphasis on the objective and systematic nature of the research process. The quantitative researcher is not merely looking at what is happening but rather watching with a trained eye for certain specific events that were identified following a review of previous research. To be rigorous, observations must fulfil the following four conditions:

- the observations undertaken are consistent with the study's specific objectives
- there is a standardised and systematic plan for observation and recording of data
- all of the observations are checked and controlled
- the observations are related to scientific concepts and theories.

Observation is particularly suitable as a data collection method in complex research situations that are best viewed as total entities and that are difficult to measure in parts, such as studies dealing with nursing practice, social interactions or group processes. In addition, observational methods can be the best way to operationalise some variables of interest in nursing studies, particularly individual characteristics and conditions, such as traits and symptoms, verbal and non-verbal communication behaviours, activities, skill attainment or environmental characteristics.

Observational methods can be distinguished also by the role of the observer; that is, the amount of interaction or communication between the observer and those being observed. Each of the following four basic types of observational roles is distinguishable by the amount of involvement by the observer/researcher:

- complete participant
- participant as observer
- observer as participant
- complete observer (Gold cited in Kennedy, 1999).

Participant observation is a commonly used observational technique where the researcher functions as a part of a social group to study the group in question. This approach is grounded in anthropology and sociology, as well as in ethnography where the researcher becomes immersed in the field or research setting (see Chapter 12 for further discussion). Distinction between the mixed participant observer roles above relates to the research setting and purpose, as well as the clinical experience of the investigator, and may change during the course of the fieldwork. This may also lead to role strain and conflict for the nurse researcher, as evidenced by a narrative on the observation of an intensive care unit as a learning environment for registered nurses (Kite, 1999). The limitations associated with this type of observation include participant reactivity, particularly the Hawthorne effect (the distortion created when the subjects change behaviour because they are being observed).

Although rarely used in clinical research today because of ethical concerns and the requirement for informed participant consent, concealment can be used in observational studies. Concealment of the observer refers to whether the subjects know that they are being observed. An intervention can also be employed where the observer provokes actions from those who are being observed. When a researcher is concerned that the subjects' behaviour will change as a result of being observed, the type of observation most commonly employed is that of concealment without intervention. In this case the researcher watches the subjects without their knowledge of the observation and he or she does not provoke or stimulate a reaction. Often such concealed observations use hidden television cameras, audiotapes or one-way mirrors. However, as noted above, observing subjects without their knowledge may violate requirements for informed consent and, therefore, researchers face ethical problems with this type of approach. Consent to participate in the research study is still a requirement, even though concealment may be used to ensure reliable data collection. The researchers will need to justify to their institutional ethics committee why concealment is necessary. If they can argue that there is no other way to collect the data and the data collection procedure is unlikely to have negative consequences for the subjects, the study may be approved. Sometimes, approval may be given to inform subjects after the observation and allow them the opportunity to refuse to have their data included in the study and to discuss any questions they might have. This process is called debriefing.

Observations may be structured or relatively unstructured. Structured observations, such as the tools used to examine work activities within an intensive care unit (ICU) (Marasovic, Kenney, Elliott & Singhusake, 1997), involve specifying in advance what behaviours or events are to be observed and preparing data forms for record keeping, such as categorisation systems, checklists and rating scales. Whichever system is employed, the observer watches the subject and then marks on the recording form what was seen. When observations are undertaken by more than one observer, then adequate training and inter-rater reliability (discussed in Chapter 21) is required to ensure consistency of the observations. The previous observational study used work sampling methodology and a random timer to observe the nursing activities within an ICU (Marasovic et al., 1997). At random intervals, a researcher would observe the activities of the nursing staff and list the activities on a specifically designed data collection sheet that categorised nursing care. This cost-effective method enabled the researchers to determine that a clinical information system (CIS) did not demonstrate significant benefits over paper-based documentation with regard to the frequency of nursing activities.

Participant observation has several strengths as a data collection method, the main one being that observation may be the only way for the researcher to study the variable of interest. This is particularly the case with exploration of the practice base of a discipline such as nursing (Kennedy, 1999). In addition, no other data collection method can match the depth and variety of information that can be collected when using this technique. As with all data collection methods, observation also has its limitations. Problems of reactivity and ethical concerns regarding concealment and intervention have already been highlighted. In addition, data obtained by observational techniques are vulnerable to bias of the observer. Previous experiences, attitudes, knowledge and values of the researcher can all influence the way that behaviours and events are observed (Kennedy, 1999; Kite, 1999). In general, the more the observer needs to make inferences and judgments about what is being observed, the more likely it is that distortions will occur. Thus, in judging the adequacy of observational methods from a quantitative position, it is important to consider how observational tools were constructed and how the observers were trained and evaluated.

Interviews and questionnaires

Subjects in a study often have information that can only be obtained by researchers asking the subject. Such questions may be asked verbally by a researcher in person or over the telephone in an interview, or they may be asked in the form of a written request such as a questionnaire. Both interviews and questionnaires require subjects to report data about their knowledge, attitudes and beliefs, but each approach has unique advantages and disadvantages. Survey research relies on questioning subjects using either interviews or questionnaires, but these methods of data collection can also be used in other types of research. No matter what type of study is conducted, the purpose of questioning subjects is to obtain information. This information may be collected directly, such as asking about a subject's level of pain, or indirectly, by using a combination of items to estimate to what degree the respondent has some trait or characteristic.

When individual items are combined to obtain an overall score, the instrument is called a scale. Scales are commonly used in nursing research and can provide a useful way of operationalising abstract concepts, for example, pain, anxiety, stress, coping, anger, comfort, or health-related quality of life (HRQOL). The term 'profile' refers to a comprehensive instrument that assesses different components of a concept within one measurement approach (e.g. the SF-36 Health Survey) (Ware, 2000). A battery is comparable to a profile with assessment of multiple components, but is derived from different original sources. The term 'index' denotes a single number that may be derived from various sources. For example, Jackson, Schmierer and Schneider (1996) developed a scale comprising 36 attitudinal and opinion statements that, when combined, produced a score that reflected an overall attitude to learning in pregnancy.

The content of an interview or questionnaire is determined from the literature. When evaluating these methods, the reader should consider the content of the individual items (questions) and the order in which they are presented. The basic standard for evaluating individual items in an interview or questionnaire is that the item must be written so that the intent of the question and the nature of the information sought are clear to the respondent. Each item must ask only one question, be grammatically correct, free of jargon and value-laden terms, not open to alternative interpretations, and written in language understandable to the respondents. One way to determine whether questions are understandable to the target respondents is to pilot test the instrument in a similar population. Statistical procedures such as factor analysis can also be used to demonstrate the reliability and validity of such instruments (see Chapters 21 and 23 for further discussion).

Items used in questionnaires may be open-ended or close-ended. Open-ended items are used when the researcher wants the subjects to respond in their own words or when the researcher does not know all of the possible alternative responses. An example of an open-ended question is presented in Box 18.1.

Close-ended items are used when there are a fixed number of alternative responses. Close-ended questions can take many forms, including fixed response, multi-choice formats and lists of items that subjects are asked to rank. Fixed-response items can be used for questions requiring a dichotomous 'yes' or 'no' response, or when there are categories such as language spoken at home, highest educational level, or employment status. Structured, fixed-response items are best used when the question has a limited number of responses and the respondent is asked to choose the response closest to their preferred answer. Fixed-response items have the advantage of simplifying the respondent's task and the researcher's analysis, but they may miss some important information about the subjects. A Likert Scale is an example of a fixed-response format. Likert Scales are lists of statements on which respondents indicate, for example, whether they 'strongly agree', 'agree', 'disagree' or 'strongly disagree'. The use of a four-point scale is an example of a forced-response item, although inclusion of a neutral category, such as 'neither agree nor disagree', can provide respondents with another option. The use of the neutral category, however, may create a limitation in the data as it can be the most frequent response but is difficult to interpret. Including a neutral response creates an odd-point scale. Likert Scales are commonly constructed as 4-point, 5-point, 7-point or 10-point scales. An example of a 5-point scale is illustrated in Box 18.1. Open-ended questions allow the respondents to answer in their own words. The respondent may also choose to leave the item blank, and therefore provide no information for the researcher. Unstructured open-ended response formats allow a greater range of responses to be collected and use a technique called content analysis to interpret the information. A quantitative approach to content analysis uses previously identified categories to list the open-ended responses so that the information can be coded and examined in a numerical format (similar to the close-ended format). See Chapter 9 for discussion of qualitative content analysis.

BOX 18.1 Examples of close-ended and open-ended questions

Close-ended: Likert-type scale

How satisfied are you with your learning in this current research subject?

1. Very satisfied
2. Moderately satisfied
3. Undecided
4. Moderately dissatisfied
5. Very dissatisfied

To what extent do the following factors contribute to your current level of satisfaction?

	Not at all	Very little	Somewhat	Moderate amount	A great deal
Subject content	1	2	3	4	5
Learning process	1	2	3	4	5
Related readings	1	2	3	4	5
Student activities	1	2	3	4	5
Assessments	1	2	3	4	5

Close-ended

On average, how many clients do you see in the community health centre in a day?

1. 1–4
2. 5–9
3. 10–14
4. 15–19
5. 20 or more

How would you characterise the pace of your midwifery clinic?

1. Too slow
2. Slow
3. About right
4. Busy
5. Too busy

Closed-ended: analogue scale (Linear Analogue Scale—LAAS)

Mark on the scale below the amount of anxiety you are now in.

1	2	3	4	5	6	7	8	9	10
No anxiety									Extreme anxiety

Open-ended

Are there incentives that the Australian College of Critical Care Nurses ought to provide for members that are currently not being offered?

All methods that involve self-reports share a problem with accuracy. There is often no way of knowing whether the responses are true. For example, people are known to respond to questions in a way that makes a favourable impression; this response style is known as social desirability. Because there is no way to tell whether the respondent is telling the truth or responding in a socially desirable way, the researcher must assume that the respondent is telling the truth.

Questionnaires and interviews also have some specific purposes, advantages and disadvantages. Questionnaires and paper-and-pencil instruments are most useful when there is a finite set of questions to be asked and the researcher can be assured of the clarity and specificity of the items. If questionnaires are too long or complicated, they are less likely to be completed; this relates to respondent burden. Interviews, either face-to-face or by telephone, are best used when the researcher may need to clarify the task for the respondent or is interested in obtaining sensitive or personal information. Telephone interviews may also allow the researcher to reach more respondents than face-to-face interviews.

A study used a combination of scales, checklists and open-ended questions to measure the burnout level of New Zealand nursing staff working in a paediatric unit (Watson & Feld, 1996). Distress was measured using the Maslach Burnout Inventory, the Nursing Situations Questionnaire and Hopkins Symptom Checklist-21, and measured coping using the Ways of Coping Checklist. Additional information giving depth and context to individual responses was obtained by including open-ended questions. This use of multiple measures gives a more complete picture than the use of just one measure.

Both face-to-face and telephone interviews offer some advantages over questionnaires. All things being equal, interviews are better than questionnaires because the response rate is almost always higher and this helps to eliminate bias in the sample. Respondents seem to be less likely to hang up the telephone or to close the door in an interviewer's face than to throw away a questionnaire. Another advantage of the interview is that children, some people with disabilities, and those who are unable to write, may be unable to fill out a questionnaire but could participate in an interview. With an interview, the data collector knows that the subject is responding. When questionnaires are mailed, someone other than the subject could be supplying the responses. Investigation of sensitive or intimate information is an interesting issue. Some participants may prefer the relative anonymity and indirect nature of a questionnaire about moral, cultural or ethico-legal issues (e.g. religious beliefs, sexual behaviour, substance use). However, the direct two-way communication and a developing rapport of an interview may improve the quality and rate of responses to these types of questions.

Advantages of questionnaires include:

- being less expensive to administer than interviews, as the latter may require the hiring and training of interviewers, and transcription of the interviews
- no researcher being present assures no interviewer bias is possible
- a larger sample can be accessed to enable increased generalisability of results.

Records or other available documentation

All of the data collection methods previously discussed illustrate the ways that nurse researchers gather new data to study phenomena of interest. Records and other available documents or data are 'secondary' sources, and include hospital records, care plans, clinical databases, and census or population data (see the Australian Institute of Health and Welfare website for examples of available data—http://www.aihw.gov.au/). These sources are used to answer specific primary research questions, and this process is equivalent to approaches used in historical research (see Chapter 10). Primary studies may also use existing data as well as primary sources. For example, Daly and colleagues (2000) used existing patient medical records to obtain clinical and socio-demographic data about participants in their study investigating the health status and coping ability of survivors of acute myocardial infarction. Other data in this study were then collected by questionnaire in repeated measures after discharge from hospital. Existing information can be also re-examined and synthesised to provide new and additional information as for systematic reviews or meta-analyses (see Chapters 5 and 6).

Using available data has certain advantages. Because the data collection step of the research process is sometimes the most difficult and time-consuming, the use of available records enables significant time-saving. If records have been kept in a similar manner over time, as with State perinatal databases (which collect information about all births), analysis of these records allows for the examination of trends over time.

Various government privacy acts protect the rights of individuals who may be identified in records. As a result, healthcare institutions may be reluctant to allow researchers to have access to their medical records, unless the information is able to be provided in a format that does not allow an individual to be identified (thus preserving anonymity). Another problem that may affect the quality of available data is whether the records available are representative of all of the possible records; if not, the researcher may have a problem of a biased sample. Often there is no way to tell whether the records have been saved in a biased manner, and the researcher has to make an intelligent estimation of their accuracy. Current policies on storage of subject data in Australia are available from the NHMRC (http://www.nhmrc.gov.au). It may be difficult for a research consumer or primary researcher to uncover these types of subtle biases. Despite these potential limitations, health records and other available data constitute a rich source for study.

CONSTRUCTION OF NEW INSTRUMENTS

As discussed earlier, researchers sometimes cannot locate an instrument or method with acceptable reliability and validity to enable measurement of the variable of interest. This is often the case when testing a part of a nursing theory or when evaluating the effect of a clinical intervention. However, the development of a reliable and valid questionnaire is complex and time-consuming. The process begins with the identification of a construct, which is a concept developed for a specific research purpose. Defining the construct to be measured requires an extensive review of the literature for all tests and measures that deal with the construct. The researcher then uses this information to synthesise available knowledge so that the construct can be operationalised for measurement purposes. Instrument developers need to consider numerous issues (see Table 18.1).

TABLE 18.1 Common considerations in the development of measurement tools

CONSIDERATION	EXAMPLE/ELABORATION
The well-constructed scale, questionnaire or interview schedule should consist of an objective, standardised measure of samples of a behaviour that has been clearly defined. Observations should be made on a small but carefully chosen representative sample of the behaviour of interest.	In their study of acute confusion, Neelon et al. (1996) based the tool on a thorough review of previous literature, clinical bedside observations and clinical consultants in establishing selected factors as being representative of 'acute confusion in hospitalised older patients', as it had been defined.
The tool should be *standardised*; that is, a set of uniform items and response possibilities that are uniformly administered and scored.	In the study by Neelon et al. (1996), evaluation of the confusion scale consisted of objective assessment by research nurses in various settings, using specific criteria and ratings for the observed behaviours. Without these criteria, evaluations would be based on the nurses' subjective impressions, which may have varied significantly between observers and conditions.

The items of a measurement tool should be unambiguous, concise, exact statements with only one idea per item. Negative stems or items with negatively phrased response possibilities that result in a double negative may cause ambiguity in meaning and scoring.	In constructing a tool to measure job satisfaction, a nurse researcher constructs the following item, 'I never feel that I don't have time to provide good nursing care'. The response format consists of 'Agree', 'Undecided', and 'Disagree'. It is possible that a response of 'Disagree' may not reflect the respondent's true intent, because of the confusion that is created by the double negatives in the statement.
The type of items used in any one test or scale should be restricted to a limited number of variations. Subjects who are expected to shift from one kind of item to another may fail to provide a true response as a result of the distraction of making such a change.	Mixing true-or-false items with questions that require a yes-or-no response and items that provide a response format of five possible answers increases the likelihood of measurement error.
Items should not provide irrelevant clues. Unless carefully constructed, an item may furnish an indication of the expected response or answer. In addition, the correct answer or expected response to one item should not be given by another item.	An item that provides a clue to the expected answer may contain value words that convey cultural expectations, such as, 'A good wife enjoys caring for her home and family'.
The items of a measurement tool should not have unnecessarily complex or exact operations. In addition, the difficulty of an item should be appropriate to the level of the subjects being assessed. Limiting each item to one concept or idea helps to accomplish this objective.	A test constructed to evaluate learning in an introductory course in research methods may contain an item that is inappropriate for the designated group, such as, 'A non-linear transformation of data to linear data is a useful procedure before testing a hypothesis of curvilinearity'.
The diagnostic, predictive or measurement value of a tool depends on the degree to which it serves as an indicator of the broad construct or concept. Items should reflect the operational definition of the construct. The extent to which the test items appear to accomplish this objective is an indication of the validity of the instrument.	Two nurse researchers, A and B, are studying the construct of patient satisfaction. Each has defined this construct in a different way. Consequently, the measurement tool that each nurse devises will include different questions. The questions on each tool will reflect the construct for patient satisfaction as defined by each researcher.
The instrument should adequately cover the defined behaviour. The primary consideration is whether the number and nature of items in the sample are adequate. If there are too few items, the accuracy or reliability of the measure must be questioned. In general, there should be a minimum of ten items for each independent aspect of the construct.	Very few people would be satisfied with an assessment of such traits as intelligence if the scales were limited to three items.
The measuring instrument must prove its worth empirically through tests of reliability and validity (see Chapter 21).	A researcher should demonstrate to the reader that the instrument is accurate and measures what it purports to measure.

Once the construct is defined, individual items can be developed. The researcher usually develops more items than are needed to address each aspect of the construct or sub-construct. Items are evaluated by a panel of experts in the field, to ensure that the researcher has addressed the issue of whether the items measure what they are intended to measure. During the process of item validation, the number of items will be decreased, as some items will not fit as intended and will be discarded. In this phase the researcher needs to ensure consistency among the items, as well as consistency in testing and scoring procedures by using factor and item analyses. Finally, the researcher administers or pilot tests the new instrument by giving it to a group of people who are similar to those who will be studied in the larger investigation. The purpose of this analysis is to determine the quality of the instrument as a whole (reliability and validity), as well as the ability of each individual item to discriminate between respondents (variance in item response) (see Chapter 21).

It is important that researchers who invest significant amounts of time in instrument development publish their findings (e.g. Fisher, King & Tague, 2001; Green et al., 1988). This type of research serves not only to introduce other researchers to the instrument but also to ultimately enhance the field, because our ability to conduct meaningful research is supported by our ability to measure important variables in a reliable and valid way. The following example presents the development of a questionnaire about subjects' assessment of the seriousness of diabetes (Dunning & Martin, 1996). The following steps were taken in the development process:

1. The construct to be measured was defined, that is, there was an assessment of the seriousness of diabetes.
2. Sixteen draft items were formulated including both close-ended and open-ended questions.
3. The items were assessed for validity—the researchers convened a panel of six experts in diabetes management, questionnaire development, psychology, statistics and epidemiology to critique the questionnaire.
4. Instructions were developed for respondents and users.
5. A pilot study was conducted with 25 respondents to test the questionnaire in the population in which it was to be used.
6. Estimations were made from analysis of pilot study responses, including test–retest reliability (stability) using a correlation of subjects' responses to the same questions over time and internal reliability using Cronbach's alpha.

In another example, an 'Attitudes to learning in pregnancy scale' was developed and tested (Jackson et al., 1996), using statements designed under six themes and distributed randomly throughout the form:

1. education through the antenatal period
2. consequences of pregnancy
3. decision-making in pregnancy
4. midwife's role in antenatal education
5. learning in pregnancy
6. information given during pregnancy.

A factor analysis was conducted to determine whether items were grouped empirically under each of the six themes. The next step was an item analysis of the revised sub-scales to demonstrate their reliability, and finally, Pearson's correlation was used to examine associations between the sub-scales. All of these analytical steps were used to demonstrate the reliability and validity of the new scale. Having conducted these analyses, the authors were confident that the scale measured attitudes to learning in pregnancy in a repeatable way.

EVALUATING DATA COLLECTION METHODS

Evaluating the adequacy of data collection methods from research papers is often challenging for nursing research consumers, as the instrument(s) used is/are not usually provided in the paper for inspection, and the reader may not feel confident about judging the adequacy of the method without reviewing it. Readers may need to check the reference list of the paper and obtain any other papers which describe or test the instrument.

A number of questions can be considered when examining the research method (see criteria in Box 18.2). The paper should adequately describe the methods and data collection procedures (as well as the psychometric properties—reliability, validity, responsiveness; of the instruments used—discussed in Chapter 21).

BOX 18.2 Criteria for evaluating data collection methods

1. Are all of the data collection instruments clearly identified and described?
2. Is the rationale for their selection given?
3. Is the method used appropriate to the problem being studied?
4. Is the method used appropriate to the clinical situation?
5. Are the data collection procedures similar for all subjects?

Physiological measurement

1. Is the instrument used appropriate and consistent with the research problem?
2. Is a rationale given for why a particular instrument was selected?
3. Is there a provision for evaluating the reliability, validity, responsiveness of the instrument and those who use it?

Observational methods

1. Were the observations performed using the principles of informed consent?
2. How were any observers trained to minimise any bias?
3. Was there an observers' guide?
4. Were the observers required to make inferences about what they observed?
5. Is there any reason to believe that the presence of the observers affected the behaviour of the subjects?

Questionnaires

1. Is the instrument (questionnaire) adequately described to assess whether it addresses the concept of interest?
2. Is there evidence that subjects were able to complete the responses?
3. Is there a clear indication that the subjects understood the questionnaire?
4. Are the majority of the items appropriately close-ended or open-ended?

Records and other available documents or data

1. Are the records used appropriate to the problem being studied?
2. Are the data examined in such a way as to provide new information rather than summarising current information?
3. Is there any indication of selection bias in the available records?

All studies should have clearly identified data collection methods. The conceptual and operational definitions of each important variable should be presented. It may be relevant for the researcher to provide a rationale for the particular method chosen. For example, if the study dealt with frail elderly patients, the researcher may explain that a questionnaire was deemed to be an unreasonable task for such participants, so an interview was chosen. If a questionnaire was used, justification of why this procedure was used in preference to an interview should be clear. Consider whether the method was appropriate to the clinical situation. For example, does it make sense to interview patients in the intensive care unit or recovery room when their cognition may be impaired?

Once all relevant variables are defined appropriately, the method and data collection procedure can be examined. For studies using physiological measurement, it is important to determine whether the instrument was appropriate to measure the concept under investigation. The rationale for selecting a particular instrument should be given, as well as an evaluation of the accuracy of the instrument and the operators who used it when collecting data.

Several considerations are important when reading studies that use observational methods. Who were the observers and how were they trained? Is there any reason to believe that different observers saw events or behaviours differently? Remember that the more inferences the observers are required to make, the more likely it is that there will be differences in their observations. Also consider the problem of reactivity: in any observational situation, the possibility exists that the presence of an observer could change the behaviour of the subjects, thus leading to bias. Finally, consider whether the observational procedure was ethical. The reader needs to consider whether subjects were informed that they were being observed, whether any intervention was performed and whether subjects had agreed to be observed.

Interviews and questionnaires should be clearly described to allow the reader to decide whether the variables were adequately operationalised. Sometimes the researcher will cite the original report that used the tool and the reader may wish to read this study before deciding if the tool was appropriate for the present study. The respondents' task should be clear. Thus provision should be made for the subjects to understand both their overall responsibilities and the individual items. Who were the interviewers in the interview situation? Does the researcher explain how they were trained to decrease any interviewer bias?

Available data are subject to potential bias, and the research report should present evidence that addresses the authenticity and accuracy of the primary records. In addition, the reader should be aware of the problems with selective survival of records. The researcher may not have an unbiased sample of all of the possible records in the area under investigation, and this may have an effect on the validity of the results. Finally, the reader should consider the data collection procedure. Is any assurance provided that all of the subjects received the same information? In addition, it is important to try to determine whether all of the information was collected in the same way for all of the subjects in the study.

Once you have decided that the data collection method used was appropriate to the problem and the procedures were appropriate to the population studied, the reliability and validity of the instruments themselves need to be considered. These issues are discussed in Chapter 19.

KEY POINTS

- Data collection methods are both objective and systematic. The methods of a study provide the operational definitions of the relevant variables. A critical evaluation of data collection methods should emphasise the appropriateness, objectivity and consistency of the method employed.
- Types of data collection methods include physiological, observational, interviews, questionnaires and available data or records. Each method has strengths and limitations.
- Physiological measurements are methods that use technical instruments to collect data about patients' physical or biological status. Such instruments are particularly suited to the study of the effectiveness of nursing care and the ways to improve the provision of nursing care. Physiological measurements aim to be objective, precise and sensitive.
- Observational methods are frequently used in nursing research when the variables of interest deal with events or behaviours. Scientific observation requires preplanning, systematic recording, and controlling observations. Observational methods enable collection of data in many types of situations. Observation also has potential limitations of reactivity, concealment, or biased observation.
- Interviews and questionnaires are the most commonly used data collection methods in nursing research. Both have the purpose of asking subjects to report data about themselves. Open-ended and close-ended questions may be used when asking subjects questions in either approach. The form of the question should be clear to the respondent, free of bias and grammatically correct.
- Questionnaires are particularly useful when there are a finite number of questions to be asked and the researcher is sure that the questions are clear and specific. Items can be combined into scales that provide an estimate of the degree to which the respondent possesses some trait or characteristic. Questionnaires are much less costly in time and money to administer to a large number of subjects, but interviews enable clarification of responses and two-way communication with the respondents.
- Records and available data are an important source for research data. The use of available data may save the researcher considerable time and money when conducting a study. This data collection method reduces problems with both reactivity and ethical concerns. However, records and available data are subject to problems of availability, authenticity and accuracy.

CRITICAL THINKING CHALLENGES

- 'Physiological measurements are objective, precise and sensitive.' Discuss this statement and comment on the factors that might impact on their validity and reliability.
- A student in your class asks a nurse researcher why research assistants who participate in a clinical research study as data collectors need to be trained. What important factors or rationale would you offer to support the establishment of inter-rater reliability?
- Observational methods are frequently used in nursing research. What are the advantages and disadvantages of using this method of data collection?

Additional resources

Butz, A.M. & Alexander, C. (1991). Use of health diaries with children. *Nursing Research*, 40, 59–61.

Cowan, M.J. (1995) Measurement of heart rate variability. *Western Journal of Nursing Research*, 17, 32–48.

Kite, K. (1999). Participant observation, peripheral observation or apart-icipant observation? *Nurse Researcher*, 7(1), 45–55.

Kvale, S. (1996). *InterViews: an introduction to qualitative research interviewing*. Sage, Thousand Oaks, California.

Macnee, C.L. & Talsma, A. (1995). Development and testing of the barriers to cessation scale. *Nursing Research*, 44(4), 214–19.

Minichiello, V., Aroni, R., Timewell, E. & Alexander, L. (1997). *In-depth interviewing*. (2nd ed.). Longman, Melbourne.

Morse, J.M. (1991). Approaches to qualitative–quantitative methodological triangulation. *Nursing Research*, 40, 120–23.

Reineck, C. (1991). Nursing research instruments: pathway to resources. *Applied Nursing Research*, 4, 34–45.

Santamaria, N., Daly, S., Addicott, R. & Clayton, L. (2001). The development, validity and reliability of the Hospital in the Home dependency scale (HDS). *Australian Journal of Advanced Nursing*, 18(4), 8–14.

Shyu, Y.H. (2000). Development and testing of the Family Caregiving Factors Inventory (FCFI) for home health assessment in Taiwan. *Journal of Advanced Nursing*, 32(1), 226–34.

Weinert, C. & Burman, M. (1996). Nurturing longitudinal samples. *Western Journal of Nursing Research*, 18, 360–64.

19
CHAPTER

Observational designs and methods

Doug Elliott and Lillian Hayes

LEARNING OUTCOMES

After reading this chapter the student should be able:

- Distinguish the differences between observational and interventional designs.
- Describe the overall purpose of observational designs.
- List the advantages and disadvantages of surveys and each type of descriptive design and interrelationship design.
- Discuss relational inferences versus causal inferences as they relate to non-experimental designs.
- Identify the criteria used to critique observational designs.
- Apply the critiquing criteria to the evaluation of observational research designs as they appear in research reports.

Key terms

after-only design
bias
case-control study
cohort study
confounders
correlational study
cross-sectional analysis (CSA)
descriptive/exploratory surveys
design
incidence
odds ratio (OR)
numbers needed to treat (NNT)
prevalence
prospective studies
relative risk (RR)
retrospective studies
study base
variable

INTRODUCTION

Quantitative research methods enable the researcher to manipulate numerical data to answer research questions and draw inferences from their findings. A vast array of methods and measurement instruments to assist in the conduct of research are available for quantitative approaches. Study objectives, questions or hypotheses, and their links to probability or non-probability samples, have been discussed in Chapter 17, and data collection methods common to quantitative designs were discussed in Chapter 18. This chapter introduces the research consumer to a range of observational designs that researchers can use for a variety of nursing, midwifery, public health or epidemiological questions.

One of the fundamental purposes of scientific research in any profession is to determine cause-and-effect relationships. In nursing, for example, we are concerned with developing effective approaches to supporting patients through their health crisis, and for maintaining and restoring wellness. Testing such nursing interventions to determine how well they actually work—that is, evaluating the outcomes in terms of efficacy and cost-effectiveness—is accomplished by using experimental, quasi-experimental or observational (non-experimental) designs. Interventional designs differ from non-experimental designs in one important way: the researcher actively seeks to bring about a desired effect from a specific intervention. Experimental and quasi-experimental studies are also important to consider in relation to research utilisation. It is the findings of such studies that provide the validation of clinical practice and rationale for changing specific aspects of practice. These designs provide a higher level of evidence than observational studies or other forms of evidence (see Chapter 6 for levels of evidence).

Experimental designs are particularly suitable for testing cause-and-effect relationships because they help eliminate potential confounding or extraneous variables that influence the findings (threats to validity) (see Chapter 17). However, most research in nursing is not experimental, because unlike the physical sciences, nursing continues to identify the complex concepts and relationships that are the exclusive province of nursing science. In addition, an experimental design requires that all of the relevant variables have been defined so that they can be manipulated, controlled or studied. With the very complex nature of nursing, this requirement cannot always be met.

OBSERVATIONAL RESEARCH DESIGNS

Observational (non-experimental) designs are used in studies in which the researcher wishes to construct a picture of a phenomenon or explore events, people or situations, as they naturally occur in the environment. The aim of a non-experimental design is therefore to observe and identify variables of interest and explore relationships.

It was previously noted that many phenomena of interest to nurses do not lend themselves to experimental designs. For example, nurses studying pain may be interested in the amount and quality of pain, the measurement of pain and its variations, and patient responses and experiences. However, an investigator would not design an experimental study that would potentially intensify a patient's pain just to study the pain experience. Instead, the researcher would examine the factors that contribute to the variability in a patient's post-operative pain experience using a non-experimental design.

Non-experimental research designs also work from a clear, concise problem statement that is based on a theoretical framework. Even though the researcher does not actively manipulate the variables, the concepts of control and rigour should be considered as much as possible. Figure 19.1 illustrates a continuum for quantitative research designs, although there is some disagreement about how to classify non-experimental studies.

FIGURE 19.1 Continuum of quantitative research designs

Non-experimental ⟶ Quasi-experimental ⟶ Experimental

For the purposes of discussion, this chapter will consider descriptive/exploratory survey studies and correlational studies, and epidemiological methods as presented in Box 19.1.

BOX 19.1 Summary of observational research designs

1. Descriptive/exploratory survey studies
2. Correlational studies
3. Epidemiological studies
   - cross-sectional
   - longitudinal studies
   - case-control (ex-post facto) studies
   - cohort (prediction) studies—retrospective and prospective

These categories are somewhat flexible and other sources may classify observational studies in a different way. Some studies fall exclusively within one of these categories, whereas other studies have characteristics of more than one category. In addition, epidemiological methods include randomised treatment studies, but these designs are discussed in the following chapter. This section will introduce the various types of observational designs, including the advantages and disadvantages, their use in nursing, issues of causality, and the critical review process as it relates to observational research.

Descriptive/exploratory survey studies

The broadest category of observational designs is the survey. These studies are sub-classified as descriptive or exploratory research designs. Surveys collect detailed descriptions of existing variables and use the data to justify and assess current conditions and practices or to make more informed decisions to improve healthcare practices. In these designs, investigators attempt only to relate one variable to another; they do not attempt to determine causation or the direction of the effect. Readers of research will find that the terms 'exploratory', 'descriptive' and 'survey' are used either alone, interchangeably or together to describe the design of a study. Investigators use this design to search for accurate information about the characteristics of particular subjects, groups, institutions or situations, or about the frequency of a phenomenon's occurrence, particularly when little is known about the phenomenon within the positivist paradigm.

Data in survey research can be collected by either a questionnaire or an interview (see Chapter 16). The types of variables of interest can be classified as opinions, attitudes or facts. One study explored opinions, attitudes and expectations of critical care nurses regarding the implementation of a clinical information system in a general ICU (Marasovic, Kenney, Elliott & Sindhusake, 1997). Studies such as this provide the basis for further investigation into this area and also for the development of educational programs for nurses that will meet their practice needs.

Most studies also collect demographic data. Facts include attributes of individuals that are a function of their membership in society; such as gender, income level, political and religious affiliations, ethnicity, occupation and educational level. In the Marasovic et al. (1997) study, data about the age, speciality qualifications, experience, and educational status of the participants were collected to describe the sample in relation to the population of nurses from which they were drawn (generalisability).

Descriptive/exploratory survey studies are also used to determine differences between variables. An example of a descriptive or exploratory survey examined nurses' views on continuing competence (Pearson & Fitzgerald, 2001). Most respondents favoured a signed declaration of competence, with random audits. This study did not manipulate variables but assessed perceptions of nurses' views on professional competence that could guide future intervention studies.

There are both advantages and disadvantages when using survey research. Two major advantages are that a great deal of information can be obtained from a large population in a fairly economical manner, and that survey research information can be surprisingly accurate. If a sample is representative of the population (see Chapter 17), a relatively small number of subjects can provide an accurate picture of the population. There are several disadvantages of descriptive/exploratory survey studies. First, the information obtained in a survey tends to be brief and superficial: breadth rather than depth of information is emphasised. Second, conducting a survey requires a great deal of expertise in a variety of research areas, including sampling techniques, questionnaire construction, interviewing and data analysis, so as to produce a reliable and valid study. Third, large-scale surveys can be time-consuming and costly.

Correlational studies

In contrast to survey research, investigators also endeavour to trace the relationships or differences between variables that will provide a deeper insight into a phenomenon. These studies enable examination of the relationship between pairs of variables, as well as a comparison between groups, and are classified as correlational studies. In a correlational study an investigator examines the relationship between two or more variables. The researcher is testing whether the variables relate or co-vary, that is, as one variable changes, does a related change occur in the other variable? The researcher using this design is interested in quantifying the strength of the relationship between the variables, as well as the direction of the relationship—that is, the association between variables may be direct or inverse.

It should be emphasised that correlation designs do not test a cause-and-effect relationship—that is, whether one variable causes measurable changes in another variable. When reviewing a correlational study, the reviewer should identify the variables and their relationship the researcher is testing and consider whether the implied relationship is consistent with the conceptual framework and hypotheses being tested. Correlational studies offer researchers and research consumers the following advantages:

- an increased flexibility when investigating complex relationships among variables
- an efficient and effective method of collecting a large amount of data about an issue of interest
- a potential foundation for future, interventional studies
- a framework for exploring the relationship between variables that is inherently not able to be changed or manipulated.

However, there are some limitations to the design, including:

- the researcher is unable to manipulate the variables of interest
- the researcher does not employ randomisation in the sampling procedures because of using pre-existing groups and therefore generalisability is decreased
- the researcher is unable to determine a causal relationship between the variables because of the lack of manipulation, control and randomisation.

One of the most common misuses of a correlational design is the researcher's conclusion that a causal relationship exists between the variables. However, the inability to draw causal statements should not lead the research consumer to conclude that a non-experimental correlational study is an irrelevant design. It is a very useful design for clinical research studies because many of the phenomena of clinical interest are beyond the researcher's ability to manipulate, control and randomise. For instance, a researcher interested in studying the grief experiences of women who have recently miscarried could not randomly assign subjects to grief and non-grief groups. As well as ethical issues, the experience of a miscarriage is a naturally occurring process and, as such, cannot be manipulated. Examination of people's experiences or responses to a life event is best answered using qualitative methods.

EPIDEMIOLOGICAL APPROACHES

Epidemiology is a science that encompasses certain methods and a distinct body of knowledge. In many areas of nursing, clinicians employ aspects of epidemiological methods and utilise epidemiological knowledge. One definition of epidemiology is 'The study of the distribution and determinants of health related states or events in specified populations, and the application of this study to control of health problems' (Last, 1995, p. 55.). The Greek background of the term (*epi* = upon, *demos* = people and *logos* = science) highlights that the focus of epidemiology is populations rather than individuals. This is one aspect of epidemiology that makes it different from other healthcare research.

In epidemiology, 'population' refers to a group of people who share some common characteristic. In a broader sense, the term population could also refer to hospitals, diagnostic samples or health records. For example, the characteristic may be geographically defined (people residing in New South Wales), gender defined (females or males or both), or clinically defined (patients undergoing a specific procedure or in a specific unit). The research questions being asked determine the common characteristic of the population.

Epidemiology, while historically concerned with disease, is now concerned with all states of health from wellness to illness, and with the distribution, or the patterns associated with, these states. There is a basic assumption that health related states are not random events, and that patterns such as time, place and person provide clues to the determinants of these states. As more is known about the determinants (be they biological, social, physical, cultural or behavioural), steps can be taken to promote good health, prevent illness and provide the best management of illness and disease.

Epidemiological approaches commonly use a time perspective as part of their design. Investigators in epidemiological studies are concerned not only with the existing status and interrelationship of phenomena but also with changes that result from elapsed time.

The following types of study designs will be discussed: cross-sectional analysis (CSA); case-control; and longitudinal cohort studies. The study types vary in terms and strength of causality (see Box 19.2).

BOX 19.2 Strength of causality for observational designs in rank order

1. Cohort—retrospective or prospective
2. Case-control with well-defined study base
3. Case-control with poorly defined study base
4. Cross-sectional analysis
5. Ecological/before–after study

Other than the randomised controlled trial (RCT), which is an experimental interventional design (see Chapter 20), a well designed cohort study provides the strongest evidence of causality.

Nursing and epidemiology

Nursing has had a long and varied association with epidemiology. The role of epidemiology in nursing was recognised by Florence Nightingale, who was the first nurse to utilise epidemiological methods and knowledge to enhance and evaluate her nursing practice and improve the health of her patients. Nightingale recognised the importance of keeping accurate records, using statistics to examine these records, and presenting data in such a way ('polar diagrams') to argue a case for and achieve reform in healthcare practices. Mortality rates eloquently identified the impact of the devastation of disease and injuries on soldiers during the Crimean War (1854–1856) and highlighted the effect of improving the hospital environment (sanitary conditions). Nightingale also used these methods to illustrate that in England during peace-time, the mortality rates for soldiers ('army at home') aged 20–35 years, were twice that of a comparable male civilian population ('English male population') (Cohen, 1984, p. 104). This comparative study led to a Royal Commission on the Health of the Army. Nightingale used her epidemiological skills in a variety of settings from hospital to community, to identify the magnitude of a problem and to evaluate the effectiveness of interventions. She compared groups to identify possible causal factors.

Comparisons of groups is a basic epidemiological strategy to find out the 'who, what, where, when and how' of diseases causation. 'Who does and does not become sick?', 'Under what particular circumstances?', 'Where is illness found or not found?', 'When was the time and place of onset?', and 'How does illness affect groups?' are the questions of interest.

Today, nurses working in a variety of settings ask similar questions to those asked by Nightingale. Who has the health problem? What is the magnitude of the heath problem? What caused the health problem? Do interventions work? These are all questions that epidemiological methods may help to answer. The role and application of epidemiology in nursing has been well recognised in community and public health nursing (PAHO Advisory Committee on the Teaching of Community Nursing, 1976), and is now being recognised in other clinical nursing areas. For example, Murphy (1992) stressed the importance of clinical epidemiology in her editorial that discussed the application of science to the art of nurse-midwifery. Infection control nurses have also long used surveillance skills in their practice.

More recently, the debate on evidence-based nursing has seen a call for nurses to be more 'epidemiologically informed' and to recognise the complementary nature of quantitative and qualitative research (Cullum, 1998; Mulhall, 2000). Nevertheless, epidemiology has a major role to play in evidence-based nursing (Closs & Cheater, 1999) (see Chapter 6). As an example of epidemiological methods, a diabetic nurse consultant was interested in the impact of rural isolation on the utilisation of healthcare services related to diabetes care. A descriptive study analysed routinely collected health data (Medicare data) to help answer this research question (Overland, Yue & Mira, 2001).

Basic epidemiological concepts

There are a number of important concepts in epidemiology, but only two will be considered here: the natural history of a disease, and prevention.

The natural history of disease

The natural history of disease refers to the processes whereby diseases occur and progress in humans—that is, the stages of disease from onset, through the pre-symptomatic stage, to the signs and symptoms, to resolution (its final clinical end points). Epidemiology contributes to the understanding of this natural process from the risk factors that predispose individuals to disease to predicting the progression and duration of the disease.

Prevention

The goals of epidemiology include the prevention, control, and where possible the eradication, of disease and injury. How these goals are achieved depends, in part, on what is known about the natural history of a disease (stages of disease) and the identification of where in this process interventions may be effectively implemented. The identification of risk factors allows for intervention before the occurrence of disease (primary prevention). For example, smoking is a known risk factor for lung cancer; therefore, an early intervention in health promotion is to reduce exposure to cigarette smoke. It is not always possible to intervene before changes take place, however it may be possible to detect the disease early (secondary prevention). Screening is the most common form of secondary prevention (e.g. mammography, for the early detection of breast cancer). Not all diseases are able to be detected at an early stage. The aim of prevention in the later stages is, where possible, to arrest the disease process, limit disability, and rehabilitate (tertiary prevention) or provide palliation.

Epidemiological study designs

As noted earlier, epidemiological studies are either observational or experimental—the latter is discussed in Chapter 20. Observational studies from an epidemiological position are categorised as descriptive or analytic (experimental studies are also classified as analytic, but are discussed in the following chapter). Analytic studies use inferential statistics (see Chapter 23) to infer a causal relationship between two or more variables of interest. Table 19.1 highlights these broad categorisations and commonly used epidemiological study types. Many terms are used to describe the same type of study and some of these synonyms are included in Table 19.1 as a reference.

TABLE 19.1 Epidemiological study types

STUDY TYPES	ALTERNATIVE NAMES/SYNONYMS
OBSERVATIONAL	
Descriptive	
Cross-sectional survey	Prevalence Disease frequency survey Health survey
Prospective Cross-sectional ecological surveys Longitudinal ecological studies	Repeated cross-sectional incidence
Analytic	
Ecological	Correlational
Before–after	
Cross-sectional analytic	
Case-control	Retrospective study Case comparison study Case history study Case referent study
Cohort	Prospective Concurrent Follow-up Incidence Longitudinal
Historical cohort	Retrospective cohort study Historical prospective study Nonconcurrent prospective cohort study
EXPERIMENTAL	
Randomised controlled trails (RCT)	Clinical trials—randomised controlled clinical trials
Field trials	Randomised controlled field trials
Community trials	Community intervention studies

Box 19.3 lists some epidemiological terms to become familiar with as a research consumer.

BOX 19.3 Epidemiological terms

Independent variable is referred to as the *study factor* or the *exposure*.

Dependent variable is referred to as the *outcome factor*.

Extraneous variable may be an *extraneous factor* and a *confounder*.

The *study base* is 'the persons (or person time) in which the outcome of interest is observed' (Last, 1995).

The *study population* is 'the group selected for investigation' (Last, 1995).

Directionality is the 'order in which the outcome factor (i.e. disease) and study factor (i.e. exposure) are investigated. (Gerstman, 1998, p. 140).

The three common observational designs in epidemiological research are cross-sectional, cohort, and case-control; they differ according to timing and directionality of the study. If the exposure and the outcome factor are measured at around the same point in time, the study is cross-sectional (i.e. there is no direction). Cohort studies are forward looking, from exposure to outcome, while case-control studies are backward looking from outcome to exposure (see Figure 19.2).

FIGURE 19.2 Design dimension, directionality and timing

Observational design type	Directionality
Cross-sectional	No direction ↕
Cohort	Forward →
Case-control	Backward ←

Timing refers to the occurrence of the study outcome and the exposure in relation to when the data were actually collected. If the occurrence was before the beginning of the study, the design is historical. An example of this is when pre-existing records are examined or study subjects recall previous events. If the events occur during the study period, it is said to be concurrent. When some of the data are historic and some of the information is concurrent, the timing is described as mixed. The following figure illustrates this in relation to the cohort study design (see Figure 19.3).

FIGURE 19.3 Timing of data collection in cohort designs

	Past		Present		Future
Historical	E ⟶	O			
Concurrent			E ⟶	O	
Mixed		E	⟶	O	

E = exposure
O = outcome

The type of epidemiological study used depends on the questions that need to be answered. Research questions or study objectives are either concerned with causality or the magnitude of a health problem. Causality questions include identification of the determinants of health states, identification of the risk factors, and assessing the effectiveness of interventions. Magnitude questions include: 'What proportion of the population have a disease or condition?'; 'Is this changing over time?'; 'How common is the health problem?'; 'Does this problem or condition vary from one area to another?'; and 'Which people are most affected by this problem?'.

Descriptive studies

Descriptive studies are used to answer magnitude questions in epidemiology. They identify patterns of health states in defined human populations. Health states are related to basic characteristics of the person, such as age, sex, social class, occupation and income, geographic location (where the health event occurs) and time (seasonal variations and time). Such studies may be used to identify groups at high risk. This descriptive information is important in alerting clinicians to what types of persons may be affected by disease, and where and when the disease will occur. Some disease outbreaks are seasonal (e.g. meningococcal meningitis) and are known to affect certain age groups in particular locations. Descriptive studies help with planning health services and generating hypotheses about the determinants of health states. Routinely collected data, such as mortality data, are frequently used in descriptive studies. Descriptive studies do not make comparisons between groups and are not concerned with causality.

Cross-sectional descriptive studies

Health surveys involve measurement of a health characteristic in a population at a given point in time. They may involve the selection of a representative sample of the total population of interest, particularly if the population is large. The study measures the prevalence of the outcome of interest. For example, a survey of school children may be used to determine their knowledge, attitudes and behaviours in relation to substance use. Advantages of this design include being quick, easy and cheap to conduct, and the ability to generate hypotheses. Disadvantages include the inability to test hypotheses, and no temporal relationship between the variables. Repeated cross-sectional studies (also then a longitudinal study) follow a group of people for a period of time during a series of studies to help describe the natural history of disease or behaviour (e.g. to answer the question 'How many women recently diagnosed with breast cancer will die in the next five years?').

Cross-sectional analytic studies

Cross-sectional studies examine data at one point in time, that is, data are collected on only one occasion with the same subjects rather than on the same subjects at several points in time. Thus, the outcome factor and the study factor are measured simultaneously in the population of interest. The lack of time as a factor provides weak evidence of causality, as it is difficult to determine the temporal relationship between the outcome and the study factor.

In a study by Bucknall and Thomas (1997), data were collected on only one occasion from a group of critical care nurses to investigate how the nurses perceived problems associated with their decision-making in the critical care environment. This design is appropriate for the study question, as the researchers are interested in decision-making at one point in time—there is no necessity for repeated measures.

Brooks and colleagues also used a cross-sectional design to examine the health outcomes of survivors of a critical illness (Brooks, Bauman, Daffurn & Hillman, 1995; Brooks, Kerridge, Hillman, Bauman & Daffurn, 1997). A sample of 113 patients was examined at 12–18 months post-discharge and compared with a community sample of 117 subjects. The findings demonstrated significant differences in health status between the two groups. However, it was not established that the two groups were similar in age, chronic illness, or health status prior to the patients' ICU admissions. In addition, no pre-illness health status was measured for the ICU patients for comparison with their post-discharge health status and quality of life.

Another cross-sectional study approach is to simultaneously collect data on the variables of interest from different cohort groups. An excellent example of a cross-sectional study with different age cohort groups compared the influence of age, coping behaviour and self-care on psychological, social and physiological adaptation in pre-adolescents and adolescents with diabetes (Grey, Cameron & Thurber, 1991). This study focused on children aged 8–18 years with insulin-dependent diabetes mellitus, and their parents. Several questionnaires were completed at one point in time. Differences between pre-adolescent and adolescent groups were found after analysis.

Cross-sectional studies are less time consuming, less expensive and thus more manageable for the researcher. Because large amounts of data can be collected at one point, the results are more readily available. In addition, the confounding variable of maturation, resulting from the elapsed time, is not presented. However, the investigator's ability to establish an in-depth developmental assessment of the interrelationships of the phenomena being studied is lessened. Thus the researcher is unable to determine whether the change that occurred was related to the change that was predicted, because the same subjects were not followed over a period of time. In summary, cross-sectional studies look at a broad perspective of a cross-section of the population at a specific point in time. In contrast, longitudinal studies begin in the present and end in the future.

Case-control studies

Case-control subjects are selected on the basis of the study outcome (characteristic) they do or do not exhibit. The direction of the study is from the study outcome to the cause or the exposure. Individuals with the outcome (disease or condition) of interest are identified as the 'cases'. The cases are then matched with 'controls', who are a sample of people who are similar to the cases, but do not have the outcome of interest. The controls come from the same 'study base' as the cases. Detailed past histories, particularly in relation to possible risk factors (exposure), are taken from both groups. The histories are examined to see if the cases have been more exposed to the suspected causative factor (exposure) than the controls. There will be a problem of selection bias if the cases are not from a well defined (in time and place) study base. Case-control studies are described as having a poorly defined study base if controls do not come from the same study base as the cases.

The advantages of the case-control design are similar to those in the correlational design, with the additional benefit of a higher level of control than a correlational study. For example, in a cigarette smoking study, a group of non-smokers' lung tissue samples are compared with samples of smokers' lung tissue. This comparison enables the researcher to establish that there is a differential effect of cigarette smoking on lung tissue.

However, the researcher remains unable to draw a causal linkage between the two variables, and this inability is the major disadvantage of this design. In addition, incidence cannot be measured within the study base. Another disadvantage is the problem of an alternative hypothesis being the reason for the documented relationship. If the researcher obtains data from two existing groups of subjects, such as one that has been exposed to cigarette smoking and one that has not, and the data support the hypothesis that smoking is related to lung cancer, the researcher cannot be sure whether smoking or some extraneous variable is the real cause of the occurrence of the cancer.

Finding naturally occurring groups of subjects who are similar in all respects except for their exposure to the variable of interest is very difficult. There is always the possibility that the groups differ in some other way, such as exposure to some other lung irritants such as asbestos, which can affect the findings of the study and produce spurious results. The researcher must attempt to match controls to the cases for characteristics such as age, gender or procedure. Consequently, the critical reader of such a study needs to cautiously evaluate the conclusions drawn by the investigator in relation to measurement error (see Chapter 21).

Retrospective studies

Retrospective (ex-post facto) studies are where the dependent variable has already been affected by the independent variable and the investigator attempts to link present events to events that have occurred in the past. The term 'retrospective' is primarily used by epidemiologists, whereas the term 'ex-post facto' is preferred by social scientists. When researchers explain causality or the factors that determine the occurrence of events or conditions, an experimental design is preferred. However, they cannot always manipulate the independent variable or use random assignment. In cases in which experimental designs cannot be employed, a retrospective cohort study may be used. Ex-post facto literally means, 'from after the fact'. Ex-post facto studies are also known as causal–comparative studies or comparative studies. Note that many elements of epidemiological research are similar to quasi-experimental designs because they explore differences between variables (Campbell & Stanley, 1963). However, interventions occur outside the researcher's control in the majority of epidemiological designs.

In ex-post facto studies a researcher hypothesises that a predictor variable (cigarette smoking) is related to and is a determinant of a study variable (lung cancer). The presumed cause is not manipulated and subjects are not randomly assigned to groups. Rather, a group of subjects who have experienced cigarette smoking in a normal situation is located and a control group of subjects who have not is chosen. The behaviour, performance or condition (evidence of lung cancer), of the two groups are compared to determine whether the exposure to smoking had the effect predicted by the hypothesis. In practical terms, this design is equivalent to the case-control design described previously.

Cohort studies

The direction of a cohort study is from the exposure to the outcome, or cause to effect. That is, a group of people are followed over a period of time, and the incidence of the study outcome is observed in relation to exposure to possible causes/risk factors. A disadvantage of such studies is the time period and high costs involved, as there may be a considerable time lag between time of exposure and subsequent study outcome. This may be partly overcome in a historical cohort study if some of the data of individuals exposed in the past are available for use.

Cohort designs can be used to examine relationships both retrospectively and prospectively. Prospective (longitudinal) studies explore presumed causes, presumed differences or presumed relationships and move forward in time to the presumed effect. To test this hypothesis, the investigator would draw a sample of subjects who did and who did not have the condition (exposure) of interest. The occurrence of the outcome of interest in both groups would then be analysed.

In another situation a researcher may wish to study the development of a particular health outcome. In this type of study the investigator selects the participants from a population known to be free of the health outcome under study and classifies the participants according to whether they have one or more factors (independent or explanatory variables) presumably related to the outcome. These participants, who are frequently referred to as a cohort, are then studied over a period, ranging from months to years, to determine who develops the health outcome. The Framingham heart study examined the effect of blood pressure, cholesterol levels, smoking, exercise and other variables, on the development of coronary artery disease in a cohort of healthy men, at specified intervals over a period of years (e.g. Margolis et al., 1974; Peeters et al., 2002).

Repeated measures (longitudinal) studies

In contrast to a cross-sectional design, longitudinal studies collect data from the same group at different points in time. For instance, the investigator conducting the study with diabetic children could elect to use a longitudinal design. In that case the investigator could collect yearly data and follow the same children over a number of years to compare changes in the variables at different ages. By collecting data from each subject at yearly intervals, a longitudinal perspective of the diabetic process is accomplished.

There are many advantages and disadvantages of cross-sectional and longitudinal designs. When assessing the appropriateness of a cross-sectional study versus a longitudinal study, the research consumer should first assess what the goal of the researcher was in relation to the theoretical framework. The advantages of a longitudinal study are that each subject is followed separately and thereby serves as his or her own control, and increased depth of responses can be obtained and early trends in the data can be investigated. The researcher can assess changes in the variables of interest over time and both relationships and differences can be explored between variables. The disadvantages inherent in a longitudinal design must also be considered, including the long duration of data collection, threats to internal validity such as 'testing' and 'mortality' (loss to follow-up), and the influence of confounding variables. Subjects in such a study may also respond in a socially desirable way that they believe is congruent with the investigators' expectations (the 'Hawthorne effect') (see page 273). These realities make a longitudinal design costly in terms of time, effort and money. However, despite the pragmatic constraints imposed by a longitudinal study, the researcher should proceed with this design if the theoretical framework supports a longitudinal developmental perspective.

Randomised controlled trials

Randomised controlled trials are also used in epidemiological research. In this experimental method, individuals are randomly allocated to receive treatment or intervention (study factor) or not in order to determine the effects of the treatment or intervention. These studies provide the strongest evidence of cause and effect. Community trials involve the random allocation of groups to the intervention of control exposure. Chapter 20 discusses these and other experimental designs in more detail.

Error

While observational studies aim to accurately measure the occurrence of the study outcome (health-related state), nurses need to be aware that there are a number of potential sources of error—random error and bias. Random error is where variations in measurements are due to chance. Bias is the effect of interference at any stage of the study that produces results that differ from the true value in a systematic way. There are three common sources of bias:

- selection
- measurement
- confounding.

Selection bias

Selection bias occurs when there are systematic differences between those selected to participate in a study and those not selected for the study. If groups are being compared, they should be similar in attributes except with respect to the study factor, and the subject's selection process should ensure this. Study validity is compromised if the people who volunteer or who are willing to participate in a study are different to those who do not volunteer or decline to participate. Convenience samples such as the use of hospital-based controls in a case-control study may not be reflective of the referent population. A probability sampling method is one way of overcoming this problem (see Chapter 17).

Measurement bias

Measurement bias is the systematic error in measures of effect or association due to inaccurate measurement of study factors, study outcome and confounders. The subject, the observer and the measurement instrument have the potential to contribute to inaccurate measurements (see Chapter 21).

Confounding

Confounding bias is a distortion of the measurement of the effect of the study factor or exposure on the study outcome because of an extraneous factor. Confounding bias only occurs if the extraneous factor is an independent risk factor for the study outcome, is associated with the study factor, and is not an intervening variable (see Figure 19.4).

FIGURE 19.4 Influence of confounding bias

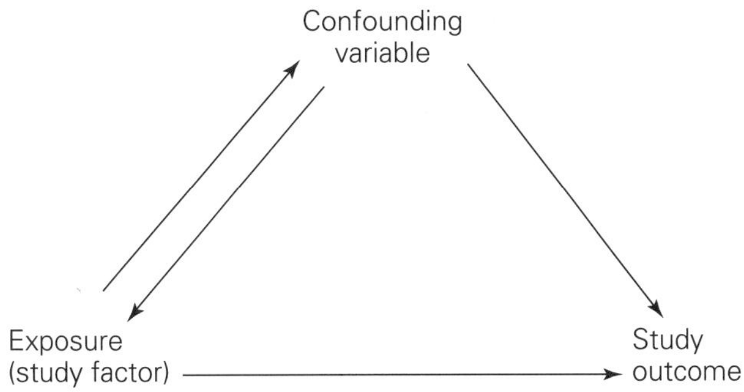

Measurement

In order to make statements about the distribution and determinants of health-related states and events, it is necessary to use measures of frequency and association which permit comparisons between populations or sub-groups within a population. Common measures used in descriptive studies include:

- rates, e.g. mortality rates, morbidity, etc.
- prevalence, i.e. the proportion of a population with the disease
- incidence, i.e. the proportion of a population developing the disease over a period of time.

Many of the measures of disease or health status are expressed as a rate.

Rates

A rate is a measure of a (demographic) event in a defined population in a specified period of time. For example, rates for the number of infant deaths in a local government area in NSW in 1998 are illustrated in Box 19.4.

BOX 19.4 Calculating rates of disease

$$\text{Rate} = \frac{\text{specified event in a specified period of time}}{\text{defined population in a specific period of time}} \times \text{constant multiplier}$$

$$\text{Rate} = \frac{\text{Numerator}}{\text{Denominator}} \times \text{constant}$$

The constant multiplier may be 100 to make a percentage, or 10^n such as 1000 and 100,000. This produces a rate that is a manageable number—for example, 8 infant deaths per 1000 live births per year rather than 0.008 infant deaths per year.

Example: In a NSW local government area there were 16 infant deaths and 2000 live births over a 12-month period.

$$\text{Infant Mortality Rate} = \frac{\text{Number of deaths in a year of children less than 1 year of age}}{\text{Number of live births in the same year}} \times 1000$$

$$\text{Infant Mortality Rate} = \frac{16}{2000} \times 1000$$

$$= \text{8 infant deaths per 1000 live births in one year}$$

The defined population may also be expressed as the population at risk of experiencing an event in a specified period of time. There are three aspects of a rate to consider:

- What is the denominator?
- What is the numerator?
- What is the period of time (time dimension)?

In the infant mortality example given above, the denominator was live births, the numerator was deaths in children less than one year of age, and the period of time was one year.

Data presentation

Data from epidemiological studies can often be displayed in two-way tables (also known as two-by-two tables or fourfold tables). These tables are a convenient way of ordering categorical study data so that results such as the appropriate measures of association can be calculated (see Table 19.2). In the cross tables and associated formulas that follow:

a = Exposed and diseased
b = Exposed and non-diseased
c = Not exposed and diseased
d = Not exposed and non-diseased
N = Overall total

TABLE 19.2 Two by two table format for data presentation

	OUTCOME FACTOR		
STUDY FACTOR	Diseased	Non-diseased	TOTAL
Exposed	*a*	*b*	*a* + *b*
Not exposed	*c*	*d*	*c* + *d*
TOTAL	*a* + *c*	*b* + *d*	*N*

In a cohort study, the marginal totals for the exposed (*a* + *b*) and the non-exposed (*c* + *d*) are known (i.e. the row totals). As the study progresses, the outcome factor becomes known, and at the end of the study the internal cells become known. The Relative Risk (also known as the Risk Ratio) is then derived using the following formula:

$$\text{Relative Risk (RR)} = \frac{\text{Cumulative incidence in the exposed group}}{\text{Cumulative incidence in the unexposed group}}$$

$$\text{RR} = \frac{a / (a + b)}{c / (c + d)}$$

Conversely, in a case-control study, the row totals are not known, as the true values of all the exposed ($a + b$) and the unexposed ($c + d$) and the total population (N) are not known. However, the column totals are known, that is, the number of subjects with the study outcome (the cases) ($a + c$), and those without the study outcome ($b + d$). A relative risk cannot be calculated because of these unknown values.

A measure of strength of association for case-control studies is the Odds Ratio (OR). This is the ratio of the odds of exposure in the diseased, divided by the odds of exposure in the non-diseased. Using the notation in Table 19.2 above:

$$\text{Odds Ratio (OR)} = \frac{a / c}{b / d}$$

$$= \frac{a \times d}{b \times c}$$

A number of other parameters can also be derived (see Table 19.3).

TABLE 19.3 Derived epidemiological parameters

PARAMETER	FORMULA
The Relative Risk (RR): also the ratio of the experimental event rate over the control event rate	$\text{RR} = \frac{\text{EER}}{\text{CER}}$
The Absolute Risk Reduction (ARR): the difference between the experimental and control event rates	ARR = EER – CER
Numbers needed to treat (NNT): a statistic that provides an indication of the numbers of patients to be treated to prevent a bad outcome	$\text{NNT} = \frac{1}{\text{ARR}}$

The latter provides some evidence of what constitutes a clinical important change in the continuous measure: NNT = 1/experimental rate, i.e. the control rate (see Chapters 6 and 23 for further discussion).

CAUSALITY IN OBSERVATIONAL RESEARCH

A concern of researchers and research consumers is the issue of causality. Researchers are interested in explaining cause-and-effect relationships. Historically, researchers have said that only experimental research can support the concept of causality. For example, nurses are interested in discovering what causes anxiety in many settings. If the causes can be uncovered, then perhaps interventions can be developed that would prevent or decrease the anxiety. Causality makes it necessary to order events chronologically, that is, if in a randomly assigned experiment, a life or health event (e.g. stress) occurs before a response (e.g. anxiety), and those in the stressed group were anxious whereas those in the unstressed group were not anxious, an hypothesis of stress causes anxiety can be supported by empirical observations. If these results were found in a non-experimental study where some subjects underwent the stress of surgery and were anxious, and others did not have surgery and were not anxious, it could be proposed that an association or relationship exists between the stressor (surgery) and anxiety. However, a causal relationship can only be said to occur if supported by the results of a well designed experimental study.

There are also many variables like anxiety that nurse researchers wish to study that cannot be manipulated because of ethical or practical reasons. Yet there is a need to have studies that can assert a causal sequence. In light of this need, many nurse researchers are using several analytical techniques that explain relationships among variables to establish causal links. These techniques are called causal modelling and associated causal analysis techniques (Aaronson, Frey & Boyd, 1988; Asher, 1983; Boyd, Frey & Aaronson, 1988; Ferketich & Verran, 1984; Verran & Ferketich, 1984). The reader of research will also find the terms 'path analysis', 'LISREL' (Linear Structural Relation Analysis), 'analysis of covariance structures' and 'structural equation modelling' (SEM) used to describe these techniques (Pedhazur & Schmelkin, 1991). See Chapter 23 for further discussion of these techniques.

CRITICAL REVIEW OF OBSERVATIONAL DESIGNS

Criteria for the review of observational designs are presented in Box 19.5. The first step in critiquing observational research is to determine which type of design was used in the study. Often a statement describing the design of the study appears in the Abstract and in the Methods section of the report. If such a statement is not present, the reader should examine the paper closely for evidence of which type of design was employed. The reader should be able to discern that either a survey or interrelationship design was used, as well as the specific sub-type.

Factors that actually influence changes in the outcome (or dependent) variable are often ambiguous in observational designs. As with all complex phenomena, multiple factors can contribute to variability in the subjects' responses. When an experimental design is not used for controlling some of these extraneous variables that can influence results, the researcher must strive to provide as much control of them as possible within the context of a non-experimental design. When it has not been possible to randomly assign subjects to treatment groups as an approach to controlling an independent variable, the researcher may use a strategy of matching subjects for identified variables, as in a case-control study. For example, in a study of infant birth weight, pregnant women could be matched on variables such as weight, height, smoking habits, drug use and other factors that might influence birth weight. The independent variable of interest—type of prenatal care—would then be the major difference in the groups. The reader would then feel more confident that the only real difference between the two groups was the differential effect of the independent variable, because the other factors in the two groups were theoretically the same. However, the reader should remember also that there may be other influential variables that were not matched, such as income, education and diet. Extraneous and confounding variables represent a major influence on the interpretation of a non-experimental study, because they impose limitations on the generalisability (external validity) of the results.

BOX 19.5 Criteria for evaluating observational designs

1. What is the research statement for the study?
2. Is the design experimental, quasi-experimental or non-experimental?
3. What specific observational design is used in the study?
4. Is the problem one of a cause-and-effect relationship?
5. Is the method used appropriate to the problem?
6. Which specific observational design is utilised in the study?
7. Based on the theoretical framework, is the rationale for the type of design evident?
8. How is the design congruent with the purpose of the study?
9. Is the design appropriate for the research problem and data collection methods?
10. What is the internal and external validity?
11. Does the researcher present the findings in a manner that is congruent with the utilised design?
12. Does the research go beyond the relational parameters of the findings and erroneously infer cause-and-effect relationships between the variables?
13. Are there any reasons to believe that there are alternative explanations for the findings?
14. Where appropriate, how does the researcher discuss the threats to internal and external validity?
15. How does the author deal with the limitations of the study?

KEY POINTS

- Observational (non-experimental) research designs are used to construct a picture or description of events as they naturally occur. The major difference between non-experimental and experimental research is that in non-experimental designs the independent variable is not actively manipulated by the investigator.
- Observational designs can be classified as either survey studies or interrelationship studies; both are descriptive and exploratory in nature.
- Survey research collects detailed descriptions of existing phenomena and uses the data either to justify current conditions and practices or to make more intelligent plans for improving them.
- Interrelationship studies endeavour to explore the interrelationships between variables that provide deeper insight into the phenomena of interest.
- Non-experimental research designs do not enable the investigator to establish cause-and-effect relationships between the variables. Consumers must be wary of non-experimental studies that make causal claims about the findings unless a causal modelling technique is used.
- Correlational and epidemiological studies are examples of interrelationship studies; some may enable prediction of an event in relation to an exposure of the intervention.

- Non-experimental designs provide the least amount of control. Extraneous and confounding variables represent a major influence on the interpretation of a non-experimental study because they impose limitations on the validity of the study and generalisability of the results and, as such, should be fully assessed by the critical reader.
- The critical review process is directed towards evaluating the appropriateness of the selected non-experimental design in relation to factors such as the research problem, theoretical framework, hypothesis, methodology and data analysis and interpretation.

CRITICAL THINKING CHALLENGES

- Discuss which types of observational designs could be used to examine the work activities for nurses in a community health service.
- The group assignment for your research subject is to critique an assigned quantitative study. To proceed, you must first decide on the design to be used: you think it is an ex-post facto design; the others in the group think it is an experimental design because it has several explicit hypotheses. How would you convince them that you are correct?

Additional resources

Atwood, J.R. & Taylor, W. (1991). Regression discontinuity design: alternative for nursing research. *Nursing Research*, 40, 312–15.

Brown, S.J. (1999). *Knowledge for health care practice: a guide to using research evidence*. Philadelphia, Saunders.

Chalmers, I. & Altman, D.G. (1995). *Systemic reviews*. London, BMJ Publishing Group.

Cook, T.D. & Campbell, D.T. (1979). *Quasi-experimentation: design and analysis issues for field settings*. Chicago, Rand-McNally.

Creswell, J.W. (1994). *Research design: qualitative and quantitative approaches*. Thousand Oaks, California, Sage.

Dunning, T. & Martin, M. (1996). Developing a questionnaire: some methodological issues. *Australian Journal of Advanced Nursing*, 14, 31–38.

Frank-Stromberg, M.F. ed. (1992). *Instruments for clinical nursing research*. Boston, Jones and Bartlett.

Glass, G., McGaw, B. & Smith, M. (1981). *Meta-analysis in social research*. Newbury Park, California, Sage.

Jacobson, B.S. & Meininger, J.C. (1990). Seeing the importance of blindness. *Nursing Research*, 39, 54–57.

Jarman, H., Jacobs, E., Walter, R., Witney, C. & Zielinski, V. (2002). Allowing the patient to sleep: flexible medication times in an acute hospital. *International Journal of Nursing Practice*, 8, 75–80.

Miller, D. (1991). *Handbook of research design and social measurement*. (5th ed.). Newbury Park, California, Sage.

Minnick, A. et al. (1995). An analysis of posthospitalisation telephone survey data. *Nursing Research*, 44, 371–75.

Pelletier, D., Gallagher, R., Mitten-Lewis, S., McKinley, S. & Squire, J. (2002). Australian implantable defibrillator recipients: quality-of-life issues. *International Journal of Nursing Practice*, 8, 68–74.
Polivka, B.J. & Nickel, J.T. (1992). Case-control design: an appropriate strategy for nursing research. *Nursing Research*, 41, 250–53.
Waltz, C.F. & Bausell, R.B. (1991). *Nursing research, design, statistics and computer analysis.* Philadelphia, FA Davis.
Weinert, C. & Burman, M. (1996). Nurturing longitudinal samples. *West Journal of Nursing Research*, 18, 360–64.

20
CHAPTER

Interventional designs and methods

Doug Elliott

LEARNING OUTCOMES

After reading this chapter the student should be able to:

- List the criteria necessary for inferring cause-and-effect relationships.
- Distinguish the differences between experimental, quasi-experimental and non-experimental designs.
- Describe the use of experimental and quasi-experimental designs for evaluation research.
- Critically evaluate the findings of selected studies that test cause-and-effect relationships.

Key terms

after-only design
antecedent
contamination
control
dependent variable
design
experiment
extraneous variable
independent variable
manipulation
non-equivalent control group design
prospective studies
quasi-experiment
randomisation
retrospective studies
Solomon four-group design

INTRODUCTION

Experimental designs are particularly suitable for testing a causal hypothesis (cause-and-effect relationship) between an intervention or treatment and an outcome, because they help eliminate potential alternative explanations (threats to validity) for the study findings. To infer causality requires that the following three criteria be met:

- the causal (independent/explanatory) variable and effect (dependent/outcome) variable must be associated with each other
- the cause must precede the effect
- the relationship must not be able to be explained by another (extraneous) variable or variables.

When reviewing studies that use experimental and quasi-experimental designs, the primary focus is on assessing the validity of the finding that the intervention (independent variable) caused the desired effect on the outcome (dependent) variable. The validity of the findings and conclusion depend on how well the researcher has controlled the other variables that may explain the relationship between the explanatory and outcome variables. The focus of this chapter is to explain how the various types of experimental designs and quasi-experimental designs control and limit any bias from extraneous variables.

EXPERIMENTAL DESIGN

An experiment is a scientific investigation that makes observations and collects data according to explicit criteria and protocol. A true experiment has three identifying properties:

- randomisation
- control
- manipulation.

These properties allow for other explanations of the phenomenon to be ruled out and thereby provide the strength of the design for testing cause-and-effect relationships. The concepts of control, randomisation and manipulation and their application to experimental design are sometimes confusing. To see the way these properties allow researchers to have confidence in the causal inferences they make by allowing them to rule out other potential explanations, the use of these properties will be discussed using the paper by Small, Lumley, Donohue, Potter and Waldenström (2000) as an example (see Appendix D). The researchers designed a randomised controlled trial (RCT) to study the effects of a debriefing session compared with standard postnatal care for women after operative birth in Australia.

Randomisation

Randomisation, or random assignment to study groups, involves the distribution of subjects to either the experimental or control group on a purely random, or chance, basis. That is, each subject has an equal and known probability of being assigned to any group. Random assignment may be done individually or by groups. Random assignment to experimental or control groups allows for the minimisation or elimination of any systematic bias in the groups for attributes that may affect the dependent variable being studied. The procedure for randomisation assumes that any important intervening variables will be equally distributed between the groups and minimises variance. Note that random assignment to groups is different from random sampling as discussed in Chapter 17.

An example of random assignment is found in the study by Small and colleagues (2000), where women were randomly allocated to either a midwife-led debriefing session (i.e. the intervention or experimental group) or standard care (i.e. the control group). The outcome variables of the study, maternal depression and health status at six months post-partum, were compared between the two groups to determine the effects of the intervention. Women interested in participating in the study were randomly assigned to either standard care (control group) or midwife-led debriefing (experimental group). This means that all of the women who met the study criteria had an equal chance of being assigned to the control group or the experimental group.

The use of random assignment to groups helps ensure that the two study groups are comparable on pre-existing factors that might affect the outcome of interest. Note that the researchers checked for equivalence of the groups at pre-test, that is, whether the procedure of random assignment did, in fact, produce groups that were similar (see Table 2 of the Small et al. paper). Characteristics examined included clinical (type of operative birth, parity) and demographic variables (age, marital status, education level, English language usage, family income), and the researchers concluded that the two study groups were comparable (Small et al., 2000, p. 1045).

Control

Control is the introduction of one or more constants into the experimental situation. Control is acquired by manipulating the causal or independent variable, by randomly assigning subjects to a group, by very carefully preparing experimental protocols (as discussed in Chapter 8) and by using comparison groups. In experimental research the comparison group is the control group, or the group that receives the usual care or treatment, rather than the innovative experimental one under investigation.

In the study by Small and colleagues (2000), as well as randomisation, control was also exerted by the use of exclusion criteria (e.g. insufficient English, unwell baby or mother, early discharge) for participants in the study. Characteristics of participants (n = 1041) were also compared with non-participants (n = 2294); in this study, respondents were more likely to be older, married, better educated, with higher incomes, better English skills, and have private health insurance (Small et al., 2000, p. 1045). Readers need to examine these differences between subjects and non-subjects when considering the issue of generalisability.

Control groups may, as in the example described above, be a separate group of subjects, although in some longitudinal or cross-over research designs, the subjects act as their own controls. For instance, a study of two different methods of precannulation skin disinfection in patients with end-stage renal disease (Wellard & Palaster, 1996) compared the incidence of inflammation of cannulation sites following disinfection with either povidone iodine or chlorhexidine and alcohol solution. Because of the limited number of renal unit patients available to participate in the study, and to eliminate the effect of factors such as age, gender, immune status and concurrent medical treatment on the outcome, both treatments were administered to each subject. The effect of the two treatments on each subject was observed, thus each patient acted as a member of both the experimental (chlorhexidine and alcohol solution) and control (povidone iodine solution) groups.

The strength of the experimental design lies in its ability to help the researcher to control the effects of any extraneous variables that might constitute threats to internal validity, such as selection, history and maturation (see Chapter 17). Such extraneous variables can be either antecedent or intervening. The antecedent (preceding) variable occurs before the study but may affect the dependent variable and confuse the results. Factors such as age, gender, socio-economic status and health status might be important antecedent variables in nursing and midwifery research, because they may affect dependent variables such as recovery time and the ability to integrate healthcare behaviours. Antecedent variables that might have affected the dependent variables in the study by Small and colleagues (2000) include age, parity, English language and educational level. Random assignment to groups helps to ensure that groups are similar on these variables so that differences in the dependent variable may be attributed to the experimental treatment. It should be noted, however, that the researcher should check and report how the groups actually compared on such variables. An intervening variable occurs during the course of the study and is not part of the study, but it affects the dependent variable. An example of an intervening variable that might affect the outcomes of this study (Small et al., 2000) could be media reports of debriefing sessions on maternal morbidity in a birth centre in a nearby region that could influence women's attitudes about the usefulness of debriefing.

Manipulation

The intervention group or treatment group receives manipulation of the explanatory variable, while the control group does not. The intervention (independent variable) might be a treatment, a teaching plan or a medication. It is the effect of this manipulation that is measured to determine the result of the experimental treatment. Studies using true experimental designs in clinical settings are called randomised controlled trials (RCTs), reflecting the high level of control imposed and the importance of randomisation in gaining evidence for causation.

The degree of control exerted over the intervention and experimental conditions is illustrated by the detailed description in the Small et al. (2000) paper of the debriefing intervention. This helps to ensure that all members of the experimental group receive similar treatment and assists the reader in understanding the nature of the experimental treatment. The control group provides a comparison against which the experimental group can be judged. In this study, the model of care provided—a midwife-led debriefing session of up to one hour in duration, or standard maternity care—was manipulated. Despite exerting clear and careful control over the debriefing intervention, the investigators found that midwife-led debriefing after operative birth were ineffective in reducing the prevalence of maternal depression or improving health status at six months post-partum, and may have contributed to emotional health problems for some women (Small et al., 2000).

Types of experimental designs

There are several different experimental designs (Campbell & Stanley, 1963). Each is based on the classic design called the true experiment presented in Figure 20.1, A. Note that subjects have been randomly assigned to the experimental group or control group. The experimental treatment is given only to those in the experimental group and the pretests and post-tests are those measurements of the dependent variables that are made before and after the experimental treatment is performed. All true experimental designs have subjects randomly assigned to groups, have an experimental treatment introduced to some of the subjects and have the effects of the treatment observed. Designs vary primarily in the number of observations that are made and how the treatment is introduced.

FIGURE 20.1 Comparison of experimental designs

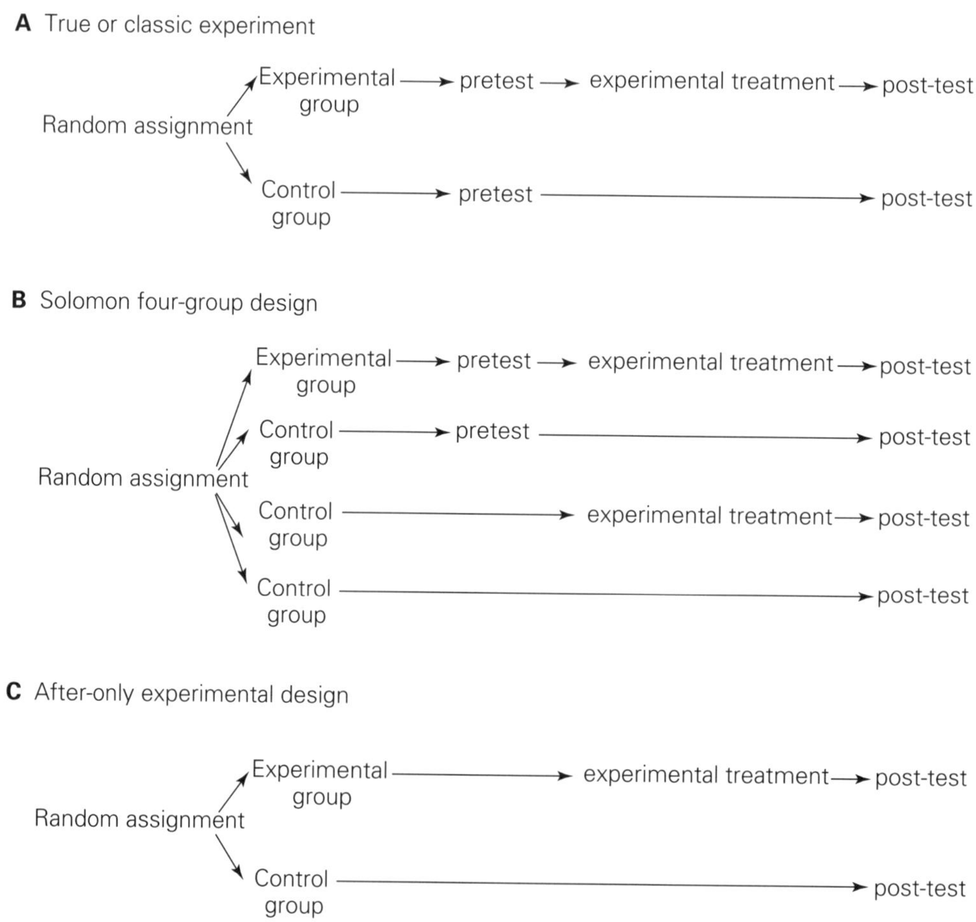

As shown, subjects are randomly assigned to the two groups, experimental and control, so that any antecedent variables are controlled. Then pretest measures or observations are usually made so that the researcher has a baseline for determining the effect of the independent variable. The researcher then introduces the intervention to one of the groups and measures the dependent variable again to see whether it has changed. The control group gets no experimental treatment but is also measured for comparison with the experimental group. The degree of difference between the two groups at the end of the study indicates the confidence the researcher has that a causal link exists between the independent and dependent variables.

For example, nursing and medical researchers wanted to find out if primary care delivered by nurse practitioners was as effective as that delivered by physicians. A randomised trial, in which 1316 patients were randomly allocated to either a nurse practitioner or a physician, was used to help answer this research question. The nurse practitioner and physician were similar in that they had the same authority and responsibilities. The study found that in an ambulatory care situation their patient outcomes were comparable (Mundinger et al., 2000).

As random assignment and the control inherent in this design minimise the effects of many threats to internal validity, it is a strong design for testing cause-and-effect relationships. However, the design is not perfect. Some threats cannot be controlled in true experimental studies. Mortality effects are often a problem in such studies, because people tend to drop out of studies that require their participation over an extended period (also called loss to follow-up). If there is a difference in the number of people who drop out of the experimental group from that of the control group, a mortality effect might explain the findings. Testing is also a problem in these studies, because the researcher is usually giving the same instrument twice and subjects tend to score better the second time just by doing the test. Researchers can get around this problem in one of two ways: they might use different forms of the same test for the two measurements; or they might use a more complex experimental design called the Solomon four-group design.

The Solomon four-group design, shown in Figure 20.1, B, has two groups that are identical to those used in the classic experimental design. In addition, two additional groups, an experimental after-group and a control after-group, are included. As the figure illustrates, all four groups have randomly assigned subjects as in all experimental studies. However, the addition of these last two groups helps to rule out testing threats to internal validity that the before and after groups may experience. Suppose a researcher is interested in the effects of some counselling on chronically ill patients' self-esteem, but just taking a measure of self-esteem may influence how the subjects report themselves. For example, the items might make the subjects think more about how they view themselves so that the next time they fill out the questionnaire, their self-esteem might appear to have improved. In reality, however, their self-esteem may be the same as it was before; it just looks different because they took the test before (called testing, which is a threat to internal validity—see Chapter 17). The use of this design with the two groups that do not receive the pretest allows for evaluating the effect of the pretest on the post-test in the first two groups. Although this design helps to evaluate the effects of testing, the threat of mortality remains a problem as with the classic experimental design.

Another frequently used experimental design is the after-only design, shown in Figure 20.1, C. This design, which is sometimes called the post-test-only control group design, is composed of two randomly assigned groups, but neither group is pretested or measured, unlike in the true experimental design. Again, the independent variable is introduced to the experimental group and not to the control group. The process of randomly assigning the subjects to groups is assumed to be sufficient to ensure a lack of bias so that the researcher can still determine whether the treatment created significant differences between the two groups. This design is particularly useful when testing effects are expected to be a major problem and the number of available subjects is too limited to use a Solomon four-group design.

Field and laboratory experiments

Experiments can also be classified by setting. Field experiments and laboratory experiments share the properties of control, randomisation and manipulation, and they use the same design characteristics, but they are conducted in different environments. Laboratory experiments take place in an artificial setting that is created specifically for the purpose of research. In the laboratory the researcher has almost total control over the features of the environment, such as temperature, humidity, noise level and subject conditions. On the other hand, field experiments are as the name implies—experiments that take place in some real, existing social setting such as a hospital unit, clinic or community where the phenomenon of interest actually occurs. Because most experiments in the nursing literature are field experiments and control is such an important element in conducting experiments, it is obvious that studies conducted in the field are subject to treatment contamination by factors specific to the setting that the researcher cannot control. However, studies conducted in the laboratory are by nature 'artificial', because the setting is created for the purpose of research. Although laboratory experiments have stronger internal validity than field work studies, they suffer more from problems with external validity. For example, a subject's behaviour in the laboratory may be quite different from the person's behaviour in the real world—a dichotomy that presents problems in generalising findings from the laboratory to the real world. When research reports are read, then, it is important to consider the setting of the experiment and what impact it might have on the findings of the study.

Consider the study of different precannulation skin preparation in patients undergoing haemodialysis (Wellard & Palaster, 1996). This study could have been done in a laboratory using animals, which would have allowed complete control over the external environment of the study, a variable that might be important in studying the potential for infection of cannulation sites. However, there is no guarantee that the results found in a study in a laboratory would be applicable to haemodialysis patients in hospital settings, so the study would lose some external validity.

Advantages and disadvantages of the experimental design

As previously discussed, experimental designs are the most appropriate for testing cause-and-effect relationships. This is because of the design's ability to control the experimental situation. Therefore it offers better evidence that, when the independent variable is manipulated in a specific way, certain outcomes can be expected. Such studies are important because one of nursing's major research priorities is documenting outcomes to provide a basis for changing or supporting current nursing practice. An Australian multi-site clinical trial (Botti et al., 1998) compared the effect of bandaging versus no bandaging on bruising, discomfort and morbidity following femoral puncture for cardiac catheterisation. The study revealed that no bandaging was associated with smaller bruise size, the occurrence of earlier post-procedure bleeding, and recovery, thus allowing earlier discharge compared with patients who had their puncture sites bandaged. The findings of this study have already changed clinical practice in the healthcare agencies in which the study took place and have the potential to be applied in many other settings. These experimental studies and others allow nurses and midwives to anticipate in a scientific manner the outcomes of their actions and provide the basis for effective high quality and evidence-based clinical practice.

However, experimental studies are not the designs most commonly used in nursing research (Cullum, 1997). Experimentation assumes that all of the relevant variables involved in a phenomenon have been identified and are measurable. For many areas of nursing research, this simply is not the case and descriptive studies need to be completed before experimental interventions can be applied.

In addition, identification of the variables important in predicting outcomes of nursing care does not mean that they are able to be manipulated in an experimental situation. For example, the ethics of a researcher who tried to randomly assign groups for the study of the effects of cigarette smoking and asked the experimental group to smoke two packs of cigarettes a day would be seriously questioned. It is also potentially true that such a study would not work, because non-smokers randomly assigned to the smoking group would be unlikely to comply with the research task. This situation is therefore managed using the notion of intention to treat, where results are analysed by the initial assigned group, even though individuals may not comply with the requirements of a particular study group. Thus, even when a researcher plans to conduct a true experiment, subjects dropping out of the study or other factors may, in effect, make the study a quasi-experiment. This was the case in a study where subjects were randomly assigned to either a training program for promoting positive parent–child interactions or a comparison group (Gross, Fogg & Tucker, 1995). Because subjects dropped out of the experimental group due to the time involved, the authors treated their study as a quasi-experimental study.

Another limitation with experimental designs is that they may be difficult or impractical to perform in nursing practice settings. It may be quite difficult to randomly assign patients on a hospital floor to different groups when they might talk to each other about the different treatments (this is called subject contamination—see Chapter 17). Experimental procedures may also be disruptive to the usual routine of the setting. If several nurses are involved in administering the experimental program, it may be impossible to ensure that the program is administered in the same way to each subject (a lack of control in implementing the study protocol). Finally, just the act of being studied may influence the results of a study. This is called the Hawthorne effect. As discussed in Chapter 17, this effect means that merely because subjects know that they are subjects in a study, they may consequently perform or answer questions differently.

Because of these problems in carrying out true experiments, researchers frequently turn to other types of research designs to evaluate cause-and-effect relationships. Such designs, because they look like experiments but lack some of the control of the true experimental design, are called quasi-experiments.

QUASI-EXPERIMENTAL DESIGNS

Quasi-experiments are research designs in which the researcher initiates an experimental treatment but some characteristic of a true experiment is lacking—either control or randomisation. However, like experiments, quasi-experiments involve manipulation in the introduction of an experimental treatment. Compared with the true experimental design, quasi-experiments are similar in their utilisation. Both types of designs are used when the researcher is interested in testing cause-and-effect relationships. However, the basic problem with the quasi-experimental approach is a weakened confidence in making causal assertions. Because of the lack of some controls in the research situation, quasi-experimental designs are subject to contamination by many, if not all, of the threats to internal validity, as discussed in Chapter 17.

Types of quasi-experimental designs

There are many different quasi-experimental designs. Only the ones most commonly used in nursing research are discussed in this chapter. Refer back to the true experimental design shown in Figure 20.1, A and compare it with the non-equivalent control group design shown in Figure 20.2, A. Note that this design looks exactly like the true experiment except that subjects are not randomly assigned to groups.

FIGURE 20.2 **Comparison of quasi-experimental designs**

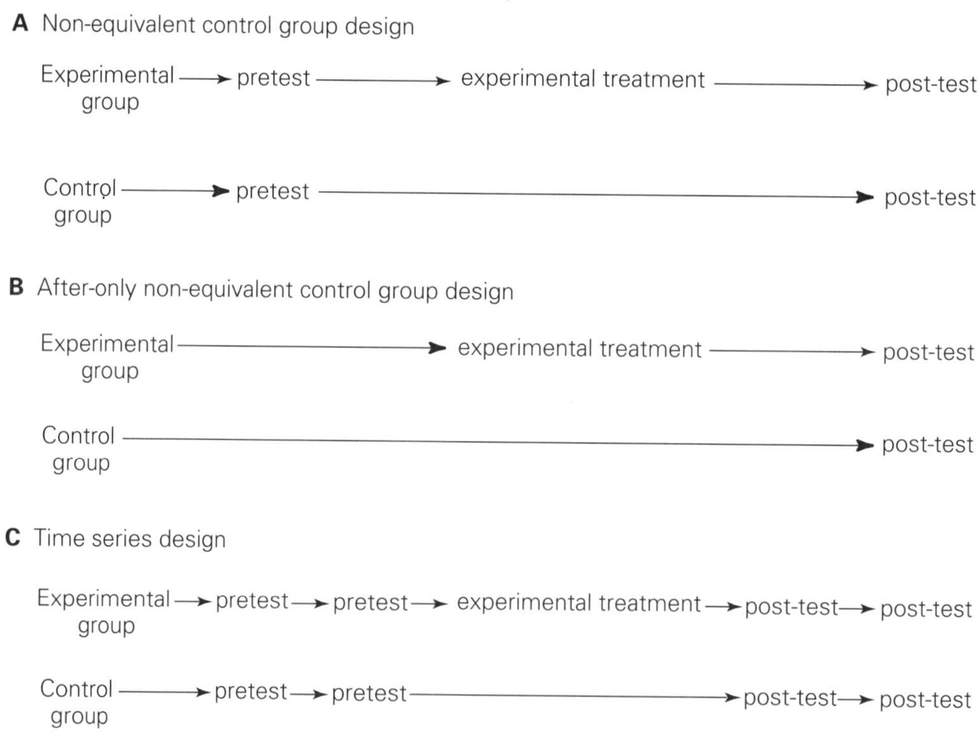

Suppose a researcher is interested in the effects of a new diabetes education program on the physical and psycho-social outcome of patients newly diagnosed with diabetes. If conditions were right, the researcher might be able to assign subjects randomly to either the group receiving the new program or the group receiving the usual program, but for any number of reasons, that design is not possible. A difficulty is where patients on the same unit have to receive both experimental and control interventions, without any overlap. The potential for subject contamination needs to be considered by the researcher, who has two choices: to abandon the experiment or to conduct a quasi-experimental study. To conduct a quasi-experiment, the researcher might find a similar unit that has not been introduced to the new program and study the newly diagnosed diabetic patients who are admitted to that unit as the comparison group. There would be no random assignment of patients by the researcher in this context, thus reflecting a quasi-experimental design.

A classic Australian study by Hodge et al. (1990) used a non-equivalent control group design to study the effectiveness of the Norton Scale assessment tool in the care of hospitalised patients. The study investigated whether incorporating the use of the tool into nursing assessment of patients would identify patients at risk of developing pressure areas and lead to earlier and more effective intervention by the nurses caring for those patients. Random assignment of patients could have resulted in data contamination because nurses caring for patients would have had to change their method of patient assessment of the patient according to whether the patient was in the experimental group (Norton Scale assessment) or the control (standard care) group. To prevent data contamination, data were collected sequentially. All of the control group data were collected over a three-month period, which was followed by staff education about the Norton Scale assessment tool. The experimental group data were collected over the next three months. This design clearly lacks randomisation of subjects to groups and is therefore quasi-experimental. Although the design is not as strong as a true experiment, it was the most practical way to collect data in the clinical area to credibly answer the research question. The two major limitations with the design were that the environment may have changed in the time that control and experimental group data were collected, and that the patient sample may not have been equivalent at the beginning of the data collection period, thereby weakening any comparison made between the groups.

Despite limitations, the non-equivalent control group design is commonly used in nursing research. Threats to internal validity (such as selection, maturation, testing and mortality) are possible with this design (see Chapter 17). However, the design is relatively robust, because the gathering of the data at the time of the pretest allows the researcher to compare the equivalence of the two groups on important antecedent variables before the independent variable is introduced. In the previous example (Hodge et al., 1990), the researchers demonstrated that the control and experimental groups were equivalent in respect to age and gender but did not compare other characteristics that might have affected the development of pressure ulcers. Any differences found between the two groups of variables could be controlled statistically in data analysis comparing the control and experimental groups.

However, suppose that the researcher did not think to measure specific characteristics of the subjects before the introduction of the new treatment, but later decided that it would be useful to have data demonstrating the effect of the program. Perhaps, for example, a third party asks for such data to determine whether the extra cost of the new teaching program is justified. Sometimes the outcomes simply cannot be measured before the intervention, as with prenatal interventions that are expected to impact on birth outcomes. The study that could be conducted would be the after-only non-equivalent control group design, shown in Figure 20.2, B. This design is similar to the after-only experimental design, but randomisation is not used to assign subjects to groups. This design makes the assumption that the two groups are equivalent and comparable before the introduction of the independent variable. Thus the soundness of the design and the confidence that we can put in the findings depend on the soundness of this assumption of pre-intervention comparability. Often it is difficult to support the assertion that the two non-randomly assigned groups are comparable at the outset of the study, because there is no way of assessing its validity.

In the example of the teaching program for patients with newly diagnosed diabetes, measuring the subjects' motivation after the teaching program would not tell us whether their motivations differed before they received the program and it is possible that the teaching program would motivate individuals to learn more about their health problem. Therefore the researcher's conclusion that the teaching program improved physical status and psycho-social outcome would be subject to the alternative conclusion that the results were an effect of pre-existing motivations (selection effect) in combination with greater learning in those so motivated (selection–maturation interaction). Nonetheless, this design is frequently used in nursing research because there are often limited opportunities for data collection and because it is particularly useful when testing effects may be problematic. Consider again the example of the experiment conducted by Small and colleagues (2000). Suppose that they had not randomly assigned the women to the debriefing intervention during postnatal care, but rather took all women before a certain time point and assigned them to the control group and then assigned all new women to the experimental group. The study would then be an example of an after-only non-equivalent control group design. Had the authors chosen to conduct the study with this design and found the same results, they would have been less confident of the findings because selection effects may have been a strong influence on the outcomes.

One approach used by researchers when only one group is available is to study that group over a longer period. This quasi-experimental design is called a time series design and it is illustrated in Figure 20.2, C. Time series designs are useful for determining trends. To rule out some alternative explanations for the findings of a one-group pretest–post-test design, researchers can measure the phenomenon of interest over a longer period and introduce the experimental treatment some time during the course of the data collection period. Even with the absence of a control group, the broader range of data collection points helps to rule out threats to validity, such as history effects. Obviously, the earlier hypothetical example of teaching patients with diabetes will not lend itself to this design, because there is not access to patients before their diagnosis.

How a time-series design would strengthen causal conclusions is provided in a study that compared primary nursing and team nursing by studying units using team nursing and after conversion to primary nursing (Gardner, 1991). Data on quality of care, impact on nursing staff and cost were collected once before the transition of the care delivery model and twice after. There were no comparison units that were not changing, so there was no control group available. It is, however, difficult to be confident that the outcomes described are the result of actual change in nursing care delivery rather than the development of the profession or changes in patient mix. If the author had more data from before the transition, showing that there was not a trend, it would strengthen the conclusion that the increased quality of care and decreased cost were caused by the change in nursing delivery systems. The use of a time series design would weaken the alternative explanation that the changes occurred because of something else that happened during the study period. However, the threat to validity (testing) is a concern with these designs because measures are repeated so many times.

Advantages and disadvantages of quasi-experimental designs

The range of potential threats to validity when interpreting the results of studies using quasi-experimental studies must be considered in balance with their benefits. Quasi-experimental designs are used because they are practical, feasible and generalisable. In addition, these designs are more adaptable to the real-world practice setting than controlled experimental designs. Finally, for some hypotheses, these designs may be the only way to evaluate the effect of the independent variable of interest.

The weakness of a quasi-experimental approach relates to the inability to make clear cause-and-effect inferences. However, if the researcher can rule out any plausible alternative explanations for the findings, such studies can lead to furthering knowledge about causal relationships. Researchers have several options for evaluating these alternative explanations. They may control them a priori by design or by statistical analysis. In some cases, clinical or practical knowledge of the problem and the patient population can suggest that a particular explanation is not plausible. Nonetheless it is important to replicate such studies to support the causal assertions developed through the use of quasi-experimental designs.

The literature on cigarette smoking is an example of how findings from many studies, both experimental and quasi-experimental, can be linked to establish a causal relationship. A large number of well controlled experiments with laboratory animals randomly assigned to smoking and non-smoking conditions have documented that lung disease will develop in smoking animals. Although such evidence is suggestive of a link between smoking and lung disease in humans, it is not directly transferable because animals and humans are different. And we cannot randomly assign humans to smoking and non-smoking groups for ethical and other reasons. So researchers interested in this problem have to use quasi-experimental designs to test their hypotheses about smoking and lung disease. Several different quasi-experimental designs have been used to study this problem and all have had similar results—that there is a causal relationship between cigarette smoking and lung disease. Note that the combination of results from both experimental and quasi-experimental studies led to the conclusion that smoking causes cancer, because the studies together meet the causal criteria of relationship, timing and lack of an alternative explanation. This process is labelled a systematic review (see Chapter 5). Nonetheless, the tobacco industry continues to argue that because the studies on humans are not true experiments, there may be another explanation (extraneous variables) for the relationships that have been established. For example, they suggest that the tendency to smoke is linked to the tendency for lung disease to develop and smoking is merely an unimportant intervening variable. The evidence from studies to determine whether the cause-and-effect relationship needs to be evaluated carefully to establish whether what is postulated is believable.

CRITICAL REVIEW OF EXPERIMENTAL AND QUASI-EXPERIMENTAL DESIGNS

As discussed earlier, various designs for research studies differ in the amount of control the researcher has over the antecedent and intervening variables that may affect the results of the study. True experimental designs offer the most possibility for control, and pre-experimental designs offer the least possibility for control. Quasi-experimental designs fall somewhere in between. Research designs must balance the needs for internal validity and external validity to produce useful results (see Chapter 15). In addition, judicious use of design requires that the chosen design be appropriate to the problem, free of bias and capable of answering the research question in an ethical fashion. Questions that should be posed when reading studies that test cause-and-effect relationships are listed in Box 20.1. All of these questions should help the reader to judge whether it can be confidently believed that a causal relationship exists.

BOX 20.1 Criteria for evaluating experimental and quasi-experimental designs

1. What design is used in the study?
2. Is the design experimental or quasi-experimental?
3. Is the problem one of a cause-and-effect relationship?
4. Is the method used appropriate to the problem?
5. Is the design suited to the setting of the study?

Experimental designs

1. What experimental design is used in the study and is it appropriate?
2. How are randomisation, control and manipulation applied?
3. Are there any reasons to believe that there are alternative explanations for the findings?
4. Are all threats to validity, including mortality, addressed in the report?
5. Regardless of whether the experiment was conducted in the laboratory or a clinical setting, are the findings generalisable to the larger population of interest?

Quasi-experimental designs

1. What quasi-experimental design is used in the study and is it appropriate?
2. What are the most common threats to the validity of the findings of this design?
3. What are the plausible alternative explanations and have they been addressed?
4. Are the author's explanations of threats to validity acceptable?
5. What does the author say about the limitations of the study?
6. Are there other limitations related to the design that are not mentioned?

For studies in which either experimental or quasi-experimental designs are used, first identify the type of design used. Often a statement describing the design of the study appears in the Abstract and in the Methods section of the paper, but this is not always the case. If a statement is not present, the reader should examine the paper for evidence of the following three characteristics: control, randomisation and manipulation. If all are present, the design is probably experimental. On the other hand, if the study involves the administration of an experimental treatment but does not involve the random assignment of subjects to groups, the design is quasi-experimental. Next, determine which specific type of design has been used. Answering these questions enables a beginning critique, as each design has its inherent threats to validity. The next question to ask is whether the researcher is answering a solution to a cause-and-effect problem. If so, the study is suited to these designs. Finally, consider the conduct of the study in the setting. Is it realistic to think that the study could be conducted in a clinical setting without some contamination?

The most important question to ask as you read experimental studies is, 'What else could have happened to explain the findings?'. It is important that the author provides adequate accounts of how the procedures for randomisation, control and manipulation have been carried out. The paper should include a sufficient description of the procedures for random assignment so that the reader may determine just how likely it would have been for any one subject to be assigned to a particular group. The description of each of the major variables (independent; dependent; intervening) should also be detailed. This information helps the reader to decide if it is possible that the treatment given to some subjects in the experimental group might have been different from what was given to others in the same group. In addition, threats to validity, such as testing and study mortality, should be addressed. Otherwise there is the potential for the findings of the study to be in error and less believable to the reader.

The question of potential alternative explanations or threats to internal validity for the findings is even more important when critically evaluating a quasi-experimental study, because quasi-experimental designs cannot control all plausible alternative explanations. A well written report of a quasi-experimental study will systematically review potential threats to the validity of the findings. The reader's work is then to decide if the author's explanations make sense.

KEY POINTS

- Two types of design commonly used in nursing research to test hypotheses about cause-and-effect relationships are experimental designs and quasi-experimental designs. Both are useful for the development of nursing knowledge because they test the effects of nursing actions and lead to the development of prescriptive theory.
- True experiments are characterised by the ability of the researcher to control extraneous variation, to manipulate the independent variable and to randomly assign subjects to research groups.
- Experiments conducted either in clinical settings or in the laboratory provide the best evidence in support of a causal relationship because the following three criteria can be met: 1) the independent and dependent variables are related to each other; 2) the independent variable chronologically precedes the dependent variable; and 3) the relationship cannot be explained by the presence of a third variable. However, the experiments may have little basis in clinical reality.
- Researchers frequently turn to quasi-experimental designs to test cause-and-effect relationships, because there are many times when experimental designs are impractical or unethical within the clinical setting.

- Quasi-experiments may lack either the randomisation or comparison group characteristics of true experiments or both of these factors. Their usefulness in studying causal relationships depends on the ability of the researcher to rule out plausible threats to the validity of the findings, such as history, selection, maturation and testing effects.
- The overall purpose of reviewing studies is to assess the validity of the findings and to determine whether these findings are worth incorporating into the nurse's personal practice and/or as the evidence base for current institutional clinical practices.

CRITICAL THINKING CHALLENGES

- Discuss the barriers to nurse researchers meeting the three criteria of a true experimental design.
- How is it possible to have a research design that includes an experimental treatment intervention and a control group, yet is not considered a true experimental study?
- Argue your case for supporting or not supporting the following claim, and include examples with your reasons: A study that does not use the 'purest' design (that is, true experimental design) does not decrease the value of the study, even though it may decrease the utility of the findings.
- You are beginning a clinical placement on a surgical step-down unit. The nurses completed a research-based practice protocol for patient-controlled analgesia (PCA), which will be implemented in the near future. What are the advantages and disadvantages of developing a research study to test the effectiveness of this protocol? Discuss whether an experimental design or a non-experimental design could be used.

Additional resources

Anastasi, A. (1988). *Psychological testing.* (6th ed.). New York, Macmillan.

Atwood, J.R. & Taylor, W. (1991). Regression discontinuity design: alternative for nursing research. *Nursing Research*, 40, 312–15.

Chalmers, I. & Altman, D.G. (1995). *Systemic reviews.* London, BMJ Publishing Group.

Cook, T.D. & Campbell, D.T. (1979). *Quasi-experimentation: design and analysis issues for field settings.* Chicago, Rand-McNally.

Creswell, J.W. (1994). *Research design: qualitative & quantitative approaches.* Thousand Oaks, Sage.

Hunt, R., Fazekas, B., Thorne, D. & Brooksbank, M. (1999). A comparison of subcutaneous morphine and fentanyl in hospice cancer patients. *Journal of Pain & Symptom Management*, 18, 111–19.

King, M.T., Hall, J., Caleo, S., Gurney, H.P. & Harnett, P.R. (2000). Home or hospital? An evaluation of the costs, preferences, and outcomes of domiciliary chemotherapy. *International Journal of Health Services*, 30, 557–79.

Walker, S.B., Cleary, S. & Higgins, M. (2001). Comparison of the FemoStop device and manual pressure in reducing groin puncture site complication following coronary angioplasty and coronary stent placement. *International Journal of Nursing Practice*, 7, 366–75.

Weinert, C. & Burman, M. (1996). Nurturing longitudinal samples. *Western Journal of Nursing Research*, 18, 360–64.

21
CHAPTER

Assessing instrument psychometrics

Doug Elliott

LEARNING OUTCOMES

After reading this chapter the student should be able to:

- Discuss how measurement error can affect the outcomes of a research study.
- Discuss the purposes of reliability, validity and responsiveness.
- Discuss the concepts of stability, equivalence and homogeneity as they relate to reliability.
- Compare and contrast the estimates of reliability.
- Define validity.
- Discuss the approaches used to examine construct validity.
- Identify the criteria for evaluating the reliability and validity of measuring instruments.
- Evaluate the reliability and validity of measuring instruments.

Key terms

consistency
content analysis
equivalence
inter-rater reliability
Kuder-Richardson (KR-20) coefficient
parallel or alternate form reliability
random error
reliability
responsiveness
split-half reliability
stability
systematic error (constant error)
test–retest reliability
validity

INTRODUCTION

This chapter examines the complex issues related to the psychometric assessment of measuring instruments. The various ways that researchers collect quantitative information from and about people participating in their studies will be discussed, along with some tools for evaluating the selection, utilisation and practicality of the various methods of collecting data. In addition, the important considerations of psychometric measurement of instruments (such as questionnaires), and their reliability, validity and responsiveness, will be addressed.

PSYCHOMETRIC PROPERTIES OF INSTRUMENTS

Measurement of nursing phenomena is a major focus for researchers using quantitative methods. Unless measurement tools validly and reliably reflect the concepts of the theory being tested and concepts being measured, conclusions drawn from the empirical studies will be invalid and will not advance the development of nursing theory and practice. Issues of reliability, validity and, to a lesser extent, responsiveness, are of central concern to both the researcher and research consumer. From either perspective, the measurement tools that are used in a research study must be evaluated in terms of the extent to which reliability and validity have been established. Many constructs are relevant to nursing knowledge and a growing number of established measurement instruments are available to researchers that have been developed within nursing or other disciplines. However, investigators may face the challenge of developing new instruments and, as part of that process, establishing the reliability and validity of those tools. The growing importance of measurement issues, tool development and related issues such as reliability and validity are reflected in many nursing journals. Researchers must evaluate the instruments selected to be certain that they are valid and reliable measures; that is, the instruments accurately operationalise the constructs being tested, as defined by the researcher.

The research consumer, when reading studies must independently assess the reliability and validity of the instruments used to determine the soundness of instrument selection in relation to the constructs under investigation. Invalid measures produce invalid estimates of the relationships between variables, thus affecting internal validity. The use of invalid measures also produces inaccurate generalisations to the populations being studied, thus affecting external validity and the ability to apply research findings in clinical practice. As such, the assessment of reliability and validity is an extremely important skill the critical reader of nursing research needs to develop.

This section examines the major types of instrument reliability and validity, and demonstrates the applicability of these concepts to the development, selection and evaluation of measurement tools in nursing research. Regardless of whether a new or already developed measurement tool is used in a research study, evidence of reliability and validity is of crucial importance to the research investigator and evaluator. Box 21.1 identifies several resources that research consumers can use to access and evaluate the reliability and validity of measurement instruments used in research studies.

BOX 21.1 Selected resources for accessing and evaluating the psychometric properties of measurement instruments

Health and Psychosocial Instruments (HaPI) Behavioral Measurement Database Services
http://www.lib.utexas.edu/subject/ss/psyc/hapi.html

Quality of life assessment in medicine
http://www.qlmed.org/LIST/index.html
- List of 800 instruments, covering specific dimensions, therapy, conditions or illnesses.
- Some information including contacts for copyright purposes.
- Some links to sites.

Online Journal of Knowledge Synthesis for Nursing
http://www.nursingsociety.org/ojksn/toc.html
- Integrative reviews and summaries of research on clinical topics.
- Full-text articles.

Virginia Henderson International Nursing Library
Sigma Theta Tau Honor Society of Nursing
http://www.stti.iupui.edu/library/
Includes the following (US-based databases):
- Registry of nurse researchers.
- HIV/AIDS knowledge base.
- Registry of research projects.
- Registry of research results.

Sigma Theta Tau International Nursing Honor Society
http://www.nursingsociety.org
http://www.stti.iupui.edu/library/

CINAHL Information Systems
http://www.cinahl.com/
- Access to searches for instruments used in nursing and 17 allied health disciplines.

MEASUREMENT ERROR

Researchers are concerned about whether scores that were obtained for a sample of subjects were consistent and true measures of the behaviours for that population of interest, and thus an accurate reflection of the real differences between individuals. The extent of variability in test scores that is attributable to error rather than a true measure of the behaviours is the error variance.

An observed test score that is derived from a set of items actually consists of the true score plus error (see Figure 21.1). The error may be either chance error or random error, or it may be what is known as systematic error. Validity is concerned with systematic error, whereas reliability is concerned with random error. Chance errors or random errors are unsystematic in nature and difficult to control, such as a respondent's anxiety level at the time of testing. Random errors are a result of a transient state in the subject, in the context of the study or in the administration of the instrument. For example, perceptions or behaviours that occur at a specific point in time, such as anxiety, are known as a transient state or transient characteristic and are often beyond the awareness and control of the observer. Another example of random error is in the measurement of infant weight (Alsop-Shields & Alexander, 1997), where random errors could occur with different nurses weighing the same infant and obtaining different measurements (inter-observer error or inter-rater error) or the same nurse obtaining different weights on repeated weighing of the same infant (intra-observer error).

FIGURE 21.1 Components of observed scores

Observed scores =	**True variance +**	**Error variance**	
Actual score obtained	Consistent, hypothetical stable or true score	Chance/random error	Systematic error
		■ Transient subject factors	■ Consistent instrument, subject or environment factors
		■ Instrumentation variations	
		■ Transient environment factors	

Systematic error or constant error is measurement error that is attributable to relatively stable characteristics of the study population that may bias their behaviour and/or cause incorrect instrument calibration. Such error has a systematic biasing influence on the subjects' responses and thereby influences the validity of the instruments. Level of education, socio-economic status, social desirability, response set or other characteristics may influence the validity of the instrument by altering measurement of the 'true' responses in a systematic way.

For example, a subject who wants to please the investigator may constantly answer items in a socially desirable way, thus making the estimate of validity inaccurate. Systematic error also occurs when an instrument is improperly calibrated. Consider a set of scales, such as those used in Alsop-Shields and Alexander's (1997) study of errors that can occur when weighing infants. If the scales were incorrectly calibrated and consistently weighed each infant at 500g less than their actual body weight, the scale would be quite reliable (that is, capable of reproducing a stable repeatable measurement), but the results would be incorrect and thus invalid.

PERFORMANCE CHARACTERISTICS OF AN INSTRUMENT

As already mentioned, the psychometric properties of an instrument include the following concepts:

- reliability
- validity
- responsiveness.

The purpose of testing dictates the type of analytical test used to establish reliability and validity, and the reader needs to be familiar with these purposes and the results obtained from the analyses (see Figure 21.2). The following subsections examine each property separately.

FIGURE 21.2 Performance characteristics of a measuring instrument

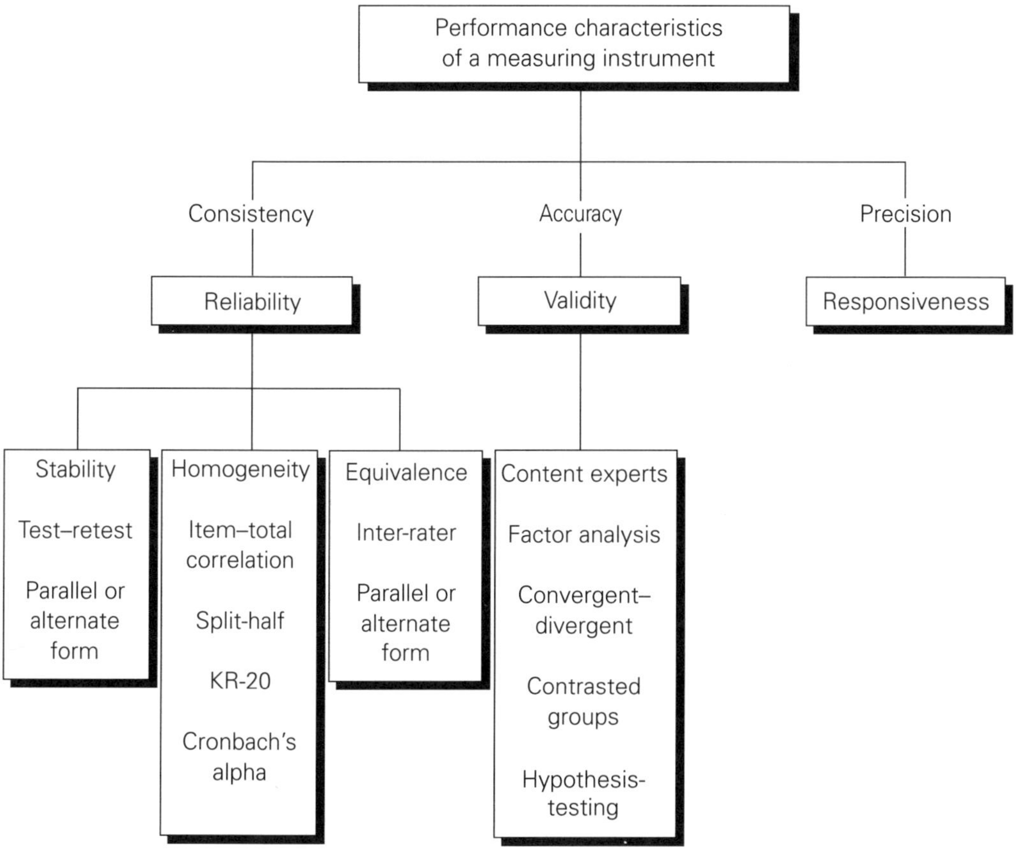

RELIABILITY

Reliable people are people whose behaviour can be relied on to be consistent and predictable. Reliability of a research instrument likewise is defined as the extent to which the instrument yields the same results on repeated measures. Reliability is then concerned with consistency, precision, stability, equivalence and homogeneity. When asking questions about the validity of an instrument, the researcher and the critical reader will also ask the question, 'How reliable is the instrument?'. A reliable instrument is one that can produce the same results if the behaviour is measured again by the same scale. In other words, if the same instrument is used on more than one occasion to measure a set of behaviours that ordinarily remain relatively constant, similar results would be expected if the tool is reliable.

The three main attributes of a reliable scale are stability, homogeneity and equivalence. The stability of an instrument is the instrument's ability to produce the same results with repeated testing. The homogeneity of an instrument means that all the items in a tool measure the same concept or characteristic. An instrument exhibits equivalence if the tool produces the same results when similar or parallel instruments or procedures are used. Each of these attributes and the means to estimate them will be discussed. But before they are discussed, an understanding of how to interpret reliability is essential.

Reliability coefficient interpretation

Because all the attributes of reliability are concerned with the degree of consistency between scores that are obtained at two or more independent times of testing, they are often expressed in terms of a correlation coefficient. The reliability coefficient ranges from 0 to 1, and expresses the relationship between the error variance, true variance and the observed score. A zero correlation indicates that there is no relationship. When the error variance in a measurement instrument is low, the reliability coefficient will be closer to 1. The closer to 1 the coefficient is, the more reliable the tool. For example, a reliability coefficient of a tool is reported to be 0.89. This tells you that the error variance is small and the tool has little measurement error. However, if the reliability coefficient of a tool is reported to be 0.49, the error variance is high and the tool has a problem with measurement error. For a tool to be considered reliable, a level of 0.70 or higher is considered to be acceptable. The interpretation of the reliability coefficient depends on the purpose of the study and the instrument. There are seven major tests of reliability that can be used to calculate a reliability coefficient. The test(s) used depend on the nature of the tool, and are listed below as they relate to the attributes of stability, equivalence and homogeneity (see Table 21.1). The reader should ensure that the method of reliability testing that the researcher uses is consistent with the investigator's aim and the type of measure used.

TABLE 21.1 Measures used to test reliability

ATTRIBUTE	TEST	PURPOSE
Stability	Test–retest reliability	Tests consistency on repeated measures of the instrument
	Parallel (alternate form)	Tests consistency of two sets of instrument items
Homogeneity	Item to total correlation	Tests individual items against total instrument
	Split-half reliability	Tests consistency of the items
	KR-20 coefficient	Used with dichotomous response levels
	Cronbach's α	Used with Likert-type response levels
Equivalence	Inter-rater reliability	Tests consistency of two or more observers

Stability

An instrument exhibits stability when the same results are obtained on repeated administration of the instrument. Researchers are concerned with the stability of an instrument so as to measure a construct consistently over a period of time. For example, one would expect personality traits or characteristics to remain relatively constant or stable over time. Stability of measurements over time is important when an instrument is used in a repeated-measures longitudinal study. For example, when measuring the health status of patients following coronary artery graft surgery over six months post-discharge, several functional domains measured by 15D were stable over time—vision, hearing, eating, speech, elimination, mental function and depression (see Figure 21.3 below).

FIGURE 21.3 Mean 15D scores for cardiac surgical patients

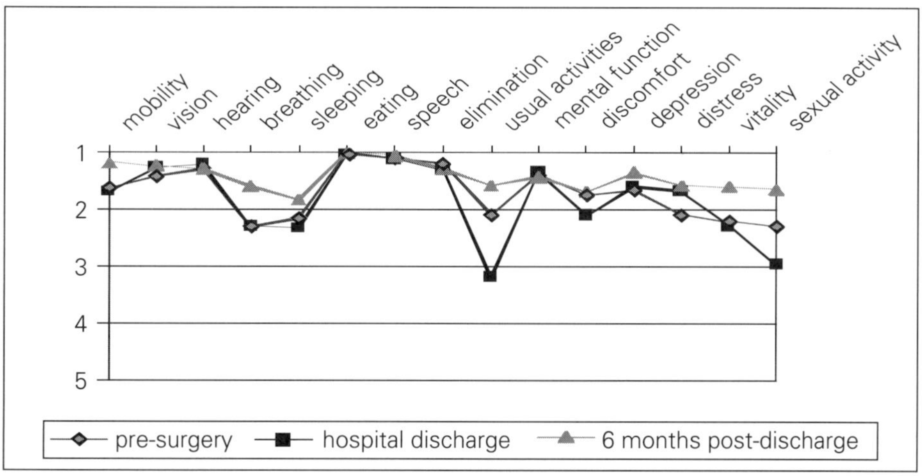

Notes:
1: full function
5: minimal function

Reported another way, there were no statistically significant differences for those concepts when measured repeatedly and examined by one-way analysis of variance (ANOVA) (see Chapter 23). Also note that the scores are close to the ceiling of the instrument (in this case, '1'), which relates to a limitation of responsiveness (precision) for concepts with small response ranges (i.e. 5-point Likert Scale); this effect can occur at either end of the scale, and is termed the floor and ceiling effect (see the 'Responsiveness' section on pages 345–46 later in this chapter for further discussion).

Stability is also a consideration when the researcher is conducting an intervention study that is designed to affect an alteration in a specific variable. In this case, the instrument is administered before, and again after, the change intervention has been completed. The tests used to estimate stability are test–retest and parallel or alternate form.

Test–retest reliability

Test–retest reliability is the administration of the same instrument to the same subjects under similar conditions on two or more occasions. Scores on the repeated testing are compared and expressed as a correlation coefficient, usually a Pearson's r (see Chapter 22). The interval between repeated administrations varies and depends on the construct being measured, but should be a sufficient timeframe to minimise any bias related to 'testing'.

Parallel or alternate form

Parallel or alternate form reliability is applicable if two comparable forms of the same instrument measuring the same construct exist. It is like test–retest reliability, in that the same individuals are tested within a specific time interval, but it differs because a different form of the same instrument is given to the subjects on the second testing. Parallel forms or tests contain the same types of items that are based on the same domain or construct, but wording of the items is different. The development of parallel forms is desired if the instrument is intended to measure a variable for which a researcher believes that 'testing' will be a problem. In practice, it is difficult to develop alternate forms of an instrument when one considers the many issues required to validate an instrument. When alternate forms of an instrument yield a high correlation, then stability is demonstrated. This approach is also used to examine the equivalence of two instruments.

Homogeneity

Internal consistency or homogeneity test whether the items within the scale reflect or measure the same construct (concept). This means that the items within the scale correlate or are complementary to each other. A uni-dimensional scale is one that measures one construct. The Life Support Preferences Questionnaire (LSPQ) (Beland & Froman, 1995), a tool that measures attitudes about life support decisions, is an example of a uni-dimensional scale. Homogeneity is assessed using one of four methods: item to total correlations; split-half reliability; Kuder-Richardson (KR-20) coefficient; or Cronbach's alpha. The purpose for each approach is listed in Table 21.1 and is discussed further below.

Item to total correlations

Item to total correlations measure the relationship between each of the items and the total scale. When item to total correlations are calculated, a correlation for each item on the scale is generated. Items that do not achieve a high correlation may be deleted from the instrument. Usually in a research study, not all the item to total correlations are reported unless the study is a report of how the researcher developed the tool (a methodological study). Typically the lowest and highest correlations are reported, or a table may present analysis of all items tested (e.g. Fisher, King & Tague, 2001).

The aim is to eliminate items that have too low a correlation (e.g. < 0.30), and to accept other items that measure the same concept without being redundant. If item to total correlations are found to be too high (e.g. > 0.70), there is redundancy, as a specific item is measuring the same dimension as the total instrument (see Table 21.2). That is, they overlap rather than complement each other. This is unlike the other measures of reliability in which a higher correlation is generally a desirable finding.

TABLE 21.2 Hypothetical example of item–total correlations

ITEM	ITEM TO TOTAL CORRELATION	COMMENT
1	0.5096	Keep item
2	0.7455	Correlation > 0.70 therefore delete redundant item
3	0.4479	Keep item
4	0.4369	Keep item
5	0.2939	Correlation < 0.30 therefore delete item
6	0.4016	Keep item

In a study that measured student nurses' readiness for self-directed learning, 10 items were deleted from the initial scale, as the item to total correlation was less than 0.30. This resulted in a final instrument with 40 items (Fisher, King & Tague, 2001).

Split-half reliability

Split-half reliability involves dividing the items of a scale into two halves and making a comparison between them. The halves may be odd numbered items and even numbered items, or a simple division of the first from the second half, or items may be randomly selected. The split-half provides a measure of consistency in terms of sampling the content. The contents of both halves are assumed to be comparable and a correlation coefficient is calculated. If the scores for the two halves are approximately equal, the instrument is considered reliable.

Kuder-Richardson coefficient

The Kuder-Richardson (KR-20) coefficient is the estimate of homogeneity used for instruments that have a dichotomous response format; that is, a format in which the question asks for a 'yes/no' or a 'true/false' response. The technique yields a correlation that is based on the consistency of responses to all the items of the instrument.

Cronbach's alpha

The most commonly used test of internal consistency for an instrument is Cronbach's alpha. Many tools used to measure psycho-social variables and attitudes have a Likert Scale response format. A Likert Scale format asks the subject to respond to a question on a scale of varying degrees of intensity between two extremes. The two extremes are anchored by responses such as 'strongly agree' to 'strongly disagree' or 'no anxiety' to 'extreme anxiety'. The points between the two extremes may range from 1 to 5 or 1 to 10. Subjects are asked to circle the response closest to how they feel. Cronbach's alpha compares each item in the scale simultaneously with all other items. An alpha level of > 0.70 demonstrates acceptable internal consistency. From the previous example of a study measuring nurses' readiness for self-directed learning, Cronbach's alpha values for the total item pool (n = 40), and sub-scales self management (n = 13), desire for learning (n = 12) and self control (n = 15), were 0.92, 0.86, 0.85 and 0.83 respectively, as reported by Fisher, King and Tague (2001, p. 520). These results demonstrated acceptable internal consistency of the instrument.

Equivalence

Equivalence is the consistency or agreement among observers using the same measurement instrument, or among alternate forms of an instrument. An instrument demonstrates equivalence when two or more observers have a high percentage of agreement of an observed behaviour. Thus, there are two methods to test equivalence: inter-rater reliability and alternate or parallel form. The procedures for assessing equivalence using parallel forms are the same as those for assessing stability (see the section on 'Parallel or alternate form' on page 338).

Inter-rater reliability

Measurement instruments that use direct observations and systematic recording of variables from more than one observer need to be tested for inter-rater reliability. To accomplish inter-rater reliability, two or more individuals should make an observation or one observer should observe the behaviour on several occasions. The observers should be trained to observe and record the behaviour in a standard, consistent manner. In the method of direct observation of behaviour, the consistency or reliability of the observations between observers is extremely important. When establishing inter-rater reliability, it is the reliability or consistency of the observers rather than the reliability of the instrument that is tested. Inter-rater reliability is expressed as a percentage of agreement between scorers or as a correlation coefficient between the scores assigned to the observed behaviours.

Botti et al. (1998) used two different methods to measure puncture site bruise size in patients following coronary angiography. This was done because previous studies indicated that inter-rater reliability for measurement of bruises using a tape measure was high when haematomas were less than 50 cm^2 but low for larger bruises. As a consequence, a more reliable method that traced the bruise outline onto a transparent film was used to measure large haematomas.

VALIDITY

Validity is the most fundamental consideration in instrument development, and refers to the degree to which current evidence and theory support the performance of instruments (American Educational Research Association, American Psychological Association & National Council on Measurement in Education, 1999). Thus, measurement (instrument) validity is the extent to which an instrument measures what it was designed to measure; a valid instrument truly reflects the concept of interest. Validity is the appropriate, meaningful and useful interpretation of test scores in relation to the purpose of a study (Goodwin, 1997). Measurement validity should not be confused with study validity, which relates to the rigour of the study approach (internal validity) and the generalisability of the study findings to the wider population of interest (external validity) (see Chapter 17). Measurement validity is not dichotomous, but more of a continuum, where there is continuing and stronger evidence developed for the validity of an instrument as more studies examine the instrument.

A valid measure correctly measures the construct of interest. However, a measure can be reliable but not valid. A valid instrument that is supposed to measure anxiety does so; it does not measure some other construct, such as stress. Consider that a researcher wanted to measure anxiety in patients by measuring their body temperatures. The researcher could obtain highly accurate, consistent and precise temperature recordings, but such a measure could not be a valid indicator of anxiety. Thus the high reliability of an instrument (in this case, a thermometer) is not necessarily congruent with evidence of validity. However, for an instrument to be considered valid, it must demonstrate reliability. An instrument cannot validly measure the attribute of interest if it is erratic, inconsistent and imprecise; that is, if it demonstrates poor reliability.

Measurement validity has previously been viewed as having the major subtypes: content validity; criterion-related validity; and construct validity. Recent articles, various texts and other resources still use these terms as well as others to describe the concept of validity. In examples related to internet sources, the database PsycINFO replaced the terms 'concurrent', 'construct', 'factorial' and 'predictive validity' with the encompassing term 'statistical validity' in 2000. In the CINAHL database, specific definitions still exist for content validity, criterion-related validity and construct validity (http://gateway1.ovid.com/ovidweb).

However, this artificial distinction was confusing, as the types were interrelated with an overlap of approaches evident during evaluation. The current view of measurement validity focuses on the central unitary concept of construct validity, with varying levels of evidence to support the validity of a specific instrument (American Educational Research Association, American Psychological Association & National Council on Measurement in Education, 1999). Thus, 'construct' validity is the central theme or overarching concept under which the differing approaches reside (Goodwin, 1997).

A research consumer will want to evaluate whether sufficient evidence of validity is present and whether the type of validity is appropriate to the design of the study and instruments used in the study. Instrument (measurement) validity is examined according to:

- content—experts
- structure—factor analysis
- links to other variables—discriminant (convergent-divergent); criterion-related (concurrent/predictive)
- differences between groups—contrasted/known groups
- hypothesis testing.

(American Educational Research Association, American Psychological Association & National Council on Measurement in Education, 1999; Goodwin, 1997).

The establishment of construct validity is a complex process, often involving several studies and several approaches over time. For example, during development of a new instrument to examine responses in acute coronary syndrome patients, researchers examined the validity of items individually and collectively over a number of phases using exploratory interviews, expert review, factor analysis and a concurrent instrument. This multi-method testing resulted in a final 35-item instrument that measured the health domains of physical activity, insecurity, emotional reaction, dependency, diet, medication concerns and side effects (Thompson & Roebuck, 2001). The following sub-sections discuss the testing of content and associations for establishing the validity of an instrument.

Establishing evidence about the content of a measure

Content validity refers to the ability of a sample of items (within the instrument) to represent the universe of content or the domain of a given construct. The universe of content provides the framework and basis for formulating the items that will adequately represent the content. When an investigator is developing a tool and issues of content validity arise, the concern is whether the measurement tool and the items it contains are representative of the content domain the researcher intends to measure. The researcher begins by defining the concept and identifying the dimensions that are the components of the concept.

The content experts approach includes the old term 'face validity', which is a rudimentary type of validity that verified that the instrument appears to measure the concept. It is an intuitive approach to validation in which expert professionals or subjects are asked to evaluate the content of the instrument in terms of whether it appears to reflect the concept the researcher intends to measure. This procedure is useful in the tool development process in relation to determining readability and clarity of content. However, it should be considered as a beginning component and not an alternative to other forms of evidence. Dunning and Martin (1996), when developing a questionnaire to measure subjects' assessment of the seriousness of diabetes in general and of their own diabetes, began the process of establishing the validity of their instrument by convening a panel of six experts in diabetes management, questionnaire development, psychology, statistics and epidemiology. The panel reviewed the 16-item draft questionnaire to establish whether it had face validity, before the questionnaire was pilot tested.

Establishing evidence of relationships between the measure and other variables

These approaches to validation examine the instrument for properties of similarity and/or differences between other criteria measures (hence the previous term 'criterion-related validity'). A researcher may wish to examine the concurrent or predictive properties of an instrument. The concurrent approach examines the degree of correlation of two measures of the same concept administered at the same time. A high correlation coefficient indicates agreement between the two measures. This process is undertaken to assess the ability of a new instrument compared to an established instrument—the 'gold standard'. The gold standard label is attributed to an instrument or test that is the best available measurement of a concept, attitude, behaviour or physical state. Sometimes the established gold standard may be a long or complicated measurement process, and a researcher may decide to construct a shorter instrument with less respondent burden (i.e. the amount of effort and time required from the subjects).

One randomised controlled trial assessed the concurrent validity of three different psychometric measures for the concept of anxiety, in a sample of 56 patients admitted to a coronary care unit with ischaemic chest pain (Elliott, 1993). The State-Trait Anxiety Inventory (STAI) (Spielberger, 1973) has 20 items (questions); the Hospital Anxiety and Depression (HAD) Scale (Zigmond & Snaith, 1983) has seven items related to anxiety; and the Linear Analogue Anxiety Scale (LAAS) is a 10 cm line with anchor descriptors of 'no anxiety' and 'extreme anxiety'. The respondent burden was different for each instrument. The STAI had previously established validity and reliability, and therefore acted as the gold standard criterion. Correlation of instruments was assessed using Pearson's r test. The product moment correlation coefficient (Pearson's r) assesses the strength of a straight line association between two variables; in this case, paired correlations of the three instruments—STAI, HAD, LAAS (see Table 21.3). Correlation coefficients greater than 0.50 indicate a strong inter-instrument relationship, while coefficients of 0.30–0.50 and 0.10–0.30 indicate moderate and weak relationships respectively (see Chapter 23 for further discussion).

TABLE 21.3 Correlation coefficients for three instruments measuring anxiety

	HAD		LAAS	
	Pre-test	Post-test	Pre-test	Post-test
STAI	0.64	0.48	0.70	0.67
HAD	–	–	0.48	0.28
LAAS	–	–	–	–

Modified from Elliott, D. (1993). Comparison of three instruments for measuring patient anxiety in a coronary care unit. *Intensive Critical Care Nursing*, 9, 195–200; used by permission of the publisher Churchill Livingstone.

As noted in Table 21.3, the study demonstrated high correlation between the 20-item STAI and the one-item LAAS, and correlation to a lesser extent between the STAI and the HAD Scale. The HAD and LAAS demonstrated a moderate to low relationship. Thus, the simple LAAS appeared to be as effective as longer instruments when measuring anxiety in acute coronary syndrome patients in coronary care units.

Predictive validity refers to the degree of correlation between the measure of the concept and some future measure of the same concept. Because of the passage of time, the correlation coefficients are likely to be lower for predictive validity studies. Macnee and Talsma (1995) assessed predictive validity of the Barriers to Cessation Scale (BCS), a tool to measure barriers to smoking cessation. The relevant criterion to be predicted by the BCS was successful smoking cessation or relapse. Statistically significant scores for subjects who subsequently ceased smoking compared to those who relapsed into smoking provided support for the predictive validity of the BCS. Statistical analysis indicated that individuals who were quitters at eight weeks had significantly lower initial BCS scores compared to individuals who continued as smokers. Therefore, the instrument demonstrated validity in predicting which individuals would cease smoking.

Hypothesis testing approach

When hypothesis testing validity is undertaken, the investigator uses the theory or concept underlying the measurement instrument's design to develop hypotheses regarding the behaviour of individuals with varying scores on the measure. Empirical testing supports or fails to support the relationships that would be predicted among concepts and provides support for the construct validity of the instruments measuring those concepts. Data collected test the hypotheses and enable inferences about whether the rationale underlying the instrument's construction is adequate to explain the findings.

Hypothesis testing was used to examine the validity of the 25-item Family Caregiving Factors Inventory for home health assessment in a Taiwanese population (Shyu, 2000). Specifically, instrument domains (resources, expectations, task difficulty and knowledge) were examined in relation to the balance of caregivers' competing needs, and the quality of the relationship between caregiver and care receiver. The findings indicated a significant positive relationship between the domains and competing needs and the caregiving relationship. Therefore, the instrument appropriately measured the variables of interest within the hypothesised conceptual framework.

Convergent and divergent approaches

Convergent validity refers to a search for other measures of a construct when no gold standard exists. Sometimes two or more tools that theoretically measure the same construct are identified and both are administered to the same subjects. A correlational analysis is performed to assess whether each subject's scores for both instruments change in the same way, that is, when one increases so does the other. If the measures are positively correlated, convergent validity is supported. This was the case in the comparison of instruments measuring anxiety, where the STAI had a high correlation with the LAAS (0.67–0.70) and HAD (0.48–0.64) (Elliott, 1993).

Divergent validity uses measurement approaches that differentiate one construct from others that may be equivalent. Sometimes researchers search for instruments that measure the opposite of the construct. If the divergent measure is negatively related to other measures, validity for the measure is strengthened. Data from a factor analysis can also be used to determine divergent validity (also called discriminant validity).

A specific method of assessing convergent and divergent validity is the multi-trait–multi-method approach. Similar to the approaches previously described, this method involves examining the relationship between indicators that should measure the same construct, and between those that should measure different constructs (Campbell & Fiske, 1959). Anxiety, for example, can be measured by a variety of strategies, such as:

- the State-Trait Anxiety Inventory (STAI)
- heart rate and blood pressure readings
- asking the subject about anxious feelings
- observing the subject's behaviour.

The results of one of these measures could then be correlated with results of each of the others in a multi-trait–multi-method matrix (Daly & Carnwell, 2001; Waltz, Strickland & Lenz, 1991). The use of multiple measures such as self-report, observation, interview and collection of physiological data, will also decrease the effect of systematic error (see the section on 'Measurement error' on pages 333–34).

Contrasted-groups approach

When the contrasted-groups (or known-groups) approach to the development of construct validity is used, the researcher identifies two groups of individuals who are expected to score extremely high or low in the characteristic being measured by the instrument. The instrument is administered to both the high-scoring and low-scoring group and the differences in scores obtained are examined. If the instrument is sensitive to individual differences in the trait being measured, the mean performance of these two groups should differ significantly and evidence of construct validity would be supported. A *t* test or analysis of variance (ANOVA) is used to statistically test the difference between the two groups (see Chapter 23).

Factor analytical approach

This approach provides the researcher with information about the extent to which a set of items measures the same underlying construct or dimension of a construct. Factor analysis assesses the degree to which the individual items on a scale truly cluster together around one or more dimensions. Items designed to measure the same dimension should load on the same factor; those designed to measure different dimensions should load on different factors. This analysis will indicate also whether the items in the instrument reflect a single construct or several constructs.

A factor analysis carried out by Jackson et al. (1996) established the construct validity of the 'Attitudes Towards Learning in Pregnancy' Scale, an instrument developed to measure midwives' attitudes. A confirmatory factor analysis of the scale was conducted to assess the factor structure of the tool and, hence, the construct validity. Three factors—cognition, motivation and professional issues—were identified. Findings from the factor analysis indicated that the final 30 items clustered around the three identified factors or dimensions. Six items that did not load onto the three identified factors were deleted from the scale. The researchers therefore concluded that the scale measured the constructs of cognition, motivation and professional issues.

RESPONSIVENESS

Responsiveness is the ability of an instrument to detect small but clinically important changes in a patient's status (Guyatt et al., 1987; Harris & Warren, 1995). Responsive instruments demonstrate: (1) maximum change when clinically important changes in status occur; and (2) minimal change on repeated applications to stable patients. Therefore, responsiveness is the magnitude of the change in a subject's score on a measuring instrument that corresponds to a minimal clinically important difference (Guyatt et al., 1987). Responsiveness is measured by comparing instrument scores before and after a treatment of known efficacy. Effect size (change in scores due to treatment effect) can also be used to examine responsiveness, as it relates to changes in mean score to the standard deviation of baseline scores (Kazis et al., 1989) or score changes among stable patients (Guyatt et al., 1987). See Chapter 23 for further discussion of effect size.

The precision of an instrument is limited by the 'floor and ceiling effects' (i.e. the range of responses possible)—the extremes of the scale limit the responses that truly reflect the subject's status for that domain (Guyatt et al., 1993). As noted earlier, Figure 21.3 illustrates a probable ceiling effect for the health status instrument 15D. This instrument used only one item (question) per concept, and as a consequence the subjects' scores clustered primarily between 1 and 2 for most concepts. This was despite a data collection period of over six months that included measurements before and after cardiac surgery. Clearly, this instrument demonstrated a lack of precision in measuring any improvements in health status over time.

Knowledge of previous responsiveness characteristics of instruments would aid in instrument selection and allow for more accurate sample size and statistical power estimations (Deyo et al., 1991). However, assessment of responsiveness has been minimal when compared to the evaluation of reliability and validity. It is therefore often difficult to select an instrument based on its comparative responsiveness against other measures. As explained by Deyo and Carter (1992), responsiveness can be improved by:

1. increasing the number of response categories
2. disaggregation of scores within a multidimensional instrument
3. the inclusion of transition questions, and
4. the use of individualised questions.

CRITICAL ANALYSIS OF PSYCHOMETRIC PROPERTIES

Reliability and validity are the crucial aspects in the critical appraisal of a measurement instrument. Criteria for the critical evaluation of psychometric properties are presented in Box 21.2. An effective critique includes establishing the instrument's level of reliability and validity and comparing the setting to the context under investigation. In a research report the reliability and validity for each measure should be presented. If these data have not been presented, the reviewer must seriously question the merit and use of the tool and the study's results.

BOX 21.2 Criteria for evaluating psychometric properties of instruments

1. Was an appropriate method used to test the reliability of the instrument?
2. Is the reliability of the instrument adequate?
3. Was an appropriate method(s) used to test the validity of the instrument?
4. Is the validity of the instrument adequate?
5. If the sample from the developmental stage of the tool was different from the current sample, were the reliability and validity recalculated to determine if the tool is still adequate?
6. Are strengths and weaknesses of instrument reliability and validity appropriately addressed in the Discussion, Limitations or Recommendations sections of the paper?
7. Is the precision or responsiveness of the instrument discussed in relation to clinically important differences?

It is the ethical responsibility of the critical reader to question the reliability and validity of instruments used in research studies and to examine the findings in light of the quality of the instruments used and the data presented. The following discussion highlights key areas related to reliability and validity that should be evident to the reader of a research article.

Appropriate reliability tests should have been performed by the developer of the measurement tool and included by the current user in the research report. If the initial standardisation sample and the current sample have different characteristics, the reader would expect that: (1) a pilot study for the present sample would have been conducted to determine if the reliability was maintained; or (2) a reliability estimate was calculated on the current sample (e.g. Elliott, 1997; Kyngas, Skaar-Chandler & Duffy, 2000; Shyu, 2000).

The researcher determines the type of reliability procedures used in the study, depending on the nature of the instrument and how it will be used. For example, if the instrument is to be administered twice, the reader might consider that test–retest reliability should be used to establish the stability of the tool. Although unlikely in practice, if an alternate form has been developed for use in a repeated-measures design, evidence of alternate form reliability should be presented to determine the equivalence. If the degree of internal consistency among the items is relevant, an appropriate test of internal consistency should be presented. In some instances more than one type of reliability will be used and the research consumer should determine whether all are appropriate. For example, the Kuder-Richardson formula implies that there is a single right or wrong answer, making it inappropriate to use with scales that provide a format of three or more possible responses. In such cases another method, such as Cronbach's coefficient alpha, is more appropriate. Another important consideration is the acceptable level of reliability, which varies according to the type of test. Coefficients of reliability of 0.70 or higher are generally desirable. The validity of an instrument is limited by its reliability, that is, less confidence can be placed in scores from tests with low reliability coefficients.

Satisfactory evidence of validity is probably the most difficult aspect for the reviewer to ascertain, but it is this that is most likely to fall short of meeting the required criteria. Validity studies are time-consuming, as well as complex, and researchers may settle for presenting minimal validity data. Therefore the reader should closely examine the item content of a tool when evaluating its strengths and weaknesses and try to find evidence of its validity. However, articles may not include the instrument, or provide only a few sample items available for review. In this case, the reviewer may need to review other articles that examine the instrument.

The reader would also expect to see the strengths and weaknesses of instrument reliability, validity and possibly responsiveness, presented in the Discussion, Limitations and/or Recommendations sections of a research article. In this context the reliability and validity might be discussed in relation to other tools devised to measure the same variable. The relationship of the findings to strengths and weaknesses in instrument reliability and validity would be another important discussion point. Finally, recommendations for improving future studies in relation to instrument reliability, validity and responsiveness should be proposed in the article.

The areas of reliability, validity and responsiveness are complex, and perhaps difficult for the beginning research consumer to undertake with confidence. The guidelines presented in this chapter enable the systematic assessment of the psychometric aspects of the study. Discussing these issues with colleagues is also a useful approach to assist research consumers in critically appraising the merits and shortcomings of existing, as well as newly developed, instruments that are reported in the nursing literature. Such exchanges promote the understanding of the basic concepts of psychometrics as well as the exploration of alternative methods of observation and the use of reliable and valid tools in clinical practice.

KEY POINTS

- Reliability and validity are crucial aspects of conducting and evaluating research.
- Validity refers to whether an instrument measures what it is purported to measure and it is a crucial aspect of evaluating a tool.
- The choice of a validation method is important and is made by the researcher on the basis of the characteristics of the measurement tool in question and its utilisation.

- Reliability examines the stability, homogeneity and equivalence of a measuring instrument, using tests such as test–retest, parallel or alternate form, split-half, item to total correlation, Kuder-Richardson, Cronbach's alpha and inter-rater reliability.
- The selection of a method for establishing reliability will depend on the purpose of the study, the characteristics of the instrument, and the testing method used for collecting data from the representative sample.

CRITICAL THINKING CHALLENGES

- Discuss the various approaches to establishing validity that would enable a reviewer to have a high level of confidence in a tool.
- What are the major tests of reliability? Is it necessary to establish more than one measure of reliability for each instrument used in a study? Which test do you think is the most important measure of reliability? Include examples in your answer.
- Is it possible to have a valid instrument that is not reliable? Is the reverse possible? Support your answer with references to instruments you might use in the clinical setting with your patients/clients.
- The researchers in an article you are reading state that the validity and reliability of the instruments used in their study were established at an acceptable level. Their study was published in a refereed journal. You are unfamiliar with these instruments. You believe that to critically review this section of the report it is necessary to find out how the validity and reliability of these instruments were determined and the criteria used to determine acceptability. How would you proceed? Include in your discussion how you could use technology to help you; support your position with examples.

Additional resources

Brown, S.J. (1999). *Knowledge for health care practice: a guide to using research evidence.* Philadelphia, Saunders.

DeKeyser, F.G. & Puch, L.C. (1990). Assessment of the reliability and validity of biochemical measures. *Nursing Research*, 39, 314–17.

Hutchinson, S. & Wilson, H.S. (1992). Validity threats in scheduled semistructured research interviews. *Nursing Research*, 41, 117–19.

Jennings, B.M. & Rogers, S. (1989). Managing measurement error. *Nursing Research*, 38, 186–87.

Jones, E.J. & Kay, M. (1992). Instrumentation in cross-cultural research. *Nursing Research*, 41, 186–88.

Knapp, T.R. & Brown, J.K. (1995). Ten measurement commandments that often should be broken. *Research in Nursing and Health*, 18, 465–69.

Laschinger, H.K.S. (1992) Intraclass correlations as estimates of interrater reliability in nursing research. *Western Journal of Nursing Research*, 14, 246–51.

Munro, B.H. (2001). *Statistical methods for health care research.* (4th ed.). Philadelphia, Lippincott.

Nunnally, J.C. (1978). *Psychometric theory.* New York, McGraw-Hill.

22
CHAPTER

Descriptive data analysis

Zevia Schneider

LEARNING OUTCOMES

After reading this chapter the student should be able to:

- Define descriptive statistics.
- State the purposes of descriptive statistics.
- Identify the levels of measurement in a research study.
- Identify the statistical procedures appropriate for each level of measurement.
- Describe a frequency distribution, a histogram and a polygon.
- Critically analyse the descriptive statistics used in published research studies.
- Determine if both statistically supported and statistically non-supported findings are discussed.
- Determine whether the results are objectively reported and include generalisations and limitations.

Key terms

central tendency

correlation

descriptive statistics

generalisability

kurtosis

levels of measurement

normal curve

standard deviation

variance

z score

INTRODUCTION

Statistical procedures are used to give organisation and meaning to numerical data. Procedures that allow researchers to describe, organise and summarise raw data are known as descriptive statistics. Statistical methods that allow researchers to estimate how reliably they can make predictions and generalise their findings based on the data are known as inferential statistics. This chapter and the next are designed to provide an understanding of statistical procedures commonly used in nursing research. This chapter focuses on the understanding and evaluation of descriptive statistical procedures and the next chapter discusses inferential statistical procedures (see Chapter 23).

There are many ways to describe data, from simple to sophisticated: the purpose of descriptive statistics is to order and summarise the data. As mentioned in Chapter 8, the design, data collection and data analysis strategies used depend on the research question. In the main, there are two important reasons for using descriptive statistics. The first refers to the graphical and numerical techniques for organising and interpreting the data—that is, the organisation of the data into various figures (e.g. pie charts, histograms, scatter diagrams, tables, line graphs). Such graphical and numerical techniques enable trends and differences to be noted, and the calculation of simple statistics, such as frequency count, percentages and proportions of scores. The second use for descriptive statistics is to condense or reduce large quantities of numerical information into meaningful units. Data can be condensed and summarised using statistics like measures of central tendency (mode, median and mean), and measures of variability (range, semi-interquartile and standard deviation), and some correlational techniques, such as scatter plots). The research consumer does not need detailed knowledge of how to calculate these statistics but does need an understanding of their meaning, use, presentation and limitations. However, when developing a research proposal for the conduct of a project, investigators clearly need to understand the use of a particular set of techniques for data analysis. To evaluate the appropriateness of the statistical procedures used in a study, the research consumer should first develop an understanding of the levels of measurement that are appropriate for each statistical technique.

LEVELS OF MEASUREMENT

Measurement is the assignment of numbers to objects or events according to certain rules (Pedhazur & Schmelkin, 1991). Every event that is assigned a specific number must be similar to every other event assigned that number. The measurement level is determined by the nature of the object or event being measured. Levels of measurement in ascending order are nominal, ordinal, interval and ratio (with the acronym NOIR). The higher the level of measurement, the greater the flexibility the researcher has in choosing statistical procedures. Every attempt should be made to use the highest level of measurement possible so that the maximum amount of information will be obtained from the data, as highlighted in Table 22.1.

TABLE 22.1 Levels of measurement

MEASUREMENT	DESCRIPTION	MEASURES OF CENTRAL TENDENCY	MEASURES OF VARIABILITY
Nominal	Classification	Mode	Modal percentage, range, frequency distribution
Ordinal	Relative rankings	Mode, median	Range, percentile, semi-quartile range, frequency distribution
Interval	Rank ordering with equal intervals	Mode, median, mean	Range, percentile, semi-quartile range, standard deviation
Ratio	Rank ordering with equal intervals and absolute zero	Mode, median, mean	All

Figure 22.1 highlights the types of descriptive statistics possible for each level of measurement.

FIGURE 22.1 Descriptive statistics decision path

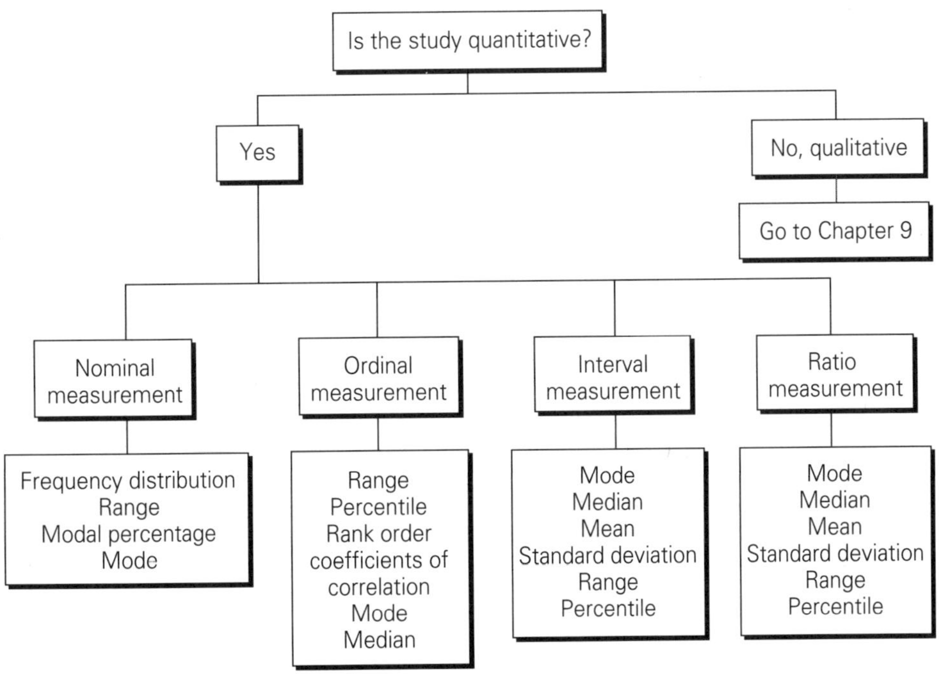

Nominal measurement

Nominal measurement is used to classify objects or events into discrete categories; but data are neither measured nor ordered. For example, male subjects may be assigned the number 1 and female subjects the number 2. The assignment of these numbers indicates that the categories of male and female are different and exclusive; and the object or event either has the characteristic or does not have it. The numbers assigned to each category are nothing more than labels (names), and therefore cannot be arithmetically manipulated; they do not give the reader any more information about the nature of the difference, they simply give a name to a category. Nominal level measurement can be used to categorise a sample on such information as gender, hair colour, marital state, country of birth, occupation and religious affiliation. Dracup et al.'s study (1997) of Australian patients' delay in response to heart attack symptoms provides an example of nominal level measurement to describe the mode of transport to hospital:

Private car/other	n = 123 (39%)
Ambulance	n = 194 (61%)

Gerdtz and Bucknell (2000) used nominal data to describe the demographic characteristics of their sample: location, type of emergency service, hospital type, appointment level, education level, educational requirements specific to triage, and experience. The nominal level of measurement allows the least amount of mathematical manipulation—frequencies and proportions. The main statistical procedure for nominal data is chi-square (χ^2).

Ordinal measurement

Ordinal numbers convey additional information to nominal measurement. Ordinal measurement is used to show the relative ranking of objects or events. The numbers assigned to each category can be compared and a member of a higher category can be said to have more of an attribute than one in a lower category. The intervals (space) between numbers on the scale are not necessarily equal, nor is there an absolute zero. For example, student nurses may be invited to place their clinical placement in order of preference on a Likert-type scale numbering 1 to 5, where number 1 is assigned to the most enjoyed placement and number 5 to the least enjoyed placement. Similarly, ordinal measurement is used to formulate class rankings where one student can be ranked higher or lower than another. However, the difference in actual score between students may differ widely.

Hofmeyer and Cecchin (2001) used a 5-point Likert Scale to determine the issues affecting students' ability to achieve their study goals. An example of one question was 'Have you had doubts about your academic ability?'. The range of possible scores used in this study was from 1 to 5, where 1 referred to 'not at all' and 5 referred to 'serious problem'. The limitation of ordinal measurement is that the intervals between the ranked categories cannot be treated as equal.

In a study investigating a paucity of published nursing research, Hicks (1995) developed an 'attitude to research' scale using Likert-type items. The ordinal scale for each attitude statement was: strongly agree; agree somewhat; don't know; disagree somewhat; and strongly disagree. Ordinal scales add 'greater than' or 'less than' to the measurement process. Mathematical manipulation of data is limited. However, in addition to what is possible with nominal data, medians, percentiles and rank order coefficients of correlation can also be calculated.

Interval measurement

In an interval scale, the differences between scores or measures can be treated as equal, as there is a specific numerical distance between each of the levels. However, the zero point remains arbitrary. For example, interval measurements are used in measuring temperatures on the Celsius scale. The distances between degrees are equal, but the zero point is arbitrary, reflecting the freezing point of water, which is not the same as having no heat. The Intelligence Quotient (IQ) is another variable that is treated as an interval scale.

In many areas of psychometric testing, including nursing and the social sciences, there is much controversy over the classification of the level of measurement of intelligence, aptitude and personality tests, with some regarding these measurements as ordinal and others seeing them as interval. The research consumer needs to be aware of this controversy and to look at each study individually in terms of how the data are analysed (Knapp, 1990; Knapp, 1993). Interval level data allow some manipulation like addition and subtraction, but they do not necessarily allow multiplication and division. Examples of interval variables are test scores, age, population size of a town or country, and the number of years of education one has completed. In these examples two values can be identified by comparison: Are they different and exclusive? (nominal); Is one value greater than another? (ordinal); Is there an equal numerical distance between intervals of the scale? (interval).

Ratio measurement

Ratio measurement shows ranking of events or objects on scales with equal intervals and absolute zeros; the zero point makes the ratio of scale values meaningful. This is the highest level of measurement, but it is usually achieved only in the physical sciences and in describing characteristics of samples. Physical scales measuring height, weight, distance, pulse and blood pressure can usually be treated as ratio scales. Because there is a zero point in ratio scales, one can state that 'a baby weighing 4 kilograms is twice as heavy as one weighing 2 kilograms'. Examples of ratio measurement used to describe characteristics of the women in Waldenström and Nilsson's study (1994) include: age, measured in years; and total length of gestation, measured in weeks. All mathematical procedures can be performed on data from ratio scales. Therefore the use of any statistical procedure is possible as long as it is appropriate to the design of the study.

Frequency distribution

One of the most basic ways of organising data is in a frequency distribution. In a frequency distribution the number of times each event occurs is counted or the data are grouped and the frequency of each group is reported. Although not always reported, it is usually the first step researchers undertake when exploring and categorising their data. A lecturer reporting the results of an examination could report the number of students receiving each grade or could group the grades and report the number in each group. Table 22.2 illustrates the results of an examination given to a class of 51 students. The results of the examination are reported in several ways. The columns on the left give the raw data tally and the frequency for each grade, whereas the columns on the right give the grouped data tally and grouped frequencies.

TABLE 22.2 Frequency distribution

INDIVIDUAL			GROUP		
SCORE	TALLY	FREQUENCY	SCORE	TALLY	FREQUENCY
90	|	1	>89	|	1
88	|	1			
86	|	1	80–89	卌 卌 卌	15
84	卌 |	6			
82	||	2	70–79	卌 卌 卌	23
80	卌	5		卌 |||	
78	卌	5			
76	|	1	60–69	卌 卌	10
74	卌 ||	7			
72	卌 ||||	9	<59	||	2
70	|	1			
68	|||	3			
66	||	2			
64	||||	4			
62	|	1			
60		0			
58	|	1			
56		0			
54	|	1			
52		0			
50		0			
Total		51			51

Mean, 73.1; standard deviation, +12.1; median, 74; mode, 72; range, 36 (54–90).

In a study on violence in New South Wales emergency departments (Lyneham, 2000), frequency distribution was used to illustrate the types and frequency of violence directed at emergency nurses in the department, types of security devices per region, and number of responses per department location. Waldenström and Nilsson (1994) present data showing the number of women in the experimental and control groups breastfeeding for up to 12 months after the birth of their baby. The number of women breastfeeding is shown grouped by intervals of one month for the two groups being compared. When data are grouped, it is necessary to define the size of the group or the interval width so that no score will appear twice in the same group. The grouping of the data in Table 22.2 prevents overlap; each score falls into only one group: that is, scores above 89; 80–89; 70–79; 60–69; and below 59. The interval widths should not be too large; very large interval widths lead to loss of data information and may obscure patterns in the data.

Figure 22.2 demonstrates an example of an histogram and a frequency polygon. The two examples are similar in that both plot scores against frequency. The greater the number of points plotted, the smoother the resulting graph. The shape of the resulting graph allows for observations that will further describe the data, particularly in terms of normal distribution.

FIGURE 22.2 Frequency distributions—A, histogram; B, frequency polygon

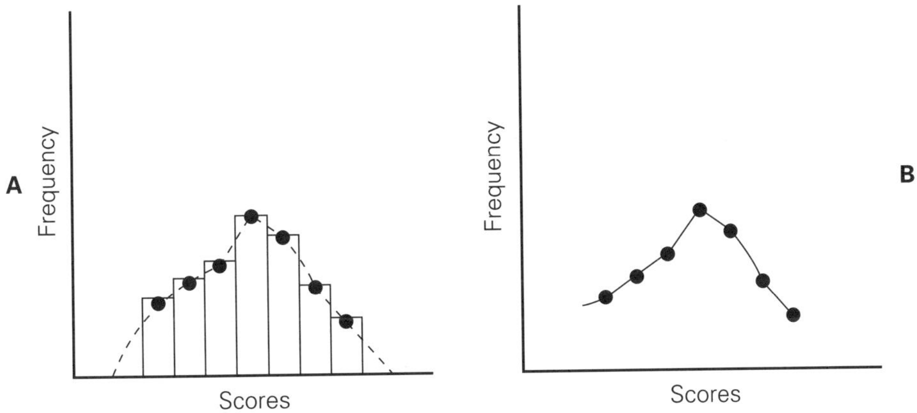

MEASURES OF CENTRAL TENDENCY

A measure of central tendency is a single central score that enables us to summarise the distribution of a data set. Measures of central tendency describe the centre of a distribution of scores. The three measures most commonly used to describe the central point of a distribution are the mode, the median and the mean. The mode refers to the numerical score that occurs with the greatest frequency in a distribution; the median is that point on a scale where half the scores fall above and half fall below; and the mean is the average score. These measures summarise members of a sample and are therefore also known as summary statistics and are sample specific. Because they are sample specific, they change with each sample. Table 22.3 illustrates hospice patients and their caregivers' concerns about analgesics. It also lists means (the arithmetic average of all scores) and standard deviations (a measure of variability discussed later in this chapter on page 361) for each sub-scale and the total score on the instrument used (Ward, Berry & Misiewicz, 1996). These scores represent the average of each sub-score and the total score and the amount of variation in each group on each of the reported scores.

TABLE 22.3 Illustration of data reporting instrument scores

SCALE	PATIENT	CAREGIVER	*t*
Fear of addiction	2.34 (1.39)	2.26 (1.18)	–0.35
Fatalism about pain relief	1.29 (1.05)	0.96 (1.01)	–1.80
Concern about drug tolerance	1.39 (1.35)	1.27 (1.25)	–1.41
Desires to be a good patient	1.73 (1.59)	0.83 (1.00)	–3.20*
Concern about side effects	2.50 (1.00)	2.57 (0.83)	0.35
Fear of injections	1.52 (1.27)	1.97 (1.64)	1.50
Concern about distracting MD	1.67 (1.28)	1.06 (1.09)	–2.15
Concern pain signifies disease progress	2.59 (1.39)	2.68 (1.53)	0.32
BQ total score	1.94 (0.85)	1.80 (0.61)	–0.92

From Ward, S.E., Berry, P.E & Misiewicz, H. (1996). Concerns about analgesics among patients and family caregivers in a hospice setting. *Research in Nursing Health*, 19, 205–11. This material is used by permission of John Wiley & Sons, Inc.

*$p < 0.01$.

Summary statistics may also be reported in narrative form as illustrated by the following excerpt from Burns and Adams' (1997) study of the accuracy of alcohol history taking by nurses and doctors:

> *Patients' scores on the AUDIT screening questionnaire*
> Of the 489 patient records that were analysed in 1994, 27% did not have completed AUDIT forms. The modal score for AUDITs that were completed was 0 (that is, the most frequently cited consumption category was non-drinker). Of those who scored more than zero, as Figure 1 demonstrates, the mode was 1.0 and the median AUDIT score was 4.0; a safe level of drinking for both males and females.

The characteristics of a sample in a study are described in terms of summary statistics. The mean test score reported in Table 22.2 ($\bar{X}$ = 73.1) is an example of such a statistic. If a different group of students was given the same test, it is likely that the mean would be different. Following is a more in-depth discussion of the mode, the median and the mean.

Mode

The mode is the most frequently occurring score in a frequency distribution and is the only measure of central tendency when the data are nominal; however, it can be used with all levels of measurement (see Table 22.1 and the example from Burns and Adams, 1997, above). A distribution can have more than one mode. The number of modes contained in a distribution is called the modality of the distribution. Figure 22.3, A, and Figure 22.4 illustrate unimodal or one-peak distributions. Figure 22.3, B, demonstrates a bimodal or two-peaked distribution. Multimodal distributions having two or more peaks are shown in Figure 22.3, B and D.

FIGURE 22.3 Symmetrical distributions

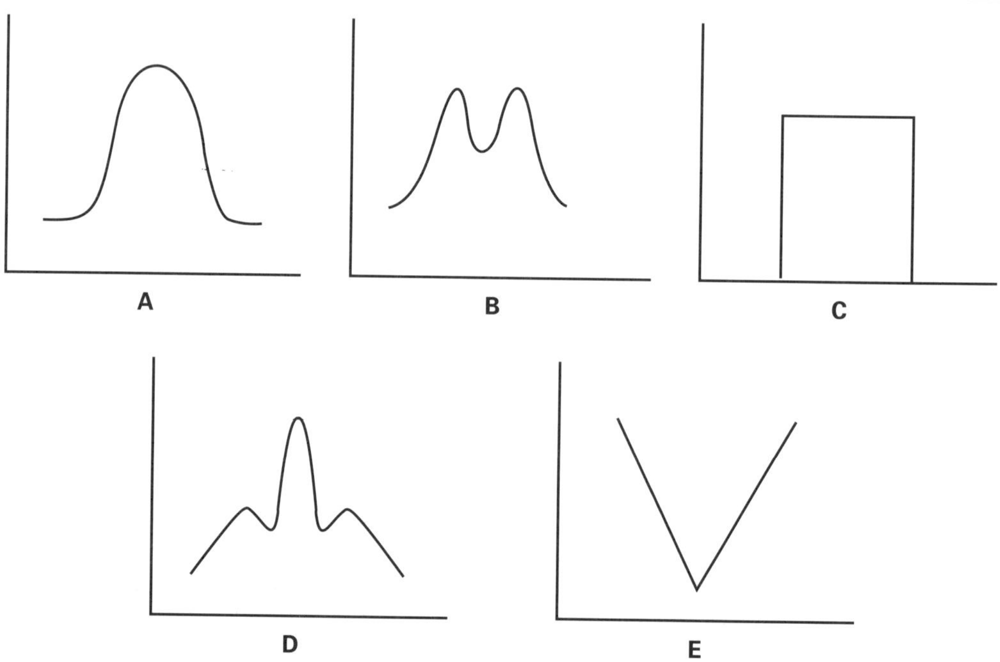

Table 22.4 illustrates how the change in a few scores can change the modality of a distribution from unimodal to bimodal. Since the mode takes account of only the most frequently occurring scores, it is not always a useful measure of central tendency.

TABLE 22.4 Measures of central tendency

SCORE	FREQUENCY	MEASURE
35	𝍸	
36	𝍸 |||	Mode
37	||||	Median, mean
38	𝍸	
39	𝍸	
40	𝍸 |	
35	𝍸	
36	𝍸 |||	Mode
37	|||	Mean
38	||||	Median
39	𝍸 |||	Mode
40	𝍸	

Median

The median is the middle score or the score where 50% of the scores are above it and 50% of the scores are below it. In a set of an odd number of scores, the median is the middle score; in a set of an even number of scores, the median is the average of the two middle scores. For ordinal scale data, either the mode or the median can be used, however, the median retains more information about the distribution of scores by taking the rank order of the values into account. The median is not sensitive to extremes in high and low scores. In the series of scores in Table 22.2 the twenty-sixth score will always be the median regardless of the highest or lowest scores. It is best used when the data are skewed (see the section called 'Normal distribution' on pages 358–59) and the researcher is interested in the 'typical' score. For example, if age is a variable and there is a wide range of ages that may affect the mean, it would be appropriate to also report the median. The median is easy to find by either inspection or calculation and can be used with ordinal or higher level data, as shown in Table 22.1.

Mean

The mean is the arithmetical average of all the scores and is used with interval or ratio data (see Table 22.1), and is the only measure that reflects and is affected by, all scores in the distribution. In a group of scores (e.g. age, income, height, test results), the mean (average) is calculated by adding all the scores and dividing the total by the number of scores in the group. The mean is the most widely used measure of central tendency and, of the three measures of central tendency, it is the most constant or least affected by chance. The larger the sample size, the less affected the mean will be by a single extreme score. In Table 22.4, the mean is the least affected by the change in the distribution from unimodal to bimodal.

If the distribution is symmetrical and unimodal, the mean, median and mode will coincide. If the distribution is skewed, the mean will be pulled in the direction of the long tail of the distribution. With a skewed distribution, all three statistics should be reported. For example, national incomes in Australia and New Zealand are skewed. The mean wage differs from the median wage because the large salaries are so much greater than the low salaries.

NORMAL DISTRIBUTION

The concept of the normal distribution is a theoretical one, based on the observation that data from repeated measures of some interval or ratio level data group themselves about a midpoint in a distribution in a manner that closely approximates the normal curve (also called Gaussian distribution), as illustrated in Figure 22.4. The vertical line or *Y*-axis represents the frequency of occurrences, that is, the values. The base line or *X*-axis shows values of the scores increasing in number from left to right. In addition, if the means of a large number of samples of the same interval or ratio data are calculated and plotted on a graph, that curve also approximates the normal curve. This tendency of the means to approximate the normal curve is termed the sampling distribution of the means. The mean of the population is derived from the means of the sampling distribution (see Chapter 23).

FIGURE 22.4 Normal distribution (mesokurtosis) with associated standard deviations

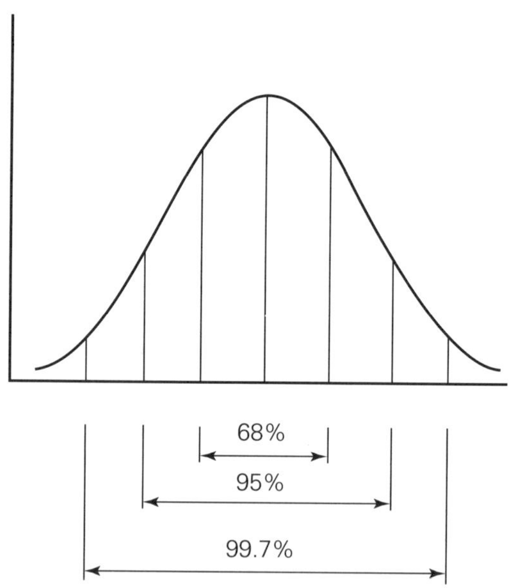

A normal distribution is bell-shaped; symmetrical about the mean and is unimodal. The mean, median and mode are equal. Most of the values are clustered around the mean with smaller frequencies moving away from the mean or centre on either side. A characteristic of the normal curve is that a fixed percentage of the scores falls within a given distance of the mean. As shown in Figure 22.4, about 68% of the scores or means will fall within 1 standard deviation (SD) of the mean; 95% will fall within 2 SD of the mean; and 99.7% will fall within 3 SD of the mean. The mean and the standard deviation are known as the parameters of a normal distribution. The mean provides the central point of the distribution and the standard deviation determines the spread.

Skewness

Not all samples of data approximate the normal curve. Some samples are non-symmetrical and have the peak off-centre. If one tail is longer than the other, the distribution is described in terms of skew. In a positive skew, the bulk of the data are at the low end of the range and there is a longer tail pointing to the right or the positive end of the graph. Individual income has a positive skew, with most individuals in the low-to-moderate range and very few in the upper range. The mean in a positive skew is to the right of the median. In a negative skew the bulk of the data are in the high range and there is a longer tail pointing to the left or the negative end of the graph. Age at death in Australia has a negative skew because most deaths occur at older ages. In a negative skew, the mean is to the left of the median. Figure 22.5 illustrates positive and negative skews. In each diagram the peak is off-centre and one tail is longer.

FIGURE 22.5 Skewed distributions—A, positive skew; B, negative skew

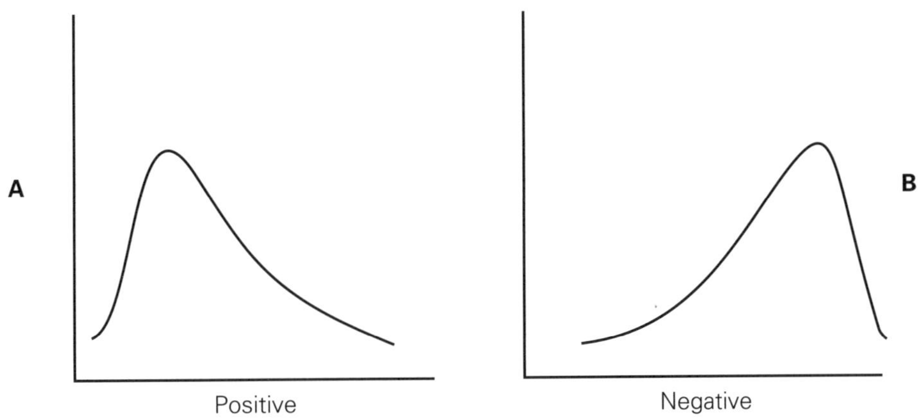

Symmetry

When the two halves of a distribution are folded over and they can be superimposed on each other, the distribution is said to be symmetrical—in other words, the two halves of the distribution are mirror images of each other. The overall shape of the distribution does not affect symmetry. Although the shapes in Figure 22.3 are different, they are all symmetrical; however, only Figure 22.2, A, approximates the normal curve. In addition, symmetry and modality are independent. Figure 22.3, A, is unimodal and symmetrical, while the graphs in Figure 22.5 are skewed.

Kurtosis

Kurtosis is related to the peakness or flatness of a distribution. The peakness or flatness of a distribution is related to the spread of the data. The further the data are spread out on a scale, the flatter the peak. The distribution that peaks sharply is called leptokurtic, whereas a broad, flat distribution is called platykurtic. Figure 22.6 illustrates kurtosis. Neither the leptokurtic nor the platykurtic distributions approximate the normal curve or mesokurtic distribution.

FIGURE 22.6 **Kurtosis—A, leptokurtosis; B, platykurtosis**

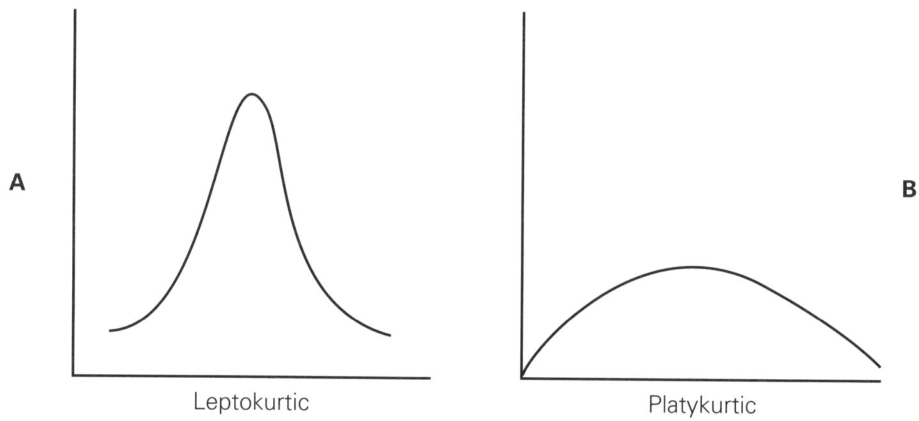

MEASURES OF VARIABILITY OR DISPERSION

Variability or dispersion is concerned with the spread of the data. Samples with the same mean could differ in both distribution (kurtosis) and skew. Variability measures answer the questions, 'Is a sample homogeneous or heterogeneous?' or 'Are the samples similar or different?'. If a researcher measures oral temperatures in two samples—one sample drawn from a healthy population and one sample from a population hospitalised with an infectious illness—it is possible that the two samples will have a similar mean temperature. However, it is likely that there will be a wider range of temperatures in the hospitalised sample than in the healthy sample. Measures of variation describe the extent to which individuals or scores in the sample vary. The most common measures used are the range, variance, standard deviation and semi-quartile range.

Range

The range is the simplest and most unstable measure of variability; it is simply the difference between the highest and lowest scores. The range in Table 22.2 is 36, i.e. 90 – 54 = 36. The disadvantage of the range is that it depends upon the two extreme scores only, which may be 'outliers' (extreme cases), compared to the rest of the scores.

Variance

A strategy commonly used to permit mathematical manipulation of difference scores is to square them. Variance is a measure of variability that includes every score in the distribution rather than only two scores. Some of the scores will be greater than the mean and some smaller. When negative (smaller) scores are squared, they become positive. The squared scores are then summed. The variance then is the average or mean of the sum of squares. The following example illustrates variance:

Value	Mean	Actual deviation	Squared deviation
2	6	–4	+16
4	6	–2	+4
7	6	+1	+1
9	6	+3	+9

Sum of squares = 30
Number of values: 4
Variance = sum of squares/number of values = 30/4 = 7.5

Because the deviations from the mean are squared, it will be noted that the variance is expressed in units different from the scores. In order to convert to the original set of data it is necessary to find the square root of the variance. The value thus obtained is the standard deviation.

$$\text{Standard deviation} = \text{square root of variance} = \sqrt{7.5} = 2.7$$

Standard deviation

The standard deviation (SD) is the most frequently used measure of variability and it is based on the concept of the normal curve (see Figure 22.4). It is a measure of average deviation or distance of each score from the group mean in a normal distribution and, as such, should always be reported with the mean. It takes all scores into account and can be used to interpret individual scores. Because the mean ($\bar{X}$) and standard deviation (SD) for the examination in Table 22.2 was 73.1 ± 12.1, a student should know that 68% of the grades were between 85.2 and 61. If the student received a grade of 88, he would know he did better than most of the class, whereas a grade of 58 would indicate he did not do as well as most of the class.

In a study identifying sources of stress and job satisfaction in the nursing environment, Healy and McKay (1999) report the means, SDs and reliability coefficients of each sub-scale of the measures used in their study. The possible range in the Nursing Stress Scale was 0–120, the mean was 40.46, and the SD was 14.50. The possible range in the Job Satisfaction Scale of the Nurse Stress Index Scale was 5–20, the mean was 12.73, and the SD was 3.50. This information allows the reader to get a feel for the variation the data contain. The SD is used in the calculation of many inferential statistics. One limitation of the SD is that it is expressed in terms of the units used in the measurement and cannot be used to compare means that have different units. If researchers were interested in the relationship between height measured in centimetres and weight measured in kilograms, it would be necessary for them to convert the height and weight measurements to standard units or *z* scores.

z scores

The *z* score is used to compare measurements in standard units. *z* scores take account of the mean and SD of the distribution. Each of the scores is converted to a *z* score and then the *z* scores are used to examine the relative distance of the scores from the mean; this process is called standardising the score. The following formula will illustrate this concept:

$$z \text{ score} = \frac{\text{original value} - \text{mean}}{\text{standard deviation}}$$

Let us say the mean score on the drug calculation test was 70/100 and the standard deviation was 10. Mary's score on the test was 80. Using the above formula, from Mary's score (80) we subtract the mean (70), and divide it by the SD (10). We find then that Mary's score is 1 standard deviation above the mean. A *z* score of 1.5 means that the observation is +1.5 SD above the mean, whereas a score of –2 means that the observation is 2 SD below the mean. By using *z* scores, a researcher can compare results from scales that use different units, such as height and weight.

Many measures of variability exist. The modal frequency is the easiest to calculate, but the SD is the most useful. The SD and the semi-quartile range are unique for each sample. The SD is the most stable statistic. Most spreadsheets and all statistical software packages will calculate basic descriptive statistics including standard deviations and *z* scores. For examples of how to calculate the SD manually, see Burdess (1994), Hicks (1996), Munro (2001), Polgar and Thomas (1995), and visit the virtual statistics textbook at http://www.surfstat.newcastle.edu.au/surfstat/main/surfstat.html

Semi-quartile range

The semi-quartile range (semi-interquartile range) indicates the range of the middle 50% of the scores. It is more stable than the range, because it is less likely to be changed by a single extreme score. It lies between the upper and lower quartiles; the upper quartile being the point below which 75% of the scores fall and the lower quartile being the point below which 25% of the scores fall. The middle 50% of the scores in Table 22.2 lies between 68 and 78 and the semi-quartile range is 10. This measure is used in conjunction with the median to describe the centre and dispersion of ordinal level data or interval/ratio level data that are skewed.

Percentile

A percentile represents the percentage of cases a given score exceeds. The median is the 50% percentile and in Table 22.2 it is a score of 74. A score in the 90th percentile is exceeded by only 10% of the scores. The zero percentile and the 100th percentile are usually dropped.

CORRELATION

Correlations are used to answer the question, 'To what extent are the variables related or connected to each other?'. Correlations are used to describe associations between variables but do not provide evidence of causation. Correlations are used most commonly with ordinal or higher level data. Correlations are discussed in Chapter 23 in more detail, but here scatter plots will be illustrated as visual representations of the strength and direction of the relationship between two variables. Figure 22.7 illustrates a perfect positive correlation (which would produce a numerical correlation coefficient with a value of +1.0), a perfect negative correlation (which would produce a numerical correlation coefficient with a value of –1.0), and no correlation (which would give a value of zero).

FIGURE 22.7 Scatter plots

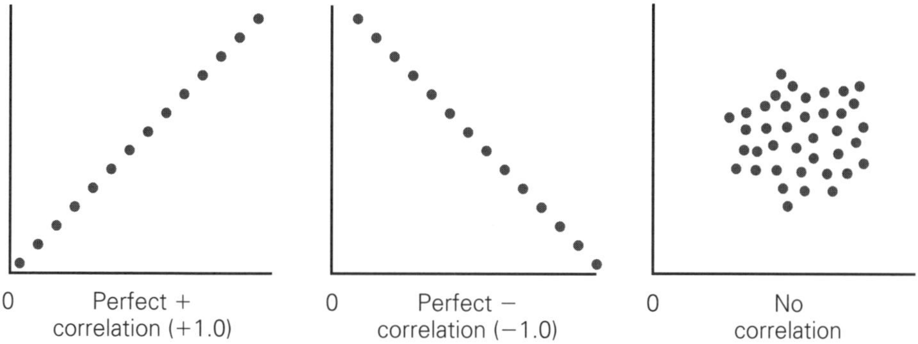

In most research, correlation results lie between the extremes of −1.0 and +1.0. The strength of the correlation is demonstrated by how closely the data points approximate a straight line. This indicates that most of the pairs of observations are behaving in the same way. In a positive correlation, the higher the score on one variable, the higher the score on the other. Temperature and pulse are positively correlated, that is, a rise in temperature is generally associated with a rise in the pulse rate. In a negative correlation, the higher the score on one measure, the lower the score on the other measure. A decrease in blood volume is generally associated with a rise in the pulse rate.

CRITERIA USED TO CRITIQUE DESCRIPTIVE STATISTICS

Students should be able to critically analyse the use of statistics in a study and make decisions about the appropriateness of the summary statistics used (see Box 22.1). For a detailed discussion on the criteria used to critique quantitative studies, read Chapter 4.

BOX 22.1 Criteria for evaluating descriptive statistics

- Were appropriate descriptive statistics used in the study?
- What level of measurement is used to measure each of the major variables?
- Is the sample size large enough to prevent one extreme score from affecting the summary statistics used?
- What descriptive statistics are reported?
- Were the descriptive statistics appropriate to the level of measurement for each variable?
- Is there sufficient information to confidently judge the results?
- If tables and graphs are used, do they agree with the text and extend it or do they merely repeat it?

Before a decision can be made as to whether the statistics employed make sense, it is important to return to the beginning of the paper and determine the purpose of the study. Although all studies use descriptive statistics to summarise the data obtained, many studies go on to use identical statistics to test specific hypotheses (see Chapter 23). If the study is an exploratory one, it is possible that only descriptive statistics will be presented, because their purpose is to describe the characteristics of a sample.

Just as the hypotheses should flow from the problem and purpose of a study, so should the hypotheses suggest the type of analysis that will follow. The hypotheses should relate to the major variables that are expected to be presented in summary form. Each of the variables in the hypotheses should be followed by appropriate descriptive information in the Results section.

After studying the hypotheses, the reader should go to the Method section. Using the operational definition provided, the level of measurement used to measure each of the variables in the hypotheses needs to be identified. From this information it should be possible to determine the measures of central tendency and variability that should be used to summarise the data. For example, it would be inappropriate to use the mean as a summary statistic for the nominal variable of gender, nationality or religion. These variables can only be reported as a frequency. The means and SDs should be provided for measurements performed at the interval or ratio levels.

Only after these aspects of the study have been examined should the results be considered. Each important variable should be summarised using an appropriate measure of central tendency and variability. Tables or graphs may be used to highlight summary data and display relationships between variables and should be clearly labelled. If grouped frequency data are presented, the groups should be logical and mutually exclusive. The size of the interval in grouped data should not obscure the pattern of the data, nor should it create an artificial pattern. Each table and figure should be referred to in the text, and each should add to the text, not merely repeat it. Table 22.4 illustrates a clearly presented table; each group is mutually exclusive and the data in the table agree with the data in the text.

The results should be written so that they are understandable to the intended audience. The audience for nursing research is the average practising nurse. Each part of the research paper must make sense in relation to the entire paper and each portion of the paper should be evaluated in relation to what has preceded it. Therefore, the evaluation of the descriptive statistics must precede the evaluation of the inferential statistics.

Box 22.2 provides a partial critique of a study by Small et al. (2000), which aimed to assess the effectiveness of a midwife-led debriefing session during the postpartum hospital stay at six months postpartum among women giving birth by caesarean section, forceps or vacuum extraction.

BOX 22.2 Critique of the statistical analysis of a study

Purpose of study:	To asses the effectiveness of a midwife-led debriefing session during the postpartum hospital stay in reducing the prevalence of maternal depression at six months postpartum among women giving birth by caesarean section, forceps or vacuum extraction; and, to reduce dissatisfaction with postpartum hospital care.
Design:	Randomised controlled trial

Hypothesis:	Null hypothesis (no difference in effects of debriefing)
Independent variable:	Debriefing session
Dependent variable:	Maternal depression
Conceptual definition:	Reduction in prevalence of depression at six months postpartum, and reduction of dissatisfaction with postpartum hospital care.
Operational definition:	Reduction in prevalence of depression at six months postpartum, and reduction of dissatisfaction with postpartum hospital care.
Measurement:	Edinburgh postnatal depression scale and the SF-36 health status measure sub-scales.
Sample size:	467 women in the debriefing group; 450 women in the standard care group.
Summary statistics:	Mean and median scores were calculated on the Edinburgh postnatal depression scale for the two groups.
Conclusion:	Reported statistics are appropriate for the research question, aims and level of measurement; sample size is large enough to prevent one score from having a large effect on the outcome.

ANALYSIS OF THE FINDINGS

The final sections of published research reports are generally titled Results and Discussion, but other topics, such as limitations of findings, implications for future research and nursing practice, recommendations and conclusions may be separately addressed or subsumed within these sections. The presentation of these areas is a function of the author's and the journal's stylistic considerations. The function of these final sections is then to bring together all aspects of the research process and to discuss, interpret and identify the limitations relevant to the investigation and thereby further nursing research.

Results

The Results section of a research report is considered to be the data-bound section of the report. It is here that the researcher presents the data: either qualitative data (in narrative form) or quantitative data (results of descriptive and inferential statistical tests). The presentation of the data analysed sets the stage for the Discussion section that follows the results. The Results section should then reflect the problem or hypothesis tested. The information from each research question or hypothesis should be sequentially presented. In quantitative studies, the tests used to analyse the data should be mentioned and the values obtained should be noted. Examples of these can be found in Table 22.5, and more detail on interpreting statistical sentences can be found in Chapter 23.

TABLE 22.5 Examples of statistical statements

STATISTICAL TEST	EXAMPLES OF REPORTED RESULTS
Mean	$\bar{X} = 118.28$
Standard deviation	$SD = 62.5$
Pearson correlation	$r = 0.39$, $p < 0.01$
Analysis of variance	$F = 3.59$, $df = 2, 48$, $p < 0.05$ F (2,48) = 3.59 $p < 0.05$
t test	$t = 2.65$, $p < 0.01$
Chi-square	$\chi^2 = 2.52$, df = 1, $p < 0.05$ χ^2 (1) = 2.52 $p < 0.05$

The Results section of a research report should contain the findings, presented in a clear, logical and concise way that answers the research questions or hypotheses posed. Any discussion or interpretation of the findings will be presented in the Discussion section of the paper. When critically appraising the Results section of the paper, the reader should keep the research question in mind and consider whether all of the relevant data have been presented to adequately answer the research questions asked.

In the study by Ward, Berry and Misiewicz (1996), the researchers developed tables to present the results visually. Table 22.6 provides demographic descriptive results about the patients and caregivers.

TABLE 22.6 Example of demographic data presentation

	PATIENTS		CAREGIVERS	
	n	%	*n*	%
Marital status				
Married	21	60%	28	80%
Not married	14	40%	7	20%
Education				
Did not complete secondary school	7	20%	1	3%
Completed secondary school	19	54%	16	46%
Studied at tertiary level	8	23%	17	48%
Missing data	1	3%	1	3%
Income				
<$29,000/year	25	71%	18	52%
>$30,000/year	6	17%	17	48%
Missing data	4	12%	—	—

Table 22.7 provides the results of testing for a relationship between patients' and caregivers' concerns about barriers to reporting pain and taking analgesics, using Pearson's correlation.

The tables allow the researchers to provide a more thorough explanation and discussion of the results. If tables and figures are used, they need to be concise. Although the text is the major mode of communicating the results, the tables and figures serve a supplementary but independent role. The role of tables and figures is to report results with some detail that the investigator does not enter into the text. This does not mean that tables and figures should not be mentioned in the text. The amount of detail that the author uses in the text to describe the specific tabled data varies with the needs of the researcher. A good table is one that meets the following criteria:

- supplements and economises the text
- has precise titles and headings
- does not repeat the text.

TABLE 22.7 Example of correlation data presentation

SUB-SCALE	ALPHA α PATIENT	CAREGIVER	CORRELATION (*r*) PATIENT/CAREGIVER
Fear of addiction	0.69	0.75	0.36
Fatalism about pain relief	0.57	0.37	0.49*
Concern about drug tolerance	0.76	0.81	0.07
Desires to be a good patient	0.82	0.80	0.26
Concern about side effects	0.58	0.71	0.15
Fear of injections	0.82	0.69	0.28
Concern about distracting MD	0.74	0.70	0.03
Concern pain signifies disease progress	0.91	0.89	0.27
BQ total score	0.82	0.90	0.13

*$p < 0.01$.

Another example of a table that meets these criteria can be found in the study by Dracup et al. (1997), which investigated the delay in seeking treatment for heart attack among Australian patients. The large number of variables included means that it is much clearer for the reader to have a table that easily and clearly summarises the results as this one does. To describe each variable in the text of the article would have been difficult to visualise and would have taken up a lot of space. The table developed by the researchers (see Table 22.8) allows the readers not only to visualise the variables quickly but also to assess the results.

TABLE 22.8 Example of significance testing presentation

VARIABLE	NUMBER OF PATIENTS (%)	MEAN HOURS	MEDIAN HOURS	INTERQUARTILE RANGE	*p*
Waited to see if symptoms would go away					0.001
No	59 (19)	6.1	1.5	0.9–3.0	
Yes	255 (81)	20.1	9.0	3.0–26.5	
Too embarrassed to ask for assistance					0.007
No	200 (63)	15.5	4.0	1.4–18.2	
Yes	115 (37)	20.8	9.8	4.2–26.3	
Worried about troubling others					0.002
No	102 (32)	14.4	1.8	1.1–9.7	
Yes	213 (68)	18.9	9.5	3.2–24.9	
Feared what might happen if sought assistance					0.005
No	97 (31)	12.9	3.5	1.3–14.4	
Yes	216 (69)	19.6	8.2	2.3–26.5	

Knew the nature of cadiac symptoms					0.001
No	225 (72)	18.4	9.5	3.0–26.7	
Yes	89 (28)	13.9	2.1	1.1–7.2	
Failed to realise the importance of symptoms					0.001
No	60 (19)	8.1	1.6	1.0–3.1	
Yes	254 (81)	19.7	9.1	3.0–26.5	

Dracup, K., McKinley, S.M. & Moser, D.K. (1997). Australian patients' delay in response to heart attack symptoms. *Medical Journal of Australia*, 166(3), 233–36.

KEY POINTS

- Descriptive statistics refer to the measures used to describe raw data. Data can be presented in tables, histograms, bar charts, pie charts, polygons and scatter plots.
- The four levels of measurements are nominal, ordinal, interval and ratio. Each has appropriate descriptive techniques associated with it.
- Measures of central tendency describe the average member of a sample. The mode is the most frequently occurring score, the median is the middle score and the mean is the arithmetical average of the scores. The mean is the most stable and useful of the measures of central tendency and, with the standard deviation, it forms the basis for many of the inferential statistics described in Chapter 23.
- The frequency distribution presents data in tabular or graphic form and allows for the calculation of observations of characteristics of the distribution of the data, including skewness, symmetry, modality and kurtosis.
- In the normal curve, sample scores and the means of large numbers of samples group themselves around the midpoint in the distribution, with a fixed percentage of the scores falling within given distances of the mean.
- In non-symmetrical distributions, the direction or the pull of the peak are described in terms of skew.
- In speaking of modality, the number of peaks is described as unimodal, bimodal or multimodal.
- The relative spread of the data is described by kurtosis.
- Each characteristic of the frequency distribution is independent.
- Measures of variability reflect the spread of the data.
- The modal percentage is the per cent of the cases in the mode.
- The range reflects the difference between the highest and the lowest scores.
- The standard deviation is the most stable and useful measure of variability for interval and ratio level data. It is derived from the concept of the normal curve.
- The analysis of the findings is the final step of a research investigation. It is in this section that the consumer will find the results reported in a straightforward manner.

- All results should be reported whether or not they support the aim of the study. Tables and figures may be used to illustrate and summarise data for presentation.
- Once the results are reported, the researcher interprets the results. In this presentation, usually titled Discussion, the consumer should be able to identify the key topics being discussed. The key topics, which include an interpretation of the results, are the limitations, implications and recommendations for future research.
- In all studies, the researcher should present limitations or weaknesses of the study. This presentation is important, because it affects the study's generalisability.

CRITICAL THINKING CHALLENGES

- Discuss the relationship between the level of measurement a researcher uses and the choice of a statistical procedure.
- What type of visual representation can be used to demonstrate the use of correlations? Use examples from clinical practice to illustrate the difference between positive and negative correlations.
- 'Nursing research studies generally present results using tables rather than graphical images or figures.' Discuss this statement, outlining the advantages and limitations of using figures to present numerical summary data.
- A student from your class tells you that she thinks it is inappropriate for the lecturer to ask the students to critique the descriptive statistics used in a study when they have not yet taken a statistics course. Would you agree or disagree with her? Defend your position.
- Support or refute the following statement: 'All results should be reported and interpreted whether or not they support the research question(s) or hypothesis(es)'.
- 'It is the Methods section and not the Results section of a paper that determines the validity of a study.' Discuss this statement in relation to both quantitative and qualitative research studies.
- Do you agree or disagree with the statement that a good study is one that raises more questions than it answers. Support your view with examples.
- Identify and discuss the usefulness of two different types of internet-based resources that you could use to assist in critiquing the findings of a study.

Additional resources

Alexy, B. (1997). Prenatal factors and birth outcomes in the public health service: a rural/urban comparison. *Research in Nursing & Health*, 20, 61–70.

Becker, P.T. (1993). A lingering identity crisis. *Research in Health & Health*, 16, 87–88.

Bergstrom, N. (1991). Scientific base for nursing practice is a goal of ANA. *Council Nursing Research*, 18(2), 1–7.

Bluman, A.G. (1995). *Elementary statistics.* (2nd ed.). Dubuque, W.C. Brown.

Downs, F.S. (1996). Research as a survival technique. *Nursing Research*, 45, 323.

Gennaro, S. & Vesseu, J. (1991). Making practice perfect. *Nursing Research*, 40, 529.
Gerdtz, M. & Bucknall, T. (2000). Australian triage nurses' decision-making and scope of practice. *Journal of Advanced Nursing*, 18(1), 24–32.
Healy, C. & McKay, M. (1999). Identifying sources of stress and job satisfaction in the nursing environment. *Australian Journal of Advanced Nursing*, 17(2), 30–34.
Kerlinger, F.N. (1986). *Foundations of behavioural research.* (2nd ed.). New York, Holt, Rinehart & Winston.
Lefort, S.M. (1993). The statistical versus clinical significance debate. *Image: the Journal of Nursing Scholarship*, 25, 57–62.
Lund, D. (1996). *Elementary statistics.* (3rd ed.). Redwood City, California, Addison Wesley.
Lyneham, J. (2000). Violence in New South Wales emergency departments. *Australian Journal of Advanced Nursing*, 18(2), 8–16.
Munro, B.H. (2001). *Statical methods for health care research.* (4th ed.). Philadelphia, Lippincott.
Patterson, E., Del Mar, C. & Najman, J. (1999). A descriptive study of nurses employed by general practitioners in south-east Queensland. *Australian Journal of Advanced Nursing*, 17(2), 13–20.
Takase, M., Kershaw, E. & Burt, L. (2000). Nurse-environment misfit and nursing practice. *Journal of Advanced Nursing*, 35(6), 819–826.
Wilton, T. & Kaufmann, T. (2001). Lesbian mothers' experiences of maternity care in the UK. *Midwifery*, 17, 203–11.

23
CHAPTER

Inferential data analysis

Zevia Schneider

LEARNING OUTCOMES

After reading this chapter the student should be able to:

- Distinguish between a parameter and a statistic.
- Discuss the purposes of inferential statistics.
- Identify those data that should be analysed using inferential statistics.
- Explain the concept of probability as it applies to the analysis of sample data.
- Distinguish between type I error and type II error and their effects on a study's outcome.
- Distinguish between parametric and non-parametric tests.
- List the commonly used statistical tests and their purposes.
- Explain the relationship between sample size and sample error.
- Critically analyse the inferential statistics used in published research studies.

Key terms

analysis of covariance (ANCOVA)
analysis of variance (ANOVA)
degrees of freedom
effect size
linear structural relationships (LISREL)
multiple analysis of variance (MANOVA)
multiple regression
path analysis
power analysis
t statistic

INTRODUCTION

It was noted in the previous chapter that descriptive statistics refer to various methods of summarising numerical data. Often, the researcher wants to do more than simply describe the data: inferential statistics enable inferences and conclusions to be drawn from those data. Statistical inference is based on probability theory and permits the generalisation from a specific sample or samples, to the entire population. Statistical inference is generally used for two purposes: to estimate the probability that statistics found in a random sample accurately reflect the population parameter; and to test hypotheses about a population. In the first instance, a parameter is a characteristic of a population, whereas a statistic is a characteristic of a sample. Statistics are used to estimate population parameters.

An example will illustrate the difference between the two. Suppose we randomly sample 100 people with diabetes and use an interval scale to study their knowledge of the disease. If the mean (average) score for these subjects is 65/100, the mean represents the sample statistic. If we could contact every person with diabetes in Australia, we could also calculate a mean, and that score would be the parameter for the population. As you know, a researcher is rarely able to study an entire population, so inferential statistics allow statements about the larger population to be made from studying a random sample drawn from that population.

Statistical inference is inductive and indirect. We draw general conclusions (inductive) about populations on the basis of specific samples tested in our experiment; it is indirect because it begins by assuming the null hypothesis (H_0), that is, that any differences are due to chance. We use the null hypothesis because statistical tests are designed to reject, rather than accept, hypotheses. The null hypothesis (also referred to as a statistical hypothesis) is the hypothesis that is actually tested by statistical methods. The null hypothesis states that there is no actual relationship between the variables and that any observed relationship or difference is merely a function of chance fluctuations in sampling. The scientific hypothesis or research hypothesis is the researcher's expectation about the outcome of a study.

HYPOTHESIS TESTING

The most common use of inferential statistics in experimental studies is hypothesis testing. Statistical hypothesis testing allows researchers to make objective decisions about the outcome of their study, and answers such questions as 'Is the difference between the two groups real?' or 'How strongly are these two variables associated with each other?'.

Watson, Town, Holbrook et al. (1997) studied the effect of a new educational program for patients with chronic obstructive pulmonary disease (COPD). Watson et al. hypothesised that the self-management plans may be effective in the long-term management of these patients. This was a scientific hypothesis, in other words, it was the hypothesis that the researchers believed would be the outcome of the study. The null hypothesis that was not explicitly stated, was that the self-management plans would not be effective.

Another example may help to clarify the difference between the null hypothesis and the scientific hypothesis. In the study by Waldenström and Nilsson (1994), the researchers wanted to know whether women who received birth centre care breastfed for longer than women who received standard maternity care. The scientific hypothesis, that women who had birth centre care would breastfeed for longer than women who had standard care, was based on the assumption that birth centre care, with its philosophy of natural childbirth, continuity of care, parental involvement, and support in labour, would have a more positive outcome for breastfeeding than standard maternity care. The researchers were interested to know whether the differences found on the various outcome variables differed significantly between the two groups.

The researchers (Waldenström & Nilsson, 1994), used the null hypothesis, that is, that there were no differences between the two groups of women, to test their scientific hypothesis. They found that the women who had birth centre care breastfed for the same length of time as women who had standard care, but had a greater incidence of sore nipples and milk stasis. In other words, the researchers found that the differences in the scores between the groups were so small that they were likely to be caused by chance alone and the null hypothesis was accepted. Note that the researchers did not reject the null hypothesis. All statistical hypothesis testing is a process of rejection or acceptance, not proof. It is impossible to prove that a scientific hypothesis is true, but it is possible to demonstrate that the null hypothesis has a high probability of being incorrect.

However, making inferences about the population from a sample involves the possibility of sampling error because we cannot assume that the sample is an exact representation of the population. Remember that random assignment does not prevent differences occurring among subjects; however, it does result in a more equal distribution of any differences across the groups in the study. So, while sampling error cannot be excluded, its probable magnitude can be calculated by using inferential statistics.

PROBABILITY AND THE LEVEL OF SIGNIFICANCE

Probability is a concept that we talk about all the time. For example, we might wonder what the chance of rain today is. But we have a difficult time defining probability, and yet it is central to our understanding of inferential statistics. Probability is given the symbol p and is expressed as a proportion between 0 (the event will not occur) and 1 (the event will occur). The probability of an event is the event's long-run relative frequency in repeated trials under similar conditions. It is the notion of repeated trials that allows researchers to use probability to test hypotheses. In other words, the statistician does not think of the probability of obtaining a single result from a single study, but rather of the chances of obtaining the same result from an idealised study that can be carried out many times under identical conditions.

The probability that is chosen to indicate that an outcome is statistically significant is called the level of significance (alpha level α). Three levels of significance can be reported: namely, the 0.05 level of significance ($\alpha = 0.05$); the 0.10 level ($\alpha = 0.10$); or the 0.01 level ($\alpha = 0.01$). The level of significance must be chosen prior to the commencement of the study, not after statistical analyses have been completed. The level of significance is the probability of making a type I error (the probability of rejecting a true null hypothesis). The minimum level of significance acceptable for all scientific disciplines, including nursing, is 0.05. If the researcher sets the alpha (α) or level of significance at 0.05, the researcher is willing to accept the fact that if the study were repeated 100 times, the decision to reject the null hypothesis would be wrong five times out of those 100 trials.

Statistical probability is based on the concept of sampling error, and inferential statistics are based on random sampling. However, even when samples are randomly selected, there is always the possibility of some errors in sampling. Therefore the characteristics of any given sample may be different from those of the entire population. Suppose a group of clinical nurses had access to a large number of patients with decubitus ulcers and wanted to find out the average length of time the ulcers would take to heal with the usual nursing care. If the nurses studied the entire population, they might obtain an average healing time of 50 days, with a standard deviation (SD) of 10 days, that is, between 40 and 60 days. Suppose too, that there were insufficient funds to study all the patients and instead the nurses conducted several consecutive studies on the group of patients. They would first sample a group of 25 patients, calculate the mean and SD, then return the sample to the main group before selecting the next sample. This process would be repeated many times and they might end up with a number of different means. If the nurses then placed the means in a frequency distribution, it might appear as in Figure 23.1: as the number of samples drawn increases, the curve will approximate the normal curve. This frequency distribution is called the sampling distribution of the means. It shows that the nurses might find that one sample's mean is 50.5 days, the next sample is 47.5 days, the next sample is 62.5 days, and so on. The tendency for statistics to fluctuate from one sample to another is called 'sampling error'.

FIGURE 23.1 Sampling distribution of the means

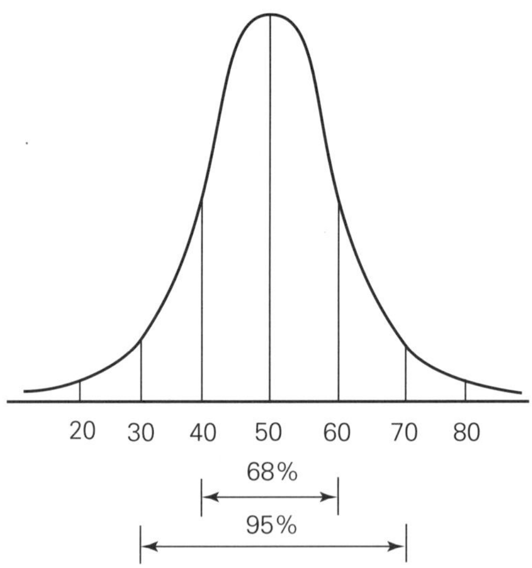

In practice, researchers do not routinely draw on consecutive samples from the same population; usually they compute statistics and make inferences based on the one sample. However, the knowledge of the properties of the sampling distribution—if these repeated samples are hypothetically obtained—permits the researcher to draw a conclusion based on one sample. This is possible because the sampling distribution of the means follows a normal curve and the mean of the sampling distribution will be the mean of the population. The fact that the sampling distribution of the means is normal tells us several important things.

When scores are normally distributed we know that 68% of the cases will fall between +1 SD and −1 SD or that the probability is 68 out of 100 that any one randomly drawn sample mean will lie within the range of values between ±1 SD. The SD of a theoretical distribution of sample means is called the standard error of the mean. The word 'error' is used because the various means that make up the distribution contain some error in their estimates of the population mean. The error is considered to be standard because it implies the magnitude of the average error, just as a standard deviation implies the average variation from one mean.

Although researchers rarely construct sampling distributions, standard error can be estimated because it bears a systematic relationship to the sample SD and the size of the sample. This tells us that increasing the size of the sample will increase the accuracy of our estimates of population parameters. The other reason that the sampling distribution is so important is that there are sampling distributions for all statistics. Researchers consult these distributions when making determinations about rejecting the null hypothesis.

95% CONFIDENCE INTERVAL

A derivation of the SD is the 95% confidence interval (95% CI). This statistic is the range around the mean (point estimate) in a sample where it can be inferred that there is a 95% chance that the 'real' difference lies between the two points. The formula is:

$$95\%\ CI = \frac{x \pm 1.96\ SD}{\sqrt{n}}$$

The following example (Figure 23.2) provides a graphical representation of the advantages of calculating the 95% CI. The physical role functioning scale

FIGURE 23.2 95% CI of physical role functioning for a sample of cardiac surgery patients

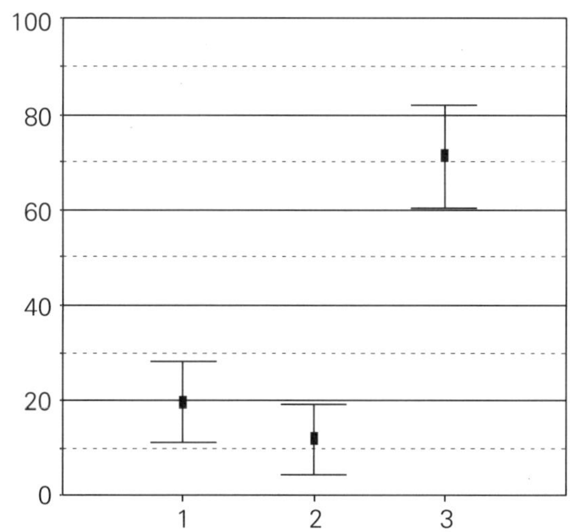

Notes:
1. pre-surgery measurement
2. hospital discharge measurement
3. six months post-discharge measurement

of SF-36 (Ware, 2000) ranges from 0–100: the higher the score, the better functioning. Figure 23.2 provides the mean score (small dark square) and the 95% interval (whisker plot) for each measurement point.

As illustrated, physical role functioning was lower at hospital discharge than prior to surgery, but at six months it was markedly improved. Note that there is overlap of the CIs between the first two scores—this means there is no statistically significant difference (i.e. the difference is > 0.05). However, as there is no overlap between the CIs for measurement 3 and the other two measures, the functioning had significantly improved at six months ($p < 0.05$). Other examples of 95% CI used in nursing or midwifery research include the studies by Small et al. (2000; see Appendix D) and Stewart et al. (1998).

ODDS RATIO

Another way of presenting probabilities is the 'odds ratio'. The odds ratio (OR) is a statistic used to assess the risk of a particular outcome. If the odds are greater than one, then the event is more likely than not to happen. In the randomised controlled trial by Small et al. (2000), the objective was to assess the effectiveness of a midwife-led debriefing session in hospital during the post-partum period in reducing maternal depression at six months. The women who participated in the trial had given birth by caesarean section, forceps or vacuum extraction. There were two groups of women: those who had a debriefing session and those who did not. The researchers found that more women in the debriefing group scored as depressed on the Edinburgh postnatal depression scale six months after birth than women having the usual post-partum care, although the difference between the groups was not significant (odds ratio = 1.24, 95% confidence interval was 0.87 to 1.77).

The odds ratio may become a more common way of presenting probabilities in nursing studies. Crichton (2001) describes the odds ratio in her paper and suggests that this measure of risk is widely used in healthcare literature, particularly epidemiology, because it can be calculated for case-control studies, in studies using logistic regression, and as a way of presenting the results of a meta-analysis.

ERRORS IN STATISTICAL INFERENCE: TYPE I AND TYPE II ERRORS

Suppose that a researcher decides to accept or reject the null hypothesis on the basis of how probable it is that the observed differences are the result of chance alone. Because data on the entire population are not available, the researcher cannot categorically assert that the null hypothesis is or is not true. It is possible, therefore, that statistical decision-making may result in incorrect decisions. There are two types of error in statistical inference: type I error and type II error. A type I error occurs when the null hypothesis is rejected when it is actually true. A type II error is the acceptance of a null hypothesis that is actually false. See Figure 23.3.

An example from Waldenström and Nilsson's (1994) study illustrates type I and type II errors. Remember that the null hypothesis of the study was that there would be no difference in breastfeeding duration between the two groups of women. The researchers found that there were no significant differences in breastfeeding duration at 2 months and 12 months after giving birth but that there were differences in complications. If the differences in complications were

FIGURE 23.3 **Outcome of statistical decision-making**

	Reality	
Conclusion of test of significance	Null hypothesis is true	Null hypothesis is not true
Not statistically significant	Correct conclusion	Type II error
Statistically significant	Type I error	Correct conclusion

truly a function of chance (perhaps this particular group of women was unusual in some way?), a type I error would occur—that is, the researchers' rejection of the null hypothesis when it is actually true. Figure 23.3 shows the relationship between the two types of error. In a practice discipline, type I errors are usually considered more serious because if the researcher says that there are differences where none are present, the potential exists for patient care to be adversely affected. As noted above, failure to reject a false null hypothesis is a type II error. Type II errors occur because of a stringent level of significance, a small sample size, or a small difference in measured effect.

POWER ANALYSIS

A related concept, power, is the probability that a study will reject a false null hypothesis. Specifically, power is $1 - \beta$, and ranges from 0 to 1. The minimal acceptable level for power is 0.80. An adequate level of power strengthens the meaning of a study's findings. Low power may be caused by hypothesis testing where small or moderate effects are evident; the phenomenon under investigation may be so complex or difficult to measure that no single study can explain a substantial portion of their variance (Polit & Sherman, 1990).

Power is influenced by the parameters:

- α level (usually set at 0.05)
- n (sample size)
- ES (effect size)

(Cohen, 1988; Rudy, 1991)

Effect size

Effect size equates to the magnitude of the effect of an intervention or treatment, compared to the control. Small effect sizes are common for nursing or psychological interventions such as muscle relaxation or music therapy. One study used these interventions in 2-minute to $3\frac{1}{2}$-minute sessions to reduce the anxiety in patients with acute coronary syndrome admitted to a coronary care unit (Elliott, 1994). The interventions resulted in an effect size of 0.19, and a related power level of 0.22, which is substantially lower than 0.80. Therefore, despite acceptance of a null hypothesis in this study, there is a high probability of a type II error.

Unfortunately, most nursing papers do not report effect sizes or the power of studies, thus making it difficult for researchers to establish appropriate sample sizes or the effect of nursing interventions. A type II error is also possible in a study that compared patient satisfaction between two models of nursing care (patient allocation and team nursing) (Wu, Courtney & Berger, 2000). A medium effect was assumed a priori but little rationale was provided for this decision, and a sample size was determined ($n = 137$). The resulting finding was acceptance of the null hypothesis for each of the three hypotheses.

Effect sizes have been calculated for a variety of parametric tests (see Table 23.1).

TABLE 23.1 Parametric tests and effect size

SAMPLE OF PARAMETRIC TESTS	EFFECT SIZE VALUES		
	SMALL	MEDIUM	LARGE
t test	0.20	0.50	0.80
ANOVA	0.10	0.25	0.40
correlation	0.10	0.30	0.50

Adapted from Cohen, 1988, pp. 40, 79, 85–87.

Various power analysis resources are available, including 'Web resources on power analysis' at http://www.im.nbs.gov/powcase/powlinks.html and a Manchester Metropolitan University site at http://149.170.199.144/resdesign/power.htm

PRACTICAL SIGNIFICANCE VERSUS STATISTICAL SIGNIFICANCE

It is important to recognise the difference between statistical significance and practical or clinical significance. When a researcher tests an hypothesis and finds that it is statistically significant, it means that the finding is unlikely to have happened by chance. In other words, if the level of significance for a sample has been set at 0.05, the odds are 19 to 1 that the conclusion the researcher reaches is correct. The conclusion would be incorrect only 5 times in 100; that is, this result would be obtained by chance alone only 5 times in 100. If, as is sometimes done, the researcher wants to have a smaller risk of rejecting a true null hypothesis, the level of significance may be set at 0.01. In this case, the researcher is willing to be wrong only once in 100 trials. The decision on how strictly the alpha level should be set depends on how important it is to not make an error. For example, if the results of a study are to be used to determine whether a great deal of money should be spent in an area of nursing care, the researcher may decide that the accuracy of the results is so important that an alpha level of 0.01 is chosen. In most studies, however, alpha is set at 0.05.

Watson et al. (1997) accepted the null hypothesis that an action plan for patients with chronic obstructive pulmonary disease (COPD) did not make a difference to a number of outcomes in their patient sample. They chose a stringent criterion for establishing what they thought would be a significant difference between the experimental and control groups: a test score difference of 5.7, which was not achieved. In the discussion, the researchers suggest that the difference they measured, although not statistically significant because of sampling bias and despite randomisation of subjects to groups, may be clinically significant. Of course, the opposite can also be true—a statistical significance may be present, but the clinical difference may be unimportant. This equates to the 'so what?' factor that all critical readers should ask.

TESTS OF STATISTICAL SIGNIFICANCE

Tests of significance may be either parametric or non-parametric. Parametric tests are used to analyse interval data or ratio scale data, and non-parametric (distribution free) tests are used for analysing nominal data and ordinal scale data. In both tests, researchers aim to discover the probability that the findings of their experiment occurred randomly by chance. There are many different statistical tests of significance that researchers use to test hypotheses. The procedure and the rationale for their use are similar from test to test. Once the researcher has chosen a significance level and collected the data, the data are used to compute the appropriate test statistic. For each test there is a related theoretical distribution that shows the probable and improbable values for that statistic. On the basis of the statistical results and the values in the distribution, the researcher either accepts or rejects the null hypothesis and then reports both the statistical result and its probability.

An example will illustrate this point. Rogers and Kashima (1998) studied responses to people with schizophrenia, comparing groups of psychiatric nurses, general nurses and lay people to clinical scenarios related to interactions with a person with schizophrenia. Participants were asked to respond to how they 'should' and then 'would' behave. A parametric test called one-way analysis of variance (ANOVA) was used to compare the 'should' responses of the three groups to determine if there was a difference in response due to group status. The reported result was written as $F(2,88) = 0.326; p = 0.72$.

The first symbol F is the abbreviation for ANOVA because the statistic calculated is known as the F ratio. In brackets are the degrees of freedom (*df*) calculated in relation to the number of groups, and the sample size used in the study. Degrees of freedom are used by the researcher in determining the critical value of F that corresponds to the preset alpha level of 0.05. (Critical value refers to the critical cut-off points for 0.05 and 0.01 levels of significance.) This value can be found in a table of F values in any general statistics text. For 2 and 88 degrees of freedom, the critical value of F is 3.15. The next value reported is 0.326. This is the calculated F ratio. If this value is greater than the critical value of F (in this case 3.15), the p value will be less than 0.05 and the researcher will conclude that there is a significant difference between groups. In this example, we can see that 0.326 is clearly less than 3.15 and the F value is 0.72, which is greater than 0.05. The researchers conclude that there is no difference in the 'should' responses between the three groups. The null hypothesis was accepted. In practical terms, statistical analysis programs calculate F statistics, the related critical value, and the statistical significance.

A simple example of what is meant by degrees of freedom may be helpful at this point. Suppose that a clinical coordinator was arranging clinical placements for ten student nurses in Year 3 of their program. The specific clinical areas the students need to experience are known. When ward placements have been allocated to nine nurses, the tenth nurse must take the last placement left. There is no 'freedom' (no choice) about the tenth nurse's placement. In other words, although there are ten student nurses (n), there are only nine ($n - 1$) degrees of freedom. This principle is true for any number of groups, that is, each group must lose one degree of freedom. In the prior example, the *df* were 2 and 88, corresponding to $k - 1$ groups and $n - 1$ subjects (3 groups − 1 = 2; 89 subjects − 1 = 88).

A study investigating nurses' research and publication activities (Hicks, 1995) analysed results using techniques of descriptive and inferential statistics. Nurses' attitudes to research were presented as a histogram (descriptive); in addition, data were subjected to chi-square χ^2 and extended chi-square analyses (inferential) to identify whether any significant relationships existed between the biographical variables on the one hand, and the attitude scale and research activity questionnaires on the other.

The format in which the statistical results are presented is commonly used in refereed journals, and once the student is familiar with this format it becomes easy to interpret reported findings from any statistical test. The abbreviations for some of the commonly used tests of difference are: *t* test (t), chi-square test (χ^2), ANOVA (F), Mann-Whitney *U* test (U) and Wilcoxon test (W).

These are the most commonly used inferential statistics. The test that is used depends on the level of the measurement of the variables in question and the type of hypothesis being studied. Basically these statistics test two types of hypotheses—that there is a difference between groups or that there is a relationship between two or more variables:

- tests of difference
  - means
  - proportions
- tests of relationships
  - associations
  - predictive relationships.

Tests of difference

Suppose a researcher using an after-only design wanted to find out if two randomly assigned groups are different after the introduction of the experimental treatment. If the measurements were at the interval level, the researcher would use the *t* test to analyse the data. If the *t* statistic was found to be high enough to be unlikely to have occurred by chance, the researcher would reject the null hypothesis and conclude that the two groups were indeed more different than would have been expected on the basis of chance alone. In other words, the researcher would conclude that the experimental treatment caused the difference (see Table 23.2).

A study by Botti et al. (1998) illustrates the use of the *t* statistic. The authors were studying the effectiveness of pressure bandaging in reducing bleeding and bruising in patients undergoing coronary angiography, and investigating the contribution that pressure bandages make to patient discomfort after angiography. They used the *t* test for unpaired samples to compare groin pain in patients who had pressure bandages applied to the puncture site, compared with patients who had no pressure bandages applied. The result was reported as $t\,(103) = 1.99$, $p < 0.05$. The *t* statistic obtained was 1.99. When compared to the critical value of *t* for 103 degrees of freedom (critical value 1.67, found in a table of critical values of *t*), the obtained value was less than 0.05, indicating a difference in groin pain between the two groups. The researchers concluded that

TABLE 23.2 Tests of differences between means

LEVEL OF MEASUREMENT	ONE GROUP	TWO GROUPS RELATED	TWO GROUPS INDEPENDENT	MORE THAN TWO GROUPS
Non-parametric				
Nominal	Chi-square	Chi-square Fisher exact probability	Chi-square	Chi-square
Ordinal	Kolmogorov-Smirnov	Sign test Wilcoxon matched pairs Signed rank	Chi-square Median test Mann-Whitney U	Chi-square
Parametric				
Interval or ratio	Correlated *t* ANOVA (repeated measures)	Correlated *t*	Independent *t* ANOVA	ANOVA ANCOVA MANCOVA

due to the increase in patient discomfort and the delay in time of onset of bleeding, pressure bandages should not be used routinely in the management of patients after coronary angiography, especially in the context of early discharge from hospital.

Another study by Botti et al. (2001) aimed to describe the incidence and occurrence of femoral artery bleeding during the first six hours after coronary angiography, and to determine whether a relationship existed between current post-angiogram observation protocols and the detection of complications. In addition to times of bleeding frequencies and vital sign measurements, means and SDs were used to compare those patients in the bleeding group with those in the non-bleeding group. The researchers state that while the use of pressure bandaging has a significant effect on the incidence and pattern of bleeding, routine vital sign measurement has no relevance in detecting local complications after angiography.

Parametric tests

Parametric tests are commonly used to examine whether the mean scores of two groups (*t* test) or three or more groups (ANOVA) are different. To use these tests, the variables must have been measured at the interval or ratio level and the groups must be independent, that is, nothing in one group helps to determine who is in the other group(s). Parametric tests have the following three attributes:

- they involve the estimation of at least one parameter
- they require measurement on at least an interval scale, and
- they make certain assumptions about the variables being studied. This last attribute assumes that variances of scores (when two or more groups are being compared) are the same among the groups, that is, normally distributed in the population. This is called homogeneity of variance.

The advantages of using parametric tests are that the mathematical calculations are more sophisticated and robust than non-parametric tests and are therefore able to provide additional information. For example, they permit analysis of interactions between two or more variables, and are usually more powerful in identifying significant differences. They are also most likely to reject the null hypothesis when it is false (less susceptible to type II errors).

As well as demonstrating differences between groups, *t* tests or ANOVA are used to determine whether random assignment to groups was effective in creating groups that were equivalent (homogenous) before the introduction of the experimental treatment. At the pre-test the researcher wants to show that there is no difference among the groups. In the study of the effects of birth centre care on breastfeeding experience and duration, Waldenström and Nilsson (1994) reported that the randomisation resulted in two groups without any statistical difference in regard to age, length of gestation, parity, civil status, ethnic background, education or attitudes to breastfeeding. The variables compared using the *t* test were measured at the interval or ratio level: age, length of gestation and education, with the remaining variables at the nominal level of measurement. If the groups had differed in age, this variable would have had to be controlled statistically in order for the researchers to conclude that their experimental program was effective. This is done using the technique of analysis of covariance (ANCOVA). ANCOVA also measures differences among group means and uses a statistical technique to equate the groups on an important variable. Another expansion of the notion of analysis of variance is multiple analysis of variance (MANOVA), which is used to determine differences in group means when there is more than one dependent variable.

Non-parametric tests

The position taken by most researchers and statisticians is that non-parametric statistics are best used when the data cannot be assumed to be at the interval level of measurement, or when the sample is small and the normality of the underlying distribution cannot be inferred. Non-parametric tests are based on fewer assumptions than parametric tests and are also less powerful, and therefore, less likely to identify significant differences. Because they are 'distribution-free', they can be used to analyse data when the distribution of the population is unknown.

When data are at the nominal level and the researcher wants to determine whether groups are proportionally different, the chi-square statistic (χ^2) is used. Chi-square is a non-parametric statistic that is used to determine whether the frequency in each category is different from what would be expected by chance. As with the *t* test and ANOVA, if the calculated chi-square value is high enough, the researcher would conclude that the frequencies found would not be expected on the basis of chance alone and the null hypothesis would be rejected. This test can be used in many different situations, but cannot be used to compare frequencies when sample size is small. In these instances, the Fisher's exact probability test is used.

When the data are ranked at the ordinal level, researchers may use several other non-parametric tests, including the Kolmogorov-Smirnov test, the sign test, the Wilcoxon matched pairs test, the signed rank test for related groups, and the median test and the Mann-Whitney *U* test for independent groups. Explanation of these tests is beyond the scope of this chapter, however, relevant readings appear in the 'Additional resources' section at the end of the chapter.

The related studies on patients' delay in response to acute coronary syndrome symptoms illustrates the use of three statistical tests. For data measured at the nominal level, the chi-square statistic was used. Data measured at the interval level included social and cognitive factors measured by the Response to Symptoms Questionnaire and data from medical records. These data were analysed using *t* tests or ANOVA, depending on the number of groups compared (Dracup, McKinley & Moser, 1997; McKinley, Moser & Dracup, 2000).

Tests of relationships

When the relationship between two or more variables is explored, statistics are used to determine the correlation or the degree of association between the variables. Tests of the relationships between variables are sometimes considered to be descriptive statistics. This is the case when they are used to describe the magnitude and direction of a relationship of two variables in a sample and the researcher does not wish to make statements about the larger population. Such statistics can also be inferential when they are used to test hypotheses about the correlations that exist in the target population (see Table 23.3).

TABLE 23.3 Tests of association

LEVEL OF MEASUREMENT	TWO VARIABLES	MORE THAN TWO VARIABLES
Non-parametric		
Nominal	Phi coefficient Point-biserial	Contingency coefficient
Ordinal	Kendall's tau Spearman rho	Discriminant function analysis
Parametric		
Interval or ratio	Pearson *r*	Multiple regression Path analysis Canonical correlation

Recall that the null hypothesis tests the relationships between variables and assumes that there is no relationship between the variables. When a researcher rejects the null hypothesis, the conclusion is that the variables are in fact related. Suppose a researcher is interested in the relationship between the age of patients and the length of time it takes them to recover from surgery. As with other statistics discussed, the study is designed to collect the appropriate data and then analyse the data using measures of association. In this example, age and length of time until recovery can be considered to be interval level measurements, and a test called the Pearson correlation coefficient (Pearson *r* or Pearson product moment correlation coefficient) would be used. Once the Pearson *r* is calculated, the distribution for this test is examined to determine whether the value obtained was likely to have occurred by chance. This is also calculated automatically in statistical analysis packages. Again, both the value of the correlation and its probability occurring by chance alone would be reported.

Correlation coefficients can range in value from –1.0 to +1.0, including zero. A zero coefficient means that there is no relationship between the variables. A perfect positive correlation is indicated by a +1.0 coefficient and a perfect negative correlation is indicated by a –1.0 coefficient (see Figure 22.7, page 363, for graphic illustrations). The example of age and length of time until recovery will illustrate the meaning of these coefficients. If there were no relationship between the age of the patient and the time he or she requires to recover from surgery, a correlation of zero would be found (with a wide scatter plot of data points). If, however, the correlation was +1.0, this would mean that the older the patient, the longer it would take him or her to recover. A negative correlation would suggest that the younger the patient, the longer it would take him or her to recover. Relationships are rarely perfect. The magnitude of the relationship is indicated by how close the correlation comes to the absolute value of 1. Thus, a correlation of +0.76 is just as strong as a correlation of –0.76, but the direction of the relationship is opposite (or inverse). As with other statistical tests of significance, the larger the sample, the greater the likelihood of finding a significant correlation. Therefore, the degrees of freedom associated with the test are also reported.

A study was designed to develop and test the validity and reliability of the 'Hospital-in-the-Home (HITH) Dependency Scale' (HDS). The HDS is designed to measure the dependency of HITH patients. One aspect of the study was to examine the concordance between the instruments values and those of HITH nurses to typical patient scenarios. The researchers (Santamaria et al., 2001) used Pearson's product moment correlation coefficient for test–retest results, scale reliability was tested by calculating item to total correlation coefficients and Cronbach's alpha for the overall scale. Alpha was also calculated for the scale if individual items were removed. A significance level of 0.05 was set for all the tests. Reporting on the reliability of the HDS, the authors found that a correlation coefficient of 0.809, $p < 0.01$ was produced on the test–retest reliability of the HDS—there was a one month interval between scores. The authors were satisfied with the test–retest correlation coefficient value and also with Cronbach's alpha of 0.72 for internal consistency of the HDS. However, they caution the reader when interpreting the results because 'the scenarios were designed to have differential values' (p. 13).

McCain and Cella (1995) conducted a cross-sectional study to examine the relationships among psychological distress, quality of life, uncertainty, coping patterns, stress and CD4+ T-lymphocyte levels. The authors found that increased negative stress was correlated significantly with lower quality of life ($r = 0.64$), suggesting that as human immunodeficiency virus-positive (HIV+) patients experienced more negative stressors, they had lower quality of life. This reflects a moderately high correlation and it indicates that approximately 41% (0.64×0.64) of the variability (r^2) in quality of life is explained by negative stressful experiences.

Nominal and ordinal data can also be tested for relationships by non-parametric statistics. When two variables are being tested that have only two levels (e.g. male/female, yes/no), the phi coefficient can be used to express relationships. When the researcher is interested in the relationship between a nominal variable and an interval variable, the point–biserial correlation is used. Spearman rho is used to determine the degree of association between two sets of ranks, as is Kendall's tau. All of these correlation coefficients may range in value from –1.0 to +1.0 (see Table 23.3).

Nursing problems are rarely so simple that they can be explained by only two variables. For studying complex relationships among more than two variables, techniques other than those so far discussed are used. In these situations a technique called multiple regression is used. Multiple regression measures the relationship between one interval level dependent variable and several independent variables; it is the expansion of correlation to include more than two variables and is used to determine which variables contribute to the explanation of the dependent variable and to what degree. For example, Morse et al. (1994) were interested in determining what factors were related to treatment-seeking behaviour of menopausal women. A number of variables—such as the women's age, marital status, education and employment status, current health status, health behaviours (smoking, using alcohol, using over-the-counter medications and exercise), stress, well-being, premenstrual complaints and past chronic health history—were analysed to see whether they, separately and together, influenced utilisation of health services. Such a study required the use of multiple regression (in this case stepwise logistic regression analysis) to answer the research question. The researchers found that there were differences between menopausal women who sought treatment and those who did not. The differences related to factors such as severity of symptoms and present and past health status.

Suppose the researchers who were studying menopause (Morse et al., 1994) were interested in not just treatment-seeking behaviour for menopausal symptoms, but also in satisfaction with treatment received. Canonical correlation is used when there is more than one dependent variable. If the data are nominal or ordinal, the contingency coefficient or discriminant function analyses are used.

Analysis of variance and Spearman correlation coefficient were used in a study investigating how first-time mothers cope with childcare while still in the maternity ward (Tarkka et al., 2000). The multi-variate method used was a stepwise regression analysis. The authors found no relationship between the mother's childbirth experience, marital status, education, socio-economic position and their ability to cope with childcare. However, a mother's state of mind and self-concept were highly significantly related to coping with childcare.

Additional techniques

More complex research problems require more sophisticated statistics. An example is path analysis. Hall et al. (1996) examined the role of self-esteem as a mediator of the effects of stressors and social resources on mothers' post-partum depressive symptoms. On the basis of a theoretical model, the authors postulated that self-esteem would be affected by stressors and life events, as well as by social resources, and that self-esteem would, in turn, affect depressive symptoms. Path analysis was used to test this mediating effect. In path analysis the researcher hypothesises the ways in which variables are related and in what order, and then tests how strong those relationships or paths are. In this study, the authors found that self-esteem mediated depressive symptoms.

A technique called LISREL (linear structural relations) tests path models made up of variables that are not actually measured. For example, a researcher might study the concept of self-esteem and use three different measures to determine the subjects' level of self-esteem. A measurement model using LISREL would be used for this purpose. As many of the variables of interest to nursing are not easily defined and measured and because we are interested in causal models, LISREL and generalised linear modelling are becoming more commonly used in nursing studies (DiIorio, Hennessy & Manteuffel, 1996; Ratcliffe, 1998).

Factor analysis is another advanced statistical test often used in nursing research to examine concepts more fully and contributes to our ability to measure concepts reliably and validly. Factor analysis takes a large number of variables and sorts them into groups that are most closely linked together. Using this technique, the variables are grouped into a factor. Many factors can be identified within one data set. In addition, factor analysis is used for instrument development and theory development. In instrument development, factor analysis is used to group individual items on a scale into meaningful factors or sub-scales. Jackson, Schmierer and Schneider (1996) were interested in testing the reliability and validity of the 'Attitudes toward learning in pregnancy' Scale. Factor analysis was used to determine whether the scale actually measured the concepts that they intended the instrument to measure.

In the development of an instrument to measure the compliance of adolescents with a chronic disease, the researchers used face validity and criterion validity, factor analyses, LISREL, correlation coefficients and Cronbach's alpha (Kyngas, Skaar-Chandler & Duffy, 2000). While developing the compliance instruments, the researchers had to delete and add items based on the statistical values or the content of the items. Further discussion of factor analysis for instrument validity occurs in Chapter 21.

Many other statistical techniques are available to nurse researchers, including the Electronic Statistics Textbook, available at http://www.statsoft.com/textbook/stathome.html Consult the sources listed in the 'Additional resources' section at the end of this chapter if you need more information or if a test not discussed is included in a study of interest to you.

CRITICAL REVIEW OF STATISTICS

Review of statistical analysis can be a complex and onerous task for a research consumer, but following a logical approach to the review will facilitate the task. Once again, the terms and language may be somewhat foreign, but continued experience and practice will de-mystify the jargon. Box 23.1 outlines the steps for reviewing the statistical analysis and results of a paper.

BOX 23.1 Criteria for a critical review of statistical analyses

- Is a null hypothesis being tested?
- Does the hypothesis indicate that the researcher is interested in testing for differences between groups or in testing for relationships?
- What is the level of measurement chosen for the independent and dependent variables?
- Does the level of measurement permit the use of parametric statistics?
- Is the size of the sample large enough to permit the use of parametric statistics?
- Is there sufficient information to decide whether the appropriate statistics were used?
- Are the statistics used appropriate to the problem, the hypothesis, the method, the sample and the level of measurement?
- What is the level of significance set for the study? Is it applied throughout the paper?
- Are the results for each of the hypotheses presented appropriately?
- Do the tables and the text agree?
- Are the results understandable?
- Is a distinction made between practical significance and statistical significance? How?

The first place to begin to critique the statistical analysis of a research report is with the hypothesis. The hypothesis should indicate what type of statistics will be used. If the hypothesis predicts that a relationship will be found, indices of correlation would be expected. If the study is experimental or quasi-experimental, the hypothesis should indicate that the author is looking for differences between means.

As the Methods section of a paper is reviewed, consider what level of measurement the author has used to assess the important variables. If the level of measurement is interval or ratio, the statistics most likely to be used will be parametric. However, if the variables are measured at the nominal or ordinal level, the statistics used should be non-parametric. Also, consider the size of the sample and remember that samples have to be large enough to permit the assumption of normality. If the sample is quite small, for example, five to ten subjects, the assumptions necessary for inferential statistics to be used may have been violated. The important question is whether sufficient justification has been provided for the statistics presented.

Next, consider the results as they are presented. There should be enough data presented for each hypothesis studied to determine whether the researcher actually examined each hypothesis. The tables should accurately reflect the procedure performed and be congruent with the text. For example, the text should not indicate that a test reached statistical significance, while the tables indicate that the probability value of the test was above 0.05. If the researcher has used analyses that are not discussed in this text, refer to a statistics text to decide whether the analysis was appropriate to the hypothesis and the level of measurement.

In addition, the results of the study should be clear enough for the average reader to determine what was done and what the results were. Finally, the author should attempt to make a distinction between practical and statistical significance. Some results may be statistically significant, but their practical importance may be doubtful. If this is so, the author should note it. Alternatively, a research report may be read that is elegantly presented, but the reader may ask 'so what?'. Such a feeling may indicate that the practical significance of the study and its findings have not been adequately explained in the report. See Chapter 4 for a more detailed discussion on how to critique quantitative studies.

KEY POINTS

- Inferential statistics are a tool to test hypotheses about populations from sample data.
- Sample distributions provide the basis for all inferential statistics. Because the sampling distribution of the means follows a normal curve, researchers are able to estimate the probability that a certain sample will have the same properties as the total population of interest.
- Inferential statistics allow researchers to estimate population parameters, test hypotheses, and to make objective decisions about the outcome of a study. Such decisions are based on the acceptance or rejection of the null hypothesis that states that there is no relationship between the variables.

- Acceptance of the null hypothesis indicates that the findings are likely to have occurred by chance. If the null hypothesis is rejected, the researcher accepts the scientific hypothesis of a relationship being present between the variables and that this relationship is unlikely to have been found by chance.
- Statistical hypothesis testing is subject to two types of error—type I and type II. Type I error occurs when the researcher rejects the null hypothesis that is actually true. Type II error occurs when the researcher accepts a null hypothesis that is actually false.
- The risk of making a type I error is controlled by setting the alpha level or level of significance. Reducing the risk of a type I error by reducing the level of significance increases the risk of making a type II error.
- The results of statistical tests are reported to be significant or non-significant. Obtaining a probability value of less than 0.05 or 0.01 (depending on the level of significance set by the researcher) indicates a statistically significant result.
- Commonly used parametric and non-parametric statistical tests include those that test for differences between means, such as the *t* test and ANOVA, and those that test for differences in proportions, such as the chi-square test.
- Tests that examine data for the presence of relationships (association) include the Pearson *r*, the sign test, the Wilcoxon matched pairs, signed ranks test, and multiple regression.
- Other statistical procedures include path analysis, LISREL and factor analysis.
- The most important aspects to consider when one critiques statistical analyses are the relationship of the statistics used to address the problem, and the design and method used in the study. Clues to the appropriate statistical test to use should stem from the researcher's hypotheses. The reader should also determine if all of the hypotheses have been presented in the paper.

CRITICAL THINKING CHALLENGES

- What assumption(s) is violated when a clinical research study uses a convenience sample and applies inferential statistics?
- What are the advantages and disadvantages of decreasing the alpha level for a study? What is the relationship between setting an alpha level and type I and type II error?
- Discuss the reasons for using non-parametric statistics in a study and their impact on the usefulness of the findings.
- Identify an internet-based resource that would assist the critical reader of a research report to determine if appropriate inferential statistics have been used.

Additional resources

Blaloch, H.M. (1972). *Causal inferences in nonexperimental research.* New York, W.W. Norton.

Bland, J.M. & Altman, D.G. (2000). The odds ratio. *British Medical Journal*, 320, 1468.

Burdess, N. (1994). *The really understandable stats book.* Australia: Prentice Hall.

Burns, R.B. (1997). *Introduction to research methods.* (3rd ed.). Melbourne, Addison-Wesley Longman.

Byrnes, M. & West, S. (2000). Registered nurses' clinical reasoning abilities: a study of self perception. *Australian Journal of Advanced Nursing*, 17(3), 18–23.

Crichton, N. (2000). Information point: Mann-Whitney test. *Journal of Clinical Nursing*, 9(4), 583.

Crichton, N. (2001). Information point: regression analysis. *Journal of Clinical Nursing*, 10(4), 462.

Crichton, N.J. (1998). Statistical considerations in design and analysis. In Roe, B. & Webb, C. eds, *Research and development in clinical nursing practice.* (p. 209). London, Whurr.

Davies, H.T.O., Crombie, I.K. & Tavakoli, M. (1998). When can odds ratios mislead? *British Medical Journal*, 316, 989–91.

Ferketich, S. & Muller, M. (1990). Factor analysis revisited. *Nurse Researcher*, 39, 59–62.

Hicks, C.M. (1996). *Undertaking midwifery research. A basic guide to design and analysis.* New York, Churchill Livingstone.

Knapp, T.R. (1990). Treating ordinal scales as interval scales: an attempt to resolve the controversy. *Nurse Researcher*, 39, 121–25.

Knapp, T.R. (1994). Regression analysis: what to report. *Nurse Researcher*, 43, 187–89.

Lucke, J.F. (1994). Testing the homogeneity of correlated variance from a bivariate normal distribution. *Nurse Researcher*, 43, 314–15.

Munro, B.H. (1997). *Statistical methods for health care research.* (3rd ed.). Philadelphia, Lippincott.

Nield, M. & Gocka, I. (1993). To correlate or not to correlate: what is the question? *Nurse Researcher*, 42, 294–96.

Pedhazur, E.J. (1982). Multiple regression in behavioral research. (2nd ed.). New York, Holt, Rinehart & Winston.

Polgar, S. & Thomas, S.A. (1994). *Introduction to research in the health sciences.* (3rd ed.). Melbourne, Churchill Livingstone.

Sidani, S. & Lynn, M.R. (1993). Examining amount and pattern of change: comparing repeated measures ANOVA and individual regression analysis. *Nurse Researcher*, 42, 283–86.

Women recovering from first-time myocardial infarction (MI): a feminist qualitative study

Debra Jackson, John Daly, Patricia Davidson, Doug Elliott, Elizabeth Cameron-Traub, Vicki Wade, Christine Chin and Yenna Salamonson

Although myocardial infarction (MI) is a leading cause of death and disablement for women internationally, little is known about women's recovery. This paper describes an exploratory descriptive study that was informed by feminist principles, and which aimed to explore the recovery experiences of a group of women survivors of first-time MI in the initial period following discharge from hospital. A total of 10 female survivors were interviewed using an open-ended semi-structured interview schedule administered at 7, 14 and 21 days post-hospital discharge. Findings revealed that recovery was experienced as a complex process, initially characterized by fear and uncertainty. Over the duration of the study these feelings were replaced with a more positive outlook, a return of energy, and a sense of confidence in the future. Participants identified an unmet need for reliable information which persisted over the duration of the study. The findings of this study have implications for nursing practice and research. Chief among these is the issue of effective provision of information to women following an acute MI. The importance of providing relevant information to be understood and retained by people experiencing crisis cannot be overstated. Equally important are the provision of opportunities for patients to have regular contact with health professionals to question and seek clarifying information. These findings should now be tested on larger populations.

Keywords: acute myocardial infarction, women's health, cardiac rehabilitation, recovery, illness trajectory, hospital discharge, feminist research

Journal of Advanced Nursing, 32(6), 1403–11, 2000; reprinted with the permission of the *Journal of Advanced Nursing*.

INTRODUCTION AND BACKGROUND TO THE STUDY

Despite the development in the 1970s of 'women's health' as an area of clinical practice, research and scholarship (Auer, 1990; Sawyer, 1990), little is known about many aspects of women's health. Coronary heart disease (CHD) is a case in point. It is the leading cause of death among adult women in many of the developed countries of the world (Rankin, 1995; similarly Blumenthal & Matthews, 1993; Eaker et al., 1993; Dempsey et al., 1995; Lukkarinen & Hentinen, 1998; Reeder & Hoffman, 1998) and a major cause of disability among older women (Fleury & Cameron-Go, 1997). Myocardial infarction (MI) is a particular problem for women, and this has been known at least since the publication of the Framingham study in 1979, which revealed that 40% of the women in the study experienced a second MI within 5 years, compared with 13% of men (Kannel et al., 1979). Subsequent findings by Greenland et al. (1991) suggest, even with covariate adjustments for age and comorbidities, women have significantly higher MI related mortality than men, both in hospital and the post-discharge period, and these higher female rates are observable across cultures (Tofler et al., 1987; Greenland et al., 1991).

However, Fleury and Cameron-Go (1997) note that researchers have paid little attention to the issues influencing women's recovery. Many of the current medical and nursing treatments available for women experiencing acute MI are based on research conducted with men (Cochrane, 1992). Beery (1995, p. 429) points out that the health needs of women have not received the research interest which male focused research has generated, and also suggests that 'much of what we know about women and heart disease has been pieced together and based on studies that were not planned to describe women'. The impact of variables related to biological, emotional, and socio-cultural differences between women and men, during recovery from MI are poorly understood and largely unexplored (Greenland et al., 1991). This paper reports an exploratory study which aimed to explore the recovery experiences of women survivors of first-time MI in the initial post-discharge period.

REVIEW OF THE LITERATURE

As noted above, much of the research which has had MI as a focus has been carried out on male populations, and little is known about the specific needs of women recovering from MI (Eaker et al., 1993; Rankin, 1995; Fleury & Cameron-Go, 1997; Reeder & Hoffman, 1998). Nevertheless, the available literature raises a range of concerns. Women tend to be older than men when they experience MI, they have a twofold risk of experiencing a second MI, and the likelihood of fatality is double that of men (Beery, 1995). Lifestyle related risk factors for MI are deeply rooted in women's everyday lives, e.g. risk factors related to contraceptive practices. Women may delay seeking medical assistance for symptoms of MI (Dempsey et al., 1995), are more likely to have unrecognized MI (Eaker et al., 1993), and have a poorer post-MI prognosis than men (Kannel et al., 1979; Tofler et al., 1987; Dittrich et al., 1988; Greenland et al., 1991; Eaker et al., 1993). Poorer outcomes for women are believed to be related to the older age of presentation (Dittrich et al., 1988; Eaker et al., 1993) and associated comorbidities (Wenger, 1989). However, in an examination of research focusing on the prognosis of women following MI, it is concluded that 'women were often treated less aggressively than men and had fewer referrals for diagnostic angiographies and cardiac rehabilitation' (Reeder & Hoffman, 1998, p. 80; similarly Peberdy & Ornato, 1992).

Studies of women with coronary artery disease also raise issues of concern, specifically related to gender bias in diagnosis and treatment (Hildon, 1994; Beery, 1995). Some may argue that the tendency of women to receive less aggressive treatment modalities than men is related to physiological differences between the male and female cardiovascular systems,· however, this position has been called into question (see, e.g. Tobin et al., 1987; Beery, 1995). Sharpe (1995) suggests that reduced treatment options for women are linked to the sexist and ageist attitudes of members of the health professions, while elsewhere it is stated that the reasons for gender disparity in treatment have not been fully explored (Cochrane, 1992). Greenland et al. (1991) suggest that the significantly increased mortality of women after MI makes women deserving of aggressive assessment and treatment.

The literature reveals that women are less likely to participate in cardiac rehabilitation programmes (CRPs) (Rankin, 1995; Fleury & Cameron-Go, 1997). There is evidence to suggest women are less likely to be referred for exercise rehabilitation, and those who are referred have lower attendance and higher drop-out rates than men (Eaker et al., 1993; Fleury & Cameron-Go, 1997). Eaker et al. (1993) theorize that this may be because of the fact that many programs may be designed to meet the needs of middle-aged men in full-time employment, and may be unsuitable for the needs of older women. Other factors which may be relevant in terms of women's participation include cost of classes, timing of classes, financial problems, and the presence of comorbidities (Fleury & Cameron-Go, 1997).

Women's recovery is said to differ from men's in several key areas, including a slower return to pre-MI functioning and a larger number of social support needs. Using a grounded theory approach to describe women's recovery after an acute cardiac event, Fleury et al. (1995) suggest that women's healing comprises of three stages, each having several component categories, and each describing a step in the journey to health. While this theory provides insights into women's healing, its usefulness for this current study is somewhat limited, because only four of the 13 participants were recovering from MI. The other nine women were survivors of a range of other cardiac events (Fleury et al., 1995).

While return to paid work is commonly considered an indicator of recovery post-MI, Fleury and Cameron-Go (1997) caution against applying this marker to women survivors of MI because of the older age of presentation of women, and the fact that many women do not engage in employment outside the home. Indeed, women's recovery may well be complicated by their roles as family carers. Cochrane (1992) makes the point that men may receive greater support from family during the recovery phase of illness, but women may resume normal domestic duties earlier than recommended. Participants in Boogaard's (1984) study disclosed having feelings of guilt and inadequacy at not being able to resume full domestic duties immediately on discharge from hospital. Despite early resumption of household activities, women are likely to suffer emotional problems such as anxiety and guilt because of their illness (Eaker et al., 1993). Given that women are far less likely to participate in formal CRPs, and thus are denied an important source of support, it is important that hospital nurses and other health professionals gain insight into the recovery needs of women after MI. The literature proposes rehabilitation and recovery as the ultimate aims of nursing care, and suggest that they should begin in the critical care unit, and continue out into the community (Fleury & Cameron-Go, 1997). Yet within an Australian context and internationally, little is known about the experiences of women as they recover from MI.

THE STUDY

This study aimed to explore the recovery experiences of a group of women survivors of first-time MI in the initial post-discharge period, and to contribute to the international body of evidence of the post-MI recovery experiences of women. Specific research questions were:

- What are the needs of first-time women survivors of MI in the period immediately following hospital discharge?
- Where needs are met, what is the source of support?
- What is the nature of any unmet needs?
- What are the experiential dimensions of the recovery trajectory following first-time MI?
- Where could nursing support for women survivors of first-time MI be improved to maximize health gain?

METHODS

An exploratory descriptive design was selected as appropriate to the study. Feminist research principles as described by Cook and Fonow (1986) provided a guiding framework. These five principles position gender and gender asymmetry as central to all social life; identify consciousness-raising as part of methodology; raise issues of intersubjectivity; recognize the need for ethical research practices; and, view research as having emancipatory and transformative potential. Anderson and Jack (1991) provided a feminist framework for analysis of data.

The participants

The participants were recruited using convenience sampling, from inpatients admitted to a large public hospital in Sydney, Australia. Potential participants were selected by the cardiac nurse researchers in consultation with specialist cardiac physicians. Inclusion criteria required that potential participants be female, recently been discharged from hospital following a first-time MI, able to converse fluently in the English language, and be willing to participate in the study. Following analysis of eight sets of data, data saturation was established (Streubert & Carpenter, 1995), however, two additional participants were recruited to ensure data saturation was achieved. Thus a total of 10 participants were recruited into the study. The ages of participants ranged from 43 to 77 years, with most of the women being aged in their 60s. Several of the women had comorbidities, including nonoinsulin-dependent diabetes mellitus (NIDDM) (n = 1), hypercholesteraemia (n = 4), hypertension (n = 3), left ventricular failure (LVF) (n = 1), congestive cardiac failure (n = 1), and chronic pain (n = 1), while three had no comorbidities. Maximum length of hospital stay with the MI was 7 days. Five participants were engaged in full-time employment at the time of the MI. The remainder were involved in full time domestic duties. Of the 10 participants, five were Australian born and five were immigrants.

Countries of origin for the immigrant women were New Zealand, North America, Germany, Greece and England. All participants were married and living with their spouses.

Ethical issues

Institutional ethics clearance was obtained for the research protocol at Area Health Service and University level. Participation in the study was voluntary, and no incentives were offered. In keeping with the feminist commitment to ethical research practices, consent procedures were obtained at the first contact, and participants were given the option to withdraw at each subsequent contact. Pseudonyms are used to protect participant anonymity.

Data collection

Following recruitment into the study, demographic data were gathered. Participants then took part in individual semistructured interviews guided by a schedule which has been used previously on male survivors of MI and their spouses (Thompson et al., 1995). The first contact with participants was made 3–5 days following admission to hospital, and at this time willingness to participate in the study was ascertained. Two researchers had direct contact with the participants and they conducted all the interviews. Interviews (as per Thompson et al., 1995) took place at 7, 14 and 21 days post-discharge from hospital, giving a total of four contacts, and all participants were asked the same questions. Whilst it could be argued that the time frames selected are arbitrary the researchers' intent was to capture aspects of living day-to-day for the survivors during a vulnerable period in the recovery process following MI. The interview schedule comprised of 10 questions which focused on a range of issues, including the needs of the women in the recovery period, who they turned to have, those needs met, their goals, worries and concerns, and their feelings about recovery (Thompson et al., 1995). Interviews were conducted in the homes of the participants, and ranged from 45 to 60 minutes in duration, generating approximately 28 hours of audio-taped narrative data.

Data analysis

Audio-taped interviews were transcribed and analysed drawing on a three-step method described by feminist researchers Anderson and Jack (1991), which is suitable for use when working with data derived from oral sources. The first step required that attention be paid to the moral language in the narrative text. This focused attention on the self-concept of the narrator, particularly in relation to socio-culturally accepted standards of behaviour. This step allowed researchers to respect the individuality of each participant, and permitted illumination of the standards which are used (by participants) to judge themselves, as well as make visible the standards they seek to attain. The second step required researchers to attend to what Anderson and Jack (1991) refer to as 'the meta-statements', which appeared in the narrative text of each participant. Meta-statements drew attention to contradictions between expectations and actual events, especially in terms of internal (participant) dissonance between what was expected, and what was actually stated. The third step, attending to the 'logic of the narrative' (Anderson & Jack, 1991, p. 22), involved focusing on the internal consistency of the narrative, and the interrelatedness of the themes and issues raised by participants.

Credibility of study findings

The need to demonstrate research credibility is one of the major challenges facing qualitative feminist researchers (Olesen, 1994; Jackson, 1997), and in this study, techniques for establishing rigour were addressed from the beginning of the project. Coherence, relevance, auditability, reflexivity and credibility were considered to be relevant to the current study, and these were incorporated into the research design (Sandelowski, 1986; Hall & Stevens, 1991). Coherence was initiated by carefully selecting the research methods to ensure appropriateness with the area of research. Relevance is embedded into the study because the area of research is pertinent and germane to women, and provides information with the potential to enhance women's health services. The study is auditable (as described by Sandelowski, 1986), and all major decisions are faithfully recorded. Credibility describes a sense that study findings reflect participant experiences accurately, and to establish this, steps were taken to increase the likelihood of obtaining quality data. All interviews were undertaken by the same experienced cardiac nurse researcher, so that over time, through continued and regular interaction, mutual trust was established. The frequency and nature of the encounters meant that high quality, credible data were obtained. A reflexive approach allows researchers to develop insight into their own beliefs and attitudes, and understand how these influence the construction of a study and the interpretation of findings. In this study, reflexivity and enhanced awareness were facilitated by regular and on-going discussions among members of the research team. These regular meetings provided a forum for de-briefing, and sharing ideas and concepts that arose from the narrative of the participants, and for the discussion of insights with academic and clinical colleagues. These discussions were on-going and also gave an opportunity for continued re-conceptualization and refinement of ideas.

FINDINGS

The 3 weeks following hospital discharge was revealed as a period of intense introspection, contemplation and reflection for the participants, which involved scrutinization of many previously taken-for-granted aspects of their lives. During this time, the women questioned aspects of their lifestyles that could be considered contributing factors to their perceived poor health. In the period immediately following the MI, participants expected to slow down, rest, and make major changes in their level of activity. This period was also characterized by fear, uncertainty and emotional lability. Several expected to give up their work commitments. However, by the end of the third week following hospital discharge, participants generally expected to recover their health, and be able to return to the workforce, or resume their previous activities. A lack of reliable information was revealed throughout the study period, although by the end of the third week following discharge, some of the women had started actively to seek out information from various sources. Most of the participants hoped to regain their previous state of health, while some intended to strive for a state of health and wellbeing that exceeded their pre-MI state. However, only one of the participants had begun a CRP. Detailed findings are presented below, and provide a snapshot of the women at the end of 1, 2 and 3 weeks after hospital discharge.

One week after discharge

By the end of the first week at home, there was a sense that the women had 'weathered the storm'. They had survived the MI, and the immediate recovery period. Though the women were glad to be discharged home from hospital, the immediate post-discharge period was initially characterized by internal disorder, fear and uncertainty. Fear was experienced in relation to a range of factors including fear of the future, fear of death, fear of MI recurrence, fear of participation in usual, taken-for-granted activities, and fear about the implications of the MI on their roles as family carers. For these participants, the initial post-MI period was experienced as a time of physical exhaustion, sadness, depression and emotional lability. The women expected to make some lifestyle changes, and although there was uncertainty as to the nature of these changes, all expected to relinquish something. Early in the illness trajectory, these losses were viewed as generally negative involving the loss of ability to eat freely and to participate in a range of activities. Participants made comments such as 'I have to give up work and take things quietly', 'I have to cut back my lifestyle', and 'I have to restrict my activities', which reflected the fact that the MI was associated with sadness and loss. One participant—Linda—showed the extent of her tiredness, sadness and grief when she disclosed that she had wept at least twice a day, every day, since her discharge from hospital; this was reported to be completely out of character.

The exhaustion and anxiety the women experienced was compounded by a general lack of knowledge and understanding about MI. The uncertainty they were experiencing in terms of their recovery was particularly related to care of self and colleagues, their own state of health in relation to the health of others experiencing MI, lack of confidence in the recognition of symptoms of MI, and implications for their lifestyles imposed by the MI. The women needed specific information, that was difficult to obtain. During their hospitalization they had been placed under the care of hospital medical staff and had not been in contact with their own general practitioners (GPs). Some of the women did not have a level of understanding about MI, and most had questions relating to the implications of MI on aspects of lifestyle such as diet, consumption of alcohol, and physical activity, such as exercise, occupational and domestic duties:

> I'd like to know definitely—do I need to change the way I eat? Do I need more exercise? Do I need to get the stress out of my life? Or, is this [the MI] just a physical thing that happens and none of those things are going to help? ... Each time I saw the doctor [in the hospital] I wrote down two or three questions and asked him those questions, but he seemed to, well he had things to say to me so he said those things to me and those two, my questions and his answers didn't quite mesh which led me to believe this—that there are probably no specific answers to those questions and you just have to wait and see what happens. (Beryl)

Despite preparing written questions for her doctor, Beryl had been unable, or could not recall being able to obtain satisfactory answers to her questions. In addition to having a definite need for reliable information, participants expressed a range of needs at the end of their first week at home. These needs included companionship, emotional support, help with domestic chores and activities of daily living. These needs were mostly met by partners, and other members of extended family, however, neighbours, church and other religious groups also emerged as sources of help and support.

Two weeks after discharge

By the end of the second week at home, life was much better for the participants. The feelings of sadness, depression and the emotional lability had started to lift. When talking about her emotions, Hilda made the statement that 'last week I could cry—I did cry a lot, because I couldn't do anything else. But this week I was better. I've calmed down a little bit'. The women were also feeling physically stronger, were not tiring as quickly, and they reported having greater stamina and endurance. Although feeling stronger and more able to resume their normal household duties, some of the women had started to question their role as family carers, and indicated that they would not necessarily resume taking full responsibility for running their homes. The fears relating to the future, and the fears of death which had dominated the first week home from hospital also started to resolve by the end of the second week:

> I'm not as frightened, as time goes on I get less and less frightened. Through the day I'm not frightened at all now. I'm still a little bit at night—when I go to sleep I wonder if I'll wake up the next morning but other than that I feel like I'm getting back to normal ... I'd like to say I'm starting to feel like I'm here to stay again. (Linda)

While the women were less fearful in terms of fear of imminent death, they still had worries in several areas, e.g. there was concern about effect that the illness was having on their families. Some of the women were thinking ahead to return to their paid employment and were concerned about how they were going to manage work-related stress. Others were worried about their health, and several were nervously contemplating scheduled investigative procedures (such as angiography). These procedures raised other fears, specifically fears around the possibilities that invasive treatment could be required.

Being more active and less fearful gave the women greater confidence in themselves and the future, and this was evident when they were asked to reflect on their goals. In addition to articulating their goals, the women were now able to describe their plans for achieving these goals. For example, although Maureen had stated that she had received no information on lifestyle changes post-MI from health professionals, she was in the process of developing long-term plans to improve her health, through changing her lifestyle, particularly in the areas of stress management and regular exercise. When asked where she was obtaining the information upon which to base these plans, Maureen indicated that much of it was derived from prior knowledge and informal sources:

> Probably it's a coincidence thing—having a heart attack people always talk about it, your diet or your exercise or your stress levels ... Nobody's told me specifically that this one or the other is a major or minor factor for my ownself, but I can imagine that anyone can make those changes to lifestyle and be better off so that's where I got that information from, just general sort of knowledge. (Maureen)

The women still had a need for information, and these centred around the expected recovery trajectory, modification of lifestyle, and management of chest pain, and other problems. By the end of the second week, some of the participants had consulted their own GPs. Generally the women had a high level of trust in their GPs, and this was evident in the following excerpt, in which Hilda describes an episode of chest pain:

> When I had the discomfort on Sunday, I was a bit scared. Sunday was bad, really bad, and I said I don't want to go back in hospital ... I just didn't know what to do, you know, should I ring or should I sit here and wait [for something] to happen?... I just calmed down and waited till Monday to ring up my doctor and got the patch. I had to wait till Monday—what can you do on Sunday? I didn't want to go to a different doctor and get something different, so I rang up Monday morning. (Hilda)

Although participants relied on visits to the GP for information and management of any symptoms, needs for companionship and emotional support were still primarily provided by partner, family and friends.

Three weeks after discharge

Perceptions of improved health and wellbeing continued, and by the end of the third week, the women were feeling better, stronger and more confident than in previous weeks. Now the women were saying that they felt they were going to return to pre-MI level functioning, and expressed guarded optimism for the future:

> I feel better yes for now but I do not know [about] tomorrow or next week, you know. But at this moment I'm very good. Much better from first and second week, I'm much better. Yesterday and every day, I go for a walk. (Soula)

Although the women acknowledged a sense of improvement, there were still issues related to fear and exhaustion for some. Linda was still experiencing difficulty in settling at night. Although she felt her health was improving, she was still plagued by fears and doubts at bedtime:

> At night I feel anxious, tired like and when I'm tired I don't feel so good and I think, oh am I going to wake up in the morning ... I can't describe the feeling, just lethargic. I feel like I'm so tired ... I can't explain it ... I feel that tired I'm frightened to shut my eyes cause I feel like I'll never open them again I'm so tired. It's a heavy, heaviness, that's the only way I can describe it, you know, heavy. (Linda)

It is relevant to point out that, at this stage, Linda was the only woman who had returned to work outside the home. She was engaged in cleaning work and, although she only went back 2 days during the week, she reported feeling tired, emotional and stressed as a result. Later, Linda also revealed that she was very anxious and concerned about the possibility of further investigations and surgical intervention. She had a deep fear of any type of surgery, and felt this was because of a previous traumatic surgical experience. Other participants were also contemplating a return to paid employment, and were concerned about aspects of lifestyle, and their state of health, especially the possibility of having a further heart attack. Hilda felt it was best not to dwell on this aspect:

> I am scared I will have another heart attack, but if I don't think about it, it might not happen. If you think about it constantly it could happen. You might have one because you talk yourself into it. It's best not to think about it. (Hilda)

With the passage of 3 weeks after discharge from hospital, the women were able to reflect on events in the hospital, and most expressed disappointment over the lack of information that they were given by hospital staff, although some acknowledged that the problem may have been more related to a lack of recall, or not understanding what was said to them.

Only one of the women had commenced a CRP, some of the others were uncertain of the benefits of attending such programs, and hadn't made a decision about participating. The need for information was still strong, and the women expressed informational needs in areas as diverse as dietary issues, the location of the MI, and several had questions as to any heart damage they may have sustained. Some of the women had taken it upon themselves to find out as much as possible about MI:

> I rang up MBF [a health insurance company] and the Heart Foundation and they sent me this reading material which I found really helpful and I realize that for me seeing it written on paper is probably more effective than hearing someone say it to me. So that was helpful. I read it and thought, 'oh yeah, that makes sense to me'. That made me feel better and confident for some reason. (Maureen)

Maureen later stated that having access to quality, relevant reading material, supported by telephone contact, helped her to gain understanding, and assisted her in regaining a sense of balance and perspective. By this stage of recovery, which was approximately 1 month after the MI, the women had begun to develop personal supportive networks. These networks included partners, family, friends, GPs, as well as other organizations, such as the Heart Foundation, and community and religious groups.

DISCUSSION

The initial survival period was characterized by internal disorder and involved intense introspection and reflection. Uncertainty and lack of confidence in recognizing symptoms of MI were problematic for participants, particularly early in the recovery process. After 3 weeks of hospital discharge, the participants had started to form supportive individual networks to meet their needs and had begun to develop confidence to face the future. The social and emotional needs of the women were generally met to the satisfaction of the women by a range of informal carers and existing socio-cultural networks. The key unmet need was for reliable information, and this need continued throughout the study. There was recognition by some participants that they may indeed have been provided with information by health professionals, but were unwilling to accept, or unable to recall such information. The emotional and physical crisis precipitated by the MI, and the resultant inner disorder that was experienced by the women could well affect comprehension and recall, meaning that even if information were provided, the women may have had little understanding or memory of it. For the women in this study the most successful intervention for the provision of information was the written information augmented by the availability of telephone counsellors who were able to answer questions, and provide clarifying information.

Although all the women intended to make adjustments to their lifestyles with the aim of improving health and reducing the risk of further MI, very little interest was shown in participation in formal CRPs. The reluctance of women to take part in CRPs is a documented area of concern (see, e.g. Fleury & Cameron-Go, 1997), because such programs are a source of reliable and relevant information as well as social support for those recovering from MI, and provide consumers with an opportunity to clarify and confirm any issues that may be cause concern (*sic*). Given that the overwhelming and on-going need of the women as each of the contacts was for reliable information, the issue of the role of CRPs in the provision of information is raised, as is the implications (*sic*) to the recovery of those who choose not to participate.

Implications for nursing practice and research

The findings of this study have transformative and emancipatory implications for nursing practice and research. Chief among these is the issue of effective provision of information to women. Ensuring that women have access to adequate information throughout the illness and recovery experience can help to empower them at a time when they are extremely vulnerable. The importance of providing relevant information in ways that are understood and retained by people experiencing crises cannot be overstated. Equally important is the provision of opportunities for patients to have regular contact with health professionals, to question and to seek clarifying information as required.

The reluctance of women to participate in formal CRPs is another area of concern. These programs provide valuable opportunities for social support, as well as an on-going source of health related information, and thus could be very helpful for women recovering from MI. Nurses responsible for planning and delivering these programs might seek to explore their programmes, and try to consider what changes could be made to increase women's participation. It may be that women prefer to attend all women's groups and the cost, timing and location are all issues which could influence women in their decision not to take part in these programs. Evidence suggests that the attitudes of hospital staff may have a crucial role in recruiting people into CRPs (see, e.g. Fleury & Cameron-Go, 1997). Nurses working with women survivors could ensure that women are made aware of the benefits of cardiac rehabilitation. Nurses may need to act as advocates for their women patients, to ensure that classes are affordable, accessible and available to women participants. Follow-up of women who do not complete cardiac rehabilitation could provide insights into issues surrounding the high drop-out rate of women.

Limitations to the study

Given the multicultural nature of Australian society, it is important to include the perspectives of people from minority cultures in health related research. Thus, the major limitation of the study lies with the fact that the inclusion criteria required participants be fluent in spoken English. Although five of the 10 women participating in the study were immigrants to Australia, women with little or no English were excluded from participating. In addition, all participants were married women who were living with male partners in stable domestic relationships. The perspectives of lesbian women, and women who are single, divorced, widowed, or not in stable domestic situations are not captured in this study.

CONCLUSION

MI is a leading cause of death and disablement in women, and the literature suggests that aspects of the illness experience and recovery phase of MI in women remain unexplored and poorly understood. For the women in this study, the recovery period following MI was a time of physical, psychological and social stress, and was characterized initially by fear, uncertainty and emotional lability. Changes in the women's needs and experience were discernible over time, and these were made visible by the research design, which allowed snapshots of the women at 1, 2 and 3 weeks following discharge from hospital. Findings from this study provide insights into the initial recovery period, contribute to the knowledge base of women's recovery after MI, and point to directions for further research.

References

Auer, J. (1990). Encounters with the state: co-option and reform, a case study from women's health. In Watson, S., ed., Playing the state: Australian feminist interventions (pp. 22–41). Sydney, Allen & Unwin.

Anderson, K. & Jack, D. (1991). Learning to listen: interview techniques and analyses. In Gluck, S. & Patai, D., eds, *Women's words: the feminist practice of oral history* (pp. 11–26). New York, Routledge.

Beery, T. (1995). Gender bias in the diagnosis and treatment of cardiac disease. *Heart and Lung*, 24, 427–35.

Blumenthal, S. & Matthews, K. (1993). Psychosocial aspects of cardiovascular disease in women: introduction and overview. *Annuls of Behavioural Medicine*, 15, 109–11.

Boogaard, M. (1984). Rehabilitation of the female patient after MI. *Nursing Clinics of North America*, 19, 433–40.

Cochrane, B. (1992). Acute myocardial infarction in women. *Critical Care Nursing Clinics of North America*, 4, 279–89.

Cook, J. & Fonow, M. (1986). Knowledge and women's interests: issues of epistemology and methodology in feminist sociological research. *Sociological Inquiry*, 56, 69–93.

Dempsey, S., Dracup, K. & Moser, D. (1995). Women's decision to seek care for symptoms of acute myocardial infarction. *Heart and Lung*, 24, 444–56.

Dittrich, H., Gilpin, E., Nicod, P., Cali, G., Henning, H. & Ross, J. (1988). Acute MI in women: influence of gender on mortality and prognostic variables. *American Journal of Cardiology*, 62, 1–7.

Eaker, E., Chesebro, J., Sacks, F., Wenger, N., Whisnant, J. & Winston, M. (1993). Cardiovascular disease in women. *American Heart Association Medical/Scientific Statement*, 88, 1999–2009.

Fleury, J. & Cameron-Go, K. (1997). Cardiovascular disease in women: women's rehabilitation and recovery. *Critical Care Clinics of North America*, 9, 577–85.

Fleury, J., Kimbrell, C. & Kruszewski, M.-A. (1995). Life after a cardiac event: women's experience in healing. *Heart and Lung*, 24, 474–82.

Greenland, P., Reicher-Reiss, H., Goldbourt, U., Behar, S. & the Israeli Sprint Investigators (1991). In-hospital and 1-year mortality in 1524 women after myocardial infarction: comparison with 4315 men. *Circulation*, 83, 484–90.

Hall, J. & Stevens, P. (1991). Rigor in feminist research. *Advances in Nursing Science*, 13, 16–29.

Hildon, A. (1994). Gender bias in cardiology: are women missing out on PTCA? *Australian Journal of Advanced Nursing*, 12, 6–11.

Jackson, D. (1997). Feminism: a path to clinical knowledge development. *Contemporary Nurse*, 6, 85–91.

Kannel, W., Sorlie, P. & Mcnamara, P. (1979). Prognosis after initial myocardial infarction: the Framingham study. *The American Journal of Cardiology*, 44, 53–59.

Lukkarinen, H. & Hentinen, M. (1998). Assessment of quality of life with the Nottingham Health Profile among women with coronary artery disease. *Heart and Lung* 27, 189–99.

Olesen, V. (1994). Feminisms and models of qualitative research. In Denzin, N. & Lincoln, Y., eds, *Handbook of Qualitative Research* (pp. 158–74). Thousand Oaks, Sage Publications.

Peberdy, M.-A. & Ornato, J. (1992). Coronary artery disease in women. *Heart Disease and Stroke*, 1, 315–19.

Rankin, S. (1995). Going it alone: women managing recovery from acute myocardial infarction. *Family and Community Health*, 17, 50–62.

Reeder, S. & Hoffmann, R. (1998). The prognosis for women after an acute myocardial infarction: recommendations for practice. *Dimensions of Critical Care Nursing*, 17, 75–82.

Sandelowski, M. (1986). The problem of rigor in qualitative research. *Advances in Nursing Science*, 8, 23–37.

Sawyer, M. (1990). *Sisters in suits: women and public policy in Australia* (pp. 42–54). Sydney, Allen & Unwin.

Sharpe, P. (1995). Older women and health services: moving from ageism toward empowerment. *Women and Health*, 22, 9–23.

Streubert, H. & Carpenter, D. (1995). *Qualitative research in nursing: advancing the humanistic perspective* (pp. 89–112). Philadelphia, JB Lippincott.

Thompson, D., Ersser, S. & Webster, R. (1995). The experiences of patients and their partners one month after a heart attack. *Journal of Advanced Nursing*, 22, 707–14.

Tobin, N., Wassertheil-Smoller, S., Wexler, J., Steingart, R., Budner, N., Lense, L. & Wachpress, J. (1987). Sex bias in considering coronary bypass surgery. *Annals of Internal Medicine*, 107, 19–25.

Tofler, G., Stone, P., Muller, J., Willich, S., Davis, V., Poole, W., Strauss, H., Willerson, J., Jaffe, A., Robertson, T., Passamani, E., Braunwald, E. & the Milis Study Group (1987). Effects of gender and race on prognosis after MI: adverse prognosis for women, especially Black women. *Journal of American College of Cardiology*, 9, 473–82.

Wenger, N. (1989). CHD in women: clinical syndromes, prognosis, and diagnostic testing. In Douglas, P., ed., *Heart disease in women* (pp. 62–90). Philadelphia, F.A. Davis Company.

APPENDIX B

Enabling care: working through obscurity and uncertainty. A basic social process used in selected acute care settings

Bev O'Connell

Using grounded theory methodology this study explored the process that nurses used to determine, deliver, and communicate patient care in acute care hospital settings and to assess whether or not this was congruent with the nursing process structure (O'Connell, 1998). Data were obtained from semi-structured interviews, participant field observations and in-depth audits of patient records. Textual data were managed using NUD*IST and analysed using the constant comparative method. The findings of this study revealed a number of factors that hindered nurses from using the nursing process in its current form. Instead, nurses used a basic social process termed: *Enabling Care: Working through obscurity and uncertainty.* This paper describes a basic social process used in selected acute care settings and discusses its implications for nursing practice. An understanding of this process will assist the profession to critique some nursing theories and to construct ideas of nursing practice based on current clinical realities.

Keywords: nursing theory, nursing practice, nursing care, knowing, uncertainty, delivery modes, grounded theory

---

Australian Journal of Advanced Nursing, 17(3), 32–39, 2000; reprinted with the permission of the *Australian Journal of Advanced Nursing.*

BACKGROUND

The process used to deliver patient care has been a topic of many debates in the literature (O'Connell, 1996; Meleis, 1991; Masso, 1990). Since 1967, Yura and Walsh have espoused the structured approach to patient care that was termed the nursing process. Although this process offers a systematic approach to patient care, its use has been resisted by nurse clinicians who have questioned its utility (Elliot, 1994; Prideaus, 1991). Moreover, many nurse scholars have challenged its applicability in nursing practice from a philosophical and theoretical stance (Mitchell, 1991; Lawler, 1991; Barnum, 1987). Varcoe (1996) argued that in the absence of any empirical evidence, arguments for and against the use of the nursing process remain unsubstantiated. A grounded theory study conducted by O'Connell (1998) reviewed the clinical application of the nursing process in acute care settings. It revealed that a number of contextual factors in these settings militated against its use. Specifically, the study revealed that the espoused theory of the nursing process was not the theory in use and that nurses experienced a basic social problem of being in a state of '*unknowing*'. This state of '*unknowing*' was linked to a number of factors, such as the existence of a fragmented and inconsistent method of determining and communicating patient care, and work conditions of immense change and uncertainty (O'Connell, 1998). To overcome this problem, and to determine, deliver, and communicate care nurses in this study used a basic social process termed: *Enabling Care: Working through obscurity and uncertainty.* This basic social process described in this article provides an understanding of a practice-based process used by nurses in selected acute care settings (see Figure 1).

FIGURE 1

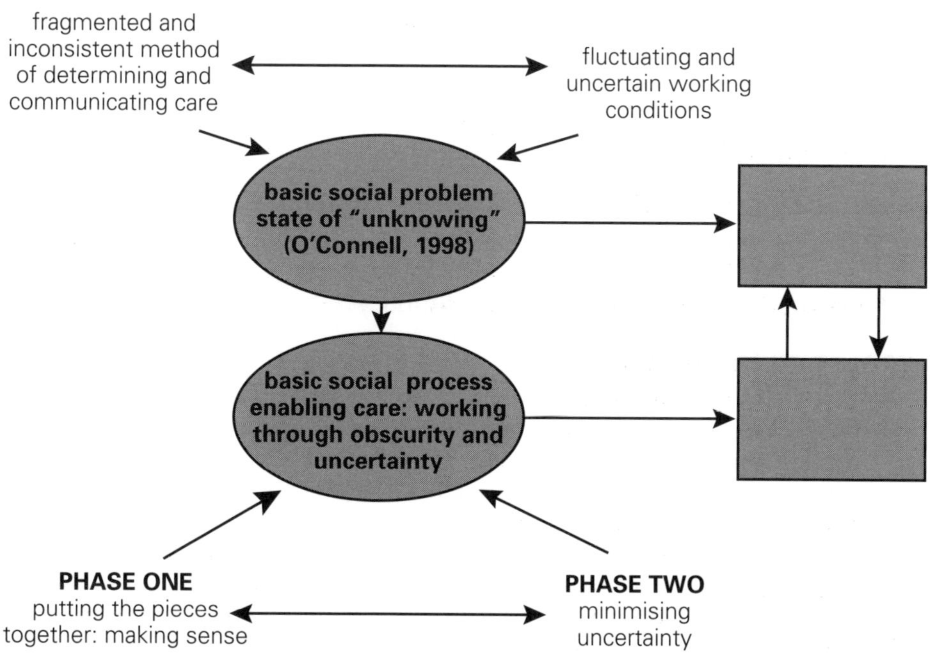

METHOD

The aim of this study was to discover and describe the process used by nurses to determine, deliver, and communicate patient care in selected acute ward settings and to provide an understanding of the contextual factors that impact on the process. Using grounded theory methodology, data were obtained from 27 semi-structured interviews with nurses who worked in a number of acute hospital settings, participant field observations conducted within five acute care settings, including informal interviews with more than 50 nurses, and in-depth analysis of patients' medical records. Theoretical sampling procedure also led to patients and patients' relatives being interviewed. These data were analysed using constant comparative analysis. This was combined with the process of memoing, diagramming, and maintaining theoretical sensitivity until saturation was achieved. The grounded theory method of open, theoretical, and selective coding was used to develop the theory (Irurita, 1996b; Glaser, 1978). To ensure credibility and trustworthiness of the emerging theory, textual data and coding were examined by other researchers. Finally, the findings were presented to approximately 20–25 experienced nurse clinicians for credibility testing.

Findings

Analysis of the data revealed a number of factors that collectively hindered nurses from knowing what to expect on a daily shift and their patients' specific nursing care needs (O'Connell, 1998). Within the context of high patient turnover, short shifts, lack of time, increased use of agency and casual nurses, increased movement of patients and nurses across wards, nurses were unable to deliver patient care using the nursing process structure. To deal with this problem, nurses in this study used a basic social process termed: *Enabling Care: Working through obscurity and uncertainty.* This basic social process had two interconnected phases that occurred simultaneously. These two phases were (1) Putting the pieces together: making sense and (2) Minimising uncertainty. Both these phases occurred in conjunction with one another (see Figure 1). The prevailing work conditions required nurses to use a number of strategies, which often conflicted with theoretical ideals of care and resulted in them becoming professionally disillusioned.

Phase one—putting the pieces together: making sense

Putting the pieces together: making sense had four sub-processes that were termed: (a) drawing on the known, (b) collecting and combining information, (c) checking and integrating information, and (d) sustaining communication.

Drawing on the known

At the start of any shift, nurses were in a state of 'unknowing', as they did not always know which patients they had been assigned or their specific care. Casual, agency and new nurses working on the ward for the first time were further disadvantaged as they did not usually know who they were working with or the ward routines. Nurses in this study were able to minimise, in part, the problem of being in a state of '*unknowing*' by *drawing on the known.*

Specifically, hospitals usually had a number of ward norms, routines, and ward specific interventions that mechanised patient care and the communication of this care. All nurses who knew these routines, regardless of whether they were permanent staff or casual staff, were able to proceed with some aspects of their work as they knew what to expect and what to do. According to Deluca (1995), nursing routines and rituals should be understood in context and while some require questioning, others assist by stopping the chaos in any acute hospital. In support, Strange (1996) adds that ritual in nursing served as a legitimating factor in nursing knowledge and should not be disregarded.

Additionally, nurses who were familiar with the equipment used and nursing patients with particular types of medical or surgical conditions were able to predict the type of patient care that would be required.

> All patients with similar diagnoses, yeah, there's a tradition, there's a standard course of events that will flow from standard diagnoses unless something happens to indicate otherwise [Int. 18].

Furthermore, knowing the patient and what to expect assisted the process of working through obscurity and uncertainty. The literature supports this finding and highlights that 'knowing the patient' is a foundational stage that assists with the planning of individualised patient care (Williams, 1998; Evans, 1996; Radwin, 1996; Irurita, 1993; Jenks, 1993; Jenny & Logan, 1992). The literature identified properties associated with 'knowing' the patient which include the nurse's experience with caring for the patient, time, and a sense of closeness between the patient and the nurse (Irurita, 1996a; Radwin, 1995; Jenny & Logan, 1992).

Collecting, combining, and pooling information

Collecting, combining and pooling information was the second subprocess used to make sense of what was happening in regard to patient care. The most commonly used mode of obtaining information was the handover. Being familiar with the patient and the nurse who was handing over was an important factor that enhanced the effectiveness of handovers for those receiving information. There was a shared, taken-for-granted trust where less clarification of information was required. Where possible and when rostering permitted, nurses had brief informal handovers with the staff members who were taking over from them. Junior nurses found this type of face-to-face personal handover very useful as it contained specifics about care that were usually missed in the general handover. For example, information that an intravenous line required the bag to be replaced.

As nurses who were handing over may have been in a state of '*unknowing*' in regard to the patient's actual care, they overcame this problem by collectively pooling and combining their patient information. Each nurse who had knowledge of a patient or a situation provided their account and collectively nurses would try to build a clinical picture of the patient and determine specific patient care. There was a lot of impromptu teaching and knowledge exchange that occurred as junior nurses asked more experienced nurses questions. While listening to tape-recorded handovers, nurses would switch the tape recorder off and discuss unclear information with each other and clarify issues where possible.

> A lot of exchange and clarification of information goes on at handover and informally. Some nurses know some patients better than others and they tend to fill the gaps. The shift coordinator who is handing over has been on annual leave and has commenced duty on an early shift. She really does not know the patients

> and within this handover she's had information confirmed from other nurses rostered on the afternoon shift, who had nursed the patient previously [Fobs. 04].

These findings concur with other studies indicating that within the handover context nurses collectively constructed a 'collaborative narrative about the patient' (Parker et al., 1992; Street, 1992). Although nurses drew on the known and pooled their knowledge about patient care with each other, there were some gaps in patient information.

Checking and integrating information

Nurses in this study constantly checked information in order to clarify (1) patient care and the accuracy of their knowledge base and judgement; and (2) whether all the care delivered was up-to-date. At any one point in time, there were a number of sources of patient information, each containing information that would form part of the story that could be used to build on already known patient information. Some sources were out dated and contained inaccurate patient information that would have to be further clarified.

> What I have done in the past with this particular person, I've gone back to them and said now I'm a bit confused as to what you meant about Mr So and So or whatever. But the other thing you do is you actually end up going around, you look in the notes and I actually go to the actual care givers who are looking after those patients. So you go to the patients themselves and just, quite surreptitiously, like you don't want to say well I don't know what's been happening to you this morning [Int. 24].

Additionally, nurses constantly asked and clarified patient care information with patients, doctors and other nurses. Many nurses stated that just looking at the patient, and/or the patient's latest observations were helpful ways of determining patient status and care, especially when the patients were unable to provide reliable information.

Sustaining communication

As nursing occurred over a 24 hour period involving a number of nurses, sustaining communication was a difficult though necessary task. The introduction of short shifts and lack of overlap time hindered nurses from communicating verbally with one another. Nurses used a number of strategies to try to sustain communication. They developed an informal written culture that compensated for an inability to use the oral communication. Nurses left each other informal reminder notes written on scrap pieces of paper left in the office, on a chart, or stuck to the patient's case notes.

> Sometimes I stick notes, actually the most effective thing I find is to actually stick notes on the front of the patient's chart [Int. 12].

Additionally, as there were many problems identified with the handover process, some nurses had developed written handover guidelines, introduced the use of various types of communication books to enhance the communication of information from doctors' rounds or changes to hospital policies and procedures (*sic*). Although this was developed to sustain and enhance communication, it increased the number of places where information was documented and complicated the communication process (see Figure 2).

FIGURE 2 **Putting the pieces together—making sense**

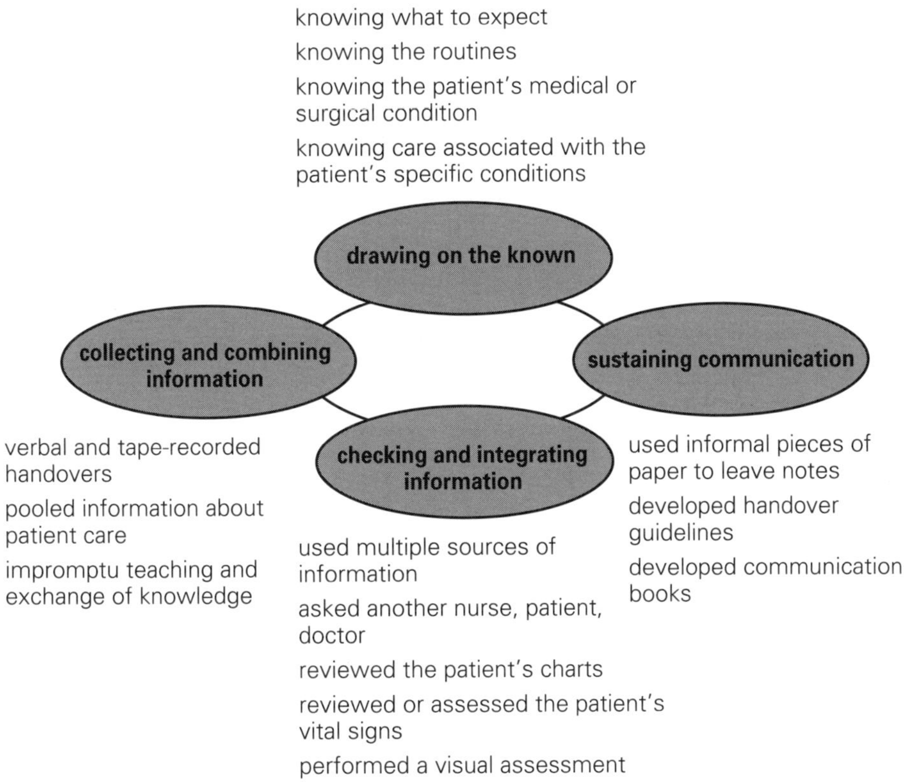

Phase two—minimising uncertainty

Minimising uncertainty had three subprocesses that were labeled: (a) adapting work practices, (b) taking control, and (c) backing-up.

Adapting work practices

Nurses worked under time constraints and constantly changing conditions of uncertainty that interrupted their work. Under these conditions, nothing seemed to be implemented in its theoretical form, as nurses were forced to modify their practices to meet certain deadlines in relation to patient care. Though they were displeased about adapting the way in which they practised, many spoke of having no choice, as taking short-cuts was seen as the only available, viable option.

> You're really rushing, you just take short cuts in order to finish on time. If you don't, then you stay back, I used to stay back all the time, but they forced me to go home on time … it's frustrating, you just have to make do [Fobs. Int. 06]

Documentation of patient information consumed a lot of nurses' time. However, this was rarely recognised formally in the system. Some nurses, due to a lack of time, would document information to comply with hospital policies rather than to communicate important information. Patient assessment data was frequently listed in the nursing care plan. This practice assisted other nurses to easily identify the patient's functional status if they were required to attend to a patient with whom they were unfamiliar. Additionally, to avoid being caught not signing the care plans at the end of a shift, some nurses signed that the care had been given at the commencement of the shift.

In order to complete the prescribed patient care, nurses compromised themselves by working unpaid overtime or by missing or taking late meal breaks. Nurses who worked the six-hour shift found it difficult to complete what they termed 'eight hours worked in six hours'.

Another strategy used to reduce the uncertainty was juggling the workload. Tasks that were a priority were performed at a set time and all other patient care was juggled around these tasks. Tasks like showering the patient may not have been prioritised as being essential and may not have been completed. Furthermore, nurses voiced concerns about being constantly interrupted and they adopted strategies to minimise this situation. For example, some patient bells would not be answered promptly, as nurses tried to complete the jobs they had commenced. Baker's (1995) findings concur with this, where she reported that nurse clinicians modified practices, not based on theory, to achieve particular goals under certain circumstances.

Taking control

Taking control was another sub-process used to minimise uncertainty. It involved:

a) controlling the care,
b) using a prompting mechanism,
c) organising the doctors, and
d) resisting change.

Controlling care

Due to the uncertain working conditions, senior nurses complained that they got 'caught' because junior and agency nurses had not completed the required tasks. Under these conditions, patients were not prepared for operating theatres, drugs were not given, and patient care was generally compromised. To try to avoid this situation, senior nurses took control and prescriptively told junior nurses how to modify their work practice (take short cuts) in order to complete their work. Shift coordinators also reallocated tasks among nursing staff to assist nurses who were falling behind. In these situations, the focus of care changed from being patient centred to being task centred. This finding supported Williams' (1998) study that nurses purposefully altered their care depending on the available time, using what she termed a process of selective focusing.

Using a prompting mechanism

Nurses were constantly interrupted while working. These interruptions often fragmented the nurses' train of thought and distracted them from their work. To overcome this, they developed several prompting mechanisms that reminded them of the jobs that needed completion. They would use a disposable paper towel to write certain tasks that needed to be performed on a particular shift. This paper towel, which was carried in their pockets, would be discarded at the end of a shift. Some nurses used a coding system of circles or stars next to the patient's name to indicate a certain procedure they had to remember. New graduate nurses would use prompts commonly used by other experienced nurses.

> On a paper towel the junior registered nurse wrote the tasks she had to do. She said it reminded her of what she has to do. This nurse had placed the obs chart and the fluid balance chart half out of the main folder, it stuck out of the folder. I asked her why she did that, she said it reminded her that the patient was on a fluid balance chart and needed observation. 'I saw night duty staff doing this and I found this helpful' [Fobs. 02).

Organising the doctors

In acute care settings, the majority of nurses' work was medically prescribed. Hence, nurses were unable to proceed with their tasks until doctors had written their orders. Doctors were rarely forthright in completing these aspects of their work and nurses often complained that they were not informed of the changes to patient care. Nurses in this study stated that they often had to ring doctors to remind them of their work and find out changes to patient care. To assist this process, some nurses had developed a communication mechanism that reminded doctors of their tasks at the start of the day. Additionally, they would purposefully try to be available to attend doctors' rounds in order to keep up with the changes to patient care. Nurses stated that they performed this role so that patients would not suffer undue interruptions to their care. This organiser or handmaiden role was inadvertently sustained as nurses were forced into maintaining this role in order to perform their job in a safe and legal way.

> If they're planning to discharge a patient you have to remind them to write the discharge drugs, you know, so that you can get them up the day before, instead of hanging around for ages, those sorts of things. But those acute things and then there's heaps and heaps of other things [you have to remind them] as well [Int. 23].

Resisting change

Nurses in this study were often described, by other nurses, as being resistant to change. Making changes to patient care or nursing practice was a difficult task to achieve. It was suggested in the data that this resistance was brought about by a motivation to reduce the uncertainty in the work place and to try to retain control.

> They [*nurses*] resist change because they like doing what they feel familiar with, what they feel comfortable with [Int. 32].

In support, Street (1992) also found that nurses resisted change. She added a different perspective stating that this resistance stemmed from nurses' lack of trust of nursing management as their changes disempowered nurses more than they empowered them.

Backing-up

As nurses experienced a social problem of being in a state of 'unknowing' and some of the subprocesses used to alleviate this problem compromised professional nursing practice, some errors occurred. As most nurses were inadvertently prone to making errors at sometime, errors that were judged to be minor were minimised by both doctors and nurses. These minimal errors were dealt with in the oral culture and not documented in the patient's notes.

Medication errors appeared to be the most frequent type of error that was covered up. When errors occurred, nurses very often discussed the incident among themselves and determined a strategy. What was reported or documented depended on the seriousness of the error. The benchmark of the measure of gravity, however, was not clear and varied across settings.

> I can remember reading in one of the patient's notes that their drug, I forgot now what drug it was, but their drug that was meant to be withheld for 24 hours in fact wasn't withheld for 24 hours, it was given. And that was written in a very convoluted fashion in the patient's notes. Nothing was handed over to us about it. There was no entry in the doctor's medical record about it. Like it was almost as if it had been entered in the nursing notes and that was the end of it. I don't know if there was an incident report filled out, but I would have assumed if an incident report was filled out that there would also be part of the entry in the medical record [Int. 22].

These findings support Baker's (1995) findings that some medication errors are redefined as not being considered as errors in some situations. She further added that errors were more likely to be reported if they were made by outsiders (casual and agency staff). While data from the current study revealed that errors were usually dealt with in the oral culture, other recent Australian studies report incidences of adverse patient events that were documented in the notes and may not have been openly discussed (Harlow, 1995; McNeil & Leeder, 1995; Wilson et al., 1995) (see Figure 3).

FIGURE 3 Minimising uncertainty

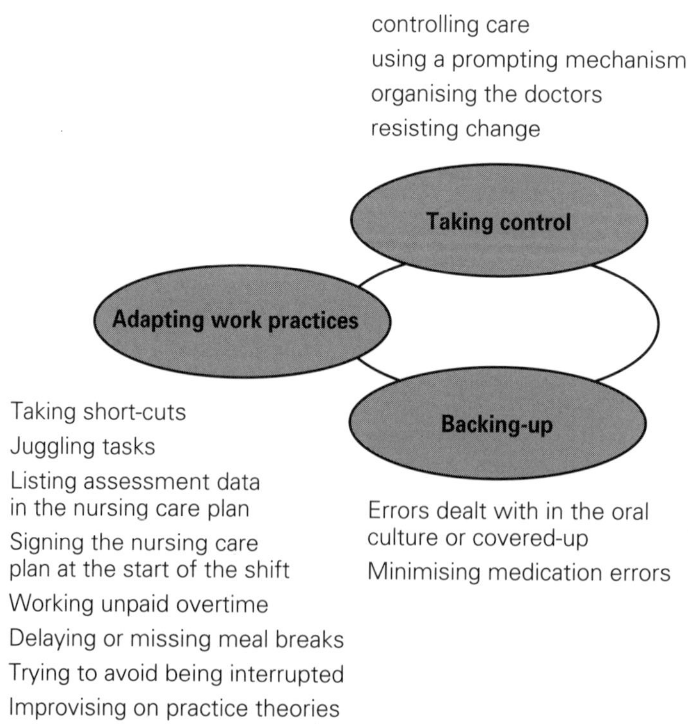

Professional disillusionment: consequence of working through obscurity and uncertainty

Nurses were dissatisfied having to work hard at delivering task-oriented care, a lack of time to spend talking to patients, and they complained of constantly struggling to complete their work. Other nurses worked unpaid overtime to compensate and stated that the situation affected them emotionally and affected their sleep pattern. Within this context, nurses became disillusioned and withdrew professionally. Some nurses resigned from nursing and spoke of 'getting out till things changed'. These findings were supported by Boon's (1997) study who found that nurses hurried work-pace resulted in less time for, what she termed, 'the essence of nursing'. This resulted in nurses withdrawing support for each other and experiencing a sense of frustration with their work. Additionally, other researchers report that the changing conditions under which nurses were required to function resulted in low morale, high turnover rates, and burnout (Droppleman & Thomas, 1996; Shindul-Rothschild et al., 1996; Shindul-Rothschild & Gordon, 1994).

IMPLICATIONS AND RECOMMENDATIONS

This study was designed to be exploratory, descriptive, and to take account of local contextual conditions. The findings should be interpreted in this context and generalisability is not claimed. This study revealed a basic social problem and a base social process used by nurses working in selected acute care settings. The theory espoused in the current study (see Figure 1), provides empirical evidence supporting Schulz and Meleis's statement that 'clinical knowledge results from engaging in the gestalt of caring, from bringing to bear multiple ways of knowing in order to solve the problems of patient care' (1988, p. 219).

The first phase of the process 'Putting the pieces together: making sense' resembles, in part, stages of diagnostic reasoning. In particular, the stages using pre-encounter data (Taylor, 1997) or pattern recognition (Crabtree, 1998) resemble the sub-process 'drawing on the known' where prior knowledge assists problem solving and the nurse being able to proceed with delivering patient care in the absence of any direction. In the current study, the process 'checking and integrating information' resembled the diagnostic reasoning process that involves collecting further information to confirm or deny hypotheses (Carnevali & Thomas, 1993). It further highlights nurses' efforts and time consumed in trying to make a decision in uncertain and changing contexts. As a key sub-process that helped optimise knowing the care was 'drawing on the known' and 'knowing what to expect', factors that enhance this state of knowing should be considered. Some strategies to consider include: making ward routines explicit for relieving staff, reducing the movement of patients and nurses across settings, and more consistency in assigning patients. Given this situation, one can question the utility of using more agency and casual nurses to fill gaps and multi-skilling nurses rather than trying to provide them with opportunities to specialise and consolidate their knowledge.

This study also highlighted the need to optimise the process of 'pooling knowledge' and 'sustaining communication'. According to Benner, Tanner and Chelsa (1997) pooling knowledge limits tunnel vision and snap judgments and therefore maximises clinical decision making. As nurses' understanding of the patient's condition and their care occurred within the context of combined knowledge from nurses, doctors, and patients, the links between these three groups need to be acknowledged and made more explicit. The reintroduction of health care teams may be one approach to strengthen these communication links and enhance this concept of 'knowing the patient'. It is also necessary to provide staff with the opportunity to have verbal handovers as they provide a forum for the exchange of patient information and nursing knowledge. It may be necessary to consider asking doctors to attend shift handovers as this may optimise the communication process. Nurses in this study spent a lot of time trying to organise the doctors. To try to minimise this problem, hospital administrators should develop duty statements for doctors to ensure that they take responsibility for their assigned tasks and develop routines that are known to the nursing staff. This will assist nurses to better plan patient care. Clearly, if nurses are able to reduce the time spent trying to clarify patient care issues and organisng the doctors, they may have more time to spend delivering patient care.

A finding of concern is that nurses worked under conditions that compromised care and professional practice. It is important for nurse leaders to take cognisance of this situation and to review workplace conditions and patient care delivery modes currently used. Team approaches to patient care need to be considered, as they enhance the processes of 'sustaining communication' and 'pooling knowledge'. Team approaches provide novice, agency, and casual nurses with the professional support they require due to their lack of experiential knowledge. Furthermore, the issue of nurses backing-up each other's work and covering-up errors is serious, as these errors may not be apparent to management or the patients and have the potential to create a false understanding of the efficacy of the care in acute care settings. It may be useful to explore the sub-process of 'backing-up' in greater depth, as it may provide insightful evidence of the quality of patient care and conditions under which quality care is able to be sustained. The nurses in this study talked about being professionally disillusioned with their working conditions. This factor needs to be explored further and strategies implemented to minimise this outcome.

Finally, this study explicated a process of nursing used by nurses in selected acute care settings. An understanding of this process will assist the critique of some nursing theories and enable the development of nursing theories informed by clinical realities.

References

Baker, H. (1995). Qualitative research conference: beyond the boundaries. Ethnomethodology in the research of nursing practice. Perth, Curtin University of Technology.

Barnum, B.J. (1987). Holistic nursing and nursing process. *Holistic Nursing Practice,* 1(3), 27–35.

Benner, P., Tanner, C. & Chelsa, C. (1997). The social fabric of nursing knowledge. *American Journal of Nursing*, 97(7), 16BBB–16DDD.

Boon, L. (1997). *Nurses' caring and the bottom line: a Canadian perspective.* Poster presented at the 9th International Nursing Research Congress. Vancouver, Canada, June.

Carnevali, D.L. & Thomas, M.D. (1993). *Diagnostic reasoning and treatment decision making in nursing.* Philadelphia, J.B. Lippincott.

Crabtree, M. (1998). Images of reasoning: a literature review. *Australian Occupational Therapy Journal*, 45, 113–23.
Deluca, E. (1995). Reconsidering rituals: a vehicle for educational change. *The Journal of Continuing Education in Nursing*, 26(3), 139–44.
Droppleman, P.G. & Thomas, S.P. (1996). Anger in nurses, don't lose it, use it. *American Nurses Journal*, 96(4), 26–31.
Elliot, T. (1994). Is it nexus, nonsense, or non-existent? A report of the use of nursing diagnosis in Australia. 2nd National Nursing Diagnosis Conference. Perth, Australia, Curtin University of Technology.
Evans, L. (1996). Knowing the patient: the route to individualised care. *Journal of Gerontological Nursing*, 22(3), 15–19.
Glaser, B.G. (1978). *Theoretical sensitivity.* California, The Sociology Press.
Harlow, P. (1995). *Report taskforce on quality in Australian health care interim report to the Hon. Dr Carmen Lawrence.* Canberra, Commonwealth Department of Human Services and Health.
Irurita, V. (1993). *From person to patient: nursing care from the patient's perspective.* Perth, Curtin University of Technology.
Irurita, V. (1996a). Preserving integrity: a theory of nursing. In Greenwood, J., ed., *Nursing theory in Australia: development and application* (pp. 263–300). Melbourne, Harper Educational.
Irurita, V. (1996b). A pathway to understanding: grounded theory in nursing. Sydney, Western Sydney Area Health Service/University of Western Nepean Flagship Nursing Research Seminars.
Jenks, J. (1993). The pattern of personal knowing in nurse clinical decision making. *Journal of Nursing Education*, 32(9), 399–405.
Jenny, J. & Logan, J. (1992). Knowing the patient: one aspect of clinical knowledge. *Image: Journal of Nursing Scholarship*, 24(4), 254–58.
Lawler, J. (1991). In search of an Australian identity. In Gray, G. & Pratt, R., eds, *Towards a discipline of nursing* (pp. 211–27). Melbourne, Churchill Livingstone.
McNeil, J. & Leeder, S. (1995). How safe are Australian hospitals? *The Medical Journal of Australia*, 16(3), 472–80.
Masso, M. (1990). Nursing process: help or hindrance? *Journal of Advanced Nursing*, 7(3), 12–16.
Meleis, A. (1991). *Theoretical nursing development and progress.* (2nd ed.) Philadelphia, J.B. Lippincott.
Mitchell, G. (1991). Nursing diagnosis: an ethical analysis. *Image: Journal of Nursing Scholarship*, 23(2), 99–101.
O'Connell, B. (1996). Nursing process: a systematic approach to patient care. In Greenwood, J., ed., *Nursing theory in Australia: development and application* (pp. 49–74). Melbourne, Harper Educational.
O'Connell, B. (1998). The clinical application of the nursing process in selected acute care settings: a professional mirage. *Australian Journal of Advanced Nursing*, 15(4), 22–32.
Parker, J., Gardner, G. & Wiltshire, J. (1992). Handover: the collective narrative of nursing practice. *Australian Journal of Advanced Nursing*, 9(3), 31–37.
Prideaus, G. (1991). Proceedings of the National Nursing Diagnosis Conference. Working with the nursing process: a question of attitude. Gold Coast, Queensland, Griffith University.
Radwin, L. (1995). Knowing the patient: a process model for individualised interventions. *Nursing Research*, 44, 364–70.

Radwin, L. (1996). Knowing the patient: a review of the research on an emerging concept. *Journal of Advanced Nursing*, 23, 1142–46.
Schultz, P. & Meleis, A. (1988). Nursing epistemology: tradition, insights, questions. *Image: Journal of Nursing Scholarship*, 20(4), 217–21.
Shindul-Rothschild, J. & Gordon, S. (1994). Single-payer versus managed competition: implications for nurses. *Journal of Nursing Education*, 33(5), 198–207.
Shindul-Rothschild, J., Berry, D. & Long-Middleton, E. (1996). Where have all the nurses gone? *American Nurses Journal*, 96(11), 25–39.
Strange, F. (1996). Handover: an ethnographic study of ritual in nursing practice. *Intensive and Critical Care Nursing*, 12, 106–12.
Street, A. (1992). *Inside nursing: a critical ethnography of clinical nursing practice*. New York, State University of New York Press.
Taylor, C. (1997). Problem solving in clinical nursing practice. *Journal of Advanced Nursing*, 26, 329–36.
Varcoe, C. (1996). Disparagement of the nursing process: the new dogma. *Journal of Advanced Nursing*, 23, 120–25.
Williams, A. (1998). The delivery of quality nursing care: a grounded theory study of nurses' perspectives. *Journal of Advanced Nursing*, 27, 808–16.
Wilson, R., Runciman, W., Gibberd, R., Harrison, B., Newby, L. & Hamilton, J. (1995). The quality in Australian health care study. *The Medical Journal of Australia*, 163, 458–71.
Yura, H. & Walsh, M. (1967). *The nursing process: assessing, planning, implementing, evaluating*. Norwalk, Appleton & Lange.

Health status, perceptions of coping, and social support immediately after discharge of survivors of acute myocardial infarction

John Daly, Doug Elliott, Elizabeth Cameron-Traub, Yenna Salamonson, Patricia Davidson, Debra Jackson, Christine Chin, Vicki Wade

BACKGROUND The period immediately after discharge from the hospital after an acute myocardial infarction is a stressful and vulnerable time about which little is known.

OBJECTIVE To explore health status, perceptions of coping, and social support among survivors of a recent myocardial infarction in the first 3 weeks after discharge from hospitals in southwestern Sydney, Australia.

METHODS A descriptive, exploratory approach with a triangulated methodology was used to assess the experiences of 38 survivors, detect patterns in these experiences, explore the health-support needs of survivors, and determine changes in health status in the first 3 weeks after discharge. Quantitative data were collected with the Medical Outcomes Study SF-36, New York Heart Association classification, Canadian Cardiovascular Society Angina Scale, and the Jalowiec Coping Scale. A semistructured interview schedule provided additional qualitative data about the experiences of the survivors.

RESULTS The health status of participants was relatively stable during the 3-week period; most had no activity limitation due to dyspnea or angina. However, the subjects' health status was considerably lower than that of their age-matched population. The most common and most effective coping strategies adopted during this period were confrontation, optimism, and self-reliance. In addition, the subjects experienced anxiety, depression, ambiguity and uncertainty, fear of recurrence of the infarction and of deterioration in health, of boredom and of inertia.

CONCLUSION These findings can help nurses in hospital and community settings assist survivors of acute myocardial infarction to prepare for and deal effectively with experiences during convalescence. (American Journal of Critical Care. 2000; 9:62-69)

American Journal of Critical Care, 9(1), 62–69, 2000; reprinted with the permission of the *American Journal of Critical Care*.

The period immediately after discharge from the hospital is a vulnerable time both physically and emotionally for survivors of myocardial infarction. This vulnerability may be accentuated by the anticipation of results of diagnostic tests and definitive revascularization strategies such as coronary artery bypass grafting or percutaneous coronary angioplasty. The recovery phase of myocardial infarction may also be affected by the trend toward shorter stays in the hospital and by the variable amount of time patients require to assimilate the meaning of a diagnosis of acute myocardial infarction (AMI). Information about health status, perceptions of coping, and social support is required for preparing patients for discharge and for timing interventions such as cardiac rehabilitation. Discrete factors such as depression are important predictors of quality of life and adoption of self-care behaviors.[1] However, data on the global experience in the period immediately after discharge are limited, particularly for Australasian patients. We did a descriptive, exploratory study of the experiences of survivors of AMI in southwestern Sydney, Australia, to provide a foundation for plans for care immediately after discharge.

Little is known about the general process of adjustment for survivors of AMI.[2,3] Specific aspects of the experience of AMI have been emphasized, with studies focusing on mortality[4] and return-to-work activities[5] or psychological constructs such as anxiety,[1,2,6–10] depression,[1,6,9–14] denial,[15,16] psychosocial status,[17,18] uncertainty,[19,20] and control.[18]

The period after discharge from the hospital is noted as a vulnerable time during which psychological morbidity is common,[3] with evidence suggesting that approximately one third of patients experience continuing anxiety and depression after AMI.[1] Wishnie et al[21] noted that psychological factors during convalescence after myocardial infarction hamper return to work and resumption of social roles and responsibilities. Scalzi et al[22] described the lack of internalization of information in the acute phase of illness. This failure to internalize information may be exacerbated by a healthcare system with decreases in resources and by shortened hospital stay. These factors have important implications for life adjustment of patients and patients' spouses and may influence morbidity and appropriate modification of life-style risk factors. Reversion to previous behaviors that are risk factors (eg, smoking and lack of exercise) may be related to anxiety and depression or may be due to lack of support or reinforcement of health-promotion strategies and resulting maladjustment after discharge.

Health-related quality of life is a concept that has gained considerable popularity in recent years, as we attempt to gain a multidimensional view of an individual's health status.[23,24] However, instruments designed to measure health-related quality of life have limited usefulness for determining the needs of the individual and diminish the importance of feelings and emotions not measured within the instruments' constructs. In addition, debate exists about the usefulness of disease-specific versus generic instruments. Despite these issues, instruments such as the Medical Outcomes Study (MOS) SF-36[25] are increasingly used in clinical research to examine health status, functional status, and quality-of-life concepts.

Although secondary prevention is important, promoting life-style changes in patients who have had an initial cardiac event is difficult.[26] Evidence is strong that a significant proportion of patients return to their previous life-styles despite cardiac rehabilitation and education.[27,28] In addition, participation rates in formalized programs are low, and a desire exists to tailor programs to the specific needs of individuals.[29] Thus, the experiences during the convalescent period immediately after hospitalization of survivors of an acute cardiac event require detailed examination to determine what issues may influence patients' recovery and compliance with life-style changes.

METHODS

A descriptive exploratory design with a triangulated methodology was used to examine the health status, coping strategies, and social support received by the survivors of an AMI. A convenience sample of patients hospitalized for AMI were enrolled in the study after approval from the health service and the university's institutional ethics committees. Participants were recruited from 3 acute care facilities in the Southwestern Sydney Area Health Service, in consultation with the primary physicians of the survivors and specialist nursing staff. Inclusion criteria required participants to be English-speaking adults who were willing to participate in the study after their hospitalization for AMI.

Data collection comprised 4 phases: in the hospital and 7, 14, and 21 days after discharge. One of the investigators made initial contact with eligible patients within 5 days of each patient's admission to the hospital with myocardial infarction. Once the patient had been informed, written consent for participation in the study was obtained, and demographic and clinical baseline data were gathered. After discharge, participants were interviewed on 3 occasions with a semistructured interview schedule[3] and completed the following instruments: MOS SF-36,[25] Cardiac Change Scale,[30] Perceived Social Support Scale,[31] Jalowiec Coping Scale,[32] New York Heart Association (NYHA) classification,[33] and Canadian Cardiovascular Society (CCVS) Angina Scale.[34] Interviews were conducted in the homes of participants by an experienced cardiac research nurse. The confidentiality of participants was maintained by using a study number as the identifier on all audiotapes, questionnaires, and interview transcripts used in the study. As specified in the consent form, no information was revealed to a participant's physician except in instances in which the participant's welfare was at risk (eg, worsening angina). When such an instance occurred, the participant was made aware of the communication with the physician, and any actions were documented. Every effort was made to facilitate appropriate referral; for example, dietary advice and counseling were offered when appropriate and were provided with the participant's consent.

Each interview lasted approximately 1 hour, including the administration of the instruments. All interviews conducted after discharge were recorded on audiotape with the consent of the research participants. After each semistructured interview, participants were given the opportunity to discuss concerns or ask questions about their recovery. Questions concerned activity level, medications, episodes of chest pain, and a number of other issues. The specialist nurse who conducted the interview was in a position to provide advice and assistance with these issues. Study participants were interviewed 7 days, 14 days, and 21 days after discharge. The MOS SF-36, NYHA classification, CCVS Angina Scale, and interview schedule were used 7 days, 14 days, and 21 days after discharge, with the addition of the Perceived Social Support Scale and Cardiac Change Scale at 7 days and 21 days after discharge.

MEASURING INSTRUMENTS

The MOS SF-36[25] is a self-reported, 36-item generic measure of health status that has been used and validated in adults in the United States, the United Kingdom, some non–English-speaking countries, and Australia.[35] Numerous health concepts are measured by the MOS SF-36: physical functioning (10 items), physical role limitations (4 items), emotional role limitations (3 items), pain (2 items), social functioning (2 items), mental health (5 items), vitality (4 items), general health perceptions (5 items), and change in health status (1 item). Raw scores are transformed to a 0 to 100 scale. Australian testing has confirmed appropriate psychometric properties, including discrimination between no illness and minor illness.[36]

The Cardiac Change Scale[30] is a 14-item self-reported measure that specifies areas of a person's life that are perceived to have changed as a result of cardiac illness. Items were based on factors commonly described in the literature as central to recovery from congestive heart disease: changes in cardiac risk factors, changes in involvement with families and friends, and changes in other factors related to recovery from illness (eg, attention to medical information, future plans, views of self). A 7-point Likert-scale response format (1 = not at all, to 7 = a great deal) is used to indicate the level of change associated with various activities. Scores range from 1 to 7. Psychometric properties were reported in only one study;[30] internal consistency was 0.92 and test–retest reliability was 0.66. In that study, criterion validity of this scale was supported by the Psychological Distress Scale but not by the Symptom Checklist. Apparently, the Cardiac Change Scale is a sensitive measure of psychological adjustment rather than of symptom reporting.

The Perceived Social Support Scale[31] is a 12-item scale with a 7-point Likert scale (1 = very strongly disagree, to 7 = very strongly agree). This scale addresses perceived support from families, friends, and significant others. Internal consistency coefficients for the total scale, and for the significant others, families, and friends subscales were reported as 0.88, 0.99, 0.87, and 0.85, respectively. In addition to the good internal consistency, the Perceived Social Support Scale has adequate stability over a 2- to 3-month period.

The Jalowiec Coping Scale[32] is a 60-item, 4-point Likert-type scale questionnaire that examines the types and frequencies of use of coping strategies. Items are classified into 8 coping styles: confrontive, evasive, optimistic, fatalistic, emotive, palliative, and supportive. Scores range from 0 to 3 for each coping style. The Jalowiec Coping Scale has been used in more than 25 studies in various clinical populations, including patients with cancer, cardiac problems, chronic pain, diabetes, gastrointestinal disorders, and psychiatric disorders.[32] Internal consistency coefficients (Cronbach α) for total use and total effectiveness of the Jalowiec Coping Scale from the results of 24 studies were 0.86 and 0.91, respectively.[32] In the study reported here, the scale was administered only once (at 7 days after discharge), because Grady and Jalowiec[32] reported stability of various coping styles during short retest intervals.

The NYHA classification[33] and CCVS Angina Scale[34] are tools for assessing functional status specifically in patients with ischemic heart disease. The NYHA classification grades level of dyspnea in relation to physical activity on a 4-point Likert-type scale, and the CCVS Angina Scale grades angina pectoris on a 4-point Likert-type scale.

DATA ANALYSIS

Descriptive statistics were used to summarize the characteristics of the study population: percentages for discrete variables, and mean and SD for continuous variables. Changes in cardiac symptoms, attitude, and health behaviors were tested by repeated analyses of variance. Changes in cardiac recovery and social support scores measured at 7 days and 21 days after discharge were compared by using a paired t test. The change in health status measured by the MOS SF-36 was investigated by using repeated-measures analysis of variance. The level of statistical significance for analyses was set at $P < .05$. All audiotaped interviews were transcribed verbatim and then subjected to thematic analysis.[37]

RESULTS

Thirty-eight participants completed the study. Table 1 describes the demographic and clinical characteristics of the sample at baseline. Mean age was 58.4 years (SD, 8.8 years), and the mean age for male participants (56 years) was 8 years younger than the mean age for female participants (64 years). About two thirds of the participants were men, and one quarter were from a non-English-speaking background. Fifty-five percent of participants were born in Australia, and the remaining 45% were from several European countries, South America, the United States, and New Zealand. The majority of participants spoke English at home (66%), but 13% spoke their language of origin, and 8% spoke both languages.

The majority (66%) had high-school education as their highest educational attainment, and more than half of the participants (53%) were still in paid employment. Participants were predominantly (70%) from a background of trade or laboring work. On hospital admission, the majority of participants had no history of AMI (94%), angina (77%), or previous coronary artery bypass graft surgery (80%). High cholesterol levels and hypertension were present in 63% and 45% of the sample, respectively. Sixty-three percent had never smoked, 34% were previous smokers, and only one person (3%) was currently a smoker.

Change in health status measured by SF-36

Figure 1 illustrates the 8 concepts related to health status measured with the SF-36 at the 3 measurement points (7 days, 14 days, and 21 days after discharge). During the period when measurements were made, some improvement in the health status concepts was apparent at each subsequent point; only general health decreased slightly between 7 and 21 days after discharge. However, the only significant difference was for emotional role functioning between 7 days and 21 days ($P = .01$). No significant correlations were evident between sex of the patient, cardiac recovery, social support, and health status.

Coping

Coping was measured at 7 days after discharge by using the Jalowiec Coping Scale. The results indicated that 3 coping styles were used most often: confrontive, optimistic, and self-reliant (Figure 2). The same 3 coping styles were also more effective than the other coping styles (Figure 3).

TABLE 1 Demographic and clinical characteristics of patients at baseline (N = 38)

CHARACTERISTIC	VALUE
Age, years	
Mean/SD	58.4/8.8
Range	45–77
Sex	
Male	26 (68)
Female	12 (32)
Language spoken at home*	
English	25 (66)
Non-English (own language)	5 (13)
Both	3 (8)
Highest educational level	
Primary school	6 (16)
High school	25 (66)
Beyond high school	7 (18)
Employment status	
Paid work	20 (53)
Home duties	2 (5)
Unemployed	1 (3)
Retired	15 (39)
CORONARY RISK FACTORS AT BASELINE	
Body mass index†	
Mean/SD	28.5/7.6
Range	19.1–49.7
Body mass index > 25	19 (50)
Hypertension	17 (45)
Hyperlipidemia	24 (63)
Diabetes	6 (16)
Smokers	1 (3)
Minimal or no regular exercise	14 (37)

Values are number (percentage) of patients unless otherwise indicated.

*Percentages do not total 100 because of missing data.
†Body mass index is calculated as weight in kilograms divided by the square of height in meters.

FIGURE 1 Health status as measured by the SF-36

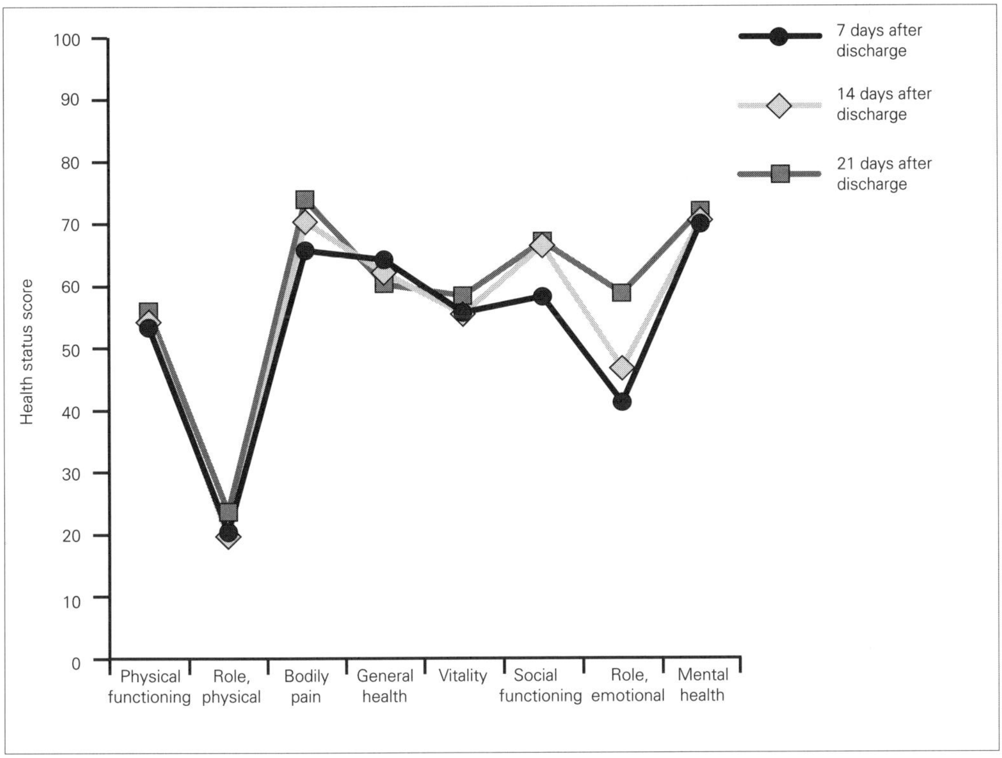

FIGURE 2 Coping styles of survivors

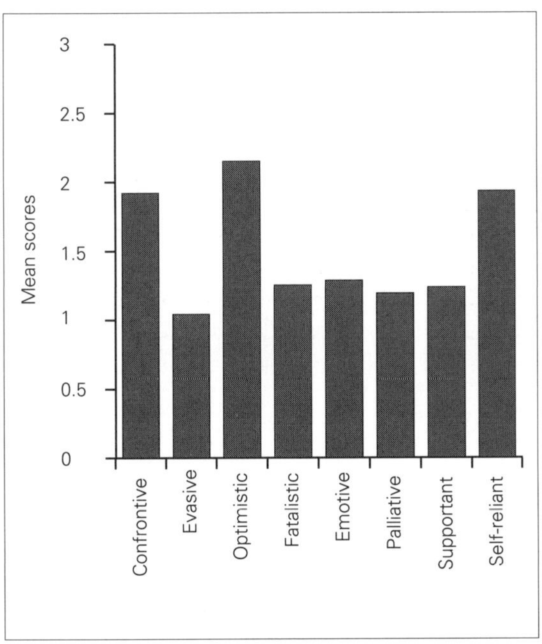

FIGURE 3 **Effectiveness of coping styles of survivors**

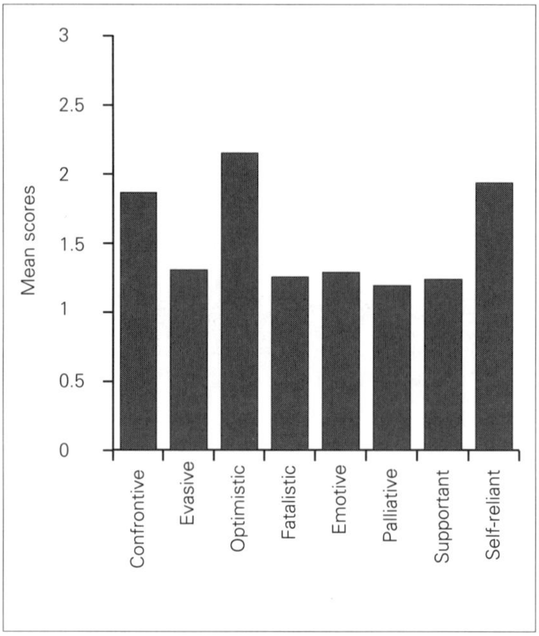

Cardiac symptoms, attitude, health behavior, social support, and cardiac recovery

Table 2 gives the changes in cardiac symptoms, attitude, and health behaviors across the study period. The percentage of survivors reporting symptoms of cardiac dysfunction measured by the CCVS Angina Scale and the NYHA classification remained about the same in the first 3 weeks (day 7 to day 21) after discharge from the hospital. The percentage of survivors reporting a significant change in their attitude about life increased from 63% at day 7 to 84% at day 21. Abstinence from smoking was maintained across the 3 measurement points after discharge, including abstinence by the survivor who had smoked at baseline. The percentage of survivors who reported that they were adhering to a low-fat diet increased through the 3 time points after discharge (from 84% to 90%). The percentage of survivors who reported that they were getting regular exercise also increased through the 3 time points (from 66% to 76%). A non-significant decrease in the mean social support score occurred from day 7 to day 21 (from 74 to 72), and the mean cardiac recovery score increased slightly (from 47 to 48) during that period, also not a significant change.

Qualitative findings

Analysis of qualitative data from the 26 male participants revealed a range of themes pertaining to coping. These themes included emphasis on anticipating resumption of valued tasks and activities and minimizing the significance of the AMI and its implications. However, data analysis also revealed flux in emotions for all of the study participants. This flux was manifested as a constellation of phenomena, including anxiety, depression, ambiguity and uncertainty, fear of recurrence of the AMI and deterioration in health, and boredom and inertia inflicted by the restrictions imposed by recovery routine. In addition, the survivors reported a struggle to integrate changes in their life-style. This struggle involved trying to deal with the required changes in diet and commitment to and compliance with exercise and other changes in life-style patterns related to cardiac rehabilitation process. Generally, to have their needs met, participants turned to their spouses or families. However, for a minority in the sample, disharmony developed in their relationships. For example, at least one participant reported that he was arguing with his spouse for the first time in their 7-year marriage. Findings suggest that this period was also stressful for the wives of survivors, because the women had to make changes to their own domestic routines, for example, in the area of food purchase and preparation.

TABLE 2 Changes in cardiac symptoms, attitude, health behavior, social support, and cardiac recovery

		DAYS AFTER DISCHARGE			
CHARACTERISTIC	**IN HOSPITAL**	**7**	**14**	**21**	***P***
Cardiac symptoms					
No angina (CCVS Angina Scale), %	42	79	66	71	<.001*
No dyspnea (NYHA classification), %	71	74	71	74	.96*
Attitude					
Significant change	NM	63	76	84	.02*
Life-style					
Significant change	NM	71	71	76	.57*
Health behavior					
Regular alcohol consumption, %	29	13	13	11	.01*
Smoking abstinence, %	97	100	100	100	.40*
Low-fat diet, %	NM	84	87	90	.69*
Regular exercise, %	63	66	68	76	.51*
Social support score, mean (SD)	NM	74.0 (13.2)	NM	72.2 (12.9)	.06†
Cardiac recovery score, mean (SD)	NM	47.1 (18.0)	NM	48.1 (19.6)	.79†

CCVS indicates Canadian Cardiovascular Society; NM, not measured; NYHA, New York Heart Association.
*Repeated-measures analysis of variance.
†Paired *t* test.

Analysis of qualitative data from the 12 female survivors revealed both similarities to and differences from the data of male survivors. Similarities included anticipating resumption of valued tasks and activities and emotional flux. As in the male survivors, this emotional flux was manifested as anxiety, depression, ambiguity and uncertainty, fear of recurrence of the AMI, and fear of further deterioration in health. Female survivors also reported a struggle to integrate changes in their life-style. Although the women also drew strength and support from family, they also reported seeking assistance with coping from other groups, such as church groups. Unlike the male survivors, the female survivors sought to allay anxiety by actively seeking information about cardiac health from organizations such as the Australian National Heart Foundation. The women did not report any marital disharmony.

DISCUSSION

Results of this study indicate relative stability in the health status of AMI survivors from 1 to 3 weeks after discharge from the hospital. Levels of health status for participants in this study were considerably lower than age-adjusted and age-matched (55–64 years old) scores from normative data for the Australian population.[38,39] In particular, participants had lower levels of physical functioning, physical role functioning, social functioning, and emotional role functioning. However, the health status scores of the participants for bodily pain, general health, vitality, and mental health, although lower than those for the comparative groups, were not considerably different. When compared with findings for a sample of participants who had illnesses and hospitalization in the preceding 12 months,[36] the findings differed slightly from the above. The scores for general health and vitality in this study were slightly higher than the scores reported by McCallum,[35] although the scores for physical functioning, physical role functioning, social functioning, and emotional role functioning were all lower than those reported by McCallum, and scores for bodily pain and mental health were similar to those reported by McCallum.

Previous researchers who examined the adjustment and experiences of survivors during the period after hospitalization for AMI found that this period is particularly stressful; uncertainty contributes to emotional distress,[20] and both emotional reactions and changes in physical condition are of concern to survivors,[40,41] resulting in the phenomenon of cardiac invalidism.[42] Family and social support and the effects of relationship dynamics were important concepts,[43,44] with positive psychosocial adjustment to cardiac disease[45] and perceived physical recovery[46] influenced by the quality of the survivor's relationship with his or her spouse.

Scherck[47] examined short-term coping in the first 3 days after a myocardial infarction and found that a variety of strategies were evident (eg, confrontive, self-reliance, optimism), with little denial apparent. This absence of denial differs from the levels of denial found in previous studies.[16] Moser and Dracup[18] examined the influence of individual perceptions of control on psychosocial recovery 6 months after an acute cardiac event. They found that persons with feelings of high control experienced less anxiety, depression, and hostility and had better psychosocial adjustment than did persons who had a low perception of control. Webster and Christman[20] reported that the postdischarge period for patients with AMI was particularly stressful, with uncertainty contributing to emotional distress and with problem-solving used in preference to effective coping strategies. Some studies examined differences between the sexes,[17] but sample sizes were often too small[48] or the percentages of women involved were insufficient for adequate comparisons to be made.[49]

Qualitative methods were used to define 4 stages of adjustment after AMI that patients pass through in striving to regain personal control; acceptance of limitations, refocusing on other life issues, and a sense of control are components of the final phase.[2] Similarly, Thompson et al[3] found 6 major themes in the first month after AMI among survivors and survivors' partners: expectations about advice and information, feelings about the future, reflections of the partner, playing down the significance of the heart attack, wanting to get back to normal, and the effect on the couple's relationship.

Implications for nursing practice

The findings of this study help elucidate the experiences during the period immediately after discharge from the hospital of survivors of an AMI and have significant implications for nursing practice. The results emphasize the importance of and the need for effective discharge planning and preparation of patients and their families for common feelings, experiences, and emotions they may experience after discharge. AMI survivors and their families also need continued healthcare support after discharge from the hospital.[44]

Recommendations for further research

This study provides useful insight into the experiences of survivors of AMI in the period immediately after discharge from the hospital. The generalizability of these results, however, is limited by convenience sampling and sample size. The study evokes the question of how much recuperative time is required before a patient returns to optimal health status after AMI. Clearly, the time frame is beyond the 3-week period after discharge examined in this study. A related issue is whether AMI survivors return to a health state similar to that of their age-matched community. Further issues to be examined include coping and adjustment of AMI survivors, particularly the elderly, who live alone without social support. It would be useful to replicate this study with a larger sample and examine the experiences of different ethnic groups. Such information would provide cardiovascular nurses with a valuable foundation for development of interventions to facilitate transition to wellness among AMI survivors in the vulnerable period after discharge from the hospital.

Acknowledgments

Funding for this study was provided by the Australian Rotary Health Research Fund.

References

1. Conn, V., Taylor, S. & Wiman, P. (1991). Anxiety, depression, quality of life, and self-care among survivors of myocardial infarction. *Issues Ment Health Nurs*, 12, 321–31.
2. Johnson, J. & Morse, J. (1990). Regaining control: the process of adjustment after myocardial infarction. *Heart Lung*, 19, 126–35.
3. Thompson, D.R., Ersser, S.J. & Webster, R.A. (1995). The experiences of patients and their partners 1 month after a heart attack. *J Adv Nurs*, 22, 707–14.
4. Fiebach, N., Viscoli, C. & Horwitz, R. (1990). Differences between women and men in survival after myocardial infarction. *JAMA*, 263, 1092–97.
5. Shanfield, S. (1990). Return to work after an acute myocardial infarction: a review. *Heart Lung*, 19, 109–17.
6. Crowe, J., Runions, J., Ebbsen, L., Oldridge, N. & Streiner, D. (1996). Anxiety and depression after acute myocardial infarction (AMI). *Heart Lung*, 25, 99–107.
7. Elliott, D. (1994). The effects of music and muscle relaxation on patient anxiety in a coronary care unit. *Heart Lung*, 23, 27–35.
8. Frederickson, N. (1989). Anxiety transmission in the patient with myocardial infarction. *Heart Lung*, 18, 617–22.

9. Malan, S. (1992). Psychosocial adjustment following MI: current views and nursing implications. *J Cardiovasc Nurs*, 6, 57–70.
10. Sykes, D. (1994). Coping with a heart attack: psychological processes. *Ir J Psychol*, 15, 54–66.
11. Frasure-Smith, N., Lesperance, F. & Talajic, M. (1993). Depression following myocardial infarction: impact on 6-month survival. *JAMA*, 270, 1819–25.
12. Schleifer, P.M., Macari-Hinson, M.M., Coyle, D.A. et al. (1989). The nature and course of depression following myocardial infarction. *Arch Intern Med*, 149, 1785–89.
13. Shively, M., Verderber, A. & Fitzsimmons, L. (1992). Depression in the post MI patient. *J Cardiovasc Nurs*, 6, 84–86.
14. Silverstone, P.H. (1987). Depression and outcome in acute myocardial infarction. *Br Med J (Clin Res Ed)*, 294, 219–20.
15. Lowery, B.J. (1991). Psychological stress, denial and myocardial infarction outcomes. *Image J Nurs Sch*, 23, 51–55.
16. Robinson, K.R. (1990). Denial in myocardial infarction patients. *Crit Care Nurse*, 10, 138–45.
17. Conn, V., Taylor, S. & Abele, P. (1991). Myocardial infarction survivors: age and gender differences in physical health, psychosocial state and regimen adherence. *J Adv Nurs*, 16, 1026–34.
18. Moser, D.K. & Dracup, K. (1995). Psychosocial recovery from a cardiac event: the influence of perceived control. *Heart Lung*, 24, 273–80.
19. Christman, N.J., McConnell, E.A., Pfeiffer, C., Webster, K., Schmitt, M. & Reis, J. (1988). Uncertainty, coping and distress following myocardial infarction: transition from hospital to home. *Res Nurs Health*, 11, 71–82.
20. Webster, K. & Christman, N. (1988). Perceived uncertainty and coping post myocardial infarction. *West J Nurs Res*, 10, 384–400.
21. Wishnie, H., Hackett, T. & Cassem, N. (1971). Psychological hazards of convalescence following myocardial infarction. *JAMA*, 215, 1291–96.
22. Scalzi, C.C., Burke, L.E. & Greenland, S. (1980). Evaluation of an inpatient educational program for coronary patients and families. *Heart Lung*, 9, 846–53.
23. Bowling, A. (1995). *Measuring disease: a review of disease-specific quality of life measurement scales.* Buckingham, England, Open University Press.
24. Fallowfield, L. (1993). Quality of life assessment in patients with heart disease. *Br Heart J*, 69, 371–72.
25. Ware, J.E. Jr, Snow, K.K., Kosinski, M. & Gandek, B. (1993). *SF-36 Health survey manual and interpretation guide.* Boston, Mass., The Health Institute, New England Medical Center.
26. Jones, D. & West, R. (1996). Psychological rehabilitation after myocardial infarction (MI): multicenter randomised trial. *BMJ*, 313, 1517–21.
27. Miller, P., Wikoff, R., McMahon, M., Garrett, M.J. & Ringel, K. (1988). Influence of nursing intervention on regimen adherence and societal adjustments postmyocardial infarction. *Nurs Res*, 37, 297–302.
28. Reid, R.D. (1995). Why don't they stay changed? *Can J Cardiol*, 11, 26A–29A.
29. *Improving cardiac care and outcomes: New South Wales policy standards for cardiac rehabilitation.* Sydney, New South Wales Dept of Health (C) 9701120.
30. Fowers, B.J. & Eisen, M. (1994). Cardiac Change Scale: a brief self-report research measure. *Curr Psychol*, 13, 185–92.
31. Blumenthal, J.A., Barefoot, J., Haney, T. & Zimet, G. (1987). Social support, type A behavior, and coronary artery disease. *Psychosom Med*, 49, 331–40.

32. Grady, K.L. & Jalowiec, A. (1995). Predictors of compliance with diet 6 months after heart transplantation. *Heart Lung*, 24, 359–68.
33. Kossman, C.E. (1964). Diseases of the heart and blood vessels: nomenclature and criteria for diagnosis. *Heart Lung*, 19, 126–35.
34. Campeau, L. (1976). Grading of angina pectoris. *Circulation*, 54, 522–23.
35. McCallum, J. (1995). The SF-36 in an Australian sample: validating a new, generic health status measure. *Aust J Public Health*, 19, 160–66.
36. McCallum, J. (1994). *The new SF-36 health status measure: Australian validity tests.* Canberra, Australian National University.
37. Smith, P. (1998). *Nursing research: setting new agendas.* London, Arnold Books.
38. Stevenson, C. (1995). Developing population norms for SF-36 from a sample survey. In *Proceedings of the health outcomes and quality of life measurement conference, Canberra, 14–15 August 1995.* Canberra, Australian Institute of Health and Welfare.
39. Williamson, M., Jorm, L., Cardona, M. & Chey, T. (1994). *Blacktown health survey 1993.* Westmead, NSW, Western Sydney Area Health Service.
40. Ford, J. (1989). Living with a history of heart attack: a human science investigation. *J Adv Nurs*, 14, 173–79.
41. Jaarsma, T., Kastermans, M., Dassen, T., Philipsen, H. (1995). Problems of cardiac patients in early recovery. *J Adv Nurs*, 21, 21–27.
42. Riegel, B.J., Dracup, K.A. & Glaser, D. (1998). A longitudinal causal model of cardiac invalidism following myocardial infarction. *Nurs Res*, 46, 285–92.
43. Hilgenberg, C. & Crowley, C. (1987). Changes in family patterns after a myocardial infarction. *Home Health Nurse*, 5 (26), 17, 30–32.
44. Riegel, B. & Dracup, K. (1992). Does overprotection cause cardiac invalidism after acute myocardial infarction? *Heart Lung*, 21, 529–35.
45. Brecht, M., Dracup, K., Moser, D. & Riegel, B. (1994). The relationship of marital quality and psychosocial adjustment to heart disease. *J Cardiovasc Nurs*, 9, 74–85.
46. Yates, B.C. (1995). The relationships among social support and short- and long-term recovery outcomes in men with coronary heart disease. *Res Nurs Health*, 18, 193–203.
47. Scherck, K. (1992). Coping with acute myocardial infarction. *Heart Lung*, 21, 327–34.
48. Ashton, K. & Saccucci, M. (1996). A follow-up study of ethnic and gender differences in cardiac rehabilitation. *Rehabil Nurs*, 21, 187–95.
49. Schuster, P. & Waldron, J. (1991). Gender differences in cardiac rehabilitation patients. *Rehabil Nurs*, 16, 248–53.

Randomised controlled trial of midwife led debriefing to reduce maternal depression after operative childbirth

Rhonda Small, Judith Lumley, Lisa Donohue, Anne Potter, Ulla Waldenström

OBJECTIVE: To assess the effectiveness of a midwife led debriefing session during the postpartum hospital stay in reducing the prevalence of maternal depression at six months postpartum among women giving birth by caesarean section, forceps, or vacuum extraction.

DESIGN: Randomised controlled trial.

SETTING: Large maternity teaching hospital in Melbourne, Australia.

PARTICIPANTS: 1041 women who had given birth by caesarean section (n = 624) or with the use of forceps (n = 353) or vacuum extraction (n = 64).

MAIN OUTCOME MEASURES: Maternal depression (score ≥ 13 on the Edinburgh postnatal depression scale) and overall health status (comparison of mean scores on SF-36 subscales) measured by postal questionnaire at six months postpartum.

RESULTS: 917 (88%) of the women recruited responded to the outcome questionnaire. More women allocated to debriefing scored as depressed six months after birth than women allocated to usual postpartum care (81 (17%) *v* 65 (14%)), although this difference was not significant (odds ratio = 1.24, 95% confidence interval 0.87 to 1.77). They were also more likely to report that depression had been a problem for them since the birth, but the difference was not significant (123 (28%) *v* 94 (22%); odds ratio = 1.37, 1.00 to 1.86). Women allocated to debriefing had poorer health status on seven of the eight SF-36 subscales, although the difference was significant only for role functioning (emotional): mean scores 73.32 *v* 78.98, t = –2.31, 95% confidence interval –10.48 to –0.84).

CONCLUSIONS: Midwife led debriefing after operative birth is ineffective in reducing maternal morbidity at six months postpartum. The possibility that debriefing contributed to emotional health problems for some women cannot be excluded.

Editorial by Kenardy.

Centre for the Study of Mothers' and Children's Health, School of Public Health, La Trobe University, Carlton Vic. 3053, Australia.

British Medical Journal, 321, 1043–47, 28 October 2000; reprinted with the permission of the *British Medical Journal*.

INTRODUCTION

Operative birth has been associated with considerable maternal morbidity, including depression, guilt, regret, loss of self esteem, prolonged pain, discomfort, infection, grief reactions, feelings of violation, dissatisfaction with care, and occasionally hostility to hospital staff.[1–6] One intervention recommended to reduce morbidity, particularly psychological morbidity, is debriefing.[3] Women are given a structured opportunity to discuss their experiences of labour and delivery with an empathic listener shortly after the birth. Debriefing has been recommended as a health promoting strategy for all women after childbirth, in recognition that even an uncomplicated birth can be traumatic[7,8] and in the belief that 'talking things through' can only prove beneficial. A recent survey of health trusts in England and Wales (response rate 183/211) found that 36% have formal arrangements in place for debriefing women after childbirth and another 26% have plans to introduce such an arrangement (S. Marchant, L. Davidson & J. Garcia, personal communication).

Outside obstetrics, psychological debriefing after traumatic events has been common for many years, despite the paucity of rigorous research evaluating its effectiveness.[9,10] Concerns about the potential for debriefing to do harm have been highlighted in the first systematic review,[11] which not only found no evidence of benefit but also reported significantly increased odds of post-traumatic stress disorder at 13 months in patients with burn trauma who had received debriefing.[12]

Only one trial included in the systematic review was in reproductive medicine. This study found that subsequent emotional adaptation after spontaneous miscarriage was not significantly influenced by debriefing.[13] Two trials of debriefing after childbirth have been reported: one small trial in the United Kingdom reported positive findings for debriefing,[8] whereas the other, larger trial from Australia found no positive effect.[14] The current study arose from an Australian population based survey that found raised rates of depression eight to nine months postpartum in women who had operative deliveries (adjusted odds ratio = 2.03) compared with women who had spontaneous vaginal deliveries.[2]

PARTICIPANTS AND METHODS

Aims

The primary aims were to reduce the prevalence of depression by one third (defined as a score of $\geqslant 13$ on the Edinburgh postnatal depression scale[15]) six months after the birth, from an expected 24% in the standard care group[2] to 16% in the debriefing group and to improve overall maternal health (as measured by mean scores on the SF-36 health status measure subscales[16]). A secondary aim was to reduce dissatisfaction with postpartum hospital care.

Sample size and study power

The sample size ($\alpha = 0.05$, two sided $\beta = 0.20$) required for the primary aim was 416 in each group. We aimed to recruit 1040 women to allow for a 5% refusal rate and a possible loss to follow up of 20%. This sample size was also more than adequate to detect a clinically important reduction in dissatisfaction with postpartum care (from 30% dissatisfied[17] to 20%).

Recruitment

Recruitment took place at one of Melbourne's three teaching hospitals from March 1996 to October 1998. Two research midwives (LD, AP) identified women who had had operative deliveries from the labour ward records and approached women on the postnatal ward at least 24 hours after the birth of their babies. We excluded women who had had stillbirths or babies weighing less than 1500 g, women with insufficient English to take part, women who were ill or whose babies were ill, and women whose private obstetricians had refused permission to approach them.

A plain language information sheet about the study was provided to women, and written informed consent was obtained from all participants. Women completed a brief questionnaire providing sociodemographic data. Each midwife carried out recruitment and debriefing for half of each week's participants.

Randomisation

We used telephone randomisation to allocate women to debriefing or standard care, with allocation determined by separate computer generated, adaptive biased coin randomisation schedules for each research midwife.

Women allocated to standard care received a brief visit from the midwife to give them a pamphlet on sources of assistance for mothers on discharge from hospital. Women allocated to debriefing also received the pamphlet, and the midwife arranged a time for the debriefing session.

Debriefing intervention

The debriefing intervention provided women with an opportunity to discuss their labour, birth, and post-delivery events and experiences. Debriefing took place before the women were discharged from hospital. Both AP and LD are midwives experienced in talking with women about birth, able to listen with empathy to women's accounts, and aware of the common concerns and issues arising for women after an operative birth. Content of the discussion was determined by each woman's experiences and concerns, and up to one hour was made available for the session.

Each debriefing session was documented by the research midwife at the end of the session using a standard reporting sheet. The information recorded included duration of debriefing session, main issues and concerns raised by the woman, themes discussed, and support provided.

Outcome assessment

The primary outcomes were the prevalence of maternal depression at six months postpartum measured by the Edinburgh postnatal depression scale and overall maternal health status measured by the SF-36. These scales were assessed by a postal questionnaire sent to all participants. We chose to assess depression at six months because we had previously found raised rates of depression in the second half year after operative birth[2] and because of other evidence of a high incidence of new cases of depression between the third and ninth month postpartum.[18,19]

The questionnaire also included detailed questions on satisfaction with care, experience of the birth, health problems, and (for women in the debriefing arm) opinion about the helpfulness of debriefing. The sequencing of the Edinburgh postnatal depression scale and the SF-36 was alternated in the questionnaires to reduce any completion order effect.

Data management and analysis

A coding schedule was developed by three of us (AP, JL, RS) with initial cross checking to ensure coding consistency. Questionnaires were then coded by one of us (AP). Data were double entered and validated. An intention to treat analysis was undertaken with SPSS PC +[20] and STATA[21] statistical packages. We used the recommended cut off for probable depression of 13 on the Edinburgh postnatal depression scale and assessed differences between the trial groups using odds ratios. Mean scores on the SF-36 subscales were compared by Student's *t* test and 95% confidence intervals.We compared women's views of their postpartum hospital care (ratings of statements about care on a seven point scale) using ordinal logistic regression to provide a cumulative odds ratio that indicated the degree of association between trial group and agreement with the statement over the whole scale.[21]

RESULTS

Recruitment and participation

Figure 1 summarises recruitment and participation and Table 1 outlines the reasons for non-participation. Response rates to the outcome questionnaire were high: 467/520 (90%) women in the debriefing arm and 450/521 (86%) in the standard care arm returned completed questionnaires (total = 917, 88% of women recruited). The difference in response rates between the two groups was not significant (odds ratio = 1.39, 95% confidence interval 0.94 to 2.07).

FIGURE 1 **Recruitment and participation of women in the trial**

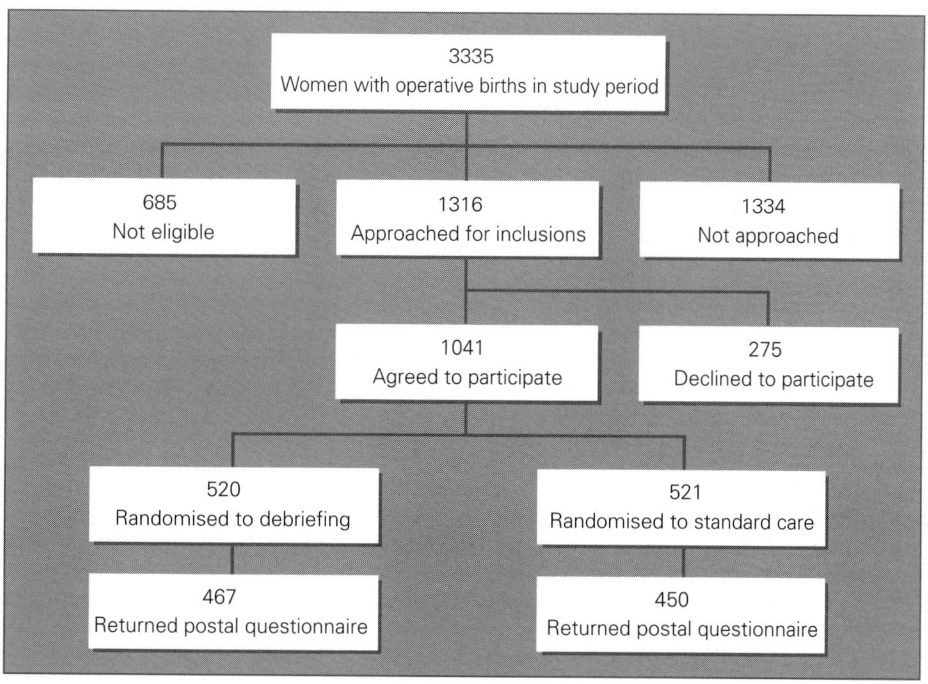

TABLE 1 Reasons for non-participation in study

REASON FOR NON-PARTICIPATION	No (%) OF WOMEN
Not eligible:	
Insufficient English	440 (19.2)
Low birthweight baby	152 (6.6)
Baby unwell	39 (1.7)
Woman unwell	39 (1.7)
Stillbirth or neonatal death	15 (0.7)
Not approached:	
Doctor had declined study participation for all his or her patients	387 (16.9)
Going home too soon to take part	376 (16.4)
Already discharged	334 (14.6)
Unavailable or too busy	145 (6.3)
Other reasons	92 (4.0)
Declined invitation to participate	275 (12.0)
Total	2294 (100)

Characteristics of study participants

Table 2 shows that the characteristics of the two study groups were comparable after randomisation. Compared with non-respondents, women who returned the outcome questionnaire were more likely to be older, married, better educated, have higher family incomes, to speak English very well if English was not their first language, and to have private health insurance.

Telephone follow up of non-respondents identified eight women who reported problems with depression. Some of the eight had received treatment, including one woman who was readmitted to hospital with probable puerperal psychosis. Two of the eight were in the debriefing group and six in the standard care group.

Maternal health outcomes

Women allocated to debriefing were not less likely to score as depressed on the Edinburgh postnatal depression scale than women allocated to standard care (Table 3). The odds of depression in the debriefing group were raised, although not significantly. The mean scores did not differ significantly between the groups ($t = 1.17$, $P = 0.24$).

Women were also asked whether 'feeling depressed or very unhappy for more than a few days' had been a problem for them in the six months since the birth. Although a higher proportion of women in the debriefing group reported depression as a problem, the difference was not significant (123/445 (28%) *v* 94/430 (22%); odds ratio = 1.37, 95% confidence interval 1.00 to 1.86).

Table 4 shows women's mean scores on the subscales of the SF-36. Women allocated to debriefing had poorer health status on seven of the eight subscales, although the difference was significant only for role functioning (emotional).

Women's views about debriefing and postpartum care

Women were positive about debriefing, with only 26/463 (6%) rating the debriefing session as 'unhelpful'; 200 (43%) rated it as 'very helpful' and 237 (51%) as 'helpful'.

TABLE 2 Characteristics of study participants

CHARACTERISTIC (TOTAL NO OF RESPONDENTS IN DEBRIEFING/ STANDARD CARE ARMS)	NO (%) IN DEBRIEFING ARM	NO (%) IN STANDARD CARE ARM
Method of operative birth (*n* = 467/450):		
Elective caesarean	125 (27)	113 (25)
Emergency caesarean	162 (35)	145 (32)
Forceps	155 (33)	162 (36)
Vacuum extraction	25 (5)	30 (7)
Parity (*n* = 467/449):		
Primiparous	284 (61)	296 (66)
Multiparous	183 (39)	153 (34)
Maternal age (years) (*n* = 466/450):		
<25	45 (10)	53 (12)
25–34	296 (64)	275 (61)
⩾35	125 (27)	122 (27)
Marital status (*n* = 467/450):		
Married	360 (77)	348 (77)
Cohabiting	83 (18)	78 (17)
Separated, divorced, or widowed	7 (1)	5 (1)
Single	17 (4)	19 (4)
Secondary education (*n* = 466/449):		
Completed year 12	306 (66)	304 (68)
Less than year 12	160 (34)	145 (32)
Tertiary education (*n* = 466/450):		
Degree or diploma	244 (52)	223 (50)
Other or none	222 (48)	227 (50)
English as first language (*n* = 467/449):		
Yes	404 (87)	372 (83)
No	63 (13)	77 (17)
English speaking ability if not first language (*n* = 63/77):		
Very good	50 (79)	55 (75)
Less than very good	13 (21)	22 (25)
Family income ($A)* (*n* = 444/427):		
⩽20 000	72 (16)	55 (13)
20 001–30 000	66 (15)	61 (14)
30 001–40 000	63 (14)	82 (19)
>40 000	243 (55)	229 (54)
Pension or benefit main income (*n* = 465/447):		
Yes	72 (15)	55 (12)
No	393 (85)	392 (88)
Health insurance (*n* = 467/449):		
Public	319 (68)	308 (69)
Private	148 (32)	141 (31)

*$1 = £0.40.

TABLE 3 Edinburgh postnatal depression scores for debriefing and standard care groups

	MEAN (SD)	MEDIAN (RANGE)	NO (%) DEPRESSED (SCORE≥13)	NO (%) NOT DEPRESSED	ODDS RATIO (95% CI)
Debriefing	7.16 (5.68)	6.00 (0–28)	81 (17)	386 (83)	1.24 (0.87 to 1.77)
Standard care	6.72 (5.50)	6.00 (0–29)	65 (14)	384 (86)	1.0

TABLE 4 Mean (SD) SF-36 scores for debriefing and standard care groups

SF-36 SUBSCALE	DEBRIEFING	STANDARD CARE	*t* TEST (95% CI FOR DIFFERENCE)
Physical functioning	86.1 (17.40)	85.73 (18.44)	0.32 (–1.96 to 2.73)
Role functioning (physical)	73.86 (35.10)	76.24 (35.29)	–1.02 (–6.98 to 2.22)
Bodily pain	77.7 (23.22)	78.6 (23.55)	–0.59 (–3.95 to 2.13)
Mental health	69.69 (18.79)	71.20 (18.14)	–1.23 (–3.91 to 0.89)
Role functioning (emotional)	73.32 (38.12)	78.98 (35.73)	–2.31 (–10.48 to –0.84)
Vitality	50.08 (22.37)	51.28 (21.79)	–0.82 (–4.07 to 1.68)
Social functioning	78.78 (24.28)	80.47 (23.69)	–1.07 (–4.80 to 1.42)
General health	72.20 (20.91)	73.22 (21.00)	–0.73 (–3.75 to 1.72)

Participation in debriefing did not affect women's views of their postpartum hospital care. In response to the question 'How satisfied are you overall with the care you and your baby received in hospital after the birth?' the proportion of women responding that they were 'very happy' was similar in both groups (133/464 (29%) debriefing *v* 124/447 (28%) standard care). Likewise only 5% (24/464) of women in the debriefing group were 'very unhappy' with their care compared with 7% (31/447) in the standard care group. There were no significant differences in ratings on the seven point scale between the two groups (cumulative odds ratio = 0.97, 95% confidence interval 0.71 to 1.26; see *BMJ*'s website for further details) or in responses to more specific statements about different aspects of postpartum hospital care.

Effect of research midwife

We also analysed the primary trial outcomes for each research midwife separately and found no differences. Analysing by research midwife also made no difference to women's views about helpfulness of the debriefing sessions or about postpartum hospital care.

DISCUSSION

This study contributes to the small number of randomised trials evaluating the effectiveness of debriefing in reducing mental health problems after traumatic events. It supports the systematic summary of current evidence by Wessely and others, which found no beneficial effect of debriefing.[11]

Nearly all women who experienced debriefing said that they found the session helpful. This finding was also reported in two other trials in which debriefing was found to be ineffective in reducing psychological problems.[13,14] Not only did we find that health outcomes for the debriefing group were no better than those for women in the standard care group, we are not able to rule out the possibility that debriefing contributed to poorer emotional health. Women allocated to debriefing were more likely to report that depression had been a problem for them in the six months since the birth, and their SF-36 scores for emotional role functioning were significantly poorer. The non-significant differences on both the Edinburgh postnatal depression scale and the SF-36 were all in the direction of women in the debriefing group faring worse (with the exception of the SF-36 physical functioning subscale).

The UK trial that found a substantial benefit from midwifery led debriefing had several methodological problems.[8] The study was designed to identify a reduction in the proportion of women scoring above seven on the hospital anxiety and depression scale (from 48% to 24%), but the analysis was of the proportion of women scoring above 10, for which the sample size planned (120) was below that required (292). In standard care more than half of women scored over 10 on both subscales, far more than in the pre-trial pilot. A 'disappointment' factor may have increased the scores of women allocated to the control group. Outcome was assessed soon after hospital discharge, and the population was atypical: 59.6% were single women.

The idea that debriefing might be ineffective or even detrimental is not new. Some authors have raised the possibility of 'secondary trauma' resulting from re-exposure to the experience during the debriefing session,[10,11] and a process of distancing the self from the experience has been suggested to be potentially adaptive.[13] Timing of the debriefing session, the people involved, the presence or absence of other factors (personality traits, social support, and individual coping styles in response both to distress and to debriefing) may also be important in determining both psychological outcome after trauma and the potential effectiveness of debriefing.[9–11,22,23]

Evidence from randomised trials is critical to the resolution of these issues. Ours was a pragmatic trial, and the intervention was designed to be incorporated within standard postpartum care if it proved effective. Debriefing was arranged during the postpartum hospital stay, and we used midwives as 'debriefers' because of their predominant role in postpartum care. The use of midwives was also important given concerns that using mental health staff for debriefing might be detrimental, unnecessarily medicalising distress.[24] Our findings, however, provide no evidence to recommend debriefing by midwives for women after operative birth as a strategy to reduce subsequent maternal depression or improve women's views of their postpartum care.

We thank all the women who participated in the trial, the nursing and medical staff at the participating hospital for their facilitation of the project, and Lyn Watson for statistical advice and assistance.

Contributors: RS drafted the grant application for the study, participated jointly in protocol design and discussion of core ideas at research team meetings, was the principal investigator for the study in its final two years, conducted the data analysis, and drafted the paper. JL initiated the study, formulated the research questions, contributed to the grant application, participated jointly in protocol design and discussion of core ideas at research team meetings, and contributed to the writing of the paper. LD contributed to the grant application and protocol design, undertook recruitment and conducted the debriefing intervention, participated in data collection and discussion of core ideas at research team meetings, and contributed to the paper. AP contributed to protocol design, undertook recruitment and conducted the debriefing intervention, participated in data collection and discussion of core ideas at research team meetings, coded all the questionnaires, and contributed to the paper. UW participated jointly in protocol design and discussion of core ideas at research team meetings, was the principal investigator for the study in its first two years, and contributed to the paper.

Funding: Research and development grants advisory committee of the Australian Commonwealth Department of Health, Housing, and Community Services.

Competing interests: None declared.

WHAT IS ALREADY KNOWN ON THIS TOPIC

Operative birth has been associated with negative psychological sequelae for women, including depression, loss of self esteem, regret, guilt, and feelings of violation

Debriefing is widely used to reduce psychological disturbance after trauma despite little evidence of its effectiveness

Debriefing is being introduced for women after childbirth with the aim of improving psychological recovery

WHAT THIS STUDY ADDS

A midwife led debriefing session after an operative delivery did not reduce subsequent maternal depression, improve overall maternal health status, or increase satisfaction with postpartum care compared with standard care

The trend in all measures of psychological wellbeing was for women in the debriefing arm to fare worse, although the difference was significant for only one measure

The results do not support the introduction of routine debriefing after an operative delivery to improve maternal emotional health

References

1. Brown, S. & Lumley, J. (1998). Maternal health after childbirth: results of an Australian population based survey. *Br J Obstet Gynaecol*, 105, 156–61.
2. Astbury, J., Brown, S., Lumley, J. & Small, R. (1994). Birth events, birth experiences and social factors in depression after birth. *Aust J Public Health*, 18, 176–84.
3. Hillan, E.M. (1992). Short-term morbidity associated with caesarean delivery. *Birth*, 19, 190–94.
4. MacArthur, C., Lewis, M. & Knox, E.G. (1991). Health after childbirth. *Br J Obstet Gynaecol*, 98, 1193–1204.
5. Fisher, J., Stanley, R. & Burrows, G. (1990). Psychological adjustment to caesarean delivery: a review of the evidence. *J Psychosom Obstet Gynaecol*, 11, 91–106.

6. Elliott, S.A. (1984). Relationship between obstetric outcome and psychological measures in pregnancy and the postnatal year. *J Reprod Inf Psychol*, 2, 18–32.
7. Ralph, K. & Alexander, J. (1994). Borne under stress. *Nursing Times*, 90, 28–30.
8. Lavender, T. & Walkinshaw, S.A. (1998). Can midwives reduce postpartum psychological morbidity? A randomized trial. *Birth*, 25, 215–21.
9. Bisson, J.I. & Deahl, M.P. (1994). Psychological debriefing and prevention of post-traumatic stress: more research is needed. *Br J Psychiatry*, 165, 717–20.
10. Raphael, B. & Meldrum, L. (1995). Does debriefing after psychological trauma work? *BMJ*, 310, 1479–80.
11. Wessely, S., Rose, S. & Bisson, J. (1999). A systematic review of brief psychological interventions ('debriefing') for the treatment of immediate trauma related symptoms and the prevention of post traumatic stress disorder. In Cochrane Collaboration. *Cochrane Library*. Issue 4. Oxford, Update Software.
12. Bisson, J.I., Jenkins, P.L., Alexander, J. & Bannister, C. (1997). Randomised controlled trial of psychological debriefing for victims of acute burn trauma. *Br J Psychiatry*, 171, 78–81.
13. Lee, C., Slade, P. & Lygo, V. (1996). The influence of psychological debriefing on emotional adaptation of women following early miscarriage: a preliminary study. *Br J Med Psychol*, 69, 47–58.
14. Hagan, R., Priest, S., Evans, S., Malmgren, S., St Jack, A., Henderson, J. et al. (1999). Stress debriefing after childbirth: maternal outcomes [abstract A84]. In *Proceedings of the third annual congress of the Perinatal Society of Australia and New Zealand, March 1999*. Parramatta, NSW, PSANZ, 95.
15. Cox, J.L., Holden, J.M. & Sagovsky, R. (1987). Detection of postnatal depression: development of the 10-item Edinburgh postnatal depression scale. *Br J Psychiatry*, 150, 782–86.
16. Ware, J.E. & Sherbourne, C.D. (1992). The MOS 36-item short-form health survey (SF-36). 1. Conceptual framework and item selection. *Med Care*, 30, 473–83.
17. Brown, S., Lumley, J., Small, R. & Astbury, J. (1994). *Missing voices. The experience of motherhood* (p. 101). Melbourne, Oxford University Press.
18. Nott, P.N. (1987). Extent, timing and persistence of emotional disorders following childbirth. *Br J Psychiatry*, 151, 523–27.
19. O'Hara, M.W. & Swain, A.M. (1996). Rates and risk of postpartum depression—a meta-analysis. *Int Rev Psychiatry*, 8, 37–54.
20. SPSS Incorporated. (1998). *SPSS for windows, version 9.0*. Chicago IL, SPSS.
21. StataCorp. (1999). *Stata statistical software; release 6.0*. College Station, TX, Stata Corporation.
22. Conlon, L., Fahy, T.J. & Conroy, R. (1999). PTSD in ambulant RTA victims: a randomized controlled trial of debriefing. *J Psychosom Res*, 46, 37–44.
23. Hobbs, M., Mayou, R., Harrison, B. & Worlock, P. (1996). Randomised controlled trial of psychological debriefing for victims of road traffic accidents. *BMJ*, 313, 1438–39.
24. Wessely, S. (1998). Commentary: reducing distress after normal childbirth. *Birth*, 25, 220–21.

Glossary

abstract A brief, comprehensive summary of a study.
accessible population A population that meets the population criteria and is available.
action research Insider research in that practitioners research their own professional actions. It requires action as part of the research process itself and is focused on the researcher's professional values rather than methodological considerations.
after-only design An experimental design with two randomly assigned groups—a treatment group and a control group. This design differs from the true experiment in that both groups are measured only after the experimental treatment.
after-only non-equivalent control group design A quasi-experimental design similar to the after-only experimental design, but subjects are not randomly assigned to the treatment or control groups.
alternate form reliability Two or more alternate forms of a measure are administered to the same subjects at different times. The scores of the two tests determine the degree of relationship between the measures.
analysis of covariance (ANCOVA) A statistic that measures differences among means of three or more groups using a technique to equate the groups under study in relation to another important variable.
analysis of variance (ANOVA) A statistic that tests whether means for three or more groups differ from each other, rather than testing each pair of means separately; ANOVA considers the variation between all groups—equivalent to the *t* test for two groups.
animal rights Guidelines used to protect the rights of animals in the conduct of research.
anonymity A research participant's protection in a study so that no one, not even the researcher, can link the subject with the information given.
antecedent variable A variable that affects the dependent variable but occurs before the introduction of the independent variable.
applied research That which tests the practical limits of descriptive theories but does not examine the efficacy of actions taken by practitioners.
assumption A basic principle assumed to be true without the need for scientific proof.
auditability The researcher's development of the research process in a qualitative study that allows a researcher or reader to follow the thinking or conclusions of the researcher.
axial coding A data analysis strategy used in the grounded theory method. It requires intense coding around a single theme.
basic research Theoretical or pure research that generates, tests and expands theories that explain or predict a phenomenon.
beneficence An obligation to do no harm and to maximise possible benefits.
benefit Potential positive outcomes of participation in research study.
bias A distortion in the data analysis results.
bracketing A process during which the researcher identifies personal biases about the phenomenon of interest to clarify how personal experience and beliefs may colour what is heard and reported.
case study method The study of selected contemporary phenomenon over time to provide an in-depth description of essential dimensions and processes of the phenomenon.
chance error Measurement error which is attributable to fluctuations in subject characteristics that occur at a specific point in time and are often beyond the awareness and control of the examiner. Also called random error.
chi-square (χ^2) A non-parametric statistic used to determine whether the frequency measured in each category is different from the frequency that would be expected by chance.
clinical audits Monitor innovations, the use of interventions, and the quality of care patients receive against agreed standards.

clinical governance Aims to ensure that strategies/systems to monitor quality of clinical practice are functioning properly, that clinical practice is improved as a result, and that clinical practitioners meet the standards as required by their professional regulatory body.
close-ended item A question that the respondent may answer within a fixed number of choices.
cluster sampling A probability sampling strategy that involves a successive random sampling of units. The units sampled progress from large to small.
collaborative evaluation (fourth generation evaluation or FGE) An approach that moves beyond process evaluation strategies to include stakeholders in the evaluation.
concealment Refers to whether the subjects know that they are being observed.
concept An image or symbolic representation of an abstract idea.
conceptual definition The general meaning of a concept.
conceptual literature Published and unpublished non-data-based material, such as reports of theories, concepts, synthesis of research on concepts or professional issues, some of which underlie reported research, as well as other non-research material.
conceptual model A set of interrelated concepts that symbolically represents a phenomenon.
concurrent validity The degree of correlation of two measures of the same concept that are administered at the same time.
confidentiality The assurance that a research participant's identity cannot be linked to the information that was provided to the researcher.
consent See informed consent.
consistency The collection of data from each subject in the study in exactly the same way or as close to the same way as possible.
constancy Methods and procedures of data collection are the same for all subjects.
constant comparative method A process of continuously comparing data as they are acquired during research using the grounded theory method.
construct An abstraction that is adapted for scientific purpose.
construct replication The use of original methods, such as sampling techniques, instruments or research design, to study a problem that has been investigated previously.
construct validity The extent to which an instrument is said to measure a theoretical construct or trait.
consumer One who actively uses and applies research findings in nursing practice.
content analysis A technique for the objective, systematic and quantitative description of communications and documentary evidence.
content validity The degree to which the content of the measure represents the universe of content or the domain of a given behaviour.
contrasted-group approach A method used to assess construct validity. A researcher identifies two groups of individuals who are suspected to have an extremely high or low score on a characteristic. Scores from the groups are obtained and examined for sensitivity to the differences. Also called known-group approaches.
control Activities or procedures used to hold uniform or constant the conditions under which a quantitative investigation occurs.
control group The group in an experimental investigation that does not receive an intervention or treatment; the comparison group.
convenience sampling A non-probability sampling strategy that uses the most readily accessible persons or objects as subjects in a study.
convergent validity A strategy for assessing construct validity in which two or more tools that theoretically measure the same construct are administered to subjects. If the measures are positively correlated, convergent validity is said to be supported.
correlation The degree of association between two variables.
correlational study A type of observational research design that examines the relationship between two or more variables.
credibility Steps in qualitative research to ensure accuracy, validity or soundness of data.
criteria to critique The criteria used for objectively and critically evaluating a research article.

critical reading An active interpretation and objective assessment of an article during which the reader is examining key concepts, ideas and justifications.
critical thinking The rational examination of ideas, inferences, principles and conclusions.
critique The process of objectivity and critically evaluating a research report's content for scientific merit and application to practice, theory or education.
Cronbach's alpha A test of internal consistency that simultaneously compares each item in an instrument to all others; a test of instrument reliability.
cross-sectional study An observational research design that looks at data at one point in time, that is, in the immediate present.
Cumulative Index to Nursing and Allied Health Literature (CINAHL) A database of journal articles and other information sources abstracted from a wide selection of nursing and allied health publications; available on CD-ROM and online, and previously in print format.
data Information systematically collected in the course of a study; the plural of datum.
database A compilation of information about a topic organised in a systematic way; available in print, online or CD-ROM formats.
data saturation A point in qualitative research when data collection can cease, as no new information from participants is being shared with the researcher; data from subsequent participants becomes repetitive; inclusion of additional participants does not result in new ideas.
deductive reasoning A logical thought process in which hypotheses are derived from theory; reasoning moves from the general to the particular.
degrees of freedom (*df*) Used to determine whether two or more scores have reached a statistical level of significance; accounts for sample size and numbers of groups being compared.
delimitations Those characteristics that restrict the population to an homogeneous group of subjects.
Delphi technique The technique of gaining expert opinion or group consensus on a subject. It uses rounds or multiple stages of data collection, with each round using data from the previous round to refine the collective opinion.
dependent variable In experimental studies the presumed effect of the independent variable or experimental variable on the outcome; also termed outcome variable.
descriptive/exploratory survey A type of observational research design that collects descriptions of existing phenomena; often used as a preliminary phase of research when little is known about concepts or relationships between variables of interest.
descriptive statistics Statistical methods used to describe and summarise sample data.
design The plan or blueprint for the conduct of a study.
direct observation A method for measuring psychological and physiological behaviours of participants.
directional hypothesis A hypothesis that specifies the expected direction of the relationship between the independent and dependent variables.
dissemination The communication of research findings through presentations and/or publications.
divergent validity A strategy for assessing construct validity in which two or more tools that theoretically measure the opposite of the construct are administered to subjects. If the measures are negatively correlated, divergent validity is said to be supported.
domains Symbolic categories that include the smaller categories of an ethnographic study.
effect size The magnitude of the effect of an intervention, compared to the control.
element The most basic unit about which information is collected.
eligibility criteria Those characteristics that restrict the sample to an homogeneous group of subjects.
emic view The natives' or insiders' view of the world.
empirical The obtaining of evidence or objective data.
equivalence Consistency or agreement among observers using the same measuring instrument or agreement among alternate forms of an instrument.
error variance The extent to which the variance in test scores is attributable to error rather than a true measure of the behaviours.
ethics The theory or discipline dealing with principles of moral values and moral conduct.

ethnographic method A qualitative research method that enables observation, interaction and description of cultural groups. The goal of the ethnographer is to understand the participants' view of their world.
ethnography A qualitative research approach designed to examine cultural behaviour.
etic view An outsider's view of another's world.
evaluation research The use of specific research methods and procedures to evaluate a program, treatment, practice or policy outcomes; analytical means are used to document the value of an activity.
evidence-based nursing Has its roots in the evidence-based medicine movement; examines the evidence base or knowledge base for practice, using a systematic approach to search and evaluate the literature.
ex-post facto study A type of observational research design that examines the relationships among the variables after the outcome of interest has occurred; retrospective measurement.
experiment A scientific investigation in which observations are made and data are collected within the context of procedural control, subject randomisation and manipulation of the independent (explanatory) variable.
experimental design A research design that has the following properties: randomisation, control and manipulation.
experimental group The group in an experimental investigation that receives an intervention or treatment.
external criticism A process used to judge the authenticity of historical data.
external validity The degree to which findings of a study can be generalised to other populations or environments.
extraneous variable A variable that interferes with the operations of the phenomena being studied, but which may not have been identified and controlled for by the researcher.
face validity A type of validity that uses an expert's opinion to judge the accuracy of an instrument.
factor analysis An approach to examining validity using a statistical procedure to determine the underlying dimensions or components of a measuring instrument, including the relationship between items (questions).
feminist research Generally agreed that it is undertaken to benefit women and is informed by feminist principles and ideals which must be visible in the research design.
field notes Different types of data collected during field work, such as observations, thoughts, interpretations of the researcher; often documented in a diary.
field work Research conducted by social researchers in a community or at a defined site.
findings Results of a study.
Fisher's exact probability test A test used to compare frequencies when samples are small and expected frequencies are less than six in each cell.
fittingness Answers the questions in qualitative research studies: Are the findings applicable outside the study situation? Are the results meaningful to the individuals not involved in the research?
formative evaluation Refers to the ongoing monitoring of the implementation of an innovation in order to understand how the objectives are being achieved so that action can be taken if modifications are required.
frequency distribution Descriptive statistical method for summarising the occurrences of events under study.
gatekeeper Individuals in an organisation who have control over a researcher's access to people or situations for the purpose of a specified study.
generalisability (generalise) The inferences that the data are representative of similar phenomena in a population beyond the studied sample.
grounded theory Theory that is constructed inductively from a base of observations of the world as it is lived by a selected group of people.
grounded theory method An inductive approach that uses a systematic set of procedures to arrive at a theory about basic social processes.
historical research method The systematic compilation of data resulting from evaluation and interpretation of facts regarding people, events and occurrences of the past.

history An internal validity threat that refers to events outside of the experimental setting that may affect the dependent variable.
holism A perspective by which social phenomena are understood in the total context of all the factors that contribute to them.
homogeneity Similarity of conditions or items; termed internal consistency; also relates to a sample of subjects with similar characteristics.
hypothesis A prediction about the relationship between two or more variables.
hypothesis testing validity A strategy for assessing construct validity in which the theory or concept underlying a measuring instrument's design is used to test hypotheses. Inferences are made based on the findings about whether the rationale underlying the instrument's construction is adequate to explain the findings.
impact evaluation Tests the performance of a program, project or innovation once it has been implemented and as soon as it has been completed.
independent variable The antecedent or the variable that has the presumed effect on the dependent variable; also termed the explanatory variable.
inductive reasoning A logical thought process in which generalisations are developed from specific observations; reasoning moves from the particular to the general.
inferential statistics A set of statistical analysis procedures that enable inferences to be drawn about a population using findings (results) from a representative sample; enables generalisability of findings.
informant A knowledgeable member of the social group being studied who provides the researcher with data about the group.
informed consent An ethical principle that requires a researcher to obtain the voluntary participation of subjects after fully informing them of the study, including any potential benefits and risks to the participant.
innovation diffusion Process by which an innovation or research findings are communicated through various channels over time among the members of a profession.
institutional ethics committee (IEC) Boards established in universities, healthcare institutions and other organisations to review research proposals involving human subjects within the institution or in programs sponsored by the institution.
instrument Used in quantitative research to measure the variables of interest, e.g. questionnaires, observational data sheets, physiological equipment, laboratory tests.
instrumentation A threat to internal validity where changes in the measurement of the variables may account for changes in the obtained measurement.
integrative research review A synthesis review of the literature on a specific concept or topic.
internal consistency A component of instrument reliability which examines the extent to which items within a scale reflect or measure the same concept.
internal criticism A process of judging the reliability or consistency of information within an historical document.
internal validity The degree to which it can be inferred that the experimental treatment, rather than an uncontrolled condition, resulted in the observed effects.
inter-rater reliability A component of reliability which examines the consistency of direct observations of the variables of interest between two or more observers; often expressed as a percentage of agreement between raters or observers.
interval Differences or intervals between points on a measuring scale; the interval between measurement points is assumed to be approximately equal.
interval measurement The level used to show rankings of events or objects on a scale with equal intervals between numbers but with an arbitrary zero (e.g. temperature using the Celsius scale).
intervening variable A variable that occurs during an experimental or quasi-experimental study that affects the dependent (outcome) variable.
intervention A treatment that is manipulated for one group but not another in an experimental design; also refers to whether or not the observer provokes actions from those who are being observed.
interviews A method of data collection in which a data collector questions a subject verbally. Interviews may be face-to-face or performed over the telephone and they may

consist of open-ended or close-ended questions; allows for two-way interaction between the researcher and participants, including clarification or questions or responses.

item to total correlation A measure of the reliability of an instrument, by examining the relationship between each of the items (questions) in a scale and the total scale.

justice The fair treatment of human subjects.

key informants Individuals who have special knowledge, status or communication skills and who are willing to teach the ethnographer about the phenomenon.

Kuder-Richardson (KR-20) coefficient The estimate of homogeneity utilised in instruments that use a dichotomous response pattern.

kurtosis The relative peakness or flatness of a distribution of scores for a particular variable.

level of significance (alpha level; α) A measure of certainty about a study's results; the level set by the researcher for assessing whether a true difference exists between sets of scores; an α level of 0.05 means that a true difference exists 95 times out of 100, that is, there is only a 5% chance that the results occurred by chance—the risk of making a type I error.

levels of measurement Categorisation of the precision with which an event can be measured and analysed—nominal, ordinal, interval and ratio.

life context The matrix of human–human–environment relationships emerging over the course of one's life.

Likert Scale An ordinal or interval measurement scale that lists statements with responses of 'strongly agree', 'agree', 'disagree' or 'strongly disagree', or scales of 1–5.

limitation Weakness of a study identified by the researcher as potentially affecting the results.

linear structural relationships (LISREL) Software developed to analyse covariance and the testing of complex causal models.

lived experience In phenomenological research a term used to refer to the focus on living through events and circumstances (pre-lingual) rather than thinking about these events and circumstances (conceptualised experience).

longitudinal study A research design in which a researcher collects data from the same group at different points in time; may be observational or interventional; also termed repeated measures studies.

manipulation The provision of some experimental treatment, in one or varying degrees, to subjects in the intervention group of an experimental study.

matching A sampling strategy used to construct matched pairs in case-control studies, using pre-established variables such as age, gender, admission diagnosis or admission period.

maturation A threat to internal validity, where developmental, biological or psychological processes that develop within an individual over time are external to the events of the study.

mean A measure of central tendency; the arithmetic average of all scores for a specific variable.

measurement The assignment of numbers to objects or events according to specific rules.

measures of central tendency Descriptive statistical procedure that describes the average characteristics of a sample, using the mathematical concepts mean, median and mode.

measures of variability Descriptive statistical procedure that describes how much dispersion there is in the distribution of a sample's data.

median A measure of central tendency; the middle score in the distribution.

mediating variable A variable that is between or occurs between an independent and dependent variable and can produce an indirect effect of the independent variable on the dependent variable.

Medline A database of medical literature; available online and on CD-ROM.

meta-analysis A statistical procedure that pools the results of multiple studies in a specific area and synthesises the data to draw some conclusions about the results of the combined studies; a quantitative data pooling component of a systematic review.

methodological research The controlled investigation and measurement of the means of gathering and analysing data.

modality The number of peaks in a frequency distribution.

mode A measure of central tendency; most frequent score in a distribution of scores.

mortality The loss of a research subject from time one data collection to time two data collection.

multiple analysis of variance (MANOVA) A test used to determine differences in means for three or more groups; used when there is more than one dependent variable.

multiple regression Measure of the relationship between one interval level dependent variable and several independent variables. Canonical correlation is used when there is more than one dependent variable.

multi-stage sampling (cluster sampling) Involves successive random sampling of units (clusters) that moves from large to small and meets sample eligibility criteria.

multi-trait–multi-method approach An approach to examining instrument validity using more than one method to assess accuracy.

network sampling (snowballing) A strategy used for locating samples difficult to access; it uses social networks and the fact that friends tend to have characteristics in common; subjects who meet the eligibility criteria are asked for assistance in getting in touch with others who meet the same criteria.

nominal measurement The lowest level of measurement used to classify objects or events into mutually exclusive categories without any relative ranking or any meaningful numerical value, e.g. gender, hair colour.

non-directional hypothesis A hypothesis that indicates the existence of a relationship between the variables but does not specify the anticipated direction of that relationship.

non-equivalent control group design A quasi-experimental design that is similar to the true experiment, but subjects are not randomly assigned to the treatment or control groups.

non-experimental research design A research design in which an investigator observes a phenomenon without manipulating the independent variable(s).

non-parametric statistics Statistics that are used when variables are measured at the nominal or ordinal level because they do not estimate population parameters, or when the distribution of scores is not normal; they involve less restrictive assumptions about the underlying distribution, but are not as powerful in detecting true differences between scores.

non-parametric tests of significance Inferential statistics that make no assumptions about the population distribution.

non-probability sampling A procedure in which elements are chosen by non-random methods.

normal curve A curve that is symmetrical about the mean and unimodal; a bell-shaped distribution of scores.

null hypothesis A statement that there is no relationship between the variables and that any relationship observed is a function of chance or fluctuations in sampling.

objective Data that are not influenced by anyone who collects the information.

objectivity The use of facts without distortion by personal feelings or bias.

open-ended item A question that the respondent may answer in his or her own words.

operational definition The measurements used to observe or measure a variable; delineates the procedures or operations required to measure a concept.

operationalisation The process of translating concepts into observable, measurable phenomena.

ordinal The level of measurement that systematically categorises data in an ordered or ranked manner, but there is no defined interval between the categories.

ordinal measurement The level used to show rankings of events or objects; numbers are not equidistant and zero is arbitrary (class ranking).

outcome evaluation An approach that questions whether the program, project or innovation has met its goals.

parallel form reliability See alternate form (reliability).

parameter A characteristic of a population.

parametric statistics Inferential statistics that involve the estimation of at least one parameter, require measurement at the interval level or above and involve assumptions about the variables being studied, including normal distribution of scores.

participant observation A research strategy by which the researcher attempts to be fully involved in the daily life of those being studied to minimise the researcher's effect and to gain understanding of the behaviours of the participants.

path analysis A statistical technique in which the researcher hypothesises how variables are related and in what order and then tests how strong those relationships or paths are.

Pearson correlation coefficient (Pearson's *r*) A statistic that reflects the degree of relationship between two interval level variables. Also called Pearson product moment correlation coefficient.

percentile A measure of rank; percentage of cases a given score exceeds.

phenomenological method A process of learning and constructing the meaning of human experience through intensive dialogue with persons who are living the experience.

phenomenological research That which is based on the investigation of the description of experience as it is lived.

phenomenology A qualitative research approach that aims to describe experience as it is lived through, before it is conceptualised.

philosophical research That which is based on the investigation of the truths and principles of existence, knowledge and conduct.

physiological measurement The use of specialised equipment to determine the physical and biological status of subjects.

population A well defined set that has certain specified properties.

power The probability that a statistical test will detect a significant difference that actually exists; rejection of a false null hypothesis.

power analysis A statistical procedure to determine the risk of a type II error—incorrect acceptance of a false null hypothesis; strengthens the meaning of a study's findings; influenced by the significance level, sample size and effect size.

predictive validity The degree of correlation between the measure of the concept and some future measure of the same concept.

primary source Scholarly literature that is written by a person(s) who developed the theory or conducted the research. Primary sources include eyewitness accounts of historic events, provided by original documents, films, letters, diaries, records, artefacts, periodicals or tapes.

probability The probability of an event is the event's long-run relative frequency in repeated trials under similar conditions.

probability sampling A procedure that uses some form of random selection when the sample units are chosen.

problem statement An interrogative sentence or statement about the relationship between two or more variables.

process consent In qualitative research, the ongoing negotiation with subjects for their participation in a study.

product testing The testing of medical devices.

program A list of instructions in a machine-readable language written so that a computer's hardware can carry out an operation; software.

propositions The linkage of concepts that lays a foundation for the development of methods that test relationships.

prospective study A study design that begins with an exploration of assumed causes and then moves forward in time to the presumed effect; can be observational or interventional.

psychometrics The theory and development of measuring instruments.

purposive sampling A non-probability sampling strategy in which the researcher selects subjects who are considered to be typical of the population.

qualitative measurement The items or observed behaviours are assigned to mutually exclusive categories that are representative of the kinds of behaviour exhibited by the subjects.

qualitative research The study of broadly stated questions about human experiences, conducted in natural settings and using descriptive, narrative data.

quantitative measurement The assignment of categories or numerical codes to items or behaviours that represent the amount of a possessed characteristic.

quasi-experimental design A study design in which random assignment is not used but the independent variable is manipulated and certain mechanisms of control are used.
questionnaires Paper and pencil or online instruments designed to gather data from individuals.
quota sampling A non-probability sampling strategy that identifies the strata of the population and proportionately represents the strata in the sample.
random selection A selection process in which each element of the population has an equal and independent chance of being included in the sample.
randomisation A sampling selection procedure in which each person or element in a population has an equal chance of being selected to either the experimental group or the control group.
range A measure of variability; difference between the highest and lowest scores in a set of sample data.
ratio The highest level of measurement that possesses the characteristics of categorising, ordering and ranking and also has an absolute or natural zero that has empirical meaning.
ratio measurement The level that ranks the order of events or objects and that has equal intervals and an absolute zero (e.g. height, weight).
reactivity The distortion created when those who are being observed change their behaviour because they know that they are being observed.
reciprocity The exchange of favours that frequently occurs when conducting field work. Researchers are 'indebted' to the social group being studied and are 'obliged' to return favours.
recommendation The application of a study to practice, theory and future research.
records Information that is collected from existing materials such as hospital records, historical documents, videotapes or other available data sources.
refereed journal (peer-reviewed journal) A scholarly journal that has a panel of external and internal reviewers or editors; the panel reviews manuscripts that are submitted for possible publication, using a standard set of scholarly criteria to judge if the manuscripts are worthy of publication.
reflexivity In social research, the process of the researcher reflecting on the effect of the presence of the researcher on the behaviour of those being studied.
reliability The consistency or constancy of a measuring instrument.
replication The repetition of a study procedure that uses different samples and is conducted in different settings.
representative sample A sample whose key characteristics closely approximate those of the population.
research The systematic, logical and rigorous enquiry into the possible relationships among particular phenomena to produce verifiable knowledge.
research base The accumulated knowledge gained from several studies that investigate a similar concept of interest.
research-based practice Nursing or midwifery practice that is based on the findings from high quality research; also called evidence-based practice.
research-based protocols Practice standards that are formulated from a systematic review of the findings from several studies.
research hypothesis A statement about the expected relationship between the variables; also known as a scientific hypothesis.
research literature The body of knowledge about a particular phenomenon, sourced from research activities.
research problem The question that is to be asked in a research study.
research utilisation A systematic method of implementing sound research-based innovations in clinical practice, evaluating the outcome and sharing the knowledge through the process of research dissemination.
respect for persons The recognition that people have the right to self-determination and to treatment as autonomous agents, that is, they have the freedom to participate or not participate in research.

retrospective study An observational research design that begins with the phenomenon of interest (dependent variable) in the present and examines its relationship to another variable (independent variable) in the past.
review of the literature An extensive, systematic and critical review of the most important published scholarly literature on a particular topic. In most cases it is not considered exhaustive.
risk Potential negative outcome(s) of participation in research study.
risk–benefit ratio The extent to which the benefits of the study are maximised and the risks are minimised such that the subjects are protected from harm during the study; an important consideration when developing and reviewing research proposals.
sample A sub-set of sampling units from a population.
sampling A process in which representative units of a population are selected for study in a research investigation.
sampling error The tendency for statistics to fluctuate from one sample to another.
sampling frame A list of all units of the population.
sampling interval The standard distance between elements chosen for the sample.
sampling unit The element or set of elements used for selecting the sample.
saturation See data saturation.
scale A self-report inventory that provides a set of responses for each item (question). A rating or score is assigned to each response.
scholarly literature Published and unpublished data-based and conceptual literature materials found in print and non-print forms.
scientific approach A logical, orderly and objective means of generating and testing ideas.
scientific hypothesis The researcher's expectation about the outcome of a study; also known as the research hypothesis.
scientific merit The degree of validity of a study or group of studies.
scientific observation Collecting data about the environment and subjects. Data collection has specific objectives to guide it, is systematically planned and recorded, is checked and controlled and is related to scientific concepts and theories.
secondary source Scholarly material written by person(s) other than the individual who developed the theory or conducted the research. Most are usually published. Often a secondary source represents a response to or a summary and critique of a theorist's or researcher's work. Examples are documents, films, letters, diaries, records, artefacts, periodicals, tapes or systematic reviews that provide a view of the phenomenon from another person's perspective.
selection bias An internal validity threat that arises when pre-treatment differences between the experimental group and the control group are present.
semi-quartile range A measure of variability; range of the middle 50% of the scores; also known as semi-interquartile range.
simple random sampling A probability sampling strategy in which the population is defined, a sampling frame is listed and a sub-set from which the sample will be chosen is selected; members randomly selected.
skew Measure of the asymmetry of a distribution of scores.
snowballing See network sampling.
social desirability The response of a subject in a manner that he or she believes will please the researcher rather than in an honest manner.
Solomon four-group design An experimental design with four randomly assigned groups: the pre-test–post-test intervention group; the pre-test–post-test control group; a treatment or intervention group with only post-test measurement; and a control group with only post-test measurement.
split-half reliability A component of reliability; an index of the comparison between the scores on one half of a test with those on the other half to determine the consistency in response to items that reflect specific content.
stability An instrument's ability to produce the same results with repeated testing.
standard deviation (SD) A measure of variability; measure of average deviation of scores from the mean.
standard error of the mean The standard deviation of a theoretical distribution of sample means; it indicates the average error in the estimation of the population mean.

statistical hypothesis An hypothesis that states that there is no relationship between the independent variables and dependent variables. The statistical hypothesis is also known as the null hypothesis.

statistical reliability An index of the interval consistency of responses to all items of a single form of measure that is administered at one time.

stratified random sampling A probability sampling strategy in which the population is divided into strata or sub-groups. An appropriate number of elements from each sub-group are randomly selected based on their proportion in the population.

symbolic interaction A theoretical perspective that holds that the relationship between self and society is an ongoing process of symbolic communication whereby individuals create a social reality.

systematic Data collection carried out in the same manner with all subjects.

systematic error That which is attributable to lasting characteristics of the subject that do not tend to fluctuate from one time to another; also called constant error.

systematic sampling A probability sampling strategy that involves the selection of subjects randomly drawn from a population list at fixed intervals.

***t* statistic** The result of a statistical test that examines whether two group means are more different than would be expected by chance. Groups may be related or independent.

target population A population or group of individuals that meet the sampling criteria.

test A self-report inventory that provides for one response to each item for which the examiner assigns a rating or score. Inferences are made from the total score about the degree to which a subject possesses whatever trait, emotion, attitude or behaviour the test is supposed to measure.

testable Variables of proposed study that lend themselves to observation, measurement and analysis.

testing A threat to internal validity; the effects of taking a pre-test on the scores of a post-test.

test–retest reliability A component of instrument reliability; administration of the same instrument twice to the same subjects under the same conditions within a prescribed time interval, with a comparison of the paired scores to determine the stability of the measure.

theoretical framework Theoretical rationale for the development of hypotheses.

theoretical sampling Used to select experiences that will help the researcher test ideas and gather complete information about developing concepts when using the grounded theory method.

theory A set of interrelated concepts, definitions and propositions that present a systematic view of phenomena for the purpose of explaining and making predictions about those phenomena.

time series design A quasi-experimental design used to determine trends before and after an experimental treatment. Measurements are taken several times before the introduction of the experimental treatment, the treatment is introduced and measurements are taken again at specified times afterwards.

triangulation A multi-method approach to examining a concept of interest; useful for checking the validity of a set of information.

true experiment Also known as the pre-test–post-test control group design. In this design, subjects are randomly assigned to an experimental or control group, pre-test measurements are performed, an intervention or treatment occurs in the experimental group and post-test measurements are performed, e.g. randomised controlled trial (RCT).

type I error The rejection of a null hypothesis that is actually true; differences between groups were detected in the study when there were no differences in the population of interest.

type II error The acceptance of a null hypothesis that is actually false; no difference was evident in the study when there were true differences in the population of interest; occurs when there is a stringent level of significance, a small sample size, or a small difference in measured effect.

validation sample The sample that provides the initial data for determining the reliability and validity of a measurement tool.

validity Determination of whether a measurement instrument actually measures what it is purported to measure.

variable A defined concept.

web browser Software program used to access the internet and world wide web (WWW).

world wide web (WWW) A conceptual group of servers on the internet, allowing unprecedented access to information sources.

z **score** Used to compare measurements in standard units; examines the relative distance of the scores from the mean.

References

Aamodt, A.M. (1989). Ethnography and epistemology: generating nursing knowledge. In Morse, J.M., ed., *Qualitative nursing research* (pp. 29–41). Maryland, Aspen Publication, Inc.

Aaronson, L.S., Frey, M.A. & Boyd, C.J. (1988). Structural equation models and nursing research: part II. *Nurse Researcher*, 37, 315–18.

Abercrombie, N., Hill, S. & Turner, B.S. (1984). *The Penguin dictionary of sociology*. Harmondsworth, Penguin Books.

ACCCN [Australian College of Critical Care Nurses]. (2002). *Competency standards for specialist critical care nurses* (2nd ed.). Carlton, ACCCN.

Adler, P. & Adler, P. (1998). Observational techniques. In Denzin, N. & Lincoln, Y., eds, *Collecting and interpreting qualitative materials*. Thousand Oaks, California, Sage Publications.

Alexy, B., Nichols, B., Heverly, M.A. & De Garzon, L. (1997). Prenatal factors and birth outcomes in the public health service: a rural/urban comparison. *Research in Nursing & Health*, 20, 61–70.

Allen, D.G. (1985). Nursing research and social control: Alternative models of science that emphasize understanding and emancipation. *Image: The Journal of Nursing Scholarship*, 17(2), 58–64.

Alsop-Shields, L. & Alexander, H. (1997). A study of errors that can occur when weighing infants. *Journal of Advanced Nursing*, 25, 587–94.

American Educational Research Association, American Psychological Association, National Council on Measurement in Education. (1999). *Standards for educational and psychological testing*. Washington, DC, American Educational Research Association.

American Nurses Association. (1985). *Guidelines for nurses in clinical and other research*. Kansas City, ANA.

American Psychiatric Association. (2000). *Diagnostic and statistical manual of mental disorders: DSM-IV*. (4th ed.). Washington, DC, American Psychiatric Association.

American Psychological Association. (2001). *Publication manual of the American Psychological Association*. (5th ed.). Washington, DC, American Psychological Association.

Anderson, K. & Jack, D. (1991). Learning to listen: interview techniques and analysis. In Gluck, D. & Patai, D., eds, *Women's words: the feminist practice of oral history*. New York, Routledge.

Annells, M. (1996). Grounded theory method: philosophical perspectives, paradigm of inquiry, and postmodernism. *Qualitative Health Research*, 6(3), 379–93.

Annells, M. (1997a). The impact of flatus upon the nursed. PhD thesis, Flinders University of South Australia, Adelaide, Australia.

Annells, M. (1997b). Grounded theory method: part 2. Options for users of the method. *Nursing Inquiry*, 4, 176–80.

Annells, M. (1997c). Grounded theory method: part 1. Within the five moments of qualitative research. *Nursing Inquiry*, 4, 120–29.

Annells, M. & Koch, T. (2001). 'The real stuff': implications for nursing of assessing and measuring a terminally ill person's quality of life. *Journal of Clinical Nursing*, 10(6), 806–12.

Artinian, B. (1998). Grounded theory research: its value for nursing. *Nursing Science Quarterly*, 11(1), 5–6.

Asher, H.B. (1983). *Causal modelling*. (2nd ed.). Beverly Hills, California, Sage.

Atkinson, P. & Hammersley, M. (1994). Ethnography and participant observation. In Denzin, N. & Lincoln, Y., eds, *Handbook of qualitative research*. Thousand Oaks, California, Sage.

Australian Bureau of Statistics. (1993). *State of health in New South Wales (1989–90)*. Canberra, Commonwealth of Australia.

Australian College of Midwives, Incorporated (ACMI). (1998). *Competency standards for midwives.* Melbourne, Australian College of Midwives Incorporated.

Australian Research Council (ARC), Australian Tertiary Institutions Commercial Companies Association, Australian Vice-Chancellors Committee, Department of Education, Training and Youth Affairs, The Department of Industry, Science and Resources, IP Australia, The National Health and Medical Research Council. (2001). *National principles of intellectual property management for publicly funded research.* Canberra, Department of Industry, Science and Resources.

Australian Vice-Chancellors Committee. (1995). *Ownership of intellectual property in universities: a discussion paper.* AVCC. Canberra. Available at http://www.avcc.edu.au

Bailey, B. & Gephart, M. (1999). Moving along with the facts: introduction to evidence-based practice—the management of constipation. In Aranda, S. & O'Connor, M. eds, *Palliative nursing: a guide to practice.* Melbourne, Ausmed Publications.

Baillie, L. (1999). Preparing adult branch students for their management role as staff nurses: an action research project. *Journal of Nursing Management*, 7(4), 225–34.

Balfour, M. & Clarke, C. (2001). Searching for sustainable change. *Journal of Clinical Nursing*, 10(1), 44–50.

Baly, M. (1996). Some pitfalls in researching documentary sources: a note for the historian of nursing. *International History of Nursing Journal*, 2(1), 70–76.

Barclay, L., Donovan, J., & Genovese, A. (1996). Men's experiences during their partner's first pregnancy: a grounded theory analysis. *Australian Journal of Advanced Nursing*, 13(3), 12–24.

Barclay, L., Everitt, L., Rogan, F., Schmied, V. & Wyllie, A. (1997). Becoming a mother—an analysis of women's experience of early motherhood. *Journal of Advanced Nursing*, 25: 719–28.

Barnason, S., Zimmerman, L., Anderson, A., Mohr-Burt, S. & Nieveen, J. (2000). Functional status outcomes of patients with a coronary artery bypass graft over time. *Heart & Lung: The Journal of Acute and Critical Care*, 29, 33–46.

Barrett, M. & Phillips, A., eds. (1992). *Destabilizing theory: contemporary feminist debates.* Cambridge, Polity Press.

Barriball, K.L. & White, A.E. (1999). Non-response survey research: a methodological discussion and development of an explanatory model. *Journal of Advanced Nursing*, 30(3), 677–86.

Bavier, A.R. (1995). Where research and practice meet. *Nurse Policy Forum*, 1(4), 20–27.

Bazeley, P. (1999). The bricoleur with a computer: piecing together qualitative and quantitative data. *Qualitative Health Research*, 9(2), 279–87.

Bazeley, P. & Richards, L. (2000). *The NVivo qualitative project book.* London, Sage.

Beck, C.T. (1992). The lived experience of postpartum depression: a phenomenological study. *Nurse Researcher*, 41(3), 166–70.

Beck, C. T. (1994). Phenomenology: its use in nursing research. *International Journal of Nursing Studies*, 31(6), 449–512.

Beck, C.T. (1996). Use of a meta-analytic database management system. *Nursing Research*, 45(3), 181–84.

Beck, C.T. & Gable, R.K. (2001). Further validation of the postpartum depression screening scale. *Nurse Researcher*, 50(3), 155–64.

Beck, C.T., Reynolds, M. & Rutowski, P. (1992). Maternity blues and postpartum depression. *Journal of Obstetric, Gynecological and Neonatal Nursing*, 21(4), 287–93.

Becker, H.S., Geer, H., Hughes, E. & Strauss, A.L. (1961). *Boys in white: student culture in medical school.* Chicago, University of Chicago Press.

Becker, P.T. (1993). A lingering identity crisis. *Research in Nursing & Health*, 16, 87–88.

Begley, A-M. (1996). Literature and poetry: pleasure and practice. *International Journal of Nursing Practice*, 2(4), 182–88.

Beland, D.K. & Froman, R.D. (1995). Preliminary validation of a measure of life support preference. *Image: The Journal of Nursing Scholarship*, 24(4), 307–10.

Bell, P.F., Daly, J. & Chang, E.M.L. (1997). A study of the educational and research priorities of registered nurses in rural Australia. *Journal of Advanced Nursing*, 25, 794–800.

Belsey, C. & Moore, J., eds. (1997). *The feminist reader: essays in gender and the politics of literary criticism.* (2nd ed.). London, Macmillan Press.
Benner, P. (1994). The tradition and skill of interpretive phenomenology in studying health, illness, and caring practices. In Benner, P., ed., *Interpretive phenomenology: embodiment, caring and ethics in health and illness.* (pp. 99–128). Thousand Oaks, California, Sage.
Bennett, B. (1998). Increasing collaboration within a multidisciplinary neurorehabilitation team: the early stages of a small action research project. *Journal of Clinical Nursing*, 7(3), 227–31.
Benoliel, J. (1996). Grounded theory and nursing knowledge. *Qualitative Health Research*, 6(3), 406–28.
Bergen, A. & While, A. (2000). A case for case studies: exploring the use of case study design in community nursing research. *Journal of Advanced Nursing*, 31, 926–34.
Bergstrom, N. (1991). Scientific base for nursing practice is a goal of ANA. *Council Nursing Research*, 18(2), 1–7.
Bessant, J. & Bessant, B. (1991). *The growth of a profession: nursing in Victoria 1930s–1980s.* Melbourne, La Trobe University Press.
Beyea, S., Farley, J.K. & Williams-Burgess, C. (1996). Teaching baccalaureate students to use research. *Western Journal of Nursing Research*, 18(2), 213–18.
Blackburn, S. (1994). *The Oxford dictionary of philosophy.* Oxford, Oxford University Press.
Blackford, J., Street, A. & Parsons, C. (1997). Breaking down language barriers in clinical practice. *Contemporary Nurse*, 6(1), 15–21.
Blumenthal, J.A., Barefoot, J., Haney, T. & Zimet, G. (1987). Social support, type A behaviour, and coronary artery disease. *Psychosomatic Medicine*, 49, 331–40.
Bogdan, R. & Taylor, S. (1975). *Introduction to qualitative research methods.* New York, John Wiley & Sons.
Borko, H., Michalec, P., Timmons, M. & Siddle, J. (1997). Student teaching portfolios: a tool for promoting reflective practice. *Journal of Teacher Education*, 48(5), 345–57.
Botti, M., Williamson, B. & Steen, K. (2001). Coronary angiography observations: evidence-based or ritualistic practice? *Heart & Lung: The Journal of Acute and Critical Care*, 30(2), 138–45.
Botti, M., Williamson, B., Steen, K., McTaggart, J. & Reid, E. (1998). The effect of pressure bandaging on complications and comfort in patients undergoing coronary angiography: a multicenter randomised trial. *Heart & Lung: The Journal of Acute and Critical Care*, 27(6), 360–73.
Boutain, D. (1999). Critical nursing scholarship: exploring critical social theory with African American studies. *Advances in Nursing Science*, 21(4), 37–47.
Bower, F. (1994). Research: outcomes must be the focus. *Image: The Journal of Nursing Scholarship*, 26, 4.
Bowles, N. (1999). The delphi technique. *Nursing Standard*, 13, 32–36.
Boyd, C.J., Frey, M.A. & Aaronson, L.S. (1988). Structural equation models and nursing research: part 1. *Nurse Researcher*, 37, 249–51.
Boyle, M., Butcher, R. & Kenney, C. (1998). Study to validate the outcome goal, competencies and educational objectives for use in intensive care orientation programs. *Australian Critical Care*, 11, 20–24.
Boyle, M., Way, P., Pinfold, M. & Lawrence, J. (2001). Comparison of the lower inflection point of the static total respiratory compliance curve with outcomes in postoperative cardiothoracic patient. *American Journal of Critical Care*, 10(6), 399–407.
Bradley, D. (1993). Competency standards for female dominated professions: a dual closure strategy? *Labour and Industry*, 5(3), 33–55.
Braunwald, E., Fauci, A.S., Isselbacher, K.J., Kasper, D.L., Hauser, S.I., Longo, D.L. & Jameson, J.L., eds. (2001). *Harrison's principles of internal medicine.* (15th ed.). New York, McGraw-Hill.
Brazier H. & Begley C. M. (1996). Selecting a database for literature searches in nursing: Medline or CINAHL? *Journal of Advanced Nursing*, 4(4), 868–75.
Brewer, J.D. (2000). *Ethnography.* Buckingham, Open University Press.
Brooks, R., Bauman, A., Daffurn, K. & Hillman, K. (1995). Post hospital outcomes following intensive care. *Clinical Intensive Care*, 6, 127–35.

Brooks, R., Kerridge, R., Hillman, K., Dauman, A. & Daffurn, K. (1997). Quality of life outcomes after intensive care: comparison with a community group. *Intensive Care Medicine*, 23, 581–86.
Bruni, N. (1994). Exploring critical ethnography: rethinking Malinowski. Paper presented to the International Nursing Research Conference (RCNA and Sigma Theta Tau), Sydney, Australia, 6–10 July.
Bucknall, T.K. (1996). Clinical decision making in critical care nursing practice: decisions, processes and influences. PhD thesis, La Trobe University, Melbourne, Australia.
Bucknall, T. & Thomas, S. (1997). Nurses' reflections on problems associated with decision making in critical care settings. *Journal of Advanced Nursing*, 25, 229–37.
Buerhaus, P.I. (1996). The value of consumer and nurse partnerships. *Nurse Policy Forum*, 2(2), 13–20.
Buerhaus, P.I., Staiger, D.O. & Auerbach, D.I. (2000a). Implications of an aging registered nurse workforce. *Journal of the American Medical Association*, 283(22), 2948–54.
Buerhaus, P.I., Staiger, D.O. & Auerbach, D.I. (2000b). Policy responses to an aging registered nurse workforce. *Nursing Economics*, 18(6), 278–84.
Burdess, N. (1994). *The really understandable stats book*. Sydney, Prentice Hall.
Burgess, R.G. (1984). *In the field: an introduction to field research*. London, George Allen & Unwin.
Burns, L. & Adams, M. (1997). Alcohol-history taking by nurses and doctors: how accurate are they really? *Journal of Advanced Nursing*, 25, 509–13.
Burr, G. (1998). Contextualising critical family needs through triangulation: an Australian study. *Intensive and Critical Care Nursing*, 14, 161–69.
Byrne, D. & McMurray, A. (1997). Caring for the dying: nurses' experiences in hospice care. *Australian Journal of Advanced Nursing*, 15(1), 4–11.
Byrne, M. (2001). Evaluating the findings of qualitative research. *Association of Operating Room Nurses Journal*, 73(3), 703–04.
Byrnes, M. & West, S. (2000). Registered nurses' clinical reasoning abilities: a study of self perception. *Australian Journal of Advanced Nursing*, 17(3), 18–23.
Cady, J., Distad, L. & Germundsen, R. (1998). Reflective practice groups in teacher induction: building professional community via experiential knowledge. *Education*, 118(3), 459, (412).
Campbell, D. & Fiske, D. (1959). Convergent and discriminant validation by the matrix. *Psychological Bulletin*, 53, 273–302.
Campbell, D.T. & Stanley, J.C. (1963). *Experimental and quasi-experimental designs for research*. Chicago, Rand McNally.
Campbell, J. & Bunting, S. (1991). Voices and paradigms: perspectives on critical and feminist theory in nursing. *Advances in Nursing Science*, 13(3), 1–15.
Carnegie, E. (1976). *Historical perspectives of nursing research*. Boston, Boston University, Nursing Archive, Special Collections.
Carnwell, R. (2000). Essential differences between research and evidence-based practice. *Nurse Researcher*, 8(2), 55–68.
Carr, E. (1961). *What is history?* London, Pelican.
Carroll-Johnson, R.M. (1992). Searching … one of the first steps of writing is to conduct a comprehensive literature search. *Oncology Nursing Forum*, 19(5), 705.
Carryer, J. (1995). Feminist research: strengths and challenges. *Contemporary Nurse*, 4(4), 180–86.
Cassell, J. (1991). *Expected miracles: surgeons at work*. Philadelphia, Temple University Press.
Castle, J. (1984). Nursing at The Wollongong Hospital 1926–1982. The University of Wollongong, NSW.
Caudell, K.A. & Gallucci, B.B. (1995). Neuroendocrine and immunological responses of women to stress. *Western Journal of Nursing Research*, 17, 672–92.
Chambers, D., Gilmore, C., Maillet, J. & Mitchell, B. (1996). Another look at competency-based education in dietetics. *Journal of the American Dietetic Association*, 96(6), 614.
Charmaz, K. (1994). The grounded theory method: an explication and interpretation. In Glaser, B., ed., *More grounded theory methodology: a reader*. Mill Valley, Sociology Press.
Charmaz, K. (1995). Between positivism and postpositivism: implications for methods. *Studies of Symbolic Interaction*, 17, 43–72.

Charmaz, K. (2000). Grounded theory: objectivist and constructivist methods. In Denzin, N. & Lincoln, Y., eds, *Handbook of qualitative research.* (2nd ed.). Thousand Oaks, California, Sage.

Charnock, Y. (2001). The nursing management of chest drains—a systematic review: The Joanna Briggs Institute for Evidence Based Nursing & Midwifery, (no. 16). Adelaide.

Cheek, J. & Rudge, T. (1995). Only connect ... feminism and nursing. In Gray, G. & Pratt, R., eds, *Scholarship in the discipline of nursing.* Melbourne, Churchill Livingstone.

Chenitz, W. & Swanson, J. (1986). *From practice to grounded theory: qualitative research.* Menlo Park, Addison Wesley.

Chesla, C. A. (1994). Parents' caring practices with schizophrenic offspring. In Benner, P., ed., *Interpretive phenomenology: embodiment, caring, ethics in health and illness.* (pp. 167–84). Thousand Oaks, California, Sage.

Chinn, P. (1995). Critique? *Advances in Nursing Science*, 181, viii–ix.

Chrisman, N.J. (1992). Review of the health and adjustment of Iranian immigrants (commentary). *Western Journal of Nursing Research*, 14, 27–28.

Ciliska D., Cullum, N. & DiCenso A. (1999). The fundamentals of quantitative measurement. *Evidence-Based Nursing*, 2, 100–01.

Ciliska, D., Cullum, N. & Marks, S. (2001). Evaluation of systematic reviews of treatment or prevention interventions. *Evidence-Based Nursing*, 4(4), 100–04.

CINAHL Information Systems, California (2002). *The CINAHL database.* Available at <http://www.cinahl.com/prodsvcs/cinahldb.htm>. Accessed 20 January 2002.

Clare, J. (1993a). A challenge to the rhetoric of emancipation: recreating a professional culture. *Journal of Advanced Nursing*, 18(7), 1033–38.

Clare, J. (1993b). Changing the curriculum—or transforming the conditions of practice? *Nurse Education Today*, 13(4), 282–86.

Closs, S. J. & Cheater F. M. (1999). Evidence for nursing practice: a clarification of the issues. *Journal of Advanced Nursing*, 30(1), 10–17.

Cluzeau, F.A. & Littlejohns, P. (1999). Appraising clinical practice guidelines in England and Wales: the development of a methodologic framework and its application to policy. *Joint Commission Journal on Quality Improvement*, 25(10), 514–521.26.

Cochrane Collaboration. http://www.cochrane.org/cochrane/cc-broch.htm (2001). Accessed 20 January 2002.

Code of Federal Regulations, USA (1983). Protection of human subjects. 45 CFR 46, OPRR Reports. (Revised 8 March).

Cohen, I.B. (1984). Florence Nightingale. *Scientific American*, 250(3), 98–107.

Cohen, J. (1988). *Statistical power analysis for the behavioral sciences.* (2nd ed.). Hillsdale, New Jersey, Lawrence Erlbaum Associates.

Cohen, J.M. & Cohen, M.J. (1980). *The Penguin dictionary of quotations.* Britain, Hazell Watson & Viney Ltd.

Colaizzi, P. (1978). Psychological research as a phenomenologist views it. In Valle, R.S. & King, M., eds, *Existential phenomenological alternatives for psychology.* New York, Oxford University Press.

Commonwealth Department of Health, Housing & Community Services. (1993). *Pathways to better health.* Canberra, Commonwealth Department of Health, Housing and Community Services.

Commonwealth Department of Health, Housing & Community Services. (1995). *Statistics on drug abuse in Australia 1994.* Canberra, Commonwealth Department of Health, Housing and Community Services.

Condon, M. & Anderson, G.C. (1990). Three methods of random assignment: comparison of balance achieved on potentially confounding variables. *Nurse Researcher*, 39(6), 376–78.

Coney, S. (1988). *The unfortunate experiment.* Auckland, Penguin.

Cook, D., Mulrow, C. & Haynes, R. (1997). Systematic reviews: synthesis of best evidence for clinical decisions. *Annals of Internal Medicine*, 126, 364–71.

Cook, D.J., Greenhold, N.L., Ellrodt, A.G. & Weingarten, S.R. (1997). The relation between systematic reviews and practice guidelines. *Annals of Internal Medicine*, 127(3), 210–16.

Cook, J. & Fonow, M. (1986). Knowledge and women's interests: issues of epistemology and methodology in feminist sociological research. *Sociological Inquiry*, 56, 69–93.
Cooper, C.D. (2000). The use of electronic mail in the research process. *Nurse Researcher*, 7(4), 24–30.
Corbin, J. & Strauss, A. (1990). Grounded theory research: procedures, canons, and evaluative criteria. *Qualitative Sociology*, 13(1), 3–21.
Corbin, J. & Strauss, A. (1996). Analytic ordering for theoretical purposes. *Qualitative Inquiry*, 2(2), 139–50.
Cormack, D.F.S. (1996). *The research process in nursing*. (3rd ed.). London, Blackwell Science.
Cowley, S. & Billings, J. R. (1999). Implementing new health visiting services through action research: an analysis of process. *Journal of Advanced Nursing*, 30(4), 965–74.
Coyne, I. (1997). Sampling in qualitative research. Purposeful and theoretical sampling: merging or clear boundaries? *Journal of Advanced Nursing*, 26(3), 623–30.
Crabtree, B. F. & Miller, W.L., eds. (1992). *Doing qualitative research*. Newbury Park, California, Sage.
Cramer, S. (1992). The nature of history: meditations on Clio's craft. *Nursing Research*, 41(1), 4–7.
Creighton, H. (1977). Legal concerns of nursing research. *Nursing Research*, 26(4), 337–40.
Crichton, N. (2001). Information point: odds ratio. *Journal of Clinical Nursing*, 10(2), 268–69.
Crigger, N.J. (1996). Testing an uncertainty model for women with multiple sclerosis. *Advanced Nursing Science*, 18(3), 37–47.
Crisp, J., Pelletier, D., Duffield, C., Nagy, S. & Adams, A. (1999). It's all in a name. When is a 'delphi study' not a delphi study? *Australian Journal of Advanced Nursing*, 16, 32–37.
Crookes, P. & Davies, S. (1998). *Research into practice: essential skills for reading and applying research in nursing and health care*. Edinburgh, Balliere-Tindall.
Cross, V. (1997). The professional development diary: a case study of one cohort of physiotherapy. *Physiotherapy*, 83(7), 375–83.
Cullum, N. (1997). Identification and analysis of randomised controlled trials in nursing: a preliminary study. *Qualitative Health Care*, 6, 2–6.
Cullum, N. (1998). Evidence based practice. *Nursing Management*, 5(3), 32–35.
Cullum, N. (2000). Evaluation of studies of treatment or prevention interventions. *Evidence-Based Nursing*, 3(4), 100–02.
Cullum, N., DiCenso, A. & Ciliska D. (1998). Evidence-based nursing: an introduction. *Evidence Based Medicine*, 3(2), 37–38.
Cutcliffe, J. (2000). Methodological issues in grounded theory. *Journal of Advanced Nursing*, 31(6), 1476–84.
Daly, J. & Chang, E.M.L. (1996). A study of clinical nursing research priorities of renal specialist nurses caring for critically ill people. *Intensive Critical Care Nursing*, 12, 45–49.
Daly, J., Chang, E.M.L. & Bell, P.F. (1996). Clinical nursing research priorities in Australian critical care: a pilot study. *Journal of Advanced Nursing*, 23(1), 145–51.
Daly, J., Elliott, D., Cameron-Traub, E., Salamonson, Y., Davidson, P., Jackson, D., Chin, C. & Wade, V. (2000). Health status, perceptions of coping and social support immediately after discharge of survivors of acute myocardial infarction. *American Journal of Critical Care*, 9(1), 62–69.
Daly, J., Elliott, D. & Chang, E. (2000). Research in nursing. In Daly, J., Speedy, S. & Jackson, D., eds, *Contexts of nursing: an introduction*. Sydney, MacLennan & Petty.
Daly, M. (1978). *Gyn/ecology: the meta-ethics of radical feminism*. Boston, Beacon Press.
Daly, W.M. & Carnwell, R. (2001). The case for a multi-method approach. *Nurse Researcher*, 8(3), 30–44.
Daniels, G., Poroch, D. & De Roach, J. (1995). Blood letting for BSL: the effects of timing and sites on blood volume. *Australian Journal of Advanced Nursing*, 12(3), 11–14.
Darbyshire, P. (1994). Understanding the life of illness: learning through the art of Frida Kahlo. *Advances in Nursing Science*, 17(1), 51–59.

Darbyshire, P. (1995a). Lessons from literature: caring, interpretation, and dialogue. *Journal of Nursing Education*, 34(5), 211–16.
Darbyshire, P. (1995b). Reclaiming 'Big Nurse': a feminist critique of Ken Kesey's portrayal of Nurse Ratched in 'One Flew over the Cuckoo's Nest'. *Nursing Inquiry*, 2(4), 198–202.
Davidson, P. & Elliott, D. (2001). Managing approaches to nursing care delivery. In Chang, E. & Daly, J., eds, *Preparing for professional nursing practice*. Sydney, MacLennan & Petty.
Davies, C. (1980). Introduction. In Davies, C., ed., *Rewriting nursing history*. Beckenham, UK, Croom Helm.
Dawes, M. (1999). Introduction to critical appraisal. In Dawes, M., Davies, P., Gray, A., Mant, J., Seers, K. & Snowball, R., eds, *Evidence-based practice: a primer for health care professionals* (pp. 47–48). Edinburgh, Churchill Livingstone.
Dawson, A. & Beanland, C. (1997). The reasons women attend childbirth education classes, Proceedings of the First Annual Congress of the Perinatal Society of Australia and New Zealand, Fremantle, Abstract P3.
Deacon, D. (1985). Political arithmetic. *Signs*, 11(1), 27–47.
Deane, W. (1999). Waiting for the dinosaurs to die. *Sydney Morning Herald*, 24 July, p. 47.
DeMarco, R., Campbell, J. & Wuest, J. (1993). Feminist critique: searching for meaning in research. *Advances in Nursing Science*, 16(2), 26–38.
Denzin, N. K. (1978). *The research act: a theoretical introduction to sociological methods*. (2nd ed.). New York, McGraw-Hill.
Denzin, N.K. & Lincoln, Y.S., eds. (1994). *Handbook of qualitative research*. Thousand Oaks, California, Sage.
Denzin, N.K. & Lincoln, Y.S. (1994). Introduction: entering the field of qualitative research. In Denzin, N. & Lincoln, Y., eds, *Handbook of qualitative research*. Thousand Oaks, California, Sage.
Department of Community Services and Health, Royal Australasian College of Physicians (1988). *Bibliography of Australian medicine and health services to 1950*. Canberra, Australian Government Publishing Service.
De Vries, S., Dunlop, M., Goopy, S., Moyle, W. & Sutherland-Lockhart, D. (1995). Discipline and passion: meaning, masochism and mythology in popular medical romances. *Nursing Inquiry*, 2(4), 203–10.
Deyo, R.A. & Carter, W.B. (1992). Strategies for improving and expanding the application of health status measures in clinical settings: a researcher–developer viewpoint. *Medical Care*, 30(5 Suppl.), MS176–86.
Deyo, R.A., Diehr, P. & Patrick, D.I. (1991). Reproducibility and responsiveness of health status measures: statistics and strategies for evaluation. *Control Clinical Trials*, 12(4 Suppl.), 142S–58S.
DiCenso, A. (2001). Clinically useful measures of the effects of treatment. *Evidence-Based Nursing*, 4(2), 36–39.
DiCenso, A., Cullum, N. & Ciliska, D. (1998). Implementing evidence based nursing: some misconceptions (editorial). *Evidence-Based Nursing*, 1(2), 38–40.
Dick, B. (1999). Sources of rigour in action research: addressing the issues of trustworthiness and credibility. Paper presented to the Conference of the Association for Qualitative Research, Melbourne, Australia, 6–10 July.
Dickenson-Hazard, N. (1995). Advancing science. *Reflections*, Fall, 2.
Dingwall, R., Rafferty, A. & Webster, C. (1988). *An introduction to the social history of nursing*. London, Routledge.
DiIorio, C., Hennessy, M. & Manteuffel, B. (1996). Epilepsy self-management: a test of a theoretical model. *Nursing Research*, 45, 211–17.
Dock, L.L. (1900). What we may expect from the law. *American Journal of Nursing*, 1, 8–12.
Downs, F.S. (1984). *A sourcebook of nursing research*. (3rd ed.). Philadelphia, FA Davis.
Downs, F.S. (1996). Research as a survival technique. *Nursing Research*, 45(6), 323.
Dracup, K., McKinley, S.M. & Moser, D.K. (1997). Australian patients' delay in response to heart attack symptoms. *Medical Journal of Australia*, 166(3), 233–36.

Draper, M. (1997). *Involving consumers in improving hospital care: lessons from Australian hospitals.* Canberra, Commonwealth Department of Health and Family Services.

Draucker, C. B. (1999). The critique of Heideggerian hermeneutical nursing research. *Journal of Advanced Nursing*, 30(2), 360–73.

Dreher, M.C. (1995). Clinical scholarship worldwide. *Reflections*, Winter, 6–7.

Droogan, J. & Cullum, N. (1998). Systematic reviews in nursing. *International Journal of Nursing Studies*, 35, 13–22.

Duffy, M.E. (1987). The research process in baccalaureate nursing education: a ten-year review. *Image: The Journal of Nursing Scholarship*, 19, 87–91.

Dunford, M., Donoghue, J. & Lazaris, M. (1999). Case presentation of nurse-managed noninvasive positive pressure ventilation in an acute ward setting. *Heart & Lung: the Journal of Acute Critical Care*, 28, 348–51.

Dunn, S. & Yates, P. (2000). The roles of Australian chairs in clinical nursing. *Journal of Advanced Nursing*, 31(1), 165–71.

Dunn, S.V., Lawson, D., Robertson, S., Underwood, M., Clark, R., Valentine, T., Walker, N., Wilson-Row, C., Crowder, K. & Herewane, D. (2000). The development of competency standards for specialist critical care nurses. *Journal of Advanced Nursing*, 31(2), 339–46.

Dunning, T. & Martin, M. (1996). Developing a questionnaire: some methodological issues. *Australian Journal of Advanced Nursing*, 14(2), 31–38.

Durdin, J. (1999). *Eleven thousand nurses.* Royal Adelaide Hospital, Adelaide, Australia.

Eaves, Y. (2001). A synthesis technique for grounded theory data analysis. *Journal of Advanced Nursing*, 35(5), 654–63.

Edell-Gustafsson, U.M., Hetter, J.E. & Aren, C.B. (1999). Sleep and quality of life assessment in patients undergoing coronary artery bypass grafting. *Journal of Advanced Nursing*, 29, 1213–20.

Elliott, D. (1993). Comparison of three instruments for measuring patient anxiety in a coronary care unit. *Intensive Critical Care Nursing*, 9, 195–200.

Elliott, D. (1994). The effects of music and muscle relaxation on patient anxiety in a coronary care unit. *Heart & Lung: The Journal of Acute and Critical Care*, 23(1), 27–35.

Elliott, D. (1999). Measuring the health outcomes of general ICU patients: a systematic review of methods and findings. *Australian Critical Care*, 12, 132–40.

Elliott, M. (1997). The Reaction Level Scale: useful tool or just another instrument? *Australasian Journal of Neuroscience*, 10(4), 6–13.

Erickson, R.S., Meyer, L.T. & Woo, T.M. (1996). Accuracy of chemical dot thermometers in critically ill adults and young children. *Image: The Journal of Nursing Scholarship*, 28(1), 23–28.

Evans, D. (2001). *Music as an intervention for hospital patients: a systematic review.* (No. 15). Adelaide, The Joanna Briggs Institute for Evidence Based Nursing & Midwifery.

Evans, D. & Chang, A. (2000). Appraising systematic reviews. *Changing practice: evidence based practice information sheets for health professionals*, 1(1), 1–6.

Evans, D., Hodgkinson, B., Lambert, L. & Wood, J. (2001). Falls risk factors in the hospital setting: a systematic review. *International Journal of Nursing Practice*, 7, 38–45.

Evans, D., Hodgkinson, B., Lambert, L., Wood, J. & Kowanko, I. (1998). *Falls in acute hospitals—a systematic review.* (No. 1). Adelaide, The Joanna Briggs Institute for Evidence Based Nursing & Midwifery.

Everell, S. & Brown, C. (1986). *Running out of patience.* AFI Distribution (film).

Evidence-Based Medicine Working Group. (1992). Evidence-based medicine. A new approach to teaching the practice of medicine. *Journal of the American Medical Association*, 268(17), 2420–25.

Farmer, A. (1999). A home-based intervention reduced out-of-hospital deaths and hospitalizations in CHF (commentary). *ACP Journal Club*, 131 (July–Aug.), 6.

Fell, J. P. (1992). The familiar and the strange: on the limits of praxis in the early Heidegger. In Dreyfus, H. L. & Hall, H., eds, *Heidegger: a critical reader* (pp. 65–80). Cambridge, Mass, Blackwell.

Ferketich, S.L. & Verran, J.A. (1984). Residual analysis for causal model assumptions. *Western Journal of Nursing Research*, 6(1), 41–60.

Fetterman, D.M. (2000). *Ethnography: step by step.* (2nd ed.). Newbury Park, Sage Publications.

Finn, J. (2001). Challenging nursing rituals with evidence. *Nursing Review: Australia's Independent Voice of Nursing*, 8 December.

Fisher, M., King, J. & Tague, G. (2001). Development of a self-directed learning readiness scale for nursing education. *Nursing Education Today*, 21, 516–25.

Flemming, K. (1998). Asking answerable questions. *Evidence-Based Nursing*, 1(2), 36–37.

Forchuk, C. & Roberts, J. (1993). How to critique qualitative research articles. *Canadian Journal of Nursing Research*, 25(4), 107–15.

Fowers, B.J. & Eisen, M. (1994). Cardiac Change Scale: a brief self-report research measure. *Current Psychology*, 13, 185–92.

Frank-Stromberg, M.F., ed. (1992). *Instruments for clinical nursing research.* Boston, James and Bartlett.

Fraser, B., ed. (1983). *Macquarie book of events.* Macquarie University, Australia, Macquarie University.

French, P. (1999). The development of evidence-based nursing. *Journal of Advanced Nursing*, 29(1), 72–78.

From charity to choice: history of the Royal Hospital for Women (film) (1997). Sydney, Royal Hospital for Women.

Fulton, Y. (1997). Nurses' view on empowerment: a critical social theory perspective. *Journal of Advanced Nursing*, 26(3), 529–36.

Gagne, E.D. (1985). *The cognitive psychology of school learning.* Boston, Little, Brown.

Gardner, K. (1991). A summary of findings of a five-year comparison study of primary and team nursing. *Nursing Research*, 40(2), 113–17.

Gatens, M. (1991). *Feminism and philosophy: perspectives on difference and equality.* Cambridge, Polity Press.

Gattuso, S. (1996). The meaning of home for older women in rural Australia. *Australian Journal on Ageing*, 15(4), 172–76.

Gelvin, M. (1989). *A commentary of Heidegger's being and time.* (rev. ed.). Illinois, Illinois University Press.

Gennaro, S., Hodnett, E. & Kearney, M. (2001). Making evidence-based practice a reality in your institution: evaluating the evidence and using the evidence to change clinical practice. *Maternal Child Nursing*, 26(5), 236–44.

Gennaro, S. & Vessey, J. (1991). Making practice perfect. *Nursing Research*, 40, 529.

Gerdtz, M. & Bucknall, T. (2000). Australian triage nurses' decision-making and scope of practice. *Australian Journal of Advanced Nursing*, 18(1), 24–33.

Gerstman, B.B. (1998). *Epidemiology kept simple.* New York, Wilry-Liss.

Giacomini, M. K. & Cook, D.J. (2000). Users' guides to the medical literature: XXIII. Qualitative research in health care. A. Are the results of the study valid? *JAMA: Journal of the American Medical Association*, 284(3), 357–62.

Glaser, B. (1978). *Theoretical sensitivity: further advances in the methodology of grounded theory.* Mill Valley, Sociology Press.

Glaser, B. (1991). In honour of Anselm Strauss: collaboration. In Maines, E., ed., *Social organisation and social process: essays in honour of Anselm Strauss.* New York, Aldine De Gruyter.

Glaser, B. (1992). *Basics of grounded theory analysis: emergence vs forcing.* Mill Valley, Sociology Press.

Glaser, B., ed. (1993). *Examples of grounded theory: a reader.* Mill Valley, Sociology Press.

Glaser, B. (1994). Introduction. In Glaser, B., ed., *More grounded theory methodology: a reader.* Mill Valley, Sociology Press.

Glaser, B. & Strauss, A. (1967). *The discovery of grounded theory: strategies for qualitative research.* New York, Aldine.

Glass, E.C. (1991). Importance of research to practice. In Matco, M.A. & Kirchhoff, K.T., eds, *Conducting and using nursing research in the clinical setting.* Baltimore, Williams & Wilkins.

Glesne, C. & Peshkin, A. (1992). *Becoming qualitative researchers: an introduction.* New York, Longman.

Godden, J., Curry, G. & Delacour, S. (1993). The decline of myths and myopia? *Australian Journal of Advanced Nursing*, 10(2), 21–28.
Godden, J. & Forsyth, S. (2000). Defining relationships and limiting power: two leaders of Australian nursing, 1868–1904. *Nursing Inquiry*, 7(1), 10–19.
Gold, R. (1958). Roles in sociological field observation. *Social Forces*, 36, 217–23. (Cited in Kennedy, C. (1999). Participant observation as a research tool in a practice based profession. *Nurse Researcher*, 7(1), 56–65.)
Goodrich, A. (1932). *The social and ethical significance of nursing: a series of addresses.* New York, MacMillan.
Goodwin, L.D. (1997). Changing conceptions of measurement validity. *Journal of Nurse Education*, 36(3), 102–07.
Gortner, S. (1990). Nursing values and science: toward a science philosophy. *Image: The Journal of Nursing Scholarship*, 22, 101–05.
Grady, K.L. & Jalowiec, A. (1995). Predictors of compliance with diet 6 months after heart transplantation. *Heart & Lung: The Journal of Acute and Critical Care*, 24, 359–68.
Grbich, C. (1999). *Qualitative research in health: an introduction.* Thousand Oaks, California, Sage.
Greco, P.J. & Eisenberg, J.M. (1993). Changing physicians' practices. *New England Journal of Medicine*, 329(17), 1271–74.
Green, D.E., Walkey, F.H., McCormick, I.A. & Taylor, J.W. (1988). Development and evaluation of a 21-item version of the Hopkins Symptom Checklist with New Zealand and United States respondents. *Australian Journal of Psychology*, 40(1), 60–70.
Green, I. & Lewis, F. (1986). *Measurement and evaluation in health education and health promotion.* Palo Alto, Mayfield Publishing.
Greenhalgh, T. (1997). *How to read a paper: the basics of evidence based medicine.* London, BMJ Publishing Group.
Greenhill, J. & Henderson, M. (1997). Report on the patient satisfaction survey: models of managing a nursing care project. Unpublished work. Nursing Research Unit, Princess Alexandra Hospital. Brisbane, Queensland.
Greenwood, J. (1994). Action research and action researchers: some introductory considerations. *Contemporary Nurse*, 3, 84–92.
Greenwood, J., Holmes, C. & Bidewell, J. (2001). Mission impossible. *Collegian*, 8(1), 8–13.
Gregg, M. & Magilvy, J. (2001). Professional identity of Japanese nurses: bonding into nursing. *Nursing and Health Sciences*, 3, 47–55.
Grey, M., Cameron, M.E. & Thurber, F.W. (1991). Coping and adaptation in children with diabetes. *Nursing Research*, 40, 144–49.
Gross, D., Fogg, L. & Tucker, S. (1995). The efficacy of parent training for promoting positive parent–toddler relationships. *Research in Nursing & Health*, 18, 489–99.
Grundy, S. (1987). *Curriculum: product or praxis?* London, Falmer.
Guba, E. & Lincoln, Y. (1981). *Effective evaluation.* San Francisco, Jossey-Bass.
Guba, E. & Lincoln, Y. (1989). *Fourth generation evaluation.* London, Sage.
Guignon, C. B. (1983). *Heidegger and the problem of knowledge.* Indianapolis, Hacket.
Gullickson, C. (1993). My death nearing its future: A Heideggerian hermeneutical analysis of the lived experience of persons with chronic illness. *Journal of Advanced Nursing*, 18, 1386–92.
Guyatt, G.H. & Rennie, D. (1993). Users' guide to the medical literature (editorial). *Journal of the American Medical Association*, 270(17), 2096–97.
Guyatt, G. H., Sackett, D. L. & Cook, D. J. (1993). Users' guides to the medical literature. II. How to use an article about therapy or prevention. A. Are the results of the study valid? Evidence-Based Medicine Working Group. *Journal of the American Medical Association*, 270(21), 2598–2601.
Guyatt, G. H., Sackett, D. L. & Cook D. (1994). J. Users' guides to the medical literature. II. How to use an article about therapy or prevention. B. What were the results and will they help me in caring for my patients? Evidence-Based Medicine Working Group. *Journal of the American Medical Association*, 271(1), 59–63.
Guyatt, G., Walter, S. & Norman, G. (1987). Measuring change over time: assessing the usefulness of evaluative instruments. *Journal of Chronic Disease*, 40, 171–78.

Habermas, J. (1972). *Knowledge and human interests.* London, Heinemann.
Habermas, J. (1984). *The theory of communicative action. Vol. 1: Reason and the rationalization of society.* Boston, Beacon Press.
Habermas, J. (1987). *The theory of communicative action. Vol. 2: Lifeworld and system: the critique of functionalist reason.* Boston, Beacon Press.
Hall, J. (1999). Marginalization revisited: critical, postmodern, and liberation perspectives. *Advances in Nursing Science*, 22(2), 88–102.
Hall, J. & Stevens, P. (1991). Rigor in feminist research. *Advances in Nursing Science*, 13(3), 16–29.
Hall, L.A., Kotch, J.B., Browne, D. & Rayens, M.K. (1996). Self-esteem as a mediator of the effects of stressors and social resources on depressive symptoms in postpartum mothers. *Nursing Research*, 45(4), 231–38.
Hall, W. & Callery, P. (2001). Enhancing the rigor of grounded theory: incorporating reflexivity and relationality. *Qualitative Health Research*, 11(2), 257–72.
Hamilton, C. (1989). Nursing now and then: one woman's memoir. *Lilith*, 6, 83–93.
Hammersley, M. & Atkinson, P. (1983). *Ethnography: principles and practice.* London, Tavistock Publications.
Hanks, P., ed. (1986). *Collins dictionary of the English language.* (2nd ed.). London, Collins.
Hanna, B. (2001). Negotiating motherhood: the struggles of teenage mothers. *Journal of Advanced Nursing*, 34(4), 456–64.
Harris, M.R. & Warren, J.J. (1995). Patient outcomes: assessment issues for the CNS. *Clinical Nurse Specialist*, 9(2), 82–86.
Hart, E. & Bond, M. (1995). *Action research for health and social care.* Buckingham, Open University Press.
Harvey, S. (1993). The genesis of a phenomenological approach to advanced nursing practice. *Journal of Advanced Nursing*, 18, 526–30.
Hawe, P., Degeling, D. & Hall, J. (1990). *Evaluating health promotion: a health worker's guide.* Sydney, MacLennan & Petty.
Hayward, R. S., Wilson, M. C., Tunis, S. R., Bass, E. B. & Guyatt G. (1995). Users' guides to the medical literature. VIII. How to use clinical practice guidelines. A. Are the recommendations valid? The Evidence-Based Medicine Working Group. *Journal of the American Medical Association*, 274(7), 570–74.
Healy, C. & McKay, M. (1999). Identifying sources of stress and job satisfaction in the nursing environment. *Australian Journal of Advanced Nursing*, 17(2), 30–35.
Healy, C.M. & McKay, M.F. (2000). Nursing stress: the effects of coping strategies and job satisfaction in a sample of Australian nurses. *Journal of Advanced Nursing*, 31(3), 681–88.
Heidegger, M. (1962). *Being and time.* (trans. J. Macquarrie & E. Robinson). Blackwell, Oxford. (Original work published 1927.)
Held, D. (1980). *Introduction to critical theory.* London, Hutchinson.
Helps, A. (Cited in Cohen, J.M. & Cohen, M.J. (1980). *The Penguin dictionary of quotations.* Britain, Hazell Watson & Viney Ltd.)
Henderson, A. & Zernike, W. (2001). A study of the impact of discharge information for surgical patients. *Journal of Advanced Nursing*, 35(3), 435–41.
Henderson, S. (2000). Patient participation determined by nurses' attitudes toward caring. *International Journal of Human Caring*, 4(1), 30–35.
Henderson, V. (1956). Research in nursing practice: when (editorial). *Nursing Research*, 4, 99.
Heslop, L., Elsom, S. & Parker, N. (2000). Improving continuity of care across psychiatric and emergency services: combining patient data within a participatory action research framework. *Journal of Advanced Nursing*, 31(1), 135–43.
Hess, J. (1995). The art of stained glass: metaphor for the art of nursing. *Nursing Inquiry*, 2(4), 221–23.
Hewitt-Taylor, J. (2002). Case study: an approach to qualitative enquiry. *Nursing Standard*, 16, 33–37.
Hicks, C. (1995). The shortfall in published research: a study of nurses' research and publication activities. *Journal of Advanced Nursing*, 21(3), 594–604.

Hicks, C.M. (1996). *Understanding midwifery research. A basic guide to design and analysis.* New York, Churchill Livingstone.
Higgens, M., Dunn, S. & Theobold, K. (2000). The patients' perception of recovery after coronary angioplasty. *Australian Critical Care*, 13(3), 83–88.
Hill Bailey, P. (1997). Finding your way around qualitative methods in nursing research. *Journal of Advanced Nursing*, 25, 18–22.
Hinshaw, A.S. (1988). The new National Centre for Nursing Research: patient care research program. *Applied Nursing Research*, 1, 2–4.
Hinshaw, A.S. (1990). National Centre for Nursing Research: a commitment to excellence in science. In McCloskey, J.C. & Grace, H.K., eds, *Current issues in nursing*. St Louis, Mosby.
Hinshaw, A.S. (1991). Interfacing nursing and biologic science. *Journal of Professional Nursing*, 7(5), 264.
Hisama, K. (2001). Patterns of Japanese clinical nursing: a historical analysis. *Journal of Clinical Nursing*, 10(4), 451–54.
Hodge, J., Mounter, J., Gardner, G. & Rowly, G. (1990). Clinical trial of the Norton Scale in acute care setting. *Australian Journal of Advanced Nursing*, 8(1), 39–46.
Hofmeyer, A. & Cecchin, M. (2001). Enactment of virtue ethics: collaboration between nurse academics and international students in questionnaire design. *Australian Journal of Advanced Nursing*, 18(3), 8–13.
Holliday, J., Lowe, J. & Outram, S. (2002). Women's experience of myocardial infarction. *International Journal of Nursing Practice*, 6, 307–16.
Holloway, I. & Wheeler, S. (1996). *Qualitative research for nurses.* Oxford, Blackwell Science.
Holmes, S. (1996). Systematic search offers a sound evidence base. *Nursing Times*, 92(4), 37–39.
Holter, I. M. & Schwartz-Barcott, D. (1993). Action research: what is it? How has it been used and how can it be used in nursing? *Journal of Advanced Nursing*, 18, 298–304.
Horsfall, J. (1997). 'Difference' and nursing research. *Contemporary Nurse*, 6(1), 40–46.
Hoskins, C. (1996). Social support and patterns of adjustment to breast cancer. *Scholarly Inquiry Nursing Practice*, 10(2), 99–123.
Hughes, K.P. (1997). Feminism for beginners. In Hughes, K.P., ed., *Contemporary Australian feminism 2.* South Melbourne, Addison Wesley Longman.
Humm, M. (1989). *The dictionary of feminist theory.* London, Harvester Wheatsheaf.
Hunt, J.M. (1996). Barriers to research utilization. *Journal of Advanced Nursing*, 23(3), 423–25.
Hunt, J.O., Hendrata, M.V. & Myles, P.S. (2000). Quality of life 12 months after coronary artery bypass graft surgery. *Heart & Lung: The Journal of Acute and Critical Care*, 29, 401–11.
Hutchinson, D. (1997). A nurse's guide to the internet. *RN*, 60(1), 46–51.
Inhorn, M.C. (1994). *Quest for conception: gender, infertility, and Egyptian medical traditions.* Philadelphia, University of Philadelphia Press.
Inquiry into the management of care of children receiving complex heart surgery at the Bristol Royal Infirmary. *Bristol Royal Infirmary Inquiry.* (July 2001). Available at <http://www.bristol-inquiry.org.uk/index.htm>. Accessed 20 January 2002.
Inwood, M. (1997). *Heidegger: a very short introduction.* Oxford, Oxford University Press.
Irurita, V. (1999a). The problem of patient vulnerability. *Collegian*, 6(1), 10–15.
Irurita, V. (1999b). Factors affecting the quality of nursing care: the patient's perspective. *International Journal of Nursing Practice*, 5, 86–94.
Jackson, D. (1997). Feminism: a path to clinical knowledge development. *Contemporary Nurse*, 6(2), 85–91.
Jackson, D. (2000). Understanding women's health through Australian women's writings: a feminist exploration. PhD thesis, Flinders University of South Australia, Adelaide, Australia.
Jackson, D., Daly, J., Davidson, T., Elliott, D., Cameron-Traub, E., Wade, V., Salomonson, Y. & Chin, C. (2000). Women recovering from first-time myocardial infarction (MI): a feminist qualitative study. *Journal of Advanced Nursing*, 32(6), 1403–11.

Jackson, D., Raftos, M. & Mannix, J. (1996). Through the looking glass: reflections on the authorship and content of current Australian nursing journals. *Nursing Inquiry*, 3(2), 112–17.
Jackson, M., Schmierer, C. & Schneider, Z. (1996). Development, refinement and future usage of the scale: attitudes toward learning in pregnancy. *International Journal of Nursing Studies*, 33(1), 36–46.
Jaeschke, R., Guyatt, G. & Sackett, D.L. (1994a). Users' guides to the medical literature. III. How to use an article about a diagnostic test. A. Are the results of the study valid? Evidence-Based Medicine Working Group. *Journal of the American Medical Association*, 271(5), 389–91.
Jaeschke, R., Guyatt, G. H. & Sackett, D.L. (1994b). Users' guides to the medical literature. III. How to use an article about a diagnostic test. B. What are the results and will they help me in caring for my patients? The Evidence-Based Medicine Working Group. *Journal of the American Medical Association*, 271(9):703–07.
Janesick, V.J. (1994). The dance of qualitative research design: metaphor, methodolatory, and meaning. In Denzin, N.K. & Lincoln, Y.S., eds, *Handbook of qualitative research*. Thousand Oaks, California, Sage.
Jenicek, M. (1997). Epidemiology: evidence based medicine and evidence based public health. *Journal of Epidemiology*, 7(4), 187–97.
Joanna Briggs Institute for Evidence Based Nursing & Midwifery. About the Institute. 18 May 2000. Available at <http://www.joannabriggs.edu.au/about.html>. Accessed 20 January 2002.
Johnson, M. (1992). A silent conspiracy: some ethical issues of participant observation in nursing research. *International Journal of Nursing Studies*, 29(2), 213–33.
Johnstone, M. (1999). *Bioethics: a nursing perspective*. (3rd ed.). Sydney, Saunders.
Karim, K. (2001). Assessing the strengths and weaknesses of action research. *Nursing Standard*, 15(26), 33–35.
Katz, J., ed. (1972). *Experimentation with human beings*. New York, Russell Sage Foundation.
Kaulfeld, J. & Kaulfeld, J. (1996). *America on-line for dummies*. Fost City, California, IDG Books Worldwide.
Kazis, L.E., Anderson, J.J. & Meenan, R.F. (1989). Effect sizes for interpreting changes in health status. *Medical Care*, 27(3 Suppl.): S178–S189.
Keddy, B., Sims, S. & Stern, P. (1996). Grounded theory as feminist research methodology. *Journal of Advanced Nursing*, 23(3), 448–53.
Keith, J.M. (1988). Florence Nightingale: statistician and consultant epidemiologist. *International Nursing Review*, 35(5), 147–49.
Kelly, D. & Simpson, S. (2001). Action research in action: reflections on a project to introduce clinical practice facilitators to an acute hospital setting. *Journal of Advanced Nursing*, 33(5), 652–59.
Kemmis, S. & McTaggart, R., eds. (1988). *The action research planner*. (3rd ed.). Geelong, Vic., Deakin University Press.
Kenardy, J. (2000). The current status of psychological debriefing (editorial). *British Medical Journal*, 321, 1032–33.
Kendall, J. (1999). Axial coding and the grounded theory controversy. *Western Journal of Nursing Research*, 21(6), 743–57.
Kennedy, C. (1999). Participant observation as a research tool in a practice based profession. *Nurse Researcher*, 7(1), 56–65.
Kerlinger, F.H. (1986). *Foundations of behavioral research*. (3rd ed.). New York, Holt, Rinehart & Winston.
Kermode, M. (1995). Patients' experiences of nursing interventions during hospitalisation with an AIDS-defining illness. *Australian Journal of Advanced Nursing*, 12(3), 20–30.
Keyzer, D.M. (2000). Nursing research in practice: the case study revisited. *Australian Journal of Rural Health*, 8, 266–80.
Kincheloe, J. & McLaren, P. (1994). Rethinking critical theory and qualitative research. In Denzin, N. & Lincoln, Y., eds, *Handbook of qualitative research*. Thousand Oaks, California, Sage.

King, K. (1994). Method and methodology in feminist research: what is the difference? *Journal of Advanced Nursing*, 20(1), 19–22.

King, M. & Wilson, K. (1998). Diabetes health care of Aboriginal people at Nunkuwarrin Yunti. *Australian Journal of Advanced Nursing*, 15(2), 26–32.

Kite, K. (1999). Participant observation, peripheral observation or apart-icipant observation? *Nurse Researcher*, 7(1), 45–55.

Kitson, A., Harvey, G. & McCormack, B. (1998). Enabling the implementation of evidence based practice: a conceptual framework. *Quality in Health Care*, 7, 149–58.

Knapp, T.R. (1990). Treating ordinal scales as interval scales: an attempt to resolve the controversy. *Nursing Research*, 39(2), 121–24.

Knapp, T.R. (1993). Treating ordinal scales as ordinal scales. *Nursing Research*, 42(3), 184–86.

Koch, T. (1994a). Establishing rigour in qualitative research: the decision trail. *Journal of Advanced Nursing*, 19, 976–86.

Koch, T. (1994b). Beyond measurement: fourth generation evaluation in nursing. *Journal of Advanced Nursing*, 20, 1148–55.

Koch, T. (1995). Interpretive approaches in nursing research: the influence of Husserl and Heidegger. *Journal of Advanced Nursing*, 21, 827–36.

Koch, T. (1996). Implementation of a hermeneutic inquiry in nursing: philosophy, rigour and representation. *Journal of Advanced Nursing*, 24(1), 174–84.

Koch, T. (2000). 'Having a say': negotiation in fourth-generation evaluation. *Journal of Advanced Nursing*, 31(1), 117–25.

Koch, T. & Harrington, A. (1998). Reconceptualising rigour: the case for reflexivity. *Journal of Advanced Nursing*, 28(4), 882–90.

Koch, T. & Kelly, S. (1999). Identifying strategies for managing urinary incontinence with women who have multiple sclerosis. *Journal of Clinical Nursing*, 8(5), 550–59.

Koch, T., Kralik, D. & Taylor, J. (2000). Men living with diabetes: minimizing the intrusiveness of the disease. *Journal of Clinical Nursing*, 9(2), 247–54.

Koch, T., Marks, J. & Moss, J. (1999). Evaluation of the Collaborative Action Program. Unpublished report. Royal District Nursing Service Research Unit. Glenside, Adelaide, South Australia.

Koch, T., Marks, J. & Tooke, E. (2001). Evaluating a community nursing service: listening to the voices of clients with an intellectual disability and/or their proxies. *Journal of Clinical Nursing*, 10(3), 352–63.

Koch, T., Zadoroznji, M., Hudson, S., Lewis, C. & Bridge, K. (1999). Career structure for South Australian nurses: developing a research agenda. *Collegian*, 6(2), 34–37.

Kondora, L.L. (1994). A Heideggerian hermeneutical analysis of survivors of incest. *Image: The Journal of Nursing Scholarship*, 25(1), 11–16.

Koniak-Griffin, D. & Brecht, M.L. (1995). Linkages between sexual risk taking, substance use and AIDS knowledge among pregnant adolescents and young mothers. *Nursing Research*, 44, 340–46.

Kowanko, I., Long, L., Hodgkinson, B. & Evans, D. (1998). *The effectiveness of strategies for preventing and treating chemotherapy and radiation induced oral mucositis in patients with cancer*. Adelaide, The Joanna Briggs Institute for Evidence Based Nursing and Midwifery.

Kralik, D., Koch, T. & Wotton, K. (1997). Engagement and detachment: understanding patients' experiences with nursing. *Journal of Advanced Nursing*, 26(2), 399–407.

Krasner, D. (1996). Using a gentler hand: reflections on patients with pressure ulcers who experience pain. *Ostomy/Wound Management*, 42(3), 20–29.

Kvale, S. (1996). *Interviews: an introduction to qualitative research interviewing*. Thousand Oaks, California, Sage.

Kyngas, H.A., Skaar-Chandler, C.A. & Duffy, M.E. (2000). The development of an instrument to measure the compliance of adolescents with a chronic disease. *Journal of Advanced Nursing*, 32(6), 1499–1506.

Lane, P., McKenna, H., Ryan, A. & Fleming, P. (2001). Focus group methodology. *Nurse Researcher*, 8(3), 45–59.

Langley, G., ed. (1989). *Animal experimentation: consensus changes*. London, MacMillan Press.

Last, J.M. (1995). *A dictionary of epidemiology.* Oxford, Oxford University Press.
Lather, P. (1991). *Getting smart: feminist research and pedagogy with/in the postmodern.* New York, Routledge.
Laupacis, A., Wells, G., Richardson, W. S. & Tugwell, P. (1994). Users' guides to the medical literature. V. How to use an article about prognosis. Evidence-Based Medicine Working Group. *Journal of the American Medical Association*, 272(3), 234–37.
Lauri, S., Lepisto, M. & Kappeli, S. (1997). Patients' needs in hospital: nurses' and patients' views. *Journal of Advanced Nursing*, 25, 339–46.
Lauri, S. & Sainio, C. (1998). Developing the nursing care of breast cancer patients: an action research approach. *Journal of Clinical Nursing*, 7(5), 424–32.
Lawler, J. (1991). *Behind the screens: nursing, somology and the problem of the body.* Melbourne, Churchill Livingstone.
Lawner, L., ed. (1975). *Letters from prison: Antonio Gramsci.* New York, Harper Colophon.
Lazarus, R.S. & Folkman, S. (1984). *Appraisal and coping.* New York, Springer.
LeFort, S.M. (1993). The statistical versus clinical significance debate. *Image: The Journal of Nursing Scholarship*, 25, 57–62.
Leininger, M. (1970). *Nursing and anthropology: two worlds to blend.* New York, Wiley.
Leininger, M. (1978). *Transcultural nursing: concepts, theories, and practices.* New York, John Wiley & Sons.
Leininger, M.M. (1985). Ethnography and ethnonursing: models and modes of qualitative data analysis. In Leininger, M.M., ed., *Qualitative research methods in nursing.* Orlando, Grune & Stratton.
Levine, F.J. (1995). Consent for research on children. *Chronicle of Higher Education*, 10 November, B1–2.
Levine, M., Walter, S., Lee, H., Haines, T., Holbrook, A. & Moyer, V. (1994). Users' guides to the medical literature. IV. How to use an article about harm. *Journal of the American Medical Association*, 271(20), 1615–19.
Lewin, K. (1946). Action research and minority problems. *Journal of Social Issues*, 2(4), 34–46.
Lewin, K. (1951). *Field theory in social science.* New York, Harper.
Lincoln, Y.S. (1992). Sympathetic connections between qualitative methods and health research. *Qualitative Health Research*, 2(4), 375–91.
Lindsey, E., Sheilds, L. & Stajduhar, K. (1999). Creating effective nursing partnerships: relating community development to participatory action research. *Journal of Advanced Nursing*, 29(5), 1238–45.
Lipson, J.G. (1992). The health and adjustment of Iranian immigrants. *Western Journal of Nursing Research*, 14, 10–24.
Lipson, J.G. (1994). Ethical issues in ethnography. In Morse, J.M., ed., *Critical issues in qualitative research methods.* Thousand Oaks, California, Sage.
LoBiondo-Wood, G. et al. (1997). The impact of transplantation on quality of life: a longitudinal perspective. *Applied Nursing Research*, 10, 26–31.
Lovibond, S.H. & Lovibond, P.F. (1995). *Manual for the depression anxiety stress scales.* Sydney, Psychology Foundation of Australia.
Lowenthal, D. (1985). *The past is a foreign country.* Cambridge, Cambridge University Press.
Lumby, J. (1995a). Re-searching the knowing through the knower. *Collegian*, 2(1), 4–15.
Lumby, J. (1995b). The power of one: the changer and the changed. In Gray, G. & Pratt, R., eds, *Scholarship in the discipline of nursing.* Melbourne, Churchill Livingstone.
Lumby, J. (1997). Liver transplantation: the death/life paradox. *International Journal of Nursing Practice*, 3(4), 231–38.
Lynaugh, J. & Reverby, S. (1987). Thoughts on the nature of history. *Nursing Research*, 36(1), 68–69.
Lyneham, J. (2000). Violence in New South Wales emergency departments. *Australian Journal of Advanced Nursing*, 18(2), 8–17.
McCain, N.L. & Cella, D.F. (1995). Correlates of stress in HIV disease. *Western Journal of Nursing Research*, 17, 141–55.
McCallin, A. (2001). Interdisciplinary practice—a matter of teamwork: an integrated literature review. *Journal of Clinical Nursing*, 10(4), 419–28.

McCalman, J. (1998). *Sex and suffering: women's health in a women's hospital.* Melbourne, Melbourne University Press.
McCarthy, L. (1999). *Conference proceedings.* Sydney, Australian Society of the History of Medicine.
McCutcheon, G. & Jung, B. (1990). Alternative perspective on action research. *Theory into Practice*, 29(3), 144–50.
McCutcheon, H.H.I. & Pincombe, J. (2001). Intuition: an important tool in the practice of nursing. *Journal of Advanced Nursing*, 35(3), 342–48.
McDonald J. & Smith J. (2001). Evidence-based health care and community nursing: issues and challenges. *Australian Health Review*, 24(3), 133–40.
McDonald, L. (2001). Florence Nightingale and the early origins of evidence-based nursing. *Evidence-Based Nursing*, 4(3), 68–69.
McElroy, A. & Sheppard, G. (1999). The assessment and management of self-harming patients in an accident and emergency department: an action research project. *Journal of Clinical Nursing*, 8(1), 66–72.
McGee, B. (1987). *The great philosophers: an introduction to Western philosophy.* Oxford, Oxford University Press.
Macintyre, S. (1986). *The Oxford history of Australia.* (vol. 4). Melbourne, Oxford University Press.
McKechnie, J.L. (general ed.). (1977). *Webster's new twentieth century dictionary of the English language, unabridged.* Cleveland, Collins+World.
McKibbon, K.A. & Marks, S. (1998a). Searching for the best evidence. Part 1: where to look. *Evidence-Based Nursing*, 1, 68–70.
McKibbon, K.A. & Marks, S. (1998b). Searching for the best evidence. Part 2: searching CINAHL and Medline. *Evidence-Based Nursing*, 1, 105–07.
Mackie, J.L. (1977). *Ethics: inventing right and wrong.* London, Pelican Books.
McKinley, S., Moser, D.K. & Dracup, K. (2000). Treatment-seeking behavior for acute myocardial infarction symptoms in North America and Australia. *Heart Lung*, 29(4), 237–47.
Macnee, C.L. & Talsma, A. (1995). Development and testing of the barriers to cessation scale. *Nursing Research*, 44(4), 214–19.
McNeill, P. (1985). *Research methods.* London, Tavistock Publications.
McNiff, J.P.L. & Whitehead, J. (1996). *You and your action research project.* London, Routledge.
McTaggart, R. (1991). *Action research: a short modern history.* Geelong, Vic., Deakin University Press.
Maggs-Rapport, F. (2001). Best research practice: in pursuit of methodological rigour. *Journal of Advanced Nursing*, 35, 373–83.
Malinowski, B. (1922). *Argonauts of the western Pacific.* London, Routledge & Kegan Paul.
Manias, E. & Street, A. (2000a). Legitimation of nurses' knowledge through policies and protocols in clinical practice. *Journal of Advanced Nursing*, 32, 1467–75.
Manias, E. & Street, A. (2000b). The handover: uncovering the hidden practices of nurses. *Intensive and Critical Care Nursing*, 16(6), 373–83.
Manias, E. & Street, A. (2001). Nurse–doctor interactions during critical care ward rounds. *Journal of Clinical Nursing*, 10(4), 442–50.
Manley, K. (1997). A conceptual framework for advanced practice: an action research project operationalizing an advanced practitioner/consultant nurse role. *Journal of Clinical Nursing*, 6, 179–90.
Mant, J. (1999). Case control studies. In Dawes, M., Davies, P., Gray, A., Mant, J., Seers, K. & Snowball, R., eds, *Evidence-based practice: a primer for health care professionals* (pp. 73–83). Edinburgh, Churchill-Livingstone.
Marasovic, C., Kenney, C., Elliott, D. & Sindhusake, D. (1997). A comparison of nursing activities associated with manual and automated documentation in an Australian ICU. *Computers in Nursing*, 15, 201–11.
Marcus, G.E. (1994). What comes (just) after 'post'?: the case of ethnography. In Denzin, N. & Lincoln, Y., eds, *Handbook of qualitative research.* Thousand Oaks, California, Sage.
Margolis, J.R., Gillum, R.F., Feinleib, M., Brasch, R.C. & Fabsitz, R.R. (1974). Community surveillance for coronary heart disease: the Framingham Cardiovascular

Disease Survey. Methods and preliminary results. *American Journal of Epidemiology, 100*, 425–36.
Marshall, B.L. (1988). Feminist theory and critical theory. *Canadian Review of Sociology and Anthropology*, 25(2), 208–30.
Marshall, P.A. (1991). Research ethics in applied medical anthropology. In Hill, C.E., ed., *Training manual in applied medical anthropology* (pp. 213–235). Washington, American Anthropological Association.
Maslach, C. & Jackson, S.W. (1986). Maslach burnout inventory manual. Palo Alto, California, Consulting Psychologists Press.
Mead, D. & Moseley, L. (2001). The use of Delphi as a research approach. *Nurse Researcher*, 8(4), 4–23.
Meah, S., Luker, K. A. & Cullum, N. A. (1996). An exploration of midwives' attitudes to research and perceived barriers to research utilisation. *Midwifery*, 12(2), 73–84.
Melia, K. (1996). Rediscovering Glaser. *Qualitative Health Research*, 6(3), 368–78.
Meyer, J. (2000). Qualitative research in health care: using qualitative methods in health related action research. *British Medical Journal*, 320(7228), 178–81.
Miller, C. (2001). Patient care information and its use by nurses: 'becoming informed'. Master's thesis, Central Queensland University, Queensland, Australia.
Miller, M.A. & Babcock, D.E. (1996). *Critical thinking applied to nursing*. St Louis, Mosby.
Miller, S. & Fredericks, M. (1999). How does grounded theory explain? *Qualitative Health Research*, 9(4), 538–51.
Milligan, R.A., Flenniken, P.A. & Pugh, L.C. (1996). Positioning intervention to minimise fatigue in breastfeeding women. *Applied Nursing Research*, 9(2), 67–70.
Minichiello, V., Aroni, R., Timewell, E. & Alexander, L. (1995). *In-depth Interviewing*. (2nd ed.). Melbourne, Longman.
Minichiello, V., Sullivan, G., Greenwood, K. & Axford, R. (1999). *Handbook for research methods in health sciences*. Sydney, Addison Wesley Longman.
Minister, K. (1991). A feminist frame for the oral history interview. In Gluck, D. & Patai, D., eds, *Women's words: the feminist practice of oral history*. New York, Routledge.
Minnick, A., Roberts, M.J., Young, W.B., Kleinpell, R.M. & Micek, W. (1995). An analysis of posthospitalization telephone survey data. *Nursing Research*, 44(6), 371–75.
Mitchell, T. & Koch, T. (1997). An attempt to give nursing home residents a voice in the quality improvement process: the challenge of frailty. *Journal of Clinical Nursing*, 6, 453–61.
Mohanty, C. (1992). Feminist encounters: locating the politics of experience. In Barrett, M. & Phillips, A., eds, *Destabilizing theory: contemporary feminist debates*. Cambridge, Polity Press.
Morison, M. & Moir, J. (1998). The role of computer software in the analysis of qualitative data: efficient clerk, research assistant or Trojan horse? *Journal of Advanced Nursing*, 28(1), 106–16.
Morse, C.A., Smith, A., Dennerstein, L., Green, A., Hopper, J. & Burger, H. (1994). The treatment-seeking woman at menopause. *Maturitas*, 18, 161–73.
Morse, J. M. (1991). Approaches to qualitative–quantitative methodological triangulation. *Nurse Researcher*, 40(1), 120–23.
Morse, J.M. & Field, P.A. (1995). *Qualitative research methods for health professionals*. (2nd ed.). Thousand Oaks, California, Sage.
Mott, S. (1996). Passing time in Clifton Court: an ethnographic study of a unit for confused older people. PhD thesis, Deakin University, Geelong, Australia.
Moyer, A., Coristine, M., Jamault, M., Roberge, G. & O'Hagan, M. (1999). Identifying older people in need using action research. *Journal of Clinical Nursing*, 8(1), 103–11.
Mulhall, A. (1996). *Epidemiology, nursing and health care*. London, MacMillan.
Mulhall, A. (2000). The case for a more epidemiologically informed nursing profession. *Nt Research*, 5(1), 65–74.
Mundinger, M.O., Kane, R.L., Lenz, E.R., Totten, A.M., Tsai, W-Y., Cleary, P.D., Friedwald, W.T., Siv, A.L. & Shelaski, M.L. (2000). Primary care outcomes in patients treated by nurse practitioners or physicians; a randomized trial. *Journal of the American Medical Association*, 283(1), 59–68.

Munro, B.H. (2001). *Statistical methods for health care research.* (4th ed.). Philadelphia, Lippincott.

Murphy, P.A. (1992). Clinical epidemiology: applying science to the art of nurse-midwifery. *Journal of Nurse Midwifery,* 37(4), 219–21.

National Centre for Biotechnology Information (NCBI). PubMed overview. National Library of Medicine/National Institute of Health. (October, 2001). Available at http://www.ncbi.nlm.nih.gov:80/entrez/query/static/overview.html Accessed 20 January 2002.

National Health and Medical Research Council (NHMRC). (1992). *Statement of human experimentation and supplementary notes.* Canberra, NHMRC.

National Health and Medical Research Council (NHMRC). (1999). *A guide to the development, implementation and evaluation of clinical practice guidelines.* Canberra, NHMRC.

National Health and Medical Research Council (NHMRC). (2000). *How to use the evidence: assessment and application of scientific evidence.* Canberra, NHMRC.

NHMRC, ARC, CSIRO, AVCC, & ARMCANZ. (1997). *Australian code of practice for the care and use of animals for scientific purposes.* (6th ed.). Canberra, AGPS.

National Institute of Nursing Research (NINR). (2001). Available at http://www.nih.gov/ninr/about/history Accessed 4 January 2002.

Neelon, V.J., Champagne, M.T., Carlson, J.R. & Funk, S.G. (1996). The NEECHAM confusion scale: construction, validation and clinical testing. *Nursing Research,* 45(6), 324–30.

New England Journal of Medicine website. Available at <http://www.nejm.org>.

New NHS Modern, Dependable–Executive Summary. Department of Health. (December 1997). Available at <http://www.doh.gov.uk/newnhs.htm>. Accessed 20 January 2002.

Newman, M., Papadopoulos, I. & Melifonwu, R. (2000). Implementation forum. Developing organisational systems and culture to support evidence-based practice: the experience of the Evidence-Based Ward Project. *Evidence-Based Nursing,* 3(4), 103–05.

Nicoll, L.H. & Ouelette, T.H. (1997). *Nurses' guide to the internet: computers in nursing.* Philadelphia, Lippincott.

Nicoll, L.H., Ouellette, T.H., Bird, D.C. & Harper, J. (1996). Bibliography database managers. *Computers in Nursing,* 14(1), 45–46.

Nightingale, F. (1863). *Notes of hospitals.* London, Longman Group.

Nixon, M., Teschendorff, J., Finney, J. & Karnilowicz, W. (1997). Expanding the nursing repertoire: the effect of massage on post-operative pain. *Australian Journal of Advanced Nursing,* 14(3), 21–26.

Nolan, A. & Hazelton, L. (1995). *The practising nurse.* Sydney, WB Saunders.

Nursing Research Section, New Zealand Nurses Organisation (NRSNZO). (2001). Available at <http://nursingresearch.co.nz/about/history>. Accessed 4 January 2002.

Nutting, M.A. (1912). *Educational status of nursing.* (Bulletin No. 7). Washington, DC, US Bureau of Education.

Nutting, M.A. (1926). *A sound economic basis for schools of nursing and other addresses.* New York, GP Putnam's Sons.

O'Brien, L. (2000). Nurse–client relationships: the experience of community psychiatric nurses. *Australian and New Zealand Journal of Mental Health Nursing,* 9, 184–94.

O'Brien, L. (2001). The relationship between community psychiatric nurses and clients with severe and persistent mental illness: the client's experience. *Australian and New Zealand Journal of Mental Health Nursing,* 10, 176–86.

Ocker, B.M. & Pawlick Plank, D.M. (2000). The research nurse role in a clinic-based oncology research setting. *Cancer Nursing,* 23(4), 286–91.

O'Connell, B. (2000). Enabling care: working through obscurity and uncertainty, a basic social process used in selected acute care settings. *Australian Journal of Advanced Nursing,* 17(3), 32–39.

Offredy, M. (2000). Advanced nursing practice: the case of nurse practitioners in three Australian states. *Journal of Advanced Nursing,* 31(2), 274–81.

Oiler Boyd, C. (1993). Philosophical foundations of qualitative research. In Munhall, P.L. & Oiler Boyd, C., eds, *Nursing research: a qualitative perspective.* (2nd ed.). New York, National League for Nursing.

Olesen, V. (1994). Feminisms and models of qualitative research. In Denzin, N. & Lincoln, Y., eds, *Handbook of qualitative research*. Thousand Oaks, California, Sage Publications.
Orlando, I.J. (1961). *The dynamic nurse–patient relationship*. New York, GP Putnam's Sons.
O'Sullivan, A.O. & Jacobson, B.J. (1992). A randomised trial of a health care program for first-time adolescent mothers and their infants. *Nursing Research*, 41(4), 210–15.
Outhwaite, W. (1994). *Habermas: a critical introduction*. Cambridge, Polity Press.
Overland, J., Yue, D.K. & Mira, M. (2001). Use of Medicare services related to diabetes care: the impact of rural isolation. *Australian Journal of Rural Health*, 9, 311–16.
Oxford Dictionary of Quotations. (1999). Oxford, Oxford University Press.
Oxman, A.D., Cook, D.J. & Guyatt, G.H. (1994). Users' guides to the medical literature. VI. How to use an overview. Evidence-Based Medicine Working Group. *Journal of the American Medical Association*, 272(17), 1367–71.
Oxman, A.D., Sackett, D.L. & Guyatt, G.H. (1993). Users' guides to the medical literature. I. How to get started. The Evidence-Based Medicine Working Group. *Journal of the American Medical Association*, 270(17), 2093–95.
Oxman, A.D., Thomson, M.A., Davis, D.A. & Haynes, R.B. (1995). No magic bullets: a systematic review of 102 trials of interventions to improve professional practice. *Cmaj*, 153(10), 1423–31.
Pagano, R.R. (1986). *Understanding statistics in the behavioural sciences*. (2nd ed.). (pp. 341–46). New York, West Publishing.
PAHO Advisory Committee on the Teaching of Community Nursing. Epidemiology in Nursing. (1976). *PAHO Bulletin*, X3, 258–65.
Palmer, I. (1977). Florence Nightingale: reformer, reactionary, researcher. *Nursing Research*, 26, 84–89.
Parker, B. & McFarlane, J. (1991). Feminist theory and nursing: an empowerment model for research. *Advances in Nursing Science*, 13(3), 59–67.
Parse, R.R. ed. (2001). *Qualitative inquiry*. Boston, Jones & Bartlett.
Pasco, G.C. (1983). Patient satisfaction in primary health care: a literature review and analysis. *Evaluation and Program Planning*, 6(1), 185–210.
Patai, D. (1991). US academics and Third World women: is ethical research possible? In Gluck, D. & Patai, D., eds, *Women's words: the feminist practice of oral history*. New York, Routledge.
Patterson, E., Del Mar, C. & Najman, J. (1999). A descriptive study of nurses employed by general practitioners in south-east Queensland. *Australian Journal of Advanced Nursing*, 17(2), 13–20.
Patton, M.Q. (1990). *Qualitative evaluation and research methods*. Newbury Park, California, Sage.
Paul, R.W. (1995). *Critical thinking: how to prepare students for a rapidly changing world*. Santa Rosa, California, Foundation of Critical Thinking.
Pearson, A. & FitzGerald, M. (2001). A survey of nurses' views on indicators for continuing competence in nursing. *Australian Journal of Advanced Nursing*, 19(1), 20–26.
Pearson, J. (1998). An exploration of the empowerment of nursing students in a clinical context. *Nursing Praxis New Zealand*, 13(3), 45–55.
Pedhazur, E. & Schmelkin, L. (1991). *Measurement, design and analysis: an integrated approach*. Hillsdale, NJ, Lawrence Erlbaum Associates.
Peele, S. (1981). Reductionism in the psychology of the eighties. *American Psychologist*, 36(8), 807–18.
Peeters, A., Mamun, A.A., Willekens, F. & Bonneux, L. (2002). A cardiovascular life history: a life course analysis of the original Framingham heart study cohort. *European Heart Journal*, 23, 458–66.
Peplau, H.E. (1952). *Interpersonal relations in nursing: a conceptual frame of reference for psychodynamic nursing*. New York, GP Putnams' Sons.
Perry, J. & Moss, C. (1989). Generating alternatives in nursing: turning curriculum into a living process. *Australian Journal of Advanced Nursing*, 6(2), 35–40.
Phillips, E.M. & Pugh, D.S. (1994). *How to get a PhD: a handbook for students and their supervisors*. (2nd ed.). London, Open University Press.

Ploeg, J. (1999). Identifying the best research design to fit the question. Part 2: qualitative designs. *Evidence-Based Nursing*, 2, 36–37.

Polgar, S. & Thomas, S.A. (1995). *Introduction to research in the health sciences.* (3rd ed.). Melbourne, Churchill Livingstone.

Polit, D.F. & Sherman, R.E. (1990). Statistical power in nursing research. *Nurse Researcher*, 39, 365–69.

Pollack, L.E. (1996). Inpatient self-management of bi-polar disorder. *Applied Nursing Researcher*, 9(2), 71–79.

Potger, K. & Elliott, D. (1994). Reproducibility of central venous pressures in supine and lateral positions: a pilot evaluation of the phlebostatic axis. He*art & Lung: The Journal of Acute and Critical Care*, 23, 285–99.

Pranulis, M.F. (1996). Protecting rights of human subjects. *Western Journal of Nursing Research*, 18(4), 474–78.

Punch, K.F. (1998). *Introduction to social research: quantitative and qualitative approaches.* Thousand Oaks, California, Sage Publications.

Quiller-Couch, A. (1954). *On the art of writing.* Cambridge, Cambridge University Press.

Rafferty, A.M., Robinson, J. & Elkan, R., eds. (1997). *Nursing history and the politics of welfare.* London, Routledge.

Raftos, M., Jackson, D. & Mannix, J. (1998). Idealised versus tainted femininity: discourses of the menstrual experience in Australian magazines that target young women. *Nursing Inquiry*, 5(3), 174–86.

Raftos, M., Mannix, J. & Jackson, D. (1997). More than motherhood? A feminist exploration of 'women's health' in papers indexed by CINAHL 1993–1995. *Journal of Advanced Nursing*, 26, 1142–49.

Ratcliffe, P. (1998). Using the 'new' statistics in nursing research. *Journal of Advanced Nursing*, 27, 132–39.

Ray, M.A. (1992). Critical theory as a framework to enhance nursing science. *Nursing Science Quarterly*, 5(3), 98–117.

Reaby, L. (1998). Breast restoration decision making: enhancing the process. *Cancer Nursing*, 21, 196–204.

Reason, P. & Bradbury, H., eds. (2001). *Handbook of action research: participative inquiry and practice.* London, Sage.

Reinharz, S. (1992). *Feminist methods in social research.* New York, Oxford University Press.

Retsas, A. (2000). Barriers to using research evidence in nursing practice. *Journal of Advanced Nursing*, 31(3), 599–606.

Reynolds, H. (1992). Henry Reynolds. *Sydney Morning Herald*, 18 April, p. 23.

Ritchie, J. (general editor). (1996). *Australian dictionary of biography.* (vol. 14). Melbourne, Melbourne University Press.

Ritzer, G. (1992). *Contemporary sociological theory.* (3rd ed.). New York, McGraw-Hill.

Robb, I.H. (1906). *Nursing: its principles and practice for hospital and private use.* (3rd ed.). Cleveland, EC Koeckert.

Roberts, J. & DiCenso, A. (1999). Identifying the best research design to fit the question. Part I: quantitative designs. *Evidence-Based Nursing*, 2, 4–6.

Rogers, B. (1993). *Diffusion of innovations.* (3rd ed.). New York, Free Press.

Rogers, M.E. (1990). Nursing: science of unitary, irreducible, human beings: update. In Barrett, E.A.M., ed., *Visions of Rogers' science-based nursing.* New York, NLN.

Rogers, T.S. & Kashima, Y. (1998). Nurses' responses to people with schizophrenia. *Journal of Advanced Nursing*, 27, 195–203.

Rose, K., Waterman, H., McLeod, D. & Tullo, A. (1999). Planning and managing research into day-surgery for cataract. *Journal of Advanced Nursing*, 29(6), 1514–19.

Ross, A.C. & Ostrow, L. (2001). Subjectively perceived quality of life after coronary artery bypass surgery. *American Journal of Critical Care*, 10, 11–16.

Rossi, P. & Freeman, H. (1993). *Evaluation: a systematic approach.* London, Sage.

Rosswurm, M.A. & Larrabee, J.H. (1999). A model for change to evidence-based practice. *Image: The Journal of Nursing Scholarship*, 31(4), 317–22.

Royal College of Nursing Australia (RCNA). (1998). *Statement on nursing research.* Royal College of Nursing, Australia.

Royle, J. A., Blythe, J., DiCenso, A., Baumann, A. & Fitzgerald, D. (1997). Do nurses have the information resources and skills for research utilization? *Canadian Journal of Nursing Administration*, 10(3), 9–30.

Rudy, E.B. (1991). Unravelling the mystique of power analysis. *Heart & Lung: The Journal of Acute and Critical Care*, 20(5), 517–22.

Rudy, E., Daly, B.J., Douglas, S., Montenegro, H.D., Song, R. & Dyer, M. A. (1995). Patient outcomes for the chronically ill: special care unit versus intensive care unit. *Nurse Researcher*, 44(6), 324–31.

Runyon, R.P. & Haber, A. (1980). *Fundamentals of behavioral science.* (4th ed.). London, Addison-Wesley Publishing Co.

Russell, C.K. (1996). Elder care recipients' care-seeking process. *Western Journal of Nursing Research*, 18, 43–62.

Russell, K.M. & Champion, V.L. (1996). Health beliefs and social influence in home safety practices of mothers with preschool children. *Image: The Journal of Nursing Scholarship*, 28, 59–64.

Russell, R.L. (1990). *From Nightingale to now: nurse education in Australia.* Sydney, Harcourt Brace Jovanovich.

Russell, R.L. (2000). Milestones in Australian nursing. In Daly, J., Speedy, S. & Jackson, D., eds, *Contexts of nursing: an introduction*. Sydney, MacLennan & Petty.

Ruthven, K.K. (1984). *Feminist literary studies: an introduction.* London, Cambridge University Press.

Sackett, D.L., Rosenberg, W.M.C., Muir Gray, J.A., Haynes, R.B. & Richardson, S. (1996). Evidence based medicine: what it is and what it isn't. *British Medical Journal*, 312(7023), 71–72.

Sackett, D.L., Straus, S.E., Richardson, W.S., Rosenberg, W. & Haynes, R.B. (2000). *Evidence-based medicine: how to practise and teach EBM.* Edinburgh, Churchill Livingstone.

St John, W. (1999). Beyond the sick role: situating community health nursing practice. *Collegian*, 6(1), 30–35.

Sanday, P.R. (1983). The ethnographic paradigm(s). In Van Maanen, J., ed., *Qualitative methodology* (pp. 19–36). Newbury Park, Sage.

Sandelowski, M. (1991). Telling stories: narrative approaches in qualitative research. *Advances in Nursing Science*, 8(3), 27–37.

Sandelowski, M. (1993). Rigor or rigor mortis: the problem of rigor in qualitative research revisited. *Advances in Nursing Science*, 16(2), 1–8.

Sandelowski, M. (1995). Qualitative analysis: what it is and how to begin. *Research in Nursing & Health*, 18, 371–75.

Santamaria, N., Daly, S., Addicott, R. & Clayton, L. (2001). The development, validity and reliability of the hospital in the Home Dependency Scale (HDS). *Australian Journal of Advanced Nursing*, 18(4), 8–14.

Saunders, J. M. (1994). Self-caring in a family unit of an HIV-positive individual. *Clinical Nursing Research*, 3(4), 334–52.

Schmitt, M.H. (1994). The connectedness of nursing research: revisiting an old issue. *Research in Nursing & Health*, 17, 319–20.

Schneider, Z. (2002). Pregnant women's experiences of models of care in some hospitals in Victoria. *Australian Journal of Advanced Nursing*, 19(3), 32–38.

Scriven, M. (1972). Pros and cons about goal free evaluation. *Evaluation comment*, 3(4), 1–5. Center for the study of evaluation, Los Angeles, University of California.

Seale, C. (1999). Quality in qualitative research. *Qualitative Inquiry*, 5(4), 465–78.

Seibold, C., Miller, M. & Hall, J. (1999). Midwives and women in partnership: the ideal and the real. *Australian Journal of Advanced Nursing*, 17(2), 21–27.

Selim, P., Bashford, C. & Grossman, C. (2001). Evidence-based practice: tap water cleansing of leg ulcers in the community. *Journal of Clinical Nursing*, 10(3), 372–79.

Seymer, L., ed. (1954). *Selected writings of Florence Nightingale.* New York, Macmillan.

Sheldon, T. (2000a). Estimating treatment effects: real or the result of chance? *Evidence-Based Nursing*, 3, 36–39.

Sheldon, T. (2000b), Statistics for evidence-based nursing. *Evidence-Based Nursing*, 3, 4–6.

Shin, K. (1999). On surviving breast cancer and mastectomy. In Madjar, I. & Walton, J. A., eds, *Nursing and the experience of illness: phenomenology in practice* (pp. 77–97). Sydney, Allen & Unwin.
Short, P. (1995). Our pictures of us. *Nursing Inquiry*, 2(4), 224–26.
Shorten, A. & Wallace, M. (1997). Evidence-based practice: the future is clear. *Australian Nursing Journal*, 4(6), 22–24.
Shorten, A., Wallace, M.C. & Crookes, P.A. (2001). Developing information literacy: a key to evidence-based nursing. *International Nursing Review*, 48, 86–92.
Shyu, Y.H. (2000). Development and testing of the Family Caregiving Factors Inventory (FCFI) for home health assessment in Taiwan. *Journal of Advanced Nursing*, 32(1), 226–34.
Sigmon, H.D., Amende, L.M. & Grady, P.A. (1996). Development of biological studies to support biobehavioural research at the National Institute of Nursing Research. *Image: The Journal of Nursing Scholarship*, 28(2), 88.
Sigsworth, J. (1995). Feminist research: its relevance to nursing. *Journal of Advanced Nursing*, 22, 896–99.
Sigurdsson, H. (2001). The meaning of being a perioperative nurse. *Association of Operating Room Nurses Journal*, 74(2), 202–17.
Silva, M.C. (1995). *Ethical guidelines in the conduct, discrimination and implementation of nursing research*. Washington, DC, American Nurses Publishing.
Simmons, L.W. & Henderson, V. (1964). *Nursing research: a survey and assessment*. New York, Appleton-Century-Crofts.
Singer, P. (1991). *Practical ethics*. London, Cambridge University Press.
Skaggs, B.G. & Yates, B.C. (1999). Quality of life comparisons after coronary angioplasty and coronary artery bypass graft surgery. *Heart & Lung: The Journal of Acute and Critical Care*, 28, 409–17.
Small, R., Lumley, J., Donohue, L., Potter, A. & Waldenström, U. (2000). Randomised controlled trial of midwife led debriefing to reduce maternal depression after operative childbirth. *British Medical Journal*, 321, 1043–47.
Smith, B., ed. (1993). *Issues and methods in research: study guide*. Adelaide, University of South Australia, Underdale Campus.
Smith, C. & Sutton, F. (1999). Best practice: what it is and what it is not. *International Journal of Nursing Practice*, 5: 100–05.
Smith, M.C. & Stullenbarger, F.A. (1991). A prototype for integrative review and meta-analysis of nursing research. *Journal of Advanced Nursing*, 16, 1272–83.
Snowball, R. (1999). Finding the evidence: an information skills approach. In Dawes, M., Davies, P., Gray, A., Mant, J., Seers, K. & Snowball, R., eds, *Evidence-based practice: a primer for health care professionals* (pp. 15–46). Edinburgh, Churchill Livingstone.
Snowdon, J. (1994). Breast cancer study monitored patients against their wishes. *Houston Chronicle*, A22, December 17.
Speedy, S. (1991). The contribution of feminist research. In Gray, G. & Pratt, R., eds, *Towards a discipline of nursing*. Melbourne, Churchill Livingstone.
Speedy, S. (1997). Nursing and feminisms: a glance backwards, a gaze forwards. *Nursing Inquiry*, 4(4), 217–18.
Spender, D. (1985). *Man made language*. (2nd ed.). London, Pandora Press.
Spielberger, C.D. (1973). *Manual for the state-trait anxiety inventory for children*. Palo Alto, California, Consulting Psychologists Press.
Spradley, J.P. (1979). *The ethnographic interview*. New York, Holt, Rinehart & Winston.
Spradley, J.P. (1980). *Participant observation*. Fort Worth, Harcourt Brace Janovich.
Spradley, J.P. & McCurdy, D.W. (1972). *The cultural experience: ethnography in complex society*. Chicago, Science Research Associates.
Stake, R. (1973). The countenance of educational evaluation. In Worthen, R. & Sanders, J., eds, *Educational evaluation: theory and practice*. Belmont, California.
Stanley, L. & Wise, S. (1993). *Breaking out again: feminist ontology and epistemology*. New York, Routledge.
Starey, N. (2001, May). What is clinical governance? *'What is?' Bulletin*, 1(12), 1–7. London, Hayward Medical Communications. Available at <http://www.evidence-based-medicine.co.uk/ebmfiles/WhatisClinGov.pdf>. Accessed 20 January 2002.

Stetler, C.B. (1994). Refinement of the Stetler/Marram model for application of research findings to practice. *Nursing Outlook*, 42(1), 15–25.
Stewart, S. & Jaarsma, T. (2001). Research in cardiovascular nursing in Europe: toward a UNITED approach. *Journal of Cardiovascular Nursing*, 16(1), 69–72.
Stewart, S., Pearson, B.A. & Horowitz, J.D. (1998). Effects of home-based intervention among patients with congestive heart failure discharged from acute hospital care. *Archives of Internal Medicine*, 158(10), 1067–72.
Stewart, S., Vandenbroek, A.J., Pearson, B.A. & Horowitz, J.D. (1999). Prolonged beneficial effects of home-based intervention on unplanned readmission and mortality among patients with congestive heart failure. *Archives of Internal Medicine*, 159(3), 257–61.
Strachan, G. (1996). *Labour of love: the history of the Nurses' Association of Queensland.* Sydney, Allen & Unwin.
Strauss, A. (1987). *Qualitative analysis for social scientists.* Cambridge, Cambridge University Press.
Strauss, A. (1993). *Continual permutations of action.* Hawthorne, Aldine de Gruyter.
Strauss, A. (1994). Awareness contexts and grounded formal theory. In Glaser, B., ed., *More grounded theory methodology: a reader.* Mill Valley, Sociology Press.
Strauss, A. (1995). Notes on the nature and development of general theories. *Qualitative Inquiry*, 1(1), 7–18.
Strauss, A. & Corbin, J. (1990). *Basics of qualitative research: grounded theory procedures and techniques.* Newbury Park, Sage.
Strauss, A. & Corbin, J. (1994). Grounded theory methodology: an overview. In Denzin, N. & Lincoln, Y., eds, *Handbook of qualitative research.* Thousand Oaks, California, Sage.
Strauss, A. & Corbin, J., eds. (1997). *Grounded theory in practice.* Thousand Oaks, California, Sage.
Strauss, A. & Corbin, J. (1998). *Basics of qualitative research: techniques and procedures for developing grounded theory.* (2nd ed.). Thousand Oaks, California, Sage.
Street, A. (1991). *From image to action: reflection in nursing practice.* Geelong, Vic., Deakin University Press.
Street, A. (1995). *Nursing replay: researching nursing culture together.* Melbourne, Churchill Livingstone.
Street, A. (1998). From soulmates to stakeholders: issues in creating quality postmodern participatory research relationships. *Social Sciences in Health*, 4(2), 119–29.
Street, A., Cuddihy, L., Wilks, D., Geladas, D., Chew, S. & Best, D. (1997). Rostering: placing the nurse in the picture. *Contemporary Nurse*, 6(3–4), 145–51.
Street, A. F. & Robinson, A. (1995). Advanced clinical roles: investigating dilemmas and changing practice through action research. *Journal of Clinical Nursing*, 10(2), 349–57.
Streubert, H. & Carpenter, D. (1995). *Qualitative research in nursing: advancing the humanistic imperative.* Philadelphia, JB Lippincott.
Stufflebeam, D. (1973). An introduction to the PDK book: educational evaluation and decision making. In Worthen, R. & Sanders, J., eds, *Educational evaluation: theory and practice.* California, Belmont.
Sturt, J. (1999). Placing empowerment research within an action research typology. *Journal of Advanced Nursing*, 30(5), 1057–63.
Suderman, E.M., Johnson, L.S., Deatrich, J.V. & Sawatzky-Dickson, D.M. (2000). Action research sets the stage to improve discharge preparation. *Pediatric Nursing*, 26(6), 571–84.
Takase, M., Kershaw, E. & Burt, L. (2001). Nurse-environment misfit and nursing practice. *Journal of Advanced Nursing*, 35(6), 819–26.
Tarkka, M-T., Paunonen, M. & Laippala, P. (2000). How first-time mothers cope with child care while still in the maternity ward. *International Journal of Nursing Practice*, 6, 97–104.
Taylor, B.J. (1992a). 'Ordinariness' in nursing: a study (part 2). *Nursing Standard*, 7, 37–40.

Taylor, B.J. (1992b). Relieving pain through ordinariness in nursing: a phenomenological account of a comforting nurse–patient encounter. *Advances in Nursing Science*, 15(1), 33–43.

Thede, L.Q. (2001). Incorporating evidence based practice into nursing practice: an introduction. *Online Journal of Knowledge Synthesis for Nursing*. Available at http://www.stti.iupui.edu/library/ojksn/e_jebpnp.html (11 June). Accessed 4 January 2002.

Thomas, J. & Retsas, A. (1999). Transacting self-preservation: a grounded theory of the spiritual dimensions of people with terminal cancer. *International Journal of Nursing Studies*, 36, 191–201.

Thomas, L.H., McColl, E., Cullum, N., Rousseau, N. & Soutter, J. (1999). Clinical guidelines in nursing, midwifery and the therapies: a systematic review. *Journal of Advanced Nursing*, 30(1), 40–50.

Thompson, D.R. & Roebuck, A. (2001). The measurement of health-related quality of life in patients with coronary heart disease. *Journal of Cardiovascular Nursing*, 16, 28–33.

Thompson, S. & Barrett, P. (1997). Summary oral reflective analysis: a method for interview data analysis in feminist qualitative research. *Advances in Nursing Science*, 20(2), 55–65.

Thomson, A. (1994). *Anzac memories*. Oxford, Oxford University Press.

Thomson, M. (1998). Closing the gap between nursing research and practice. *Evidence-Based Nursing*, 1, 7–8.

Thorne, S. & Paterson, B. (2001). Health care professional support for self-care management in chronic illness: insights from diabetes research. *Patient Education Counselling*, 42, 81–90.

Thornhill, M. & Stevens, J. (1998). Client perceptions of a rural-based cardiac rehabilitation program: a grounded theory approach. *Australian Journal of Rural Health*, 6, 105–11.

Timmerman, G.M. (1996). The art of advertising for research subjects. *Nursing Research*, 45(6), 339–40.

Titler, M., Kleiber, C., Steelman, V., Goode, C., Rakel, B., Barry-Walker, J., Small, S. & Buckwalter, K. (1994). Infusing research into practice to promote quality care. *Nursing Research*, 43, 307–13.

Tong, R. (1995). Feminist philosophy. In Audi, R., ed., *The Cambridge dictionary of philosophy*. New York, Cambridge University Press.

Tosh, J. (1999). *The pursuit of history*. (3rd ed.). London, Longman.

Underwood, M., Elliott, D., Aitken, L., Austen, D., Currey, J., Field, T., Grech, C., Kiegaldie, D., Pittard, M. & Worral-Carter, L. (1999). Position statement on postgraduate critical care nursing education. *Australian Critical Care*, 12, 160–64.

Uphall, M.J. (1992). Nursing perceptions of collaboration with indigenous healers in Swaziland. *International Journal of Nursing Studies*, 29(1), 27–36.

Uyeda, M.L., Farrell, M.J., Schneider, Z. & Millership, R. (1997). National palliative care education and training needs analysis: final report. Canberra, The Commonwealth Department of Health and Family Services. ISBN 0864446314.

Valanis, B. (1999). *Epidemiology in health care*. London, Appleton & Lange.

Van Maanen, J. (1988). *Tales of the field: on writing ethnography*. Chicago, University of Chicago Press.

van Manen, M. (1990). *Researching lived experience: human science for an action sensitive pedagogy*. London, Ontario, State University of New York Press.

Vance, C., Talbott, S., McBride, A. & Mason, D. (1985). An uneasy alliance: nursing and the women's movement. *Nursing Outlook*, 33(6), 281–85.

Verran, J.A. & Ferketich, S.L. (1984). Residual analysis for statistical assumptions of regression equations. *Western Journal of Nursing Research*, 6(1), 27–40.

Versluysen, M. (1980). Old wives' tales? In Davies, C., ed., *Rewriting nursing history*. Beckenham (UK), Croom Helm.

Wadsworth, Y. (1993). *What is participatory action research?* Melbourne, Action Research Issues Association.

Wadsworth, Y. (1997). *Everyday evaluation on the run*. Sydney, Allen & Unwin.

Wald, L.D. (1915). *House on Henry Street*. New York, Henry Holt & Co.

Waldenström, U. & Nilsson, C-A. (1994). No effect of birth centre care on either duration or experience of breast feeding, but more complications: findings from a randomised controlled trial. *Midwifery*, 10, 8–17.

Wallace, M. C., Shorten, A., Crookes, P. A., McGurk, C. & Brewer, C. (1999). Integrating information literacies into an undergraduate nursing programme. *Nurse Education Today*, 19(2), 136–41.

Walsh, K. (1999). Shared humanity and the psychiatric nurse–patient encounter. *Australian and New Zealand Journal of Mental Health Nursing*, 8(1), 2–8.

Walters, A.J. (1994). Phenomenology as a way of understanding nursing. *Contemporary Nurse*, 3(3), 134–41.

Walters, A.J. (1995a). A hermeneutic study of the experiences of relatives of critically ill patients. *Journal of Advanced Nursing*, 22, 998–1005.

Walters, A.J. (1995b). A Heideggerian hermeneutic study of the practice of critical care nurses. *Journal of Advanced Nursing*, 21, 492–97.

Walters, S. & East, L. (2001). The cycle of homelessness in the lives of young mothers: the diagnostic phase of an action research project. *Journal of Clinical Nursing*, 10(2), 171–79.

Waltz, C.F. & Strickland, O.L. (1988). *Measurement of nursing outcomes: measuring client outcomes.* (vol. 2). New York, Springer.

Waltz, C., Strickland, O. & Lenz, E. (1991). *Measurement in nursing research.* (3rd ed.). Philadelphia, FA Davis.

Ward, S.E., Berry, P.E. & Misiewiez, H. (1996). Concerns about analgesics among patients and family care-givers in a hospice setting. *Research in Nursing & Health*, 19, 205–11.

Ware, J.E. Jr. (2000). SF-36 health survey update. *Spine*, 25(24), 3130–39.

Ware, J.E. Jr, Snow, K.K., Kosinski, M. & Gandek, B. (1993). *SF-36 health survey manual and interpretation guide.* Boston, The Health Institute, New England Medical Center.

Wass, A. (2000). *Promoting health: the primary health care approach.* (2nd ed.). Sydney, Harcourt.

Wassertheil-Smoller, S. (1990). *Biostatistics and epidemiology: a primer for health professionals.* New York, Edwards Brothers, Inc.

Waterman, H. (1996). A comparison between quality assurance and action research. *Nurse Researcher*, 3(3), 58–68.

Watson, P. & Feld, A. (1996). Factors in stress and burnout among paediatric nurses in a general hospital. *Nursing Praxis in New Zealand*, 11(3), 38–46.

Watson, P.B., Town, G.I., Holbrook, N., Dwan, C., Toop, L.J. & Drennan, C.J. (1997). Evaluation of a self-management plan for chronic obstructive pulmonary disease. *European Respiratory Journal*, 10, 1267–71.

Watters, R. (2000). Regulating: the social control process registered nurses use to teach psychiatric patients about their medications. *Issues in Mental Health Nursing*, 21, 411–31.

Watts, E. (1998). The lifeworld of the ICU nurse during treatment withdrawal. Honours thesis, University of Western Sydney, Sydney, Australia.

Watts, R., Robertson, J. & Thomas, G. Review Panel. (2001). *The nursing management of fever in children—a systematic review.* (No. 14). Adelaide, The Joanna Briggs Institute for Evidence Based Nursing & Midwifery.

Webb, C. (1992). The use of the first person in academic writing: objectivity, language and gatekeeping. *Journal of Advanced Nursing*, 17(6), 747–52.

Webb, C. (1993). Feminist research: definitions, methodology, methods and evaluation. *Journal of Advanced Nursing*, 18(3):416–23.

Webb, C. & Kevern, J. (2001). Focus groups as a research method: a critique of some aspects of their use in nursing research. *Journal of Advanced Nursing*, 33(6), 798–805.

Webb, C. & Koch, T. (1997). Women's experiences of non-invasive breast cancer: literature review and study report. *Journal of Advanced Nursing*, 25, 514–25.

Webster, J. (1999). Practitioner-centred research: an evaluation of the implementation of the bedside hand-over. *Journal of Advanced Nursing*, 30(6), 1375–82.

Weedon, C. (1987). *Feminist practice and poststructuralist theory.* Oxford, Basil Blackwell Ltd.

Weedon, C. (1999). *Feminism, theory and the politics of difference.* London, Blackwell Publishers.

Wellard, S. & Palaster, L. (1996). An evaluation of two methods of pre-cannulation skin disinfection. *Australian Journal of Advanced Nursing*, 14(1), 3–7.

Westkott, M. (1990). Feminist criticism of the social sciences. In Nielson, J.M., ed., *Feminist research methods.* Boulder, Westview Press.

White, G.E. & Thomson, A.N. (1995). As every good mother should. Childhood immunisation in New Zealand: a qualitative study. *Health and Social Care*, 3, 73–82.

Whyte, W.F. (1955). *Street corner society.* Chicago, University of Chicago Press.

Wiechula, R. (2001). *Post harvest management of split thickness skin graft donor sites—a systematic review.* (No. 13). Adelaide, The Joanna Briggs Institute for Evidence Based Nursing & Midwifery.

Wiedenbach, E. (1964). *Clinical nursing: a helping art.* New York, Springer.

Wiles, V. & Daffurn, K. (2002). *There's a bird in my hand and a bear in the bed, I must be in ICU: the first pivotal years of Australian critical care nursing.* Perth, Australian College of Critical Care Nurses.

Williams, A.M. (1998). The delivery of quality nursing care: a grounded theory study of the nurse's perspective. *Journal of Advanced Nursing*, 27, 808–16.

Williams, G. & Clarke, T. (2001). A consensus driven method to measure the required number of intensive care nurses in Australia. *Australian Critical Care*, 14, 106–15.

Williams, K.S., Crichton, N. & Roe, B. (1997). Disseminating research evidence: a controlled trial in continence care. *Journal of Advanced Nursing*, 25, 691–98.

Wilmoth, M.C. (1995). Computer networks as a source of research subjects. *Western Journal of Nursing Research*, 17(3), 335–38.

Wilson, M.C., Hayward, R.S., Tunis, S.R., Bass, E.B. & Guyatt, G. (1995). Users' guides to the medical literature. VIII. How to use clinical practice guidelines. B. What are the recommendations and will they help you in caring for your patients? The Evidence-Based Medicine Working Group. *Journal of the American Medical Association*, 274(20), 1630–32.

Wimpenny, P. & Gass, J. (2000). Interviewing in phenomenology and grounded theory: is there a difference? *Journal of Advanced Nursing*, 31, 1485–92.

Woods, M. (1997). Maintaining a nursing ethic: a grounded theory of the moral praxis of experienced nurses. *Nursing Praxis New Zealand*, 12(3), 34–35.

Wolcott, H. (1992). Posturing in qualitative enquiry. In LeCompte, M., Milroy, W.L. & Priessle, J., eds, *Handbook of qualitative research in education.* San Diego, Academic Press.

Wolcott, H. (1994). *Transforming qualitative data: description, analysis and interpretation.* Thousand Oaks, California, Sage.

Wray, J. N. (1995). Remembering family breakdown: a Heideggerian hermeneutic analysis. *Addictions Nursing*, 7(2), 54–61.

Wu, M-L.W., Courtney, M. & Berger, G. (2000). Models of nursing care: a comparative study of patient satisfaction on two orthopaedic wards in Brisbane. *Australian Journal of Advanced Nursing*, 17(4), 29–34.

Wuest, J. (1995). Feminist grounded theory: an exploration of the congruency and tensions between two traditions in knowledge discovery. *Qualitative Health Research*, 5(1), 125–37.

Wuest, J. (2000). Negotiating with helping systems: an example of grounded theory evolving through emergent fit. *Qualitative Health Research*, 10(1), 51–70.

Yarandi, H.N. (1991). Planning sample sizes: comparison of factor level means. *Nurse Researcher*, 40(1), 57–58.

Yi, M. & Jezewski, M.A. (2000). Korean nurses' adjustment to hospital in the United States of America. *Journal of Advanced Nursing*, 32(3), 721–29.

Zanotti, R. (1996). Overcoming national and cultural differences within collaborative international nursing research. *Western Journal of Nursing Research*, 18(1), 6–11.

Ziemer, M.M., Cooper, D.M. & Pigeon, J.G. (1995). Evaluation of a dressing to reduce nipple pain and improve nipple skin condition in breast feeding women. *Nurse Researcher*, 44, 347–51.

Zigmond, A.S. & Snaith, R.P. (1983). The hospital anxiety and depression scale. *Acta Psychiatrica Scandinavica*, 67, 361–70.
Zwarenstein, M., Bryant, W., Bailie, R. & Sibthorpe, B. (1998). Interventions to change collaboration between nurse and doctors (Cochrane Review). The Cochrane Library.

Index